The PDR® Pocket Guide to Prescription Drugs™

Director, Clinical Services: Sylvia Nashed, PharmD

Senior Manager, Clinical Services: Nermin Shenouda-Kerolous, PharmD

Clinical Database Manager: Christine Sunwoo, PharmD

Senior Drug Information Specialist: Anila Patel, PharmD

Drug Information Specialists: Demyana Farag, PharmD; Pauline Lee, PharmD; Kristine Mecca, PharmD

Managing Clinical Editor: Julia Tonelli, MD

Editor: Sharon Strompf

Manager, Art Department: Livio Udina

Senior Director, Content Operations & Manufacturing: Jeffrey D. Schaefer

Associate Director, Manufacturing & Distribution: Thomas Westburgh

Associate Manager, Fulfillment: Gary Lew

PDR Network, LLC

Chief Executive Officer: Edward Fotsch, MD

President: Richard C. Altus

Chief Financial Officer: Dawn Carfora

Chief Technology Officer: David Cheng

Senior Vice President, Publishing & Operations: Valerie E. Berger

Senior Vice President, Sales: Jeffrey Davis

Senior Vice President, Corporate Development and General Counsel: Andrew Gelman

Senior Vice President, Marketing & Business Line Management: Barbara Senich, BSN, MBA, MPH

Publisher's Note

The drug information contained in this book is based on product labeling published in the 2012 edition of *Physicians' Desk Reference*® or supplied by the manufacturer. This information is drawn from the PDR database, which is compiled and updated on a regular basis by a staff of experienced pharmacists. While diligent efforts have been made to ensure the accuracy of each medication profile, it is essential to bear in mind that the information presented here is merely a synopsis of key points in the official product labeling, and that the complete labeling contains additional precautionary information that may be of significance in specific cases. If a profile leaves any question unanswered, be sure to consult your doctor or pharmacist for additional information.

This book does not list every possible action, adverse reaction, interaction, or precaution; all information is presented without guarantees by the authors, consultants, and publisher, who disclaim all liability in connection with its use. This book is intended only as a reference for use in an ongoing partnership between doctor and patient in the management of the patient's health. It is not a substitute for a doctor's professional judgment, and serves only as a reminder of concerns that may need discussion. All readers are urged to consult with a doctor or other healthcare provider before beginning or discontinuing use of any prescription medication or undertaking any form of self-treatment.

Brand names listed in this book are intended to represent only the more commonly used products. Inclusion of a brand name does not signify endorsement of the product; absence of a name does not imply a criticism or rejection of the product. The publisher is not advocating the use of any product described in this book, does not warrant or guarantee any of these products, and has not performed any independent analysis in connection with the product information contained herein.

Table of Contents

Tear-Out Charts

Personal Information Tracker
My Medicine Tracker

Foreword

The *PDR® Pocket Guide to Prescription Drugs*™ strives to make the many benefits of modern pharmaceuticals—as well as their possible risks—as clear and simple as can be. *The PDR Pocket Guide* spells out why each medication is prescribed, the most important information to remember about it, and then discloses its most common side effects. As a safeguard against error, this Guide also provides you with information on standard dosage recommendations and tells what to do when you miss a dose of your medication. And to help you find all these facts as quickly as possible, it lists each medication under its familiar brand name—with a cross-reference in case the medication is dispensed generically.

Still, despite the depth and detail of the information you'll find here, *The PDR Pocket Guide* is not a replacement for your doctor's advice. Rather, it serves as a reminder of the basic instructions and caveats that may be forgotten by the time you leave your doctor's office, as well as providing you with a checklist of the problems and conditions that you must be certain the doctor knows about—facts that might call for a change in your prescription. In this way, the book is designed to serve as an aid in an ongoing dialogue between you and your doctor—a collaboration necessary for any treatment to work. Just as the doctor must tell you how and why to use a particular medication, you must tell the doctor how it affects you, reporting any reactions or drug interactions you suspect you may have. And while it's up to the doctor to devise your treatment strategy, it's up to you to make sure that the right doses are administered at the right times, and that the prescribed course of therapy is completed as planned.

The *Physicians' Desk Reference®* has been providing doctors with the information needed for safe, effective drug therapy for more than 60 years. Designed especially for healthcare professionals, it presents the facts in a detailed, technical format approved by the Food and Drug Administration (FDA). To make the key facts buried in this wealth of data accessible to everyone, *The PDR Pocket Guide* strips away the medical shorthand and technical terminology, and presents the core of this information in a simple, standard format designed for maximum convenience and ease of use by the consumer. All the information you'll find in *The PDR Pocket Guide's* consumer medication profiles has been extracted from the PDR database, which is updated regularly by a staff of pharmacists and drug information specialists.

Modern drug therapy is a vast and complicated field—so complicated that, for many questions about medicines, the answer varies with each patient. *The PDR Pocket Guide to Prescription Drugs* gives you general guidelines for safe medication use. But only your doctor, evaluating the unique details of your case, can give you the exact instructions best suited for you. The goal of this book is simply to alert you to the most pertinent questions to ask, and to help clarify your doctor's answers—in short, to give you the tools you need to supervise your own medical care as effectively as possible.

We wish you good health.

Robert W. Hogan, MD
Chair, Board of Medical Consultants
Family Medicine
Southern California Permanente Medical Group
Assistant Clinical Professor
UCSD Department of Family and Preventive Medicine
San Diego, CA

How to Use This Book

Although doctors today can often work miracles with advanced technology and sophisticated medicines, it's vital for you to take an active role in managing your health. Any medicine can prove worthless (or even be harmful) if taken improperly. Likewise, you must let your doctor know if you react badly to a medication or have a condition that makes taking it dangerous. While no book is a substitute for a visit to the doctor, this guide is designed to help you use your medications safely and effectively, and to help you determine what requires further discussion with your doctor.

The book is divided into two major parts. In the first section, you'll find profiles of the more frequently prescribed medications. The second section has helpful references and an index of medications used to treat common diseases and disorders.

MEDICATION PROFILES

The profiles provide detailed information on the most frequently prescribed prescription medications. However, don't be alarmed if a medication you've been prescribed isn't among them; a number of specialized, yet valuable, medications have been omitted here due to lack of space.

The products described here are listed alphabetically by the manufacturer's brand name or the generic name. Full-profile headers appear in large, bold letters; generic cross-references are presented in smaller, bold italic type. The information that follows these names is divided into the following 12 questions:

What is this medication?
This is an overview of the major conditions for which the medication is generally prescribed.

What is the most important information I should know about this medication?
Highlighted here are key points about a medication that are especially worthwhile to know. We've placed it here for the sake of emphasis. Never regard this section as a definitive summary of the medication.

Who should not take this medication?

Some medications can be harmful under certain conditions; these are called "contraindications" and they are detailed under this question. The most common contraindication is a hypersensitivity to the medication itself. If you think one of these restrictions applies to you, alert your doctor immediately.

What should I tell my doctor before I take the first dose of this medication?

If you have any problems or conditions noted in this section that your doctor may be unaware of, be sure to bring them to his or her attention. Always tell your doctor about your complete medical history, as well as any prescription and over-the-counter products you are taking—including dietary supplements and herbs—before starting treatment with any other medication.

What is the usual dosage?

The information in this section is based on the dosage guidelines your doctor uses. Depending on your condition and medical history, your doctor may prescribe a different regimen. This information is intended only as a convenient double-check in case you suspect a misunderstanding or a typographical error on your prescription label. **Do not use this information to determine an exact dosage yourself, and do not change the dosage or stop taking your medication without your doctor's approval**.

How should I take this medication?

This section details special instructions, including how and when to take the medication, and any dietary restrictions that may apply.

What should I avoid while taking this medication?

This section gives advice on certain activities that should be avoided during treatment due to an increased risk of side effects or other potential problems. If you have any questions about the precautions in this section, talk to your doctor. Do not change your dosage or discontinue the medication on your own. Such a change might do more harm than good. Also remember that this is not a complete list of all possible medication precautions; always consult your doctor or pharmacist for more information.

What are possible food and drug interactions associated with this medication?

This section lists specific medications, classes of medications, and foods that have been known to interact with the medicine being profiled. The examples are not all-inclusive. If you're not certain whether a medication you're taking falls into one of these categories, be sure to check with your doctor or pharmacist. But never stop taking any medication without first consulting your doctor.

What are the possible side effects of this medication?

Shown here are only the most common side effects listed by the manufacturer in the drug's FDA-approved product labeling. Any medication will occasionally cause an unwanted reaction. Even the most common side effects are seen in only a small percentage of patients. **Side effects cannot be anticipated. If any develop or change in intensity, tell your doctor as soon as possible. Only your doctor can determine if it is safe for you to continue taking this medication.**

Can I receive this medication if I am pregnant or breast-feeding?

This section will tell you whether a medication has been confirmed to be safe for use during pregnancy or breastfeeding, is known to be dangerous, or is part of that large group about which clinicians are not really sure. With certain medications, the small theoretical risk they pose may be overshadowed by your need for treatment.

What should I do if I miss a dose of this medication?

Here you will find advice on what to do if you forget to take a dose. For many medications, the best option is to skip the dose you missed and return to your regular dosing schedule. Never take two doses at one time unless indicated by your doctor.

How should I store this medication?

This section provides general storage information, as well as any special requirements that may apply.

<u>OTHER FEATURES</u>

Visual Identification Guide

This full-color guide includes actual-sized photographs of the leading products discussed in the book, arranged alphabetically by brand name. Manufacturers occasionally change the color and shape of a product, so if a prescription does not match the photo shown here, check with your pharmacist before assuming there's been a mistake.

Appendix: Reference Tables

This section provides you with a number of reference tables and information that are very useful in every home.

Indices

The first index lists all brand and generic medication names alphabetically, for ease of use. The second index is the Disease and Disorder Index, which will help you to quickly identify medications that are available for a particular medical condition. Arranged alphabetically by ailment, it lists all the medications profiled in this book that are associated with a particular disease or disorder.

Abilify
Generic name: Aripiprazole

What is this medication?
Abilify is a medicine used to treat schizophrenia. This medicine is also used alone or in combination with lithium or valproate to treat manic or mixed episodes associated with bipolar disorder. In addition, Abilify is used in combination with other antidepressant medications to treat major depressive disorder. Abilify is also used to treat irritability associated with autism. Abilify is available as tablets, an oral solution, and orally disintegrating tablets called Abilify Discmelt.

What is the most important information I should know about this medication?
- Abilify can increase the risk of stroke in elderly patients. Abilify is not approved to treat psychosis in the elderly with dementia (an illness involving loss of memory, judgment, and confusion).
- Abilify can increase the risk of suicidal thoughts and behavior in children, adolescents, and young adults. Your doctor will monitor you closely for clinical worsening, suicidal or unusual behavior after you start taking Abilify or a new dose of Abilify. Tell your doctor immediately if you experience anxiety, hostility, sleeplessness, restlessness, impulsive or dangerous behavior, or thoughts about suicide or dying; or if you have new symptoms or seem to be feeling worse.
- Abilify can cause neuroleptic malignant syndrome (NMS) (a life-threatening brain disorder). NMS is a medical emergency. Tell your doctor immediately if you experience high fever, muscle rigidity, confusion, fast or irregular heartbeat, changes in your blood pressure, or increased sweating.
- Abilify can cause tardive dyskinesia (abnormal muscle movements, including tremor, shuffling and uncontrolled, involuntary movements). Tell your doctor if you experience uncontrollable muscle movements in your face, tongue, or other parts of your body.
- Abilify can cause an increase in your blood sugar levels or diabetes. Tell your doctor if you experience excessive thirst, an increase in urination, an increase in appetite, weakness, confusion,

feel sick to your stomach, or your breath smells fruity. If you have diabetes or are at risk for diabetes, monitor your blood sugar regularly, as determined by your doctor.

- Abilify can cause a sudden decrease in your blood pressure with dizziness, rapid heartbeat, and faintness. Tell your doctor if you have or have had heart problems, brain disorders (such as stroke), or other conditions that can cause low blood pressure.
- Abilify can lower the ability of your body to fight infections. Tell your doctor if you develop signs of an infection (such as a fever, sore throat, rash, or chills).
- Abilify can cause seizures. Tell your doctor if you have a history of seizures.
- Abilify can also cause difficulty when swallowing, which in turn can cause a type of pneumonia.
- If you have a condition known as phenylketonuria (an inability to process phenylalanine, a protein in your body), be aware that Abilify Discmelt orally disintegrating tablets contain phenylalanine.

Who should not take this medication?
Do not take Abilify if you are allergic to it or any of its ingredients.

Abilify is not approved for treating psychosis in the elderly with dementia (an illness involving loss of memory, judgment, and confusion).

What should I tell my doctor before I take the first dose of this medication?
Tell your doctor about all prescription, over-the-counter, and herbal medications you are taking before beginning treatment with Abilify. Also, talk to your doctor about your complete medical history, especially if you have past or current heart problems or stroke, high cholesterol, low or high blood pressure, seizures, diabetes, Alzheimer's disease, or a history of low white blood cell counts.

What is the usual dosage?
Please see general statement regarding dosage on page xii.

Schizophrenia
Adults: The recommended dose is 10 milligrams (mg) or 15 mg once a day.

Adolescents 13-17 years: The recommended dose is 10 mg once a day.

Bipolar Disorder (alone or in combination with lithium or valproate)
Adults: *Alone:* The recommended starting dose is 15 mg once a day. *With Lithium or Valproate:* The recommended starting dose is 10-15 mg once a day.

Children 10-17 years: The recommended starting dose is 2 mg once a day.

Major Depressive Disorder
Adults: The recommended starting dose is 2-5 mg once a day.

Irritability Associated with Autism
Children 6-17 years: The recommended starting dose is 2 mg once a day.

Your doctor will increase your dose as needed, until the desired effect is achieved.

If you are taking certain medications, your doctor will adjust your dose appropriately.

How should I take this medication?
- Take Abilify exactly as prescribed by your doctor. Do not change your dose or stop taking Abilify without first talking to your doctor. Take it with or without food.
- Swallow Abilify tablets whole.
- To take Abilify Discmelt tablets, open the package and peel back the foil on the blister pack. Do not push the tablet through the foil because this could damage it. Using dry hands remove the tablet and place the entire tablet on your tongue. It will dissolve rapidly.

• Do not split Abilify Discmelt tablets. It is recommended that you take Abilify Discmelt tablets without liquid. However, if needed, you can take it with liquid.

What should I avoid while taking this medication?
Do not drink alcohol while you are taking Abilify.

Do not drive, operate heavy machinery, or do other dangerous activities until you know how Abilify affects you.

Do not become over-heated or dehydrated while you are taking Abilify. Do not over-exercise. In hot weather, stay inside in a cool place if possible. Stay out of the sun and do not wear too much or heavy clothing. Drink plenty of water.

What are possible food and drug interactions associated with this medication?
If Abilify is taken with certain other drugs, the effects of either could be increased, decreased, or altered. It is especially important to check with your doctor before combining Abilify with the following: alcohol, carbamazepine, certain blood pressure medications, erythromycin, fluoxetine, grapefruit juice, itraconazole, ketoconazole, paroxetine, or quinidine.

What are the possible side effects of this medication?
Please see general statement regarding side effects on page xiii.

> **Side effects may include:** anxiety, constipation, dizziness, fatigue, feeling sleepy, headache, increased appetite, muscle stiffness, nausea, restlessness, shaking, stuffy nose, trouble sleeping, vomiting, weight gain

Can I receive this medication if I am pregnant or breastfeeding?
The effects of Abilify during pregnancy and breastfeeding are unknown. Do not breastfeed while you are taking Abilify. Tell your doctor immediately if you are pregnant, plan to become pregnant, or are breastfeeding.

What should I do if I miss a dose of this medication?
If you miss a dose of Abilify, take it as soon as you remember. However, if it is almost time for your next dose, skip the one you missed and return to your regular dosing schedule. Do not take two doses at once.

How should I store this medication?
Store at room temperature.

Abiraterone Acetate: *see Zytiga, page 1166*

Abstral
Generic name: Fentanyl

What is this medication?
Abstral is a medicine used to treat breakthrough pain in adults with cancer who are already routinely taking other opioid pain medicines around-the-clock for their constant cancer pain. Abstral is started only after you have been taking another opioid pain medicine and your body is used to it (opioid-tolerant). Abstral is a federally controlled substance because it has abuse potential.

What is the most important information I should know about this medication?
- Do not use Abstral if you are not opioid-tolerant.
- Abstral can cause life-threatening breathing problems if you are not opioid-tolerant, if you do not use Abstral exactly as prescribed by your doctor, or if a child takes Abstral by accident.
- Keep Abstral in a safe place away from children. Accidental use by a child is a medical emergency. Get emergency help immediately.
- Abstral is available only through a restricted distribution program called the TIRF REMS Access Program.
- Call your doctor or get emergency medical help immediately if you have breathing problems, drowsiness, faintness, dizziness, confusion, or any other unusual symptoms after taking Abstral.

These can be signs of an overdose. Your dose of Abstral may be too high for you. These symptoms may lead to serious problems if not treated right away. Do not take another dose of Abstral.
• If you stop taking your around-the-clock pain medicine for your constant cancer pain, you must stop using Abstral. You may no longer be opioid-tolerant. Talk to your doctor about how to treat your pain.

Who should not take this medication?
Do not use Abstral if you are allergic to it or any of its ingredients.

Do not use Abstral if you are not already taking another opioid pain medicine around-the-clock for your constant cancer pain.

Do not use Abstral if you only have pain for a short time or if your pain is from surgery, headache or migraine, or dental work.

What should I tell my doctor before I take the first dose of this medication?
Tell your doctor about all prescription, over-the-counter, and herbal medications you are taking before beginning treatment with Abstral. Also, talk to your doctor about your complete medical history, especially if you have trouble breathing or lung problems (such as asthma, wheezing, or shortness of breath), liver or kidney problems, seizures, a slow heart rate or other heart problems, low blood pressure, mental health problems, past or present alcohol or drug abuse or a family history of alcohol or drug abuse, or you have or had a head injury or brain problem.

What is the usual dosage?
Please see general statement regarding dosage on page xii.

Adults ≥18 years: The starting dose is 100 micrograms.

Your doctor will prescribe the appropriate dose for you and will increase your dose as needed, until the desired effect is achieved.

How should I take this medication?

- Take Abstral exactly as prescribed by your doctor. Do not take Abstral more often than prescribed.
- Take one dose for an episode of breakthrough cancer pain. If your breakthrough pain does not get better within 30 minutes after taking the first dose of Abstral, you can take one more dose of Abstral as instructed by your doctor. If your breakthrough pain does not get better after the second dose of Abstral, call your doctor for instructions. Do not take another dose of Abstral at this time.
- If you only need to take one dose of Abstral for an episode of breakthrough pain, you must wait 2 hours from the time of that dose to take a dose of Abstral for a new episode of breakthrough pain. If you need to take two doses of Abstral for an episode of breakthrough pain, you must wait 2 hours after the second dose to take a dose of Abstral for a new episode of breakthrough pain.

What should I avoid while taking this medication?

Do not drive, operate machinery, or do other dangerous activities until you know how Abstral affects you. Abstral can make you sleepy. Ask your doctor when it is safe to do these activities.

Do not drink alcohol while you are using Abstral. It can increase your chance of having dangerous side effects.

Do not change your dose of Abstral yourself. Your doctor will change the dose until you and your doctor find the right dose for you.

Do not suck, chew, or swallow Abstral tablets.

What are possible food and drug interactions associated with this medication?

If Abstral is used with certain other drugs, the effects of either could be increased, decreased, or altered. Abstral may interact with numerous medications. Therefore, it is very important that you tell your doctor about any other medications you are taking.

What are the possible side effects of this medication?
Please see general statement regarding side effects on page xiii.

> **Side effects may include:** constipation, dizziness, headache, nausea, shortness of breath, sleepiness, vomiting

Can I receive this medication if I am pregnant or breastfeeding?
The effects of Abstral during pregnancy are unknown. Abstral can be found in your breast milk if you take it while breastfeeding. Tell your doctor immediately if you are pregnant, plan to become pregnant, or are breastfeeding.

What should I do if I miss a dose of this medication?
Abstral should be used under special circumstances determined by your doctor (or given only as needed). You should use Abstral only when you experience breakthrough cancer pain.

How should I store this medication?
Store at room temperature.

Accupril
Generic name: Quinapril HCl

What is this medication?
Accupril is a medicine known as an angiotensin-converting enzyme (ACE) inhibitor. Accupril is used alone or in combination with other medications to treat high blood pressure or heart failure.

What is the most important information I should know about this medication?
• Accupril can cause a rare but serious allergic reaction leading to extreme swelling of your face, lips, tongue, throat, or gut (causing severe abdominal pain). You may have an increased risk of experiencing these symptoms if you have ever had an allergy to ACE inhibitor-type medicines or if you are African American. If

you experience any of these symptoms, seek emergency medical attention immediately.

- Tell your doctor if you experience lightheadedness, especially
during the first few days of Accupril therapy. If you faint, stop
taking Accupril and tell your doctor immediately.

- Vomiting, diarrhea, excessive perspiration, and dehydration may
lead to an excessive fall in your blood pressure. Tell your doctor
if you experience any of these.

- Accupril may decrease your blood neutrophil (type of blood cells
that fight infections) levels, especially if you have a collagen vascular disease (such as lupus [disease that affects the immune
system]) or kidney disease.

- Promptly report any signs of infection (such as sore throat or
fever) to your doctor.

- Accupril may not work as well in African Americans, who may
also have a higher risk of side effects. Contact your doctor if
your symptoms do not improve or if they become worse.

Who should not take this medication?

Do not take Accupril if you are allergic to it or any of its ingredients.

Do not take Accupril if you have a history of angioedema (a condition involving swelling of the face, extremities, eyes, lips, and
tongue) related to previous treatment with similar medicines.

What should I tell my doctor before I take the first dose of this medication?

Tell your doctor about all prescription, over-the-counter, and
herbal medications you are taking before beginning treatment with
Accupril. Also, talk to your doctor about your complete medical
history, especially if you have liver problems, kidney disease, or
diabetes. Tell your doctor if you have bone marrow problems or
any blood disease, any disease that affects the immune system
(such as lupus or scleroderma), collagen vascular disease, or if
you plan to have any surgery and/or anesthesia.

What is the usual dosage?

Please see general statement regarding dosage on page xii.

High Blood Pressure
Adults: The usual starting dose is 10 or 20 milligrams (mg) once a day. Your doctor will adjust your dose based on your previous blood pressure medication and will increase your dose as needed, until the desired effect is achieved.

Heart Failure
Adults: The usual starting dose is 5 mg twice a day. Your doctor may give you a higher dose depending on your needs.

If you have kidney impairment, your doctor will adjust your dose appropriately.

How should I take this medication?
• Take Accupril exactly as prescribed by your doctor.

What should I avoid while taking this medication?
Do not become pregnant while you are taking Accupril.

Do not take salt substitutes or supplements containing potassium without consulting your doctor.

Do not stand or sit up quickly when you take Accupril, especially in the morning. Sit or lie down at the first sign of dizziness, lightheadedness, or fainting.

What are possible food and drug interactions associated with this medication?
If Accupril is taken with certain other drugs, the effects of either could be increased, decreased, or altered. It is especially important to check with your doctor before combining Accupril with the following: dextran, diuretics (water pills) (such as amiloride, hydrochlorothiazide, spironolactone, or triamterene), injectable gold (sodium aurothiomalate), lithium, magnesium, nonsteroidal anti-inflammatory drugs (such as ibuprofen or naproxen), potassium supplements, salt substitutes containing potassium, or tetracycline.

What are the possible side effects of this medication?

Please see general statement regarding side effects on page xiii.

> **Side effects may include:** chest pain, cough, dizziness, fatigue, headache, low blood pressure, nausea, stomach pain, vomiting

Can I receive this medication if I am pregnant or breastfeeding?

Do not take Accupril if you are pregnant. Accupril can harm your unborn baby. Accupril can be found in your breast milk if you take it while breastfeeding. Tell your doctor immediately if you are pregnant, plan to become pregnant, or are breastfeeding.

What should I do if I miss a dose of this medication?

If you miss a dose of Accupril, take it as soon as you remember. However, if it is almost time for your next dose, skip the one you missed and return to your regular dosing schedule. Do not take two doses at once.

How should I store this medication?

Store at room temperature. Protect from light.

Acetaminophen/Butalbital/Caffeine: *see Fioricet, page 386*

Acetaminophen/Codeine Phosphate: *see Tylenol with Codeine, page 1032*

Acetaminophen/Hydrocodone Bitartrate: *see Vicodin, page 1066*

Acetaminophen/Oxycodone HCl: *see Percocet, page 778*

Acetaminophen/Tramadol HCl: *see Ultracet, page 1035*

Aciphex
Generic name: Rabeprazole Sodium

What is this medication?
Aciphex is a medicine called a proton pump inhibitor (PPI). It reduces the amount of acid in your stomach. Aciphex is used to treat gastroesophageal reflux disease and ulcers, and for long-term treatment of conditions where your stomach makes too much acid, such as Zollinger-Ellison syndrome. It is also used with other medicines to eliminate the bacteria that often cause ulcers (known as *Helicobacter pylori*).

What is the most important information I should know about this medication?
- Aciphex can cause low magnesium levels in your body. Tell your doctor immediately if you have seizures, dizziness, abnormal or fast heartbeat, jitteriness, jerking movements or shaking, muscle weakness, spasms of your hands and feet, cramps or muscle aches, or spasm of the voice box.
- Tell your doctor if you experience any symptoms of a serious allergic reaction with Aciphex (such as rash, face swelling, throat tightness, or difficulty breathing).
- People who are taking multiple daily doses of Aciphex for a long period of time may have an increased risk of fractures of the hip, wrist, or spine.

Who should not take this medication?
Do not take Aciphex if you are allergic to it, any of its ingredients, or to any other PPI.

What should I tell my doctor before I take the first dose of this medication?
Tell your doctor about all prescription, over-the-counter, and herbal medications you are taking before beginning treatment with Aciphex. Also, talk to your doctor about your complete medical history, especially if you have low magnesium levels, any allergies, or liver problems. Tell your doctor if you are pregnant, plan to become pregnant, or are breastfeeding.

What is the usual dosage?
Please see general statement regarding dosage on page xii.

Gastroesophageal Reflux Disease
Adults: The recommended dose is a 20-milligram (mg) tablet once a day for 4-8 weeks. Depending on your response, your doctor may suggest another 8 weeks of treatment.

Adolescents ≥12 years: The recommended dose is 20 mg once a day for up to 8 weeks.

Prevention of Duodenal Ulcer Due to *H. pylori* Infection
Adults: This treatment involves taking three different medications. The usual dose for the triple therapy is: Aciphex 20 mg twice a day for 7 days; amoxicillin 1000 mg twice a day for 7 days; and clarithromycin 500 mg twice a day for 7 days.

Treatment of Duodenal Ulcers
Adults: The recommended dose is one 20-mg tablet once a day after the morning meal for up to 4 weeks.

Treatment of Excess Stomach Acid (such as Zollinger-Ellison Syndrome)
Adults: The recommended dose is 60 mg once a day. Your doctor might prescribe a different dose or duration based on your condition.

How should I take this medication?
• Take Aciphex with or without food, as directed. Your doctor will tell you whether you should take Aciphex after a meal based on your medical condition. Swallow the tablets whole.

What should I avoid while taking this medication?
Do not chew, crush, or split the tablets, since this will damage them and the medicine will not work. Tell your doctor if you cannot swallow tablets whole.

What are possible food and drug interactions associated with this medication?

If Aciphex is taken with certain other drugs, the effects of either could be increased, decreased, or altered. It is especially important to check with your doctor before combining Aciphex with the following: antibiotics, atazanavir, cyclosporine, digoxin, ketoconazole, methotrexate, or warfarin.

What are the possible side effects of this medication?

Please see general statement regarding side effects on page xiii.

> **Side effects may include:** constipation, gas, headache, infection, pain, sore throat

Can I receive this medication if I am pregnant or breastfeeding?

The effects of Aciphex during pregnancy and breastfeeding are unknown. Tell your doctor immediately if you are pregnant, plan to become pregnant, or are breastfeeding.

What should I do if I miss a dose of this medication?

If you miss a dose of Aciphex, take it as soon as you remember. However, if it is almost time for your next dose, skip the one you missed and return to your regular dosing schedule. Do not take two doses at once.

How should I store this medication?

Store at room temperature, away from moisture.

Actonel

Generic name: Risedronate Sodium

What is this medication?

Actonel is a medicine used to treat or prevent osteoporosis (thin, weak bones) in women after menopause. It is also used to treat bone loss in men. Actonel is also used to prevent or treat osteoporosis caused by treatment with corticosteroid medications (such as prednisone) and to treat Paget's disease (a painful condition that weakens and deforms the bones) in men and women.

What is the most important information I should know about this medication?

- Actonel can cause irritation of your stomach and problems with your esophagus (the tube that connects your mouth and stomach).
- Actonel can lower your blood calcium levels. If you have low blood calcium levels before you start taking Actonel, it can get worse during treatment. Tell your doctor right away if you experience spasms, twitches, or cramps in your muscles; or numbness or tingling in your fingers, toes, or around your mouth as these can be symptoms of low calcium levels. Your doctor may prescribe calcium and vitamin D to help prevent low calcium levels while you are taking Actonel.
- Actonel can cause severe jaw bone problems. Your doctor should examine your mouth before you start Actonel. Your doctor may tell you to see your dentist before you start Actonel. It is important that you practice good mouth care during treatment with Actonel.
- Also, Actonel can cause bone, joint, or muscle pain or unusual fractures in your thigh bone. Tell your doctor right away if you develop pain in your hip, groin, or thigh.

Who should not take this medication?

Do not take Actonel if you are allergic to it or any of its ingredients.

Do not take Actonel if you have problems with your esophagus, low blood calcium levels, cannot stand or sit upright for at least 30 minutes.

What should I tell my doctor before I take the first dose of this medication?

Tell your doctor about all prescription, over-the-counter, and herbal medications you are taking before beginning treatment with Actonel. Also, talk to your doctor about your complete medical history, especially if you have swallowing problems, stomach or digestive problems, low blood calcium levels, plan to have dental surgery or teeth removed, kidney problems, have trouble absorbing minerals in your stomach or intestines, or if you are pregnant, plan to become pregnant, or are breastfeeding.

What is the usual dosage?

Please see general statement regarding dosage on page xii.

Osteoporosis (Prevention/Treatment)

Adults: The recommended dose is 35 milligrams (mg) once a week, 5 mg once a day, 75 mg on 2 consecutive days for a total of two tablets each month, or 150 mg once a month.

Bone Mass Increase in Men with Osteoporosis

Adults: The recommended dose is 35 mg once a week.

Steroid-Induced Osteoporosis (Prevention/Treatment)

Adults: The recommended dose is 5 mg once a day.

Paget's Disease

Adults: The recommended dose is 30 mg once a day for two months. Retreatment may be necessary.

How should I take this medication?

- Take Actonel exactly as prescribed by your doctor.
- Take Actonel in the morning at least 30 minutes before eating, drinking, or taking any other medicine. Take Actonel with 6-8 ounces (about 1 full cup) of plain water.
- Swallow Actonel tablet whole. Do not chew or suck on the tablet.
- After you take Actonel, wait at least 30 minutes before lying down. You can sit, stand, walk, and engage in normal activities like reading.

What should I avoid while taking this medication?

Do not take Actonel with mineral water, coffee, tea, soda, or juice.

Do not eat or drink (except plain water), or take any oral medications within 30 minutes of taking Actonel.

Do not lie down within 30 minutes after taking Actonel.

What are possible food and drug interactions associated with this medication?

If Actonel is taken with certain other drugs, the effects of either could be increased, decreased, or altered. It is especially important to check with your doctor before combining Actonel with the following: antacids, aspirin, nonsteroidal anti-inflammatory drugs (NSAIDs) (such as ibuprofen), or supplements or vitamins containing aluminum, calcium, iron or magnesium.

What are the possible side effects of this medication?

Please see general statement regarding side effects on page xiii.

> **Side effects may include:** abdominal (stomach) pain, allergic reactions, arthritis, back or joint pain, diarrhea, eye inflammation, headache, heartburn, infections, nausea, rash

Can I receive this medication if I am pregnant or breastfeeding?

The effects of Actonel during pregnancy and breastfeeding are unknown. Tell your doctor immediately if you are pregnant, plan to become pregnant, or are breastfeeding.

What should I do if I miss a dose of this medication?

If you miss a dose of Actonel, do not take it later in the day. Take one dose the next morning and return to your regular dosing schedule. Do not take two doses at once.

If you miss your once monthly dose, contact your doctor or pharmacist for advice.

How should I store this medication?

Store at room temperature.

Actoplus Met
Generic name: Metformin HCl/Pioglitazone HCl

What is this medication?
Actoplus Met is used to treat type 2 diabetes in addition to diet and exercise. Actoplus Met contains two medicines (pioglitazone and metformin). Actoplus Met is also available as extended-release tablets (releases medicine into your body throughout the day) called Actoplus Met XR.

What is the most important information I should know about this medication?
- Actoplus Met can cause lactic acidosis (a condition involving dangerously high levels of lactic acid in the blood). Tell your doctor if you experience any of the following symptoms: feeling very weak or tired; unusual muscle pain; unusual sleepiness; unexplained rapid breathing; unusual or unexpected stomach problems (such as nausea or vomiting); feeling cold, dizzy, or lightheaded; or suddenly having a slow or uneven heartbeat.
- Actoplus Met can cause your body to retain extra fluid, which leads to swelling and weight gain. Extra body fluid can cause or worsen heart failure. Tell your doctor right away if you experience swelling or fluid retention, especially in your ankles or legs; shortness of breath or trouble breathing, especially when you lie down; unusually fast increase in your weight; or unusual tiredness.
- Actoplus Met can cause liver problems. Tell your doctor right away if you experience nausea, vomiting, stomach pain, unusual or unexplained tiredness, loss of appetite, dark urine, or yellowing of your skin or the whites of your eyes.
- Actoplus Met can cause a diabetic eye disease called macular edema (swelling of the back of the eye). Tell your doctor right away if you have any changes in your vision. Your doctor will check your eyes regularly.
- In women, Actoplus Met can cause bones to break, usually in the hand, upper arm, or foot. Talk to your doctor about how to keep your bones healthy.
- Actoplus Met can increase your risk of developing bladder cancer. Do not take Actoplus Met if you are receiving treatment for

bladder cancer. Tell your doctor right away if you experience blood or a red color in your urine, an increased need to urinate, or pain while you urinate.

• Actoplus Met can cause low blood sugar, making you feel light-headed, dizzy, shaky, and hungry. This can happen if you skip meals, use another medicine that lowers your blood sugar, or have certain medical problems. Tell your doctor if this is a problem for you.

• Actoplus Met can increase your chance of getting pregnant if you are a premenopausal woman and do not have regular monthly periods. Talk to your doctor about receiving an adequate form of birth control while you are taking Actoplus Met.

Who should not take this medication?

Do not take Actoplus Met if you are allergic to it or any of its ingredients.

Do not take Actoplus Met if you have severe heart failure, kidney disease, diabetic ketoacidosis (a life-threatening medical emergency caused by insufficient insulin), or if you are going to receive an injection of a dye or contrast agent for an x-ray procedure.

What should I tell my doctor before I take the first dose of this medication?

Tell your doctor about all prescription, over-the-counter, and herbal medications you are taking before beginning treatment with Actoplus Met. Also, talk to your doctor about your complete medical history, especially if you have heart failure, liver or kidney problems, type 1 diabetes, macular edema, a history of diabetic ketoacidosis, or if you are going to have dye injected into a vein for an x-ray, CAT scan, heart study, or other type of scan. Tell your doctor if you drink alcohol frequently or if you are a binge drinker. Also, tell your doctor if you are a premenopausal woman who does not have periods regularly or at all.

What is the usual dosage?

Please see general statement regarding dosage on page xii.

Actoplus Met
Adults: The usual starting dose is 15/500 (15 milligrams [mg] of pioglitazone and 500 mg of metformin) or 15/850 (15 mg of pioglitazone and 850 mg of metformin) taken once or twice a day with food.

Actoplus Met XR
Adults: The usual starting dose is 15/1000 (15 mg of pioglitazone and 1000 mg of metformin) or 30/1000 (30 mg of pioglitazone and 1000 mg of metformin) taken once a day with the evening meal.

Your doctor may increase your dose as needed.

How should I take this medication?
- Take Actoplus Met exactly as prescribed by your doctor. Do not change your dose or stop taking Actoplus Met without first talking to your doctor. You should take it with food to lower the chance of getting an upset stomach.
- Swallow Actoplus Met XR tablets whole. Do not chew, cut, or crush them.
- When you take Actoplus Met XR, you may see something in your stool that looks like a tablet. This is the empty shell from the tablet after the medicine has been absorbed in your body.
- Follow your doctor's diet and exercise recommendations and test your blood sugar regularly while you are taking Actoplus Met.

What should I avoid while taking this medication?
Do not drink excessive amounts of alcohol while you are taking Actoplus Met.

Do not miss regular blood sugar testing (by yourself or your doctor).

What are possible food and drug interactions associated with this medication?
If Actoplus Met is taken with certain other drugs, the effects of either could be increased, decreased, or altered. It is especially

important to check with your doctor before combining Actoplus Met with the following: albuterol, birth control pills, blood pressure medications known as calcium channel blockers (such as nifedipine), cimetidine, corticosteroids (such as dexamethasone or prednisone), digoxin, diuretics (water pills) (such as amiloride, furosemide, hydrochlorothiazide, or triamterene), estrogen, gemfibrozil, isoniazid, morphine, nicotinic acid, phenothiazines (such as chlorpromazine), phenytoin, procainamide, pseudoephedrine, quinidine, quinine, ranitidine, rifampin, thyroid medications, trimethoprim, or vancomycin.

What are the possible side effects of this medication?
Please see general statement regarding side effects on page xiii.

> **Side effects may include:** diarrhea, dizziness, headache, low red blood cell counts, nausea, sinus infection, upper respiratory infection, upset stomach, urinary tract infection

Can I receive this medication if I am pregnant or breastfeeding?
The effects of Actoplus Met during pregnancy and breastfeeding are unknown. Do not breastfeed while you are taking Actoplus Met. Tell your doctor immediately if you are pregnant, plan to become pregnant, or are breastfeeding.

What should I do if I miss a dose of this medication?
If you miss a dose of Actoplus Met, take it with food as soon as you remember. However, if it is almost time for your next dose, skip the one you missed and return to your regular dosing schedule. Do not take two doses at once.

How should I store this medication?
Store at room temperature. Protect from moisture, excessive heat, and humidity.

Actos

Generic name: Pioglitazone HCl

What is this medication?

Actos is a medicine used to treat adults with type 2 diabetes along with diet and exercise. It can be used alone or with other diabetes medications.

What is the most important information I should know about this medication?

- Actos can cause your body to retain extra fluid, which leads to swelling and weight gain. Extra body fluid can cause or worsen heart failure. Tell your doctor right away if you experience swelling or fluid retention, especially in your ankles or legs; shortness of breath or trouble breathing, especially when you lie down; unusually fast increase in your weight; or unusual tiredness.
- Actos can cause liver problems. Tell your doctor right away if you experience nausea, vomiting, stomach pain, unusual or unexplained tiredness, loss of appetite, dark urine, or yellowing of your skin or the whites of your eyes.
- In women, Actos can cause bones to break, usually in the hand, upper arm, or foot. Talk to your doctor about how to keep your bones healthy.
- Actos can increase your risk of developing bladder cancer. Do not take Actos if you are receiving treatment for bladder cancer. Tell your doctor right away if you experience blood or a red color in your urine, an increased need to urinate, or pain while you urinate.
- Actos can cause low blood sugar, making you feel lightheaded, dizzy, shaky, and hungry. This can happen if you skip meals, use another medicine that lowers your blood sugar, or have certain medical problems. Tell your doctor if this is a problem for you.
- Actos can cause a diabetic eye disease called macular edema (swelling of the back of the eye). Tell your doctor right away if you have any changes in your vision. Your doctor will check your eyes regularly.
- Actos can increase your chance of getting pregnant if you are a premenopausal woman and do not have regular monthly

periods. Talk to your doctor about receiving an adequate form of birth control while you are taking Actos.

Who should not take this medication?

Do not take Actos if you are allergic to it or any of its ingredients.

Do not take Actos if you have severe heart failure.

What should I tell my doctor before I take the first dose of this medication?

Tell your doctor about all prescription, over-the-counter, and herbal medications you are taking before beginning treatment with Actos. Also, talk to your doctor about your complete medical history, especially if you have heart failure, type 1 diabetes, macular edema, liver problems, or if you have a history of diabetic ketoacidosis (a life-threatening medical emergency caused by insufficient insulin). Tell your doctor if you are a premenopausal woman who does not have periods regularly or at all.

What is the usual dosage?

Please see general statement regarding dosage on page xii.

Adults: The recommended starting dose is 15 milligrams (mg) or 30 mg once a day. Your doctor may increase your dose as needed.

If you have heart failure, your doctor will adjust your dose based on the severity of your condition.

How should I take this medication?

- Take Actos exactly as prescribed by your doctor. Do not change your dose or stop taking Actos without first talking to your doctor. Take it with or without food.
- Follow your doctor's diet and exercise recommendations and test your blood sugar regularly while you are taking Actos.

What should I avoid while taking this medication?

Do not miss regular blood sugar testing (by yourself or your doctor).

What are possible food and drug interactions associated with this medication?

If Actos is taken with certain other drugs, the effects of either could be increased, decreased, or altered. It is especially important to check with your doctor before combining Actos with gemfibrozil or rifampin.

What are the possible side effects of this medication?

Please see general statement regarding side effects on page xiii.

> **Side effects may include:** headache, muscle pain, respiratory tract infection, sinus infection, sore throat

Can I receive this medication if I am pregnant or breastfeeding?

The effects of Actos during pregnancy and breastfeeding are unknown. Do not breastfeed while you are taking Actos. Tell your doctor immediately if you are pregnant, plan to become pregnant, or are breastfeeding.

What should I do if I miss a dose of this medication?

If you miss a dose of Actos, take it as soon as you remember. However, if it is almost time for your next dose, skip the one you missed and return to your regular dosing schedule. Do not take two doses at once.

How should I store this medication?

Store at room temperature. Protect from light, moisture, and humidity.

Acyclovir: *see Zovirax Cream, page 1154*

Acyclovir: *see Zovirax Ointment, page 1156*

Adapalene/Benzoyl Peroxide: *see Epiduo, page 365*

Adderall

Generic name: Amphetamine Salt Combo

What is this medication?

Adderall is a medicine used to treat attention-deficit hyperactivity disorder (ADHD). This medicine can help to increase attention and decrease impulsiveness and hyperactivity in people with ADHD. Adderall is also used to treat narcolepsy (a sleep disorder characterized by excessive daytime sleepiness).

What is the most important information I should know about this medication?

- Adderall has a high potential for abuse. Taking Adderall for long periods of time may lead to extreme emotional and physical dependence. Your doctor will monitor your response and make sure you receive the correct dose. Tell your doctor if you have a history of drug or alcohol abuse.
- Adderall can cause serious heart-related and mental problems, stroke and heart attacks in adults, and increased blood pressure and heart rate. It can also cause new or worsening behavior and thought problems, bipolar illness, and aggressive or hostile behavior.
- In addition, new symptoms (such as hearing voices, believing things that are not true, or manic symptoms) can occur. Call your doctor immediately if you or your child experiences chest pain, shortness of breath, fainting, or new mental problems while taking Adderall.
- The doctor will check your child's height and weight while he/she is taking Adderall. If your child is not growing in height or gaining weight as expected, the doctor may stop this medicine.

Who should not take this medication?

Do not take Adderall if you are allergic to it or any of its ingredients. Do not take Adderall if you are very anxious, tense, or agitated.

Do not take Adderall if you have glaucoma (high pressure in the eye), heart disease, hardening of your arteries, high blood pressure, overactive thyroid, or a history of drug abuse. Also, do not use Adderall if you are taking antidepressant medications known as monoamine oxidase inhibitors (MAOIs) (such as phenelzine or tranylcypromine) or have taken them within the past 14 days.

What should I tell my doctor before I take the first dose of this medication?

Tell your doctor about all prescription, over-the-counter, and herbal medications you are taking before beginning treatment with Adderall. Also, talk to your doctor about your complete medical history, including heart problems, heart defects, high blood pressure, or a family history of these problems. Tell your doctor if you have a history of mental problems or a family history of psychosis, mania, bipolar disorder, or depression; tics or Tourette's syndrome; liver, kidney, or thyroid problems; or seizures or an abnormal brain wave test (EEG).

What is the usual dosage?

Please see general statement regarding dosage on page xii.

ADHD
Adults and children ≥6 years: The usual starting dose is 5 milligrams (mg) once or twice a day.

Children 3-5 years: The usual starting dose is 2.5 mg a day.

Narcolepsy
Adults and children ≥12 years: The usual starting dose is 10 mg a day.

Children 6-12 years: The usual starting dose is 5 mg a day.

Your or your child's doctor may increase the dose as appropriate.

How should I take this medication?
- Take Adderall exactly as prescribed by your doctor. Take it with or without food.
- Do not take Adderall late in the evening to avoid having trouble sleeping.

What should I avoid while taking this medication?

Use caution when driving, operating heavy machinery, or performing activities that require alertness.

Do not start any new medicine while you are taking Adderall without first talking to your doctor.

What are possible food and drug interactions associated with this medication?

If Adderall is taken with certain other drugs, the effects of either could be increased, decreased, or altered. It is especially important to check with your doctor before combining Adderall with the following: acetazolamide, ammonium chloride, antihistamines (such as cetirizine or loratadine), blood thinners (such as warfarin), blood pressure medications, certain antidepressants (such as desipramine or protriptyline), chlorpromazine, cold or allergy preparations containing decongestants, cryptenamine, ethosuximide, fruit juices, glutamic acid, guanethidine, haloperidol, lithium, MAOIs, meperidine, methenamine, norepinephrine, propoxyphene, reserpine, seizure medications (such as phenobarbital or phenytoin), sodium acid phosphate, sodium bicarbonate, stomach acid medicines (such as omeprazole or pantoprazole), or vitamin C.

What are the possible side effects of this medication?

Please see general statement regarding side effects on page xiii.

> **Side effects may include:** decreased appetite, dizziness, headache, nervousness, stomach ache, trouble sleeping

Can I receive this medication if I am pregnant or breastfeeding?

The effects of Adderall during pregnancy are unknown. Adderall can be found in your breast milk if you take it while breastfeeding. Do not breastfeed while you are taking Adderall. Tell your doctor immediately if you are pregnant, plan to become pregnant, or are breastfeeding.

What should I do if I miss a dose of this medication?

If you miss a dose of Adderall, take it as soon as you remember. However, if it is almost time for your next dose, skip the one you missed and return to your regular dosing schedule. Do not take two doses at once.

How should I store this medication?

Store at room temperature.

Adderall XR

Generic name: Amphetamine Salt Combo

What is this medication?

Adderall XR is a medicine used to treat attention-deficit hyperactivity disorder (ADHD). This medicine can help to increase attention and decrease impulsiveness and hyperactivity in people with ADHD. Adderall XR is an extended-release capsule. This means that it releases medicine into your body throughout the day.

What is the most important information I should know about this medication?

- Adderall XR has a high potential for abuse. Taking Adderall XR for long periods of time may lead to extreme emotional and physical dependence. Your doctor will monitor your response and make sure you receive the correct dose. Tell your doctor if you have a history of drug or alcohol abuse.
- Adderall XR can cause serious heart-related and mental problems, stroke and heart attacks in adults, and increased blood pressure and heart rate. It can also cause new or worsening behavior and thought problems, bipolar illness, and aggressive or hostile behavior.
- In addition, new symptoms (such as hearing voices, believing things that are not true, or manic symptoms) can occur. Call your doctor immediately if you or your child experiences chest pain, shortness of breath, fainting, or new mental problems while taking Adderall XR.

- The doctor will check your child's height and weight while he/she is taking Adderall XR. If your child is not growing in height or gaining weight as expected, the doctor may stop this medicine.

Who should not take this medication?

Do not take Adderall XR if you are allergic to it or any of its ingredients. Do not take Adderall XR if you are very anxious, tense, or agitated.

Do not take Adderall XR if you have glaucoma (high pressure in the eye), heart disease, hardening of your arteries, high blood pressure, overactive thyroid, or a history of drug abuse. Also, do not use Adderall XR if you are taking antidepressant medications known as monoamine oxidase inhibitors (MAOIs) (such as phenelzine or tranylcypromine) or have taken them within the past 14 days.

What should I tell my doctor before I take the first dose of this medication?

Tell your doctor about all prescription, over-the-counter, and herbal medications you are taking before beginning treatment with Adderall XR. Also, talk to your doctor about your complete medical history, including heart problems, heart defects, high blood pressure, or a family history of these problems. Tell your doctor if you have a history of mental problems or a family history of psychosis, mania, bipolar disorder, or depression; tics or Tourette's syndrome; liver, kidney, or thyroid problems; or seizures or an abnormal brain wave test (EEG).

What is the usual dosage?

Please see general statement regarding dosage on page xii.

Adults: The usual dose is 20 milligrams (mg) once a day.

Children and adolescents 6-17 years: The usual starting dose is 10 mg once a day.

Your or your child's doctor may increase the dose as appropriate.

How should I take this medication?

- Swallow your Adderall XR capsule whole with water or other liquids. Do not crush or chew it. Take it in the morning when you first wake up. Take it with or without food.
- If you cannot swallow the Adderall XR capsule whole, open the capsule carefully and sprinkle the medicine over a spoonful of applesauce. Swallow the medicine and applesauce combination right away without chewing. Follow with a drink of water or other liquid.

What should I avoid while taking this medication?

Use caution when driving, operating heavy machinery, or performing activities that require alertness.

Do not start any new medicine while you are taking Adderall XR without first talking to your doctor.

What are possible food and drug interactions associated with this medication?

If Adderall XR is taken with certain other drugs, the effects of either could be increased, decreased, or altered. It is especially important to check with your doctor before combining Adderall XR with the following: acetazolamide, ammonium chloride, antihistamines (such as cetirizine or loratadine), blood thinners (such as warfarin), blood pressure medications, certain antidepressants (such as desipramine or protriptyline), chlorpromazine, cold or allergy preparations containing decongestants, cryptenamine, ethosuximide, glutamic acid, guanethidine, haloperidol, lithium, MAOIs, meperidine, methenamine, norepinephrine, propoxyphene, reserpine, seizure medications (such as phenobarbital or phenytoin), sodium acid phosphate, sodium bicarbonate, stomach acid medicines (such as omeprazole or pantoprazole), or vitamin C.

What are the possible side effects of this medication?

Please see general statement regarding side effects on page xiii.

Side effects may include: decreased appetite, dizziness, dry mouth, fast heartbeat, headache, mood swings, nervousness, stomach ache, trouble sleeping, weight loss

Can I receive this medication if I am pregnant or breastfeeding?

The effects of Adderall XR during pregnancy are unknown. Adderall XR can be found in your breast milk if you take it while breastfeeding. Do not breastfeed while you are taking Adderall XR. Tell your doctor immediately if you are pregnant, plan to become pregnant, or are breastfeeding.

What should I do if I miss a dose of this medication?

If you miss a dose of Adderall XR, take it as soon as you remember. However, if it is almost time for your next dose, skip the one you missed and return to your regular dosing schedule. Do not take two doses at once.

How should I store this medication?

Store at room temperature.

Adipex-P

Generic name: Phentermine HCl

What is this medication?

Adipex-P is a medicine used to help reduce your appetite. Adipex-P is used for short-term (few weeks) add on treatment for weight loss based on exercise, lifestyle changes and a lower calorie diet. Adipex-P is used in patients with a body mass index (BMI) greater than or equal to 30 kg/m^2 (considerably overweight) or a BMI greater than or equal to 27 kg/m^2 (overweight) who have other risks, such as high blood pressure, diabetes, or high cholesterol.

What is the most important information I should know about this medication?

- Adipex-P has the risk of causing a rare but fatal lung disease called primary pulmonary hypertension (PPH). Tell your doctor right away if you have shortness of breath, chest pain, leg swelling, or fainting spells as these could be signs of PPH.

- Adipex-P can also cause heart problems and high blood pressure. Contact your doctor right away if you develop any new symptoms.
- Do not drive, operate heavy machinery, or participate in dangerous tasks until you know how Adipex-P affects you.
- Adipex-P can have less effect with time (tolerance). Talk to your doctor if you think Adipex-P is no longer working for you.

Who should not take this medication?

Do not take Adipex-P if you are allergic to it or any of its ingredients.

Do not take Adipex-P if you currently take or have taken antidepressant medications known as monoamine oxidase inhibitors (MAOIs) (such as phenelzine) within the past 14 days.

Do not take Adipex-P if you have heart or blood vessel problems, hyperthyroidism (an overactive thyroid gland), glaucoma (high pressure in the eye), agitated states, or a history of drug abuse.

Do not take Adipex-P if you are pregnant or are breastfeeding.

What should I tell my doctor before I take the first dose of this medication?

Tell your doctor about all prescription, over-the-counter, and herbal medications you are taking before beginning treatment with Adipex-P. Also, talk to your doctor about your complete medical history, especially if you have a history of heart disease or drug abuse; if you have high blood pressure, hyperthyroidism, glaucoma, or diabetes; or if you are pregnant, plan to become pregnant, or are breastfeeding.

What is the usual dosage?

Please see general statement regarding dosage on page xii.

Adults >16 years: The usual dose is one capsule once a day. Your doctor will prescribe the appropriate dose for you.

How should I take this medication?

- Take Adipex-P exactly as prescribed by your doctor. Take Adipex-P before breakfast or 1 to 2 hours after breakfast. You can break the tablets in half, if necessary.
- Do not take Adipex-P late at night because you can have trouble sleeping.

What should I avoid while taking this medication?

Do not drive, operate heavy machinery, or participate in dangerous tasks until you know how Adipex-P affects you.

Do not drink alcohol or take other medications for weight loss while taking Adipex-P.

What are possible food and drug interactions associated with this medication?

If Adipex-P is taken with certain other drugs, the effects of either could be increased, decreased, or altered. It is especially important to check with your doctor before combining Adipex-P with the following: alcohol, antidiabetic medications (such as insulin), certain antidepressant medications known as selective serotonin reuptake inhibitors (such as fluoxetine, fluvoxamine, paroxetine, or sertraline), MAOIs, or other medications used for weight loss.

What are the possible side effects of this medication?

Please see general statement regarding side effects on page xiii.

Side effects may include: chest pain, constipation, diarrhea, dizziness, dry mouth, fainting spells, headache, impotence, increased blood pressure, increased heart rate, intense happiness or sadness, intestinal or stomach problems, irregular heartbeat, leg swelling, rash, restlessness, shortness of breath, tremor, trouble sleeping, unpleasant taste

Can I receive this medication if I am pregnant or breastfeeding?

Do not take Adipex-P if you are pregnant. The effects of Adipex-P during breastfeeding are unknown. Tell your doctor immediately if you are pregnant, plan to become pregnant, or are breastfeeding.

What should I do if I miss a dose of this medication?

If you miss a dose of Adipex-P, take it as soon as you remember. However, if it is almost time for your next dose, skip the one you missed and return to your regular dosing schedule. Do not take two doses at once.

How should I store this medication?

Store at room temperature.

Advair Diskus

Generic name: Fluticasone Propionate/Salmeterol

What is this medication?

Advair Diskus is a combination medicine used to treat asthma and airway narrowing associated with chronic obstructive pulmonary disease (COPD), including chronic bronchitis (long-term inflammation of the lungs) and emphysema (lung disease that causes shortness of breath). Advair Diskus contains two medicines: fluticasone (decreases inflammation in the lungs) and salmeterol (relaxes muscles in the airways).

What is the most important information I should know about this medication?

- If you have asthma and use Advair Diskus, you can have an increased risk of death from asthma problems. Tell your doctor if your breathing problems worsen over time while you are using Advair Diskus. Get emergency medical care if your breathing problems worsen quickly or if you use your rescue inhaler medicine, but it does not relieve your symptoms.
- Advair Diskus must only be used if your doctor decides that your asthma is not well controlled with a long-term asthma-control

medicine, such as an inhaled corticosteroid (medicine that helps fight inflammation). When your asthma is well controlled, your doctor may tell you to stop using Advair Diskus. Your doctor will decide if you can stop Advair Diskus without loss of your asthma control. Your doctor may prescribe a different asthma-control medication for you, such as an inhaled corticosteroid.

- Children and adolescents who use Advair Diskus can have an increased risk of being hospitalized for asthma problems.
- Advair Diskus does not treat the symptoms of a sudden asthma attack. Always have a short-acting rescue inhaler (such as albuterol) to treat sudden symptoms. If you do not have a short-acting inhaler, tell your doctor to have one prescribed for you. Tell your doctor immediately if an asthma attack does not respond to the rescue inhaler or if you require more doses than usual.
- Do not use other inhaled medications similar to Advair Diskus while you are using Advair Diskus.
- Advair Diskus can cause infections in your mouth and throat. Tell your doctor if you have any redness or white colored patches in your mouth.
- Advair Diskus can increase your risk of getting pneumonia, especially if you have COPD. Call your doctor if you develop an increase in mucus production, change in mucus color, fever, chills, increased cough, or increased breathing problems.
- If you use Advair Diskus, you can have a higher risk of getting an infection. Do not expose yourself to chickenpox or measles while you are using Advair Diskus. Tell your doctor if you experience any signs or symptoms of infection (such as a fever, pain, aches, chills, feeling tired, nausea, or vomiting).
- Advair Diskus can cause a serious allergic reaction. Call your doctor right away if you experience breathing problems, hives, rash, or swelling of your face, mouth, or tongue.
- Advair Diskus can have serious effects on your heart or nervous system. Tell your doctor if you experience increased blood pressure, fast or irregular heartbeat, chest pain, shaking, or nervousness.
- Advair Diskus can cause slowed or delayed growth in children. Check your child's growth regularly during treatment with Advair Diskus.

- Cataracts (clouding of the eye's lens) or glaucoma (high pressure in the eye) can occur while you are using Advair Diskus. Tell your doctor if you experience a change in your vision.

Who should not take this medication?

Do not use Advair Diskus if you are allergic to it, any of its ingredients, or to milk proteins. Also, do not use Advair Diskus to treat an asthma attack.

What should I tell my doctor before I take the first dose of this medication?

Tell your doctor about all prescription, over-the-counter, and herbal medications you are taking before beginning treatment with Advair Diskus. Also, talk to your doctor about your complete medical history, especially if you have heart, thyroid, or liver problems; high blood pressure; seizures; diabetes; osteoporosis (thin, weak bones); or had chickenpox or measles, or have recently been near anyone with chickenpox or measles; have tuberculosis (a bacterial infection that affects the lungs), or any type of infection; cataracts or glaucoma; or are planning to have surgery. Also, tell your doctor if you take a corticosteroid medicine, seizure medications, or medicines that suppress your immune system.

What is the usual dosage?

Please see general statement regarding dosage on page xii.

Adults and children ≥4 years: The usual dose is 1 inhalation twice a day (morning and evening, approximately 12 hours apart). Your doctor will prescribe the appropriate strength for you or your child.

How should I take this medication?

- Use Advair Diskus exactly as prescribed by your doctor. Do not use Adavir Diskus more often or use more puffs than you have been prescribed.
- Rinse your mouth with water and spit it out after each dose. Do not swallow the water.

- Throw away Advair Diskus 1 month after you remove it from the foil overwrap pouch or when the dose indicator reads "0", whichever comes first.
- Please review the instructions that came with your prescription on how to properly use your inhaler.

What should I avoid while taking this medication?

You may not feel or taste the medication from your Advair Diskus when you inhale it. This does not mean that you did not get the medication. Do not repeat your inhalations even if you did not feel the medication when inhaling.

Do not stop using Adavir Diskus or other asthma medicine unless told to do so by your doctor because symptoms might get worse. Your doctor will change your medicines as needed.

Do not use a spacer device with Advair Diskus.

Do not breathe into Advair Diskus.

What are possible food and drug interactions associated with this medication?

If Adavir Diskus is used with certain other drugs, the effects of either could be increased, decreased, or altered. It is especially important to check with your doctor before combining Advair Diskus with the following: atazanavir, blood pressure/heart medications known as beta-blockers (such as propranolol), certain antidepressants (such as amitriptyline or nortriptyline), clarithromycin, diuretics (water pills) (such as furosemide or hydrochlorothiazide), indinavir, itraconazole, ketoconazole, monoamine oxidase inhibitors (MAOIs), a class of medications used to treat depression and other psychiatric conditions (such as phenelzine or tranylcypromine), nefazodone, nelfinavir, ritonavir, saquinavir, or telithromycin.

What are the possible side effects of this medication?

Please see general statement regarding side effects on page xiii.

Side effects may include: bronchitis, cough, fungal infection in your mouth and throat, headache, hoarseness and voice changes, muscle and bone pain, nausea, respiratory infections, throat irritation, vomiting

Can I receive this medication if I am pregnant or breastfeeding?

The effects of Advair Diskus during pregnancy and breastfeeding are unknown. Do not breastfeed while you are taking Advair Diskus. Tell your doctor immediately if you are pregnant, plan to become pregnant, or are breastfeeding.

What should I do if I miss a dose of this medication?

If you miss a dose of Advair Diskus, take it as soon as you remember. However, if it is almost time for your next dose, skip the one you missed and return to your regular dosing schedule. Do not take two doses at once.

How should I store this medication?

Store at room temperature, away from direct heat or sunlight.

Afluria

Generic name: Influenza Virus Vaccine

What is this medication?

Afluria is a flu virus vaccine used to immunize against certain types of influenza disease. Afluria is administered intramuscularly (injected into the muscle).

What is the most important information I should know about this medication?

- Afluria can cause an increased risk of Guillain-Barre syndrome (a disorder that causes your immune system to attack the nerves that connect your brain and spinal cord with the rest of your body).
- Afluria contains noninfectious killed viruses and cannot cause influenza.

- Afluria provides protection against illness due to influenza viruses only, and cannot provide protection against all lung illness.
- Tell your doctor immediately if you experience any side effects after you receive Afluria.
- It is recommended that you receive your flu vaccine yearly. Vaccination with Afluria may not protect all individuals who receive it.

Who should not take this medication?

Your doctor will not administer Afluria to you if you are allergic to it or any of its ingredients (including egg protein).

Your doctor will not administer Afluria to you if you had an allergic reaction to a previous dose of any flu vaccine.

What should I tell my doctor before I take the first dose of this medication?

Tell your doctor about all prescription, over-the-counter, and herbal medications you are taking before beginning treatment with Afluria. Also, talk to your doctor about your complete medical history, especially if you have an egg allergy; Guillain-Barre syndrome; a weak immune system; or are pregnant, plan to become pregnant, or are breastfeeding.

What is the usual dosage?

Please see general statement regarding dosage on page xii.

Adults and children ≥5 years: Your doctor will administer the appropriate dose for you based on your age.

How should I take this medication?

- Your doctor will administer Afluria to you.

What should I avoid while taking this medication?

Do not miss your follow-up appointments with your doctor.

What are possible food and drug interactions associated with this medication?

If Afluria is used with certain other drugs, the effects of either could be increased, decreased, or altered. It is especially important to tell your doctor if you are taking any of the following prior to treatment with Afluria: medications that weaken your immune system or any other vaccines.

What are the possible side effects of this medication?

Please see general statement regarding side effects on page xiii.

> **Side effects may include:** fever; headache; muscle pain; pain, redness, swelling, and/or tenderness at the injection site; tiredness

Can I receive this medication if I am pregnant or breastfeeding?

The effects of Afluria during pregnancy and breastfeeding are unknown. Tell your doctor immediately if you are pregnant, plan to become pregnant, or are breastfeeding.

What should I do if I miss a dose of this medication?

Afluria should be given under special circumstances determined by your doctor.

If the vaccine is for your child, do not miss the follow-up appointments with your child's doctor.

How should I store this medication?

Your doctor will store this medication for you.

Aggrastat
Generic name: Tirofiban HCl

What is this medication?
Aggrastat is a medicine used intravenously (through a vein in your arm) to treat acute coronary syndrome (condition brought on by sudden, reduced blood flow to the heart). In addition, Aggrastat is used in patients undergoing percutaneous coronary intervention (a surgical procedure to restore blood flow to blocked arteries).

What is the most important information I should know about this medication?
- Aggrastat can lead to increased bleeding (such as bleeding in your brain, heart, or bloody mucus). Your doctor will monitor you for this while you are receiving Aggrastat.

Who should not take this medication?
Your doctor will not administer Aggrastat to you if you are allergic to it or any of its ingredients, or if you have certain medical conditions that can increase your risk of bleeding.

What should I tell my doctor before I take the first dose of this medication?
Tell your doctor about all prescription, over-the-counter, and herbal medications you are taking before beginning treatment with Aggrastat. Also, talk to your doctor about your complete medical history, especially if you have kidney impairment, high blood pressure, heart disease, brain tumors, a history of bleeding or stroke, or are pregnant, plan to become pregnant, or are breastfeeding.

What is the usual dosage?
Please see general statement regarding dosage on page xii.

Adults: Your doctor will administer the appropriate dose for you intravenously, based on your body weight, condition, and whether you are taking other medications.

If you have kidney impairment, your doctor will adjust your dose appropriately.

How should I take this medication?

- Your doctor will administer Aggrastat to you and will monitor you for bleeding.

What should I avoid while taking this medication?

Do not miss any scheduled follow-up appointments with your doctor.

What are possible food and drug interactions associated with this medication?

If Aggrastat is used with certain other drugs, the effects of either could be increased, decreased, or altered. It is important to tell your doctor about any other medications you are taking.

What are the possible side effects of this medication?

Please see general statement regarding side effects on page xiii.

> **Side effects may include:** bleeding, coronary artery dissection (a tear in one of the arteries leading to your heart), decreased heart rate, dizziness, pain in your legs or pelvis, sweating, swelling

Can I receive this medication if I am pregnant or breastfeeding?

The effects of Aggrastat during pregnancy and breastfeeding are unknown. Tell your doctor immediately if you are pregnant, plan to become pregnant, or are breastfeeding.

What should I do if I miss a dose of this medication?

Aggrastat should be given under special circumstances determined by your doctor.

How should I store this medication?

Your doctor will store this medication for you.

Aggrenox
Generic name: Aspirin/Dipyridamole

What is this medication?

Aggrenox is a medicine used to lower the risk of stroke in people who have had a mini-stroke or full stroke due to a blood clot.

What is the most important information I should know about this medication?

- Aggrenox can increase the risk of bleeding. You may bleed more easily while taking Aggrenox, and it may take longer than usual to stop bleeding. Your risk is higher if you drink three or more alcoholic beverages a day. Tell your doctor right away if you experience severe headache with drowsiness, confusion or memory change, stomach pain, heartburn or nausea, vomiting blood or your vomit looks like coffee grounds, red or bloody stools, black tarry stools, or if you faint while you are taking Aggrenox.
- Aggrenox can cause new or worsening chest pain in some people with heart disease. Tell your doctor if you have new chest pain or have any change in your chest pain while you are taking Aggrenox.
- Aggrenox can cause liver problems. Tell your doctor if you experience loss of appetite, pale colored stool, stomach pain, dark urine, itching, or yellowing of your skin or whites of your eyes while you are taking Aggrenox.
- Aggrenox can cause a potentially life-threatening disease of the brain and liver if given to children or teenagers with a viral infection (such as chickenpox).
- Aggrenox can cause headaches when you first start taking the medicine. These usually go away with time. Tell your doctor if you experience headaches that you cannot tolerate while you are taking Aggrenox.

Who should not take this medication?

Do not take Aggrenox if you are allergic to it or any of its ingredients.

Do not take Aggrenox if you are allergic to nonsteroidal anti-inflammatory drugs (NSAIDs) (such as ibuprofen or naproxen).

Do not take Aggrenox if you have asthma, a constant runny nose, nasal polyps, or severe kidney failure.

Do not give Aggrenox to a child or teenager with a viral infection.

What should I tell my doctor before I take the first dose of this medication?

Tell your doctor about all prescription, over-the-counter, and herbal medications you are taking before beginning treatment with Aggrenox. Also, talk to your doctor about your complete medical history, especially if you have stomach ulcers; heart, kidney, or liver problems; low blood pressure; myasthenia gravis (loss of muscle control), or a history of bleeding problems.

What is the usual dosage?

Please see general statement regarding dosage on page xii.

Adults: The recommended dose is 1 capsule twice a day.

How should I take this medication?

- Take Aggrenox exactly as prescribed by your doctor. Take Aggrenox once in the morning and once in the evening. Take it with or without food.
- Swallow Aggrenox capsules whole. Do not crush or chew them.

What should I avoid while taking this medication?

Do not drink excessive amounts of alcohol while you are taking Aggrenox.

What are possible food and drug interactions associated with this medication?

If Aggrenox is taken with certain other drugs, the effects of either could be increased, decreased, or altered. It is especially important to check with your doctor before combining Aggrenox with the following: acetazolamide, adenosine, blood pressure/heart medications known as angiotensin-converting enzyme (ACE) inhibitors (such as enalapril or lisinopril) or beta-blockers (such as atenolol or propranolol), blood thinners (such as warfarin), diabetes medicines, diuretics (water pills) (such as furosemide), donepezil, methotrexate, NSAIDs, probenecid, rivastigmine, seizure medications (such as phenytoin or valproic acid), or sulfinpyrazone.

What are the possible side effects of this medication?
Please see general statement regarding side effects on page xiii.

> **Side effects may include:** diarrhea, headache, upset stomach

Can I receive this medication if I am pregnant or breastfeeding?
Aggrenox can harm your unborn baby if you take it during pregnancy. Do not take Aggrenox in the third trimester of your pregnancy. Aggrenox can be found in your breast milk if you take it while breastfeeding. Tell your doctor immediately if you are pregnant, plan to become pregnant, or are breastfeeding.

What should I do if I miss a dose of this medication?
If you miss a dose of Aggrenox, take it as soon as you remember. However, if it is almost time for your next dose, skip the one you missed and return to your regular dosing schedule. Do not take two doses at once.

How should I store this medication?
Store at room temperature. Protect from excessive moisture.

Albuterol Sulfate: *see Albuterol sulfate, page 46*

Albuterol Sulfate: *see Proair HFA, page 841*

Albuterol Sulfate: *see Proventil HFA, page 865*

Albuterol Sulfate: *see Ventolin HFA, page 1059*

Albuterol Sulfate/Ipratropium Bromide: *see Combivent, page 256*

Albuterol Sulfate/Ipratropium Bromide: *see Duoneb, page 338*

Albuterol sulfate

Generic name: Albuterol Sulfate

What is this medication?

Albuterol sulfate is a medicine used for the relief of bronchospasms (airway narrowing) caused by airway disease (such as asthma). Albuterol sulfate relaxes the airway muscles so that you can breathe more easily. Albuterol sulfate is available as an inhalation aerosol, inhalation solution, tablets, extended-release tablets (albuterol sulfate ER), and syrup. Albuterol sulfate aerosol is also used in the prevention of exercise-induced bronchospasms.

What is the most important information I should know about this medication?

- Tell your doctor right away if albuterol sulfate is less effective in relieving your symptoms. Also, tell your doctor if your symptoms get worse.
- Albuterol sulfate can cause heart problems, such as arrhythmias (life-threatening irregular heartbeat) or an increase in your heartbeat. Tell your doctor if you have any heart problems. Albuterol sulfate can also decrease your blood potassium levels, and this can affect your heart.
- Albuterol sulfate can cause allergic reactions or severe skin reactions. Tell your doctor right away if you experience symptoms such as itchiness, rash, angioedema (a condition involving swelling of the face, extremities, eyes, lips, and tongue), wheezing, chest tightness, or shortness of breath.

Who should not take this medication?

Do not use albuterol sulfate if you are allergic to it or any of its ingredients.

What should I tell my doctor before I take the first dose of this medication?

Tell your doctor about all prescription, over-the-counter, and herbal medications you are taking before beginning treatment with albuterol sulfate. Also, talk to your doctor about your complete medical history, especially if you have heart problems, diabetes, hyperthyroidism (an overactive thyroid gland), high blood pressure, or seizures.

What is the usual dosage?
Please see general statement regarding dosage on page xii.

The albuterol sulfate dose will depend on the severity of your condition and the type of product you are taking. Always follow the dosage prescribed by your doctor. The following is a general dosage guideline based on various manufacturer recommendations.

Inhalation Aerosol
Adults and children ≥4 years: The usual dose is 2 inhalations every 4-6 hours. In some individuals, 1 inhalation every 4 hours may be sufficient. To prevent bronchospasm due to excercise, the usual dose is 2 inhalations taken 15-30 minutes before exercise.

Inhalation Solution
Adults, children ≥12 years, and children 2-11 years and ≥15 kilograms (kg): The usual dose is 2.5 milligrams (mg) 3-4 times a day by nebulizer.

Children ≥12 years and <15 kg, and children 2-11 years: Your doctor will prescribe the appropriate dose for your child, based on their weight.

Tablets
Adults and children >12 years: The usual starting dose is 2 or 4 mg 3-4 times a day.

Children 6-12 years: The usual starting dose is 2 mg 3-4 times a day.

Extended-Release Tablets
Adults and children >12 years: The usual dose is 8 mg every 12 hours. In some individuals, 4 mg every 12 hours may be sufficient.

Children 6-12 years: The usual dose is 4 mg every 12 hours.

Syrup

Adults and children >14 years: The usual starting dose is 1 or 2 teaspoonfuls 3-4 times a day.

Children 6-14 years: The usual starting dose is 1 teaspoonful 3-4 times a day.

Children 2-5 years: Your doctor will prescribe the appropriate dose for your child, based on their weight.

If you are elderly, your doctor will adjust your dose appropriately.

How should I take this medication?

- Take albuterol sulfate exactly as prescribed by your doctor. Do not take extra doses or take it more often without asking your doctor. The effects of albuterol sulfate can last up to 6 hours.
- Swallow albuterol sulfate ER tablets whole. Do not crush, split, or chew the tablets. The effects of albuterol sulfate ER tablets should last up to 12 hours.
- If you are using the inhalation aerosol or solution, please review the instructions that came with your prescription on how to properly use your inhaler or nebulizer.

What should I avoid while taking this medication?

Do not mix other medicines with albuterol sulfate solution in the nebulizer.

Do not use albuterol sulfate solution if it changes color or becomes cloudy.

What are possible food and drug interactions associated with this medication?

If albuterol sulfate is taken with certain other drugs, the effects of either could be increased, decreased, or altered. It is especially important to check with your doctor before combining albuterol sulfate with the following: blood pressure/heart medications known as beta-blockers (such as metoprolol or propranolol), certain antidepressant medications (such as amitriptyline or phenelzine), certain diuretics (water pills) (such as furosemide or hydrochlorothiazide), digoxin, or other medications that can affect your heart (such as amphetamine or epinephrine).

What are the possible side effects of this medication?

Please see general statement regarding side effects on page xiii.

> **Side effects may include:** allergic reactions, chest pain, fast or irregular heartbeats, headache, nervousness, shakiness, worsening of bronchospasm

Can I receive this medication if I am pregnant or breastfeeding?

The effects of albuterol sulfate during pregnancy and breastfeeding are unknown. Tell your doctor immediately if you are pregnant, plan to become pregnant, or are breastfeeding.

What should I do if I miss a dose of this medication?

If you miss a dose of albuterol sulfate, take it as soon as you remember. However, if it is almost time for your next dose, skip the one you missed and return to your regular dosing schedule. Do not take two doses at once.

How should I store this medication?

Store at room temperature. Protect albuterol sulfate solution from light.

Albuterol Sulfate: see Albuterol sulfate, page 46

Albuterol Sulfate: see Proair HFA, page 841

Albuterol Sulfate: see Proventil HFA, page 865

Albuterol Sulfate: see Ventolin HFA, page 1059

Albuterol Sulfate/Ipratropium Bromide: see Combivent, page 256

Albuterol Sulfate/Ipratropium Bromide: see Duoneb, page 338

Aldactone

Generic name: Spironolactone

What is this medication?

Aldactone is a diuretic (water pill) used to treat primary hyperaldosteronism (an increase in a hormone called aldosterone which can cause an increase in blood pressure). Aldactone is also used to treat edema (swelling) caused by congestive heart failure, scarring of the liver, or a kidney disorder in which too much protein is excreted into the urine. In addition, it is used to treat high blood pressure either alone or with other diuretics or blood pressure lowering medicines. Aldactone can also be used to treat other conditions, as determined by your doctor.

What is the most important information I should know about this medication?

- Aldactone can cause high blood potassium levels. This effect may be greater in those with diabetes or kidney problems, elderly or severely ill. Your doctor will monitor you for increased blood potassium levels.
- Aldactone can cause breast enlargement in men. This is normally reversible once you stop taking the medicine. Tell your doctor if you experience this.

Who should not take this medication?

Do not take Aldactone if you are allergic to it or any of its ingredients.

Do not take Aldactone if you have high blood potassium levels, severe kidney disease, or if you are unable to produce urine.

What should I tell my doctor before I take the first dose of this medication?

Tell your doctor about all prescription, over-the-counter, and herbal medications you are taking before beginning treatment with Aldactone. Also, talk to your doctor about your complete medical history, especially if you have liver or kidney problems, high blood potassium levels, heart failure, or if you are pregnant, plan to become pregnant, or are breastfeeding.

What is the usual dosage?
Please see general statement regarding dosage on page xii.

Primary Hyperaldosteronism
Adults: Your doctor will prescribe the appropriate dose for you based on your condition.

Swelling Caused by Heart Failure, Kidney, or Liver Disease
Adults: The usual starting dose is 100 milligrams (mg) a day, either in single or divided doses.

High Blood Pressure
Adults: The usual starting dose is 50 mg-100 mg a day, either in single or divided doses.

Your doctor may adjust your dose as needed.

How should I take this medication?
• Take Aldactone exactly as prescribed by your doctor.

What should I avoid while taking this medication?
Do not take potassium supplements or eat foods with high potassium levels (such as salt substitutes) while you are taking Aldactone.

What are possible food and drug interactions associated with this medication?
If Aldactone is taken with certain other drugs, the effects of either could be increased, decreased, or altered. It is especially important to check with your doctor before combining Aldactone with the following: alcohol, barbiturates (such as phenobarbital), blood pressure medications known as angiotensin converting enzyme inhibitors (such as captopril or lisinopril), certain diuretics (such as amiloride or triamterene), corticosteroids (such as prednisone), digoxin, lithium, narcotic painkillers (such as hydrocodone or oxycodone), nonsteroidal anti-inflammatory drugs (NSAIDs) (such as ibuprofen or indomethacin), norepinephrine, or tubocurarine.

What are the possible side effects of this medication?
Please see general statement regarding side effects on page xiii.

> **Side effects may include:** blood disorders, fever, high blood potassium levels, kidney problems, mental confusion, skin rash, stomach problems

Can I receive this medication if I am pregnant or breastfeeding?

The effects of Aldactone during pregnancy are unknown. Aldactone can be found in your breast milk if you take it while breastfeeding. Do not breastfeed while you are taking Aldactone. Tell your doctor immediately if you are pregnant, plan to become pregnant, or are breastfeeding.

What should I do if I miss a dose of this medication?

If you miss a dose of Aldactone, take it as soon as you remember. However, if it is almost time for your next dose, skip the one you missed and return to your regular dosing schedule. Do not take two doses at once.

How should I store this medication?

Store at room temperature.

Alendronate Sodium: see Fosamax, page 410

Aliskiren: see Tekturna, page 973

Allopurinol: see Zyloprim, page 1159

Alphagan P

Generic name: Brimonidine Tartrate

What is this medication?

Alphagan P is an eye drop used to lower pressure in the eye in people with open-angle glaucoma or ocular hypertension (high pressure in the eye).

What is the most important information I should know about this medication?

- Alphagan P can worsen disorders associated with compromised blood flow. Tell your doctor about all your medical conditions, especially if you have severe heart disease, before beginning treatment with Alphagan P.
- Do not allow the tip of the bottle to touch your eye or any other surface, as serious eye infections may occur if your bottle becomes contaminated. Tell your doctor immediately if you experience any eye injury or infection with Alphagan P.

Who should not take this medication?

Do not use Alphagan P if you are allergic to it or any of its ingredients.

Do not use Alphagan P in children <2 years old.

What should I tell my doctor before I take the first dose of this medication?

Tell your doctor about all prescription, over-the-counter, and herbal medications you are taking before beginning treatment with Alphagan P. Also, talk to your doctor about your complete medical history, especially if you have depression, brain or heart problems, circulation problems (such as Raynaud's disease), sudden falls in your blood pressure, eye disorders, or if you had or plan to have eye surgery.

What is the usual dosage?

Please see general statement regarding dosage on page xii.

Adults and children ≥2 years: The recommended dose is 1 drop in the affected eye(s) three times a day, about 8 hours apart.

How should I take this medication?

- Apply Alphagan P exactly as prescribed by your doctor.
- If you are using Alphagan P with another eye drop, the drops should be applied at least 5 minutes apart.

What should I avoid while taking this medication?

Do not allow the tip of the bottle to touch your eye or any other surface, as this can contaminate the medication.

Do not use Alphagan P if the solution changes color or becomes cloudy.

Do not drive or operate heavy machinery until you know how Alphagan P affects you.

What are possible food and drug interactions associated with this medication?

If Alphagan P is used with certain other drugs, the effects of either could be increased, decreased, or altered. It is especially important to check with your doctor before combining Alphagan P with the following: alcohol, anesthesia, barbiturates (such as phenobarbital), blood pressure/heart medications, certain antidepressants (such as amitriptyline or phenelzine), narcotic painkillers (such as hydrocodone or oxycodone), or sedatives (such as butalbital or lorazepam).

What are the possible side effects of this medication?

Please see general statement regarding side effects on page xiii.

Side effects may include: allergic reactions, burning or itching in your eyes, changes in your vision, dry mouth, eye problems, high blood pressure, pink eye

Can I receive this medication if I am pregnant or breastfeeding?

The effects of Alphagan P during pregnancy and breastfeeding are unknown. Do not breastfeed while you are using Alphagan P. Tell your doctor immediately if you are pregnant, plan to become pregnant, or are breastfeeding.

What should I do if I miss a dose of this medication?

If you miss a dose of Alphagan P, apply it as soon as you remember. However, if it is almost time for your next dose, skip the one you missed and return to your regular dosing schedule. Do not apply two doses at once.

How should I store this medication?
Store at room temperature.

Alprazolam: see Xanax, page 1100

Alprazolam: see Xanax XR, page 1103

Altace
Generic name: Ramipril

What is this medication?
Altace is a medicine used to reduce the risk of heart attack, stroke, and death from heart problems. This medicine is also used alone or in combination with diuretics (water pills) to treat high blood pressure. It is also used to stabilize people after a heart attack by preventing heart failure.

What is the most important information I should know about this medication?
- Altace can cause a rare but serious allergic reaction leading to extreme swelling of your face, lips, tongue, throat, or gut (causing severe abdominal pain). You may have an increased risk of experiencing these symptoms if you have ever had an allergy to angiotensin-converting enzyme (ACE) inhibitor-type medicines or if you are African American. If you experience any of these symptoms, seek emergency medical attention immediately.
- Tell your doctor if you experience lightheadedness, especially during the first few days of Altace therapy. If you faint, stop taking Altace and tell your doctor immediately.
- Vomiting, diarrhea, fever, exercise, hot weather, alcohol, excessive perspiration, and dehydration may lead to an excessive fall in your blood pressure. Tell your doctor if you experience any of

these. Make sure to drink plenty of fluids when you are taking Altace.

- Altace may decrease your blood neutrophil levels (type of blood cells that fight infections), especially if you have a collagen vascular disease (such as lupus [disease that affects the immune system]) or kidney disease. Promptly report any signs of infection (such as sore throat or fever) to your doctor.

- Altace is not recommended in people with severe kidney problems.

- Patients who take a medicine for high blood pressure often feel tired or run down for a few weeks after starting treatment. Be sure to take your medicine even if you may not feel "normal." Tell your doctor if you develop any new symptoms.

- Altace may not work as well in African Americans; African Americans may also be at greater risk to have side effects. Contact your doctor if your symptoms do not improve or if they become worse.

Who should not take this medication?

Do not take Altace if you are allergic to it or any of its ingredients. Do not take Altace if you have a history of angioedema (a condition involving swelling of the face, extremities, eyes, lips, and tongue) related to previous treatment with similar medicines. Also, do not take Altace if you have a history of certain types of angioedema (such as hereditary or idiopathic).

What should I tell my doctor before I take the first dose of this medication?

Tell your doctor about all prescription, over-the-counter, and herbal medications you are taking before beginning treatment with Altace. Also, talk to your doctor about your complete medical history, especially if you have diabetes or liver or kidney problems. Tell your doctor if you have bone marrow suppression, heart disease, skin disease, severe immune system problems, lupus, or asthma, or if you are on a sodium-restricted diet. Also, tell your doctor if you have ever had an allergy or sensitivity to ACE inhibitors.

What is the usual dosage?

Please see general statement regarding dosage on page xii.

Blood Pressure
Adults: The usual starting dose without a diuretic is 2.5 milligrams (mg) once a day. Your doctor will prescribe the appropriate dose for you and will increase your dose as needed, until the desired effect is achieved.

If you have kidney or liver impairment, your doctor will adjust your dose appropriately.

Heart Attack, Stroke, and Related Complications
Adults: The initial dose is 2.5 mg once a day for 1 week, 5 mg once a day for the next 3 weeks, and then increases as tolerated to 10 mg once a day.

Heart Failure
Adults: The usual starting dose is 2.5 mg twice a day.

If you have kidney or liver impairment, your doctor will adjust your dose appropriately.

How should I take this medication?
- Swallow Altace capsules whole. You can open the capsule and sprinkle the contents on a small amount of applesauce or mixed in water or apple juice.
- Take Altace at the same time every day with or without food. Continue to use Altace even if you feel well.
- Do not take extra doses or take more often without talking to your doctor.

What should I avoid while taking this medication?
Do not become pregnant or breastfeed while you are taking Altace.

Do not become dehydrated. Drink adequate fluids while you are taking Altace.

Do not take salt substitutes or supplements containing potassium without consulting your doctor.

What are possible food and drug interactions associated with this medication?

If Altace is taken with certain other drugs, the effects of either could be increased, decreased, or altered. It is especially important to check with your doctor before combining Altace with the following: certain diuretics (such as amiloride, spironolactone, or triamterene), injectable gold, insulin and oral antidiabetic medicines, lithium, nonsteroidal anti-inflammatory drugs (such as ibuprofen or naproxen), potassium supplements, or salt substitutes containing potassium.

What are the possible side effects of this medication?

Please see general statement regarding side effects on page xiii.

> **Side effects may include:** cough, diarrhea, dizziness, fainting, liver problems, low blood pressure, nausea, rash, swelling of your face, vomiting

Can I receive this medication if I am pregnant or breastfeeding?

Do not take Altace if you are pregnant or breastfeeding. Altace can harm your unborn baby. It can be found in your breast milk if you take it during breastfeeding. Tell your doctor immediately if you are pregnant, plan to become pregnant, or are breastfeeding.

What should I do if I miss a dose of this medication?

If you miss a dose of Altace, take it as soon as you remember. However, if it is almost time for your next dose, skip the one you missed and return to your regular dosing schedule. Do not take two doses at once.

How should I store this medication?

Store at room temperature.

Altoprev
Generic name: Lovastatin

What is this medication?
Altoprev belongs to a class of medicines called "statins," which are used to lower your cholesterol when a low-fat diet is not enough. Altoprev lowers your total cholesterol and the "bad" low-density lipoprotein (LDL) cholesterol, thereby helping to prevent coronary heart disease (narrowing of small blood vessels that supply blood and oxygen to the heart).

What is the most important information I should know about this medication?
- Taking Altoprev is not a substitute for following a healthy low-fat and low-cholesterol diet and exercising to lower your cholesterol.
- Do not take Altoprev if you are pregnant, think you may be pregnant, or if you are planning to become pregnant.
- Altoprev can occasionally cause muscle pain, tenderness, or weakness. Call your doctor immediately if you notice any of these symptoms.

Who should not take this medication?
Do not take Altoprev if you are allergic to it or any of its ingredients, or if you currently have liver disease. Do not take Altoprev if you are pregnant or plan to become pregnant.

What should I tell my doctor before I take the first dose of this medication?
Tell your doctor about all prescription, over-the-counter, and herbal medications you are taking before beginning treatment with Altoprev. Also, talk to your doctor about your complete medical history, especially if you drink more than two glasses of alcohol daily, or if you have diabetes, muscle aches or weakness, or problems with your kidney, liver, or thyroid. Tell your doctor if you take medicines for any of the following: birth control, cholesterol, heart failure, HIV or AIDS, infections, or the immune system.

What is the usual dosage?

Please see general statement regarding dosage on page xii.

Adults: The usual starting dose is 20, 40, or 60 milligrams (mg) a day, taken in the evening at bedtime.

Your doctor will check your blood cholesterol levels during treatment with Altoprev and will change your dose based on the results.

For elderly patients (age ≥65 years), the starting dose is 20 mg once a day, taken in the evening at bedtime.

If you have kidney impairment or you are taking other medications, your doctor will adjust your dose appropriately.

How should I take this medication?

- Your doctor will likely start you on a low-cholesterol diet before giving you Altoprev. Stay on this diet while you are taking Altoprev.
- Swallow Altoprev tablets whole; do not chew, crush, or cut the tablets.

What should I avoid while taking this medication?

Do not drink large amounts of grapefruit juice (>1 quart a day) while you are taking Altoprev.

Avoid taking Altoprev if you are pregnant, plan to become pregnant, or are breastfeeding.

What are possible food and drug interactions associated with this medication?

If Altoprev is taken with certain other drugs, the effects of either drug could be increased, decreased, or altered. It is especially important to check with your doctor before combining Altoprev with the following: amiodarone, anti-HIV medications (such as indinavir), certain antibiotics, cholesterol-lowering medications known as fibrates (such as fenofibrate), grapefruit juice, itraconazole, ketoconazole, niacin, nefazodone, or verapamil.

What are the possible side effects of this medication?
Please see general statement regarding side effects on page xiii.

> **Side effects may include:** back pain, diarrhea, difficulty sleeping, headache, inflammation of sinuses, joint pain, muscle weakness, nausea, stomach pain

Can I receive this medication if I am pregnant or breastfeeding?
The effects of Altoprev during pregnancy and breastfeeding are unknown. Tell your doctor immediately if you are pregnant, plan to become pregnant, or are breastfeeding.

What should I do if I miss a dose of this medication?
If you miss a dose of Altoprev, take it as soon as you remember. However, if it is almost time for your next dose, skip the one you missed and return to your regular dosing schedule. Do not take two doses at once.

How should I store this medication?
Store at room temperature.

Amaryl
Generic name: Glimepiride

What is this medication?
Amaryl is used to treat adults with type 2 diabetes along with diet and exercise.

What is the most important information I should know about this medication?
- Amaryl can cause low blood sugar, making you feel lightheaded, dizzy, shaky, and hungry. This can happen if you skip meals, exercise excessively, drink alcohol, or use another medicine that lowers your blood sugar. Tell your doctor if this is a problem for you.

- Amaryl can cause allergic reactions or anaphylaxis (a serious and rapid allergic reaction that may result in death if not immediately treated). Stop taking Amaryl and tell your doctor immediately if you develop a rash, difficulty breathing, or swelling of your face, mouth, or throat.
- Amaryl can increase the risk of developing serious and possibly life-threatening heart problems compared to treatment of diabetes with diet alone or diet plus insulin. Talk to your doctor about the risks and benefits of treatment with Amaryl.

Who should not take this medication?

Do not take Amaryl if you are allergic to it or any of its ingredients.

What should I tell my doctor before I take the first dose of this medication?

Tell your doctor about all prescription, over-the-counter, and herbal medications you are taking before beginning treatment with Amaryl. Also, talk to your doctor about your complete medical history, especially if you have kidney or liver impairment, adrenal or pituitary gland problems, or if you have glucose-6-phosphate dehydrogenase (G6PD) deficiency (lack of an enzyme responsible for the breakdown of red blood cells).

What is the usual dosage?

Please see general statement regarding dosage on page xii.

Adults: The recommended starting dose is 1 milligram (mg) or 2 mg once a day. Your doctor may increase your dose as needed.

If you are elderly or have kidney impairment, your doctor will adjust your dose appropriately.

How should I take this medication?

- Take Amaryl with breakfast or the first main meal of the day.
- Follow your doctor's diet and exercise recommendations and test your blood sugar regularly while you are taking Amaryl.

What should I avoid while taking this medication?

Do not miss regular blood sugar testing (by yourself or your doctor).

Do not drive or operate machinery until you known how Amaryl affects you.

What are possible food and drug interactions associated with this medication?

If Amaryl is taken with certain other drugs, the effects of either could be increased, decreased, or altered. Amaryl may interact with numerous medications. Therefore, it is very important that you tell your doctor about any other medications you are taking.

What are the possible side effects of this medication?

Please see general statement regarding side effects on page xiii.

> **Side effects may include:** dizziness, headache, low blood sugar levels, nausea, weakness

Can I receive this medication if I am pregnant or breastfeeding?

The effects of Amaryl during pregnancy and breastfeeding are unknown. Do not breastfeed while you are taking Amaryl. Tell your doctor immediately if you are pregnant, plan to become pregnant, or are breastfeeding.

What should I do if I miss a dose of this medication?

If you miss a dose of Amaryl, take it as soon as you remember. However, if it is almost time for your next dose, skip the one you missed and return to your regular dosing schedule. Do not take two doses at once.

How should I store this medication?

Store at room temperature.

Ambien

Generic name: Zolpidem Tartrate

What is this medication?

Ambien is a medicine used for the short-term treatment of insomnia, specifically for people who have trouble falling asleep at bedtime.

Ambien is a federally controlled substance because it has abuse potential.

What is the most important information I should know about this medication?

- Ambien has abuse potential and can cause dependence. Mental and physical dependence can occur with the use of Ambien when it is used improperly for long periods of time. Keep Ambien in a safe place to prevent misuse and abuse. Selling or giving away Ambien can harm others, and is against the law. Tell your doctor if you have ever abused or have been dependent on alcohol, prescription medicines, or street drugs.
- Tell your doctor if your insomnia gets worse or is not better within 7-10 days. This may mean that there is another condition causing your sleep problem.
- Ambien can cause a serious allergic reaction. Get emergency medical help right away if you develop swelling of your tongue or throat, difficulty breathing, or nausea and vomiting.
- Ambien can cause you to get up out of bed while not being fully awake and engage in activities that you do not know you are doing (such as driving a car ["sleep-driving"], making and eating food, talking on the phone, having sex, or sleep-walking). Tell your doctor right away if you find out that you have done any of these activities after taking Ambien.
- Ambien can also cause you to have abnormal thoughts or behavior. Tell your doctor if you experience more outgoing or aggressive behavior than normal, confusion, agitation, hallucinations, worsening of your depression, or suicidal thought or actions.

Who should not take this medication?

Do not take Ambien if you are allergic to it or any of its ingredients.

What should I tell my doctor before I take the first dose of this medication?

Tell your doctor about all prescription, over-the-counter, and herbal medications you are taking before beginning treatment with Ambien. Also, talk to your doctor about your complete medical history, especially if you have a history of depression, mental illness, or suicidal thoughts; have a history of drug or alcohol abuse or addiction; have kidney or liver disease; have lung disease or breathing problems; or are pregnant, plan to become pregnant, or are breastfeeding.

What is the usual dosage?

Please see general statement regarding dosage on page xii.

Adults: The recommended dose is 10 milligrams, once a day, right before bedtime.

If you have liver impairment, your doctor will adjust your dose appropriately.

How should I take this medication?
• Take Ambien exactly as prescribed by your doctor. Take it right before you go to bed. Do not take Ambien with or right after a meal.
• Do not take Ambien unless you are able to stay in bed a full night (7-8 hours).

What should I avoid while taking this medication?

Do not drink alcohol or take other medicines to help you sleep while you are taking Ambien.

Do not drive or engage in other dangerous activities after taking Ambien until you feel fully awake.

What are possible food and drug interactions associated with this medication?

If Ambien is taken with certain other drugs, the effects of either could be increased, decreased, or altered. It is especially important to check with your doctor before combining Ambien with the following: alcohol, chlorpromazine, imipramine, ketoconazole, or rifampin.

What are the possible side effects of this medication?
Please see general statement regarding side effects on page xiii.

> **Side effects may include:** diarrhea, dizziness, drowsiness, drugged feeling

Can I receive this medication if I am pregnant or breastfeeding?
The effects of Ambien during pregnancy are unknown. Ambien can be found in your breast milk if you take it while breastfeeding. Tell your doctor immediately if you are pregnant, plan to become pregnant, or are breastfeeding.

What should I do if I miss a dose of this medication?
Ambien should be taken under special circumstances. If you miss your scheduled dose, contact your doctor or pharmacist for advice.

How should I store this medication?
Store at room temperature.

Amiodarone HCl: see Cordarone, page 265

Amitriptyline
Generic name: Amitriptyline HCl

What is this medication?
Amitriptyline is a medicine used to treat depression.

What is the most important information I should know about this medication?
- Amitriptyline can increase the risk of suicidal thoughts and behavior in children, adolescents, and young adults. Your doctor

will monitor you closely for clinical worsening, suicidal or un-usual behavior after you start taking amitriptyline or a new dose of amitriptyline. Tell your doctor immediately if you experience anxiety, hostility, sleeplessness, restlessness, impulsive or dangerous behavior, or thoughts about suicide or dying; or if you have new symptoms or seem to be feeling worse.

• Keep all follow-up visits with your doctor as scheduled. Call your doctor between visits as needed, especially if you have concerns about symptoms.

• Amitriptyline can affect your blood sugar. If you have diabetes, check your blood sugar levels regularly. Your doctor will decide if the dose of your diabetes medicine needs to be changed.

Who should not take this medication?

Do not take amitriptyline if you are allergic to it or any of its ingredients.

Do not take amitriptyline if you are currently taking other medicines known as cisapride or monoamine oxidase inhibitors (MAOIs), a class of medications used to treat depression and other psychiatric conditions (such as phenelzine or tranylcypromine). You must stop taking your MAOI at least 14 days before beginning treatment with amitriptyline.

Do not take amitriptyline if you are recovering from a heart attack.

What should I tell my doctor before I take the first dose of this medication?

Tell your doctor about all prescription, over-the-counter, and herbal medications you are taking before beginning treatment with ami-triptyline. Also, talk to your doctor about your complete medical history, especially if you have bipolar disorder, suicidal thoughts or actions, an irregular heartbeat, heart disease, liver or thyroid problems, glaucoma (high pressure in the eye), seizures, if you are unable to urinate normally, or have a history of alcohol or sub-stance abuse. Tell your doctor if you are planning to have surgery.

What is the usual dosage?

Please see general statement regarding dosage on page xii.

Adults: The recommended starting dose is 75 milligrams (mg) a day in divided doses or 50-100 mg at bedtime. Your doctor may increase your dose as needed.

Elderly and children ≥12 years: Your doctor will prescribe the appropriate dose for you.

How should I take this medication?
• Take amitriptyline exactly as prescribed by your doctor.

What should I avoid while taking this medication?
Do not change your dose or stop taking amitriptyline without first talking to your doctor. Stopping amitriptyline suddenly can cause side effects.

Do not drive or operate machinery until you know how amitriptyline affects you.

Do not start taking new medicines without first talking to your doctor.

What are possible food and drug interactions associated with this medication?
If amitriptyline is taken with certain other drugs, the effects of either could be increased, decreased, or altered. It is especially important to check with your doctor before combining amitriptyline with the following: alcohol, anticholinergics (such as ipratropium or oxybutynin), antipsychotic medications, barbiturates (such as phenobarbital), certain antidepressants (such as fluoxetine, paroxetine, or sertraline), cimetidine, disulfiram, epinephrine, ethchlorvynol, guanethidine, heart medications (such as flecainide and propafenone), local anesthetics, MAOIs, phenothiazines (such as chlorpromazine), quinidine, or thyroid medications.

What are the possible side effects of this medication?
Please see general statement regarding side effects on page xiii.

> **Side effects may include:** blood disorders, blurred vision, changes in blood pressure, confusion, constipation, diarrhea, dizziness, drowsiness, dry mouth, fatigue, hallucinations, headache, hives, impotence, increased sweating, increased urination, liver problems, loss of appetite, nausea, nightmares, restlessness, shaking, skin rash, vomiting, weakness, weight gain or loss

Can I receive this medication if I am pregnant or breastfeeding?

The effects of amitriptyline during pregnancy are unknown. Amitriptyline can be found in your breast milk if you take it while breastfeeding. Do not breastfeed while you are taking amitriptyline. Tell your doctor immediately if you are pregnant, plan to become pregnant, or are breastfeeding.

What should I do if I miss a dose of this medication?

If you miss a dose of amitriptyline, take it as soon as you remember. However, if it is almost time for your next dose, skip the one you missed and return to your regular dosing schedule. Do not take two doses at once.

How should I store this medication?

Store at room temperature. Protect from light.

Amitriptyline HCl: see Amitriptyline, page 66

Amlodipine Besylate: see Norvasc, page 699

Amlodipine Besylate/Benazepril HCl: see Lotrel, page 584

Amlodipine/Olmesartan Medoxomil: see Azor, page 123

Amlodipine/Valsartan: see Exforge, page 381

Amoxicillin

Generic name: Amoxicillin

What is this medication?

Amoxicillin is an antibiotic used to treat bacterial infections of the ear, nose, and throat; genital and urinary tract; skin; and lower (lung) respiratory tract. Amoxicillin is also used to treat uncomplicated gonorrhea. In addition, amoxicillin is used with other medicines to eliminate the bacteria that often cause ulcers (known as *Helicobacter pylori*). Amoxicillin is available as capsules, chewable tablets, oral suspension, and tablets.

What is the most important information I should know about this medication?

- Do not take amoxicillin if you are allergic to it or other similar antibiotics (such as penicillin or cephalosporins [such as cephalexin or cefdinir]). Tell your doctor right away if you take amoxicillin and you feel signs of an allergic reaction (such as a rash, swelling, or difficulty breathing).
- Diarrhea is a common problem when taking antibiotics; it usually ends when the antibiotic is stopped. Sometimes after starting treatment with antibiotics, people may develop watery and bloody stools (with or without stomach cramps and fever) even as late as two or more months after having taken the last dose of the antibiotic. Contact your doctor right away if this occurs.
- Take amoxicillin as prescribed by your doctor for the full course of treatment, even if your symptoms improve earlier. Do not skip doses. Skipping doses or not completing the full course of amoxicillin can decrease its effectiveness and can lead to the growth of bacteria that are resistant to the effects of amoxicillin.

Who should not take this medication?

Do not take amoxicillin if you are allergic to it, any of its ingredients, or other antibiotics such as penicillin or cephalosporins.

Do not take amoxicillin if you have mononucleosis (a viral illness commonly referred to as "mono" that results in weakness and fatigue for weeks or months). This can increase your risk of getting a skin rash.

Do not take amoxicillin to treat viral infections, such as the common cold.

What should I tell my doctor before I take the first dose of this medication?

Tell your doctor about all prescription, over-the-counter, and herbal medications you are taking before beginning treatment with amoxicillin. Also, talk to your doctor about your complete medical history, especially if you have allergies, kidney problems, "mono," or any infections.

What is the usual dosage?

Please see general statement regarding dosage on page xii.

Ear, Nose, Throat, Skin, Genital, and Urinary Tract Infections

Adults: For mild to moderate infections, the usual dose is 250 milligrams (mg) every 8 hours or 500 mg every 12 hours. For severe infections, the usual dose is 500 mg every 8 hours or 875 mg every 12 hours.

Children: Your doctor will prescribe the appropriate dose for your child, based on their weight.

Lower Respiratory Tract Infections

Adults: The usual dose is 500 mg every 8 hours or 875 mg every 12 hours.

Children: Your doctor will prescribe the appropriate dose for your child, based on their weight.

Gonorrhea

Adults: The usual dose is 3 grams as a single dose.

Children: Your doctor will prescribe the appropriate dose for your child, based on their weight.

H. pylori Infection

Adults: This treatment involves taking two or three different medications. The usual dose for the dual therapy is: amoxicillin

1000 mg every 8 hours for 14 days and lansoprazole 30 mg every 8 hours for 14 days. The usual dose for the triple therapy is: amoxicillin 1000 mg every 12 hours for 14 days, clarithromycin 500 mg every 12 hours for 14 days, and lansoprazole 30 mg every 12 hours for 14 days.

If you have renal impairment or are receiving dialysis, your doctor will adjust your dose appropriately.

How should I take this medication?
• Take amoxicillin exactly as prescribed by your doctor.
• Shake the oral suspension well before you or your child take the medicine. If you or your child cannot swallow the oral suspension alone, add the prescribed dose to formula, milk, fruit juice, water, ginger ale, or cold drinks. Drink the mixture right away.
• Throw away any unused amount of the oral suspension after 14 days.

What should I avoid while taking this medication?
Do not stop taking amoxicillin, even if you feel better.

What are possible food and drug interactions associated with this medication?
If amoxicilllin is taken with certain other drugs, the effects of either could be increased, decreased, or altered. It is especially important to check with your doctor before combining amoxicillin with the following: allopurinol, birth control pills, blood thinners (such as warfarin), other antibiotics (such as chloramphenicol, erythromycin, sulfamethoxazole/trimethoprim, or tetracycline), or probenecid.

What are the possible side effects of this medication?
Please see general statement regarding side effects on page xiii.

Side effects may include: diarrhea, nausea, rash, vomiting

Can I receive this medication if I am pregnant or breastfeeding?

The effects of amoxicillin during pregnancy are unknown. Amoxicillin can be found in your breast milk if you take it while breastfeeding. Tell your doctor immediately if you are pregnant, plan to become pregnant, or are breastfeeding.

What should I do if I miss a dose of this medication?

If you miss a dose of amoxicillin, take it as soon as you remember. However, if it is almost time for your next dose, skip the one you missed and return to your regular dosing schedule. Do not take two doses at once.

How should I store this medication?

Store the oral suspension in the refrigerator. Store all other forms of amoxicillin at room temperature.

Amoxicillin: see Amoxicillin, page 70

Amoxicillin/Clavulanate Potassium: see Augmentin, page 105

Amoxicillin/Clavulanate Potassium: see Augmentin XR, page 108

Amphetamine Salt Combo: see Adderall, page 25

Amphetamine Salt Combo: see Adderall XR, page 28

Amrix

Generic name: Cyclobenzaprine HCl

What is this medication?

Amrix is a muscle relaxant used in combination with rest and physical therapy to relieve symptoms associated with sudden, painful musculoskeletal conditions, such as muscle spasms.

What is the most important information I should know about this medication?

- Do not stop taking Amrix abruptly. If you do so you may develop symptoms such as nausea, headache, or discomfort.

Who should not take this medication?

Do not take Amrix if you are allergic to it or any of its ingredients.

Do not take Amrix while you are taking other medicines known as monoamine oxidase inhibitors (MAOIs) (such as phenelzine), a class of medications used to treat depression and other conditions.

Do not take Amrix if you are elderly or have an irregular heartbeat, heart failure, heart block, liver impairment, or an overactive thyroid gland, or had a recent heart attack.

What should I tell my doctor before I take the first dose of this medication?

Tell your doctor about all prescription, over-the-counter, and herbal medications you are taking before beginning treatment with Amrix. Also, talk to your doctor about your complete medical history, especially if you have liver disease, have ever had glaucoma (high pressure in the eye), or have ever been unable to urinate normally.

What is the usual dosage?

Please see general statement regarding dosage on page xii.

Adults: The recommended dose is 15 milligrams once a day. Your doctor may increase your dose as needed.

How should I take this medication?

- Take Amrix exactly as prescribed by your doctor. Take it at the same time every day.

What should I avoid while taking this medication?

Do not take Amrix for a longer period than prescribed by your doctor.

Do not take Amrix together with MAOIs or within 14 days after stopping treatment with an MAOI.

Do not drive or operate dangerous machinery until you know how Amrix affects you.

What are possible food and drug interactions associated with this medication?

If Amrix is taken with certain other drugs, the effects of either could be increased, decreased, or altered. It is especially important to check with your doctor before combining Amrix with the following: alcohol, barbiturates (such as phenobarbital), guanethidine, ipratropium or tolterodine, MAOIs, or tramadol.

What are the possible side effects of this medication?

Please see general statement regarding side effects on page xiii.

> **Side effects may include:** acne (pimples), attention disturbances, blurred vision, changes in your taste, constipation, dizziness, drowsiness, dry mouth, dry throat, fatigue, headache, nausea, shaking, throbbing heartbeat, upset stomach

Can I receive this medication if I am pregnant or breastfeeding?

The effects of Amrix during pregnancy and breastfeeding are unknown. Tell your doctor immediately if you are pregnant, plan to become pregnant, or are breastfeeding.

What should I do if I miss a dose of this medication?

If you miss a dose of Amrix, take it as soon as you remember. However, if it is almost time for your next dose, skip the one you missed and return to your regular dosing schedule. Do not take two doses at once.

How should I store this medication?

Store at room temperature.

Anaprox
Generic name: Naproxen Sodium

What is this medication?
Anaprox is a nonsteroidal anti-inflammatory drug (NSAID) used to treat rheumatoid arthritis, osteoarthritis, ankylosing spondylitis (arthritis of the spine), juvenile arthritis, tendinitis, bursitis (inflammation and pain around joints), acute gout, and pain. In addition, Anaprox is used to treat pain associated with menstrual periods. Anaprox is also available as Anaprox DS (double strength).

What is the most important information I should know about this medication?
- Anaprox can cause serious problems (such as heart attack or stroke). Your risk can increase when this medication is used for long periods of time and if you have heart disease. Tell your doctor if you experience chest pain, shortness of breath, weakness, or slurred speech.
- Anaprox can cause high blood pressure and heart failure or worsen existing high blood pressure. Tell your doctor if you experience weight gain or swelling.
- Anaprox can cause discomfort, ulcers, or bleeding in your stomach or intestines. Your risk can increase with long-term use, smoking, drinking alcohol, older age, poor health, or with certain medications. Tell your doctor immediately if you experience stomach pain or if you have bloody vomit or stools.
- Long-term use of Anaprox can cause kidney injury. Your risk can increase if you have kidney impairment; heart failure; liver problems; are taking certain medications, including diuretics (water pills) (such as furosemide or hydrochlorothiazide) or blood/heart medications known as angiotensin-converting enzyme (ACE) inhibitors (such as lisinopril); or are elderly.
- Anaprox can also cause liver injury. Stop taking Anaprox and call your doctor if you experience nausea, tiredness, weakness, itchiness, yellowing of your skin or whites of your eyes, right upper abdominal tenderness, or "flu-like" symptoms.
- Anaprox can cause a serious allergic reaction. Stop taking Anaprox and tell your doctor right away if you experience difficulty breathing or swelling of your face, mouth, or throat.

- Stop taking Anaprox and tell your doctor right away if you experience serious skin reactions, such as rash, blisters, fever, or itchiness.

Who should not take this medication?

Do not take Anaprox if you are allergic to it or any of its ingredients, or if you have experienced asthma, hives, or allergic-type reactions after taking aspirin or other NSAIDs (such as ibuprofen).

Do not take Anaprox right before or after a heart surgery called a coronary artery bypass graft (CABG).

What should I tell my doctor before I take the first dose of this medication?

Tell your doctor about all prescription, over-the-counter, and herbal medications you are taking before beginning treatment with Anaprox. Also, talk to your doctor about your complete medical history, especially if you have any of the following: allergies to medications, heart problems, history of asthma, high blood pressure, kidney or liver disease, or stomach problems, or are pregnant, plan to become pregnant, or are breastfeeding.

What is the usual dosage?

Please see general statement regarding dosage on page xii.

Rheumatoid Arthritis, Osteoarthritis, and Ankylosing Spondylitis

Anaprox
Adults: The recommended starting dose is 275 milligrams (mg) twice a day.

Anaprox DS
Adults: The recommended starting dose is 550 mg twice a day.

Pain, Menstrual Pain, Tendonitis, and Bursitis

Anaprox and Anaprox DS
Adults: The recommended starting dose is 550 mg, followed by 550 mg every 12 hours or 275 mg every 6-8 hours as required.

Acute Gout

Anaprox
Adults: The recommended starting dose is 825 mg, followed by 275 mg every 8 hours.

Your doctor will adjust your dose appropriately.

If you are elderly, or have liver or kidney problems, your doctor will adjust your dose appropriately.

How should I take this medication?
• Take Anaprox exactly as prescribed by your doctor.

What should I avoid while taking this medication?
Do not take Anaprox with other medications called Naprosyn, EC-Naprosyn, Aleve, or other medications that contain naproxen, since all these medicines contain the same active ingredient.

What are possible food and drug interactions associated with this medication?
If Anaprox is taken with certain other drugs, the effects of either could be increased, decreased, or altered. It is especially important to check with your doctor before combining Anaprox with the following: ACE inhibitors, antacids, aspirin, blood pressure/heart medications known as beta-blockers (such a propranolol), blood thinners (such as warfarin), certain antibiotics (such as trimethoprim/sulfamethoxazole or sulfisoxazole), certain antidepressants (such as fluoxetine or paroxetine), cholestyramine, diabetes medicines (such as glipizide or glyburide), diuretics, lithium, methotrexate, NSAIDs, phenytoin, probenecid, or sucralfate.

What are the possible side effects of this medication?
Please see general statement regarding side effects on page xiii.

> **Side effects may include:** constipation, diarrhea, dizziness, gas, heartburn, nausea, stomach pain, vomiting

Can I receive this medication if I am pregnant or breastfeeding?
Do not take Anaprox if you are in the late stage of your pregnancy or if you are breastfeeding. The effects of Anaprox during early pregnancy are unknown. Tell your doctor immediately if you are pregnant, plan to become pregnant, or are breastfeeding.

What should I do if I miss a dose of this medication?
If you miss a dose of Anaprox, take it as soon as you remember. However, if it is almost time for your next dose, skip the one you missed and return to your regular dosing schedule. Do not take two doses at once.

How should I store this medication?
Store at room temperature.

Anastrozole: see Arimidex, page 89

Androgel
Generic name: Testosterone

What is this medication?
Androgel is a topical gel (applied directly on the skin) that contains testosterone. Androgel is used to treat men who have low or no testosterone. This medication is available in a pump or in packets.

What is the most important information I should know about this medication?

- Androgel can transfer from your body to others. This can happen if other people come into contact with the area where you applied Androgel.
- Women and children should avoid contact with the unwashed or unclothed area where you applied Androgel. If a woman or child makes contact with the Androgel application area, that area on the woman or child should be washed well with soap and water right away.
- Androgel is flammable until dry. Let Androgel dry before smoking or going near fire or an open flame.

Who should not take this medication?

Do not use Androgel if you are allergic to it or any of its ingredients, including alcohol and soy products.

Do not use Androgel if you have known or suspected prostate cancer or breast cancer.

Women should not use Androgel.

What should I tell my doctor before I take the first dose of this medication?

Tell your doctor about all prescription, over-the-counter, and herbal medications you are taking before beginning treatment with Androgel. Also, talk to your doctor about your complete medical history, especially if you have or are suspected of having breast or prostate cancer, urinary problems due to an enlarged prostate, heart disease, sleep apnea (stopping breathing temporarily during sleep), or liver or kidney disease.

What is the usual dosage?

Please see general statement regarding dosage on page xii.

Adults: The recommended dose is 5 grams applied once a day. Your doctor will prescribe the appropriate dose for you based on your condition.

How should I take this medication?
- Apply Androgel exactly as prescribed by your doctor.
- Apply Androgel once a day, preferably in the morning. Apply it to areas (such as your shoulders, upper arms, or stomach area) that will be covered by a short sleeve t-shirt. Do not apply Androgel to your penis or scrotum (the sac located behind the penis).
- Before using Androgel for the first time, you will need to prime the pump. To prime the pump, gently push down on the pump 3 times. Do not use any Androgel that comes out while priming. Wash it down the sink or throw it in the trash to avoid accidental exposure to others.
- Depress the pump, or squeeze the entire contents from a packet, to apply the medicine directly on clean, dry, intact skin. Wash your hands with soap and water right after you apply Androgel. Let the application areas dry for a few minutes before putting on clothing.

What should I avoid while taking this medication?
Do not accidentally expose women or children to Androgel.

Do not swim or shower for at least 5 hours after you apply Androgel.

Do not apply Androgel to your genitals or to skin with open wounds or irritation.

What are possible food and drug interactions associated with this medication?
If Androgel is used with certain other drugs, the effects of either could be increased, decreased, or altered. It is especially important to check with your doctor before combining Androgel with the following: blood thinners (such as warfarin), corticosteroids (such as prednisone), or insulin.

What are the possible side effects of this medication?
Please see general statement regarding side effects on page xiii.

Side effects may include: acne (pimples), application-site irritation or redness, difficulty urinating, enlarged or painful breasts, increased urination, more erections or erections that last a long time, sleep apnea, swelling

Can I receive this medication if I am pregnant or breastfeeding?

Androgel is intended for use only by men and must not be used by women. If used during pregnancy, it can cause serious harm to the developing baby.

What should I do if I miss a dose of this medication?

If you miss a dose of Androgel, apply it as soon as you remember. However, if it is almost time for your next dose, skip the one you missed and return to your regular dosing schedule. Do not apply two doses at once.

How should I store this medication?

Store at room temperature.

Antivert

Generic name: Meclizine HCl

What is this medication?

Antivert is a medicine used to manage nausea, vomiting, and dizziness associated with motion sickness. Antivert is also used to manage vertigo (spinning feeling).

What is the most important information I should know about this medication?

- Antivert can cause drowsiness. Do not drive a car or operate dangerous machinery until you know how Antivert affects you. Also, do not drink alcohol while taking Antivert.

Who should not take this medication?

Do not take Antivert if you are allergic to it or any of its ingredients.

What should I tell my doctor before I take the first dose of this medication?

Tell your doctor about all prescription, over-the-counter, and herbal medications you are taking before beginning treatment with Antivert. Also, talk to your doctor about your complete medical history, especially if you have asthma, glaucoma (high pressure in the eye), or an enlarged prostate gland.

What is the usual dosage?

Please see general statement regarding dosage on page xii.

Motion Sickness

Adults and children ≥12 years: The recommended starting dose is 25-50 milligrams (mg) 1 hour before you will experience motion sickness. You can repeat the dose every 24 hours for the duration of the journey.

Vertigo

Adults and children ≥12 years: The recommended dose is 25-100 mg a day, in divided doses.

How should I take this medication?

• Take Antivert exactly as prescribed by your doctor.

What should I avoid while taking this medication?

Do not drive a car or operate dangerous machinery until you know how Antivert affects you.

Do not drink alcohol while taking Antivert.

What are possible food and drug interactions associated with this medication?

If Antivert is taken with certain other drugs, the effects of either could be increased, decreased, or altered. It is especially important to check with your doctor before combining Antivert with alcohol.

What are the possible side effects of this medication?

Please see general statement regarding side effects on page xiii.

> **Side effects may include:** allergic reactions, blurred vision, drowsiness, dry mouth, headache, tiredness, vomiting

Can I receive this medication if I am pregnant or breastfeeding?

The effects of Antivert during pregnancy and breastfeeding are unknown. Tell your doctor immediately if you are pregnant, plan to become pregnant, or are breastfeeding.

What should I do if I miss a dose of this medication?

Antivert should be given as needed, under certain circumstances.

How should I store this medication?

Store at room temperature.

Arcapta Neohaler

Generic name: Indacaterol

What is this medication?

Arcapta Neohaler is a medicine used for the long-term, once-a-day treatment to control symptoms associated with chronic obstructive pulmonary disease (COPD). When inhaled, Arcapta Neohaler opens up narrow air passages, allowing more oxygen to reach the lungs.

What is the most important information I should know about this medication?

- Do not use Arcapta Neohaler if you have asthma. People with asthma who use Arcapta Neohaler or similar medicines may have an increased risk of death from asthma problems.
- Arcapta Neohaler is not for initial use in sudden attacks of wheezing when fast action is needed. In other words, Arcapta Neohaler is not for "rescue therapy."

Who should not take this medication?

Do not use Arcapta Neohaler if you have asthma.

Do not use Arcapta Neohaler if you are allergic to it or any of its ingredients. Also, do not use Arcapta Neohaler if you are allergic to any milk products, such as lactose.

What should I tell my doctor before I take the first dose of this medication?

Tell your doctor about all prescription, over-the-counter, and herbal medications you are taking before beginning treatment with Arcapta Neohaler. Also, talk to your doctor about your complete medical history, especially if you have heart problems, high blood pressure, seizures, thyroid problems, or diabetes.

What is the usual dosage?

Please see general statement regarding dosage on page xii.

Adults: The recommended dose is the inhalation of the contents of 1 capsule, taken once a day, with the Neohaler device.

How should I take this medication?

- Use Arcapta Neohaler exactly as prescribed by your doctor. Arcapta is designed to be used only with the Neohaler inhalation device. Try to use the inhaler at the same time each day.
- Please review the instructions that came with your prescription on how to properly use your inhaler.

What should I avoid while taking this medication?

Do not stop using Arcapta Neohaler unless told to do so by your doctor because your symptoms can get worse.

Do not use Arcapta Neohaler more often than prescribed by your doctor.

Do not use Arcapta Neohaler with other similar medicines (such as Brovana, Foradil, or Serevent).

Arcapta is for inhalation only. Do not swallow Arcapta capsules.

What are possible food and drug interactions associated with this medication?

If Arcapta Neohaler is used with certain other drugs, the effects of either could be increased, decreased, or altered. Arcapta Neohaler may interact with numerous medications. Therefore, it is very important that you tell your doctor about any other medications you are taking.

What are the possible side effects of this medication?

Please see general statement regarding side effects on page xiii.

Side effects may include: cough, headache, nausea, runny nose, sore throat

---

Can I receive this medication if I am pregnant or breastfeeding?

The effects of Arcapta Neohaler during pregnancy and breastfeeding are unknown. Tell your doctor immediately if you are pregnant, plan to become pregnant, or are breastfeeding.

What should I do if I miss a dose of this medication?

If you miss a dose of Arcapta Neohaler, take it as soon as you remember. However, if it is almost time for your next dose, skip the one you missed and return to your regular dosing schedule. Do not take two doses at once.

How should I store this medication?

Store at room temperature. Do not store capsules in the Neohaler. Keep capsules away from moisture and light. Keep the capsules sealed until ready to use.

Aricept

Generic name: Donepezil HCl

What is this medication?

Aricept is a medicine used to treat dementia (an illness involving loss of memory, judgment, and confusion) in patients with Alzheimer's disease. Aricept is available as tablets and oral disintegrating tablets (Aricept ODT).

What is the most important information I should know about this medication?

- Aricept can cause you to develop a slow heart rate. Tell your doctor if you feel dizzy or faint.
- Aricept can also cause you to develop stomach symptoms such as nausea, vomiting, diarrhea, bleeding of your stomach or intestines, a loss of appetite, or weight loss.
- If you are planning to undergo surgery, it is important to notify your surgeon that you are taking Aricept.

Who should not take this medication?

Do not take Aricept if you are allergic to it or any of its ingredients.

What should I tell my doctor before I take the first dose of this medication?

Tell your doctor about all prescription, over-the-counter, and herbal medications you are taking before beginning treatment with Aricept. Also, talk to your doctor about your complete medical history, especially if you have any heart problems, asthma or lung disease, seizures, stomach ulcers, difficulty passing urine, liver or kidney problems, trouble swallowing tablets, or if you are pregnant, plan to become pregnant, or are breastfeeding.

What is the usual dosage?

Please see general statement regarding dosage on page xii.

<u>Mild to Moderate Alzheimer's Disease</u>

Adults: The usual starting dose is 5 milligrams (mg) once a day. Your doctor will increase your dose as appropriate.

Moderate to Severe Alzheimer's Disease

Adults: The usual starting dose is 10 mg once a day. In severe Alzheimer's disease, the usual maintenance dose is 10 mg daily. Your doctor will increase your dose as appropriate.

How should I take this medication?

- Take Aricept exactly as prescribed by your doctor. Take Aricept one time each day in the evening, just before bedtime. You can take Aricept with or without food.
- Swallow Aricept tablets whole with water. Do not split, crush, or chew the tablets.
- Aricept ODT melts on your tongue. Drink water after the tablet melts.

What should I avoid while taking this medication?

Do not skip doses of Aricept. If you missed your doses for several days, contact your doctor. Your dose may need to be lowered.

What are possible food and drug interactions associated with this medication?

If Aricept is taken with certain other drugs, the effects of either could be increased, decreased, or altered. It is especially important to check with your doctor before combining Aricept with the following: antispasmodic drugs (such as bethanechol), carbamazepine, dexamethasone, ketoconazole, nonsteroidal anti-inflammatory drugs (NSAIDs) (such as ibuprofen or naproxen), phenobarbital, phenytoin, quinidine, rifampin, or succinylcholine.

What are the possible side effects of this medication?

Please see general statement regarding side effects on page xiii.

Side effects may include: diarrhea, frequent urination, headache, loss of appetite, muscle cramps, nausea, pain, tiredness, trouble sleeping, vomiting, weight loss

---

Can I receive this medication if I am pregnant or breastfeeding?

The effects of Aricept during pregnancy and breastfeeding are unknown. Tell your doctor immediately if you are pregnant, plan to become pregnant, or are breastfeeding.

What should I do if I miss a dose of this medication?

If you miss a dose of Aricept, take it as soon as you remember. However, if it is almost time for your next dose, skip the one you missed and return to your regular dosing schedule. Do not take two doses at once.

If you have missed taking Aricept for several days, contact your doctor before taking another dose.

How should I store this medication?

Store at room temperature.

Arimidex

Generic name: Anastrozole

What is this medication?

Arimidex is a medicine used to treat hormone receptor-positive early breast cancer in women who have gone through menopause and after surgery, with or without radiation. Arimidex can be used if the breast cancer is known to be hormone receptor-positive or the hormone receptors are unknown. Arimidex can also be used to treat breast cancer in women whose disease has spread after treatment with tamoxifen.

What is the most important information I should know about this medication?

- Arimidex can cause heart disease, especially if you have a history of blockages in heart arteries (ischemic heart disease). Stop taking Arimidex and tell your doctor right away if you have chest pain or shortness of breath.

- Arimidex can cause your bones to become softer and weaker, leading to osteoporosis (thin, weak bones). This can increase your chance of fractures, especially of the spine, hip, or wrist. Your doctor will monitor your bones.

Who should not take this medication?

Do not take Arimidex if you are allergic to it or any of its ingredients.

Do not take Arimidex if you have not finished menopause, or are pregnant or plan to become pregnant. In addition, Arimidex should not be used by men or children.

What should I tell my doctor before I take the first dose of this medication?

Tell your doctor about all prescription, over-the-counter, and herbal medications you are taking before beginning treatment with Arimidex. Also, talk to your doctor about your complete medical history, especially if you have had a previous heart problem, have osteoporosis, have high cholesterol, have not finished menopause, are pregnant, plan to become pregnant, or are breastfeeding.

What is the usual dosage?

Please see general statement regarding dosage on page xii.

Adults: The recommended dose is 1 milligram (mg) once a day.

How should I take this medication?

- Take Arimidex exactly as prescribed by your doctor. You can take Arimidex with or without food.

What should I avoid while taking this medication?

Do not become pregnant or breastfeed while you are taking Arimidex.

What are possible food and drug interactions associated with this medication?

If Arimidex is taken with certain other drugs, the effects of either could be increased, decreased, or altered. It is especially important to check with your doctor before combining Arimidex with the following: medicines containing estrogen (such as birth control pills, estrogen creams, hormone replacement therapy, vaginal rings, or vaginal suppositories) or tamoxifen.

What are the possible side effects of this medication?

Please see general statement regarding side effects on page xiii.

Side effects may include: allergic reactions, back pain, bone pain, depression, hair loss, headache, high blood pressure, hot flashes, increased blood cholesterol, increased cough, joint pain, mood changes, nausea, pain, pain on the right side of your abdomen, rash, shortness of breath, skin reactions, sleep problems, sore throat, swelling, tingling or weakness in parts of your hand, vomiting, weakness, yellowing of your skin or whites of your eyes

---

Can I receive this medication if I am pregnant or breastfeeding?

Arimidex can cause harm to your unborn baby if you take it during pregnancy. The effects of Arimidex during breastfeeding are unknown. Do not take Arimidex if you are pregnant or breastfeeding. Tell your doctor immediately if you are pregnant, plan to become pregnant, or are breastfeeding.

What should I do if I miss a dose of this medication?

If you miss a dose of Arimidex, take it as soon as you remember. However, if it is almost time for your next dose, skip the one you missed and return to your regular dosing schedule. Do not take two doses at once.

How should I store this medication?

Store at room temperature.

Aripiprazole: *see Abilify, page 1*

Armour Thyroid

Generic name: Thyroid

What is this medication?

Armour Thyroid is a medicine used to treat an underactive thyroid gland (hypothyroidism). It is also used to treat or prevent certain types of goiter (an enlarged thyroid gland) and to manage thyroid cancer.

What is the most important information I should know about this medication?

- Do not use Armour Thyroid to treat obesity or weight loss.
- Armour Thyroid is a replacement therapy, so you need to take it every day for life unless your condition is temporary. Improvement in your symptoms can be seen several weeks after you start Armour Thyroid. Continue taking your medication as directed by your doctor.
- Tell your doctor immediately if you experience rapid or irregular heartbeats, chest pain, shortness of breath, leg cramps, headache, nervousness, irritability, sleeplessness, tremors, change in appetite, weight gain or loss, vomiting, diarrhea, excessive sweating, heat intolerance, fever, changes in menstrual periods, hives, or skin rash.
- Your doctor will monitor your urinary sugar levels. If you are taking an oral blood thinner (such as warfarin), your doctor will monitor your blood clotting status to determine if the dose of your blood thinner needs to be adjusted.
- Tell your doctor or dentist that you are taking Armour Thyroid before having any surgery.
- Armour Thyroid can cause partial hair loss in children during the first few months of treatment. This is usually temporary.

Who should not take this medication?

Do not take Armour Thyroid if you are allergic to it or any of its ingredients, or if you have an overactive thyroid gland. Also, do not take Armour Thyroid if your adrenal glands are not making enough corticosteroid hormone.

What should I tell my doctor before I take the first dose of this medication?

Tell your doctor about all prescription, over-the-counter, and herbal medications you are taking before beginning treatment with Armour Thyroid. Also, talk to your doctor about your complete medical history, especially if you are elderly and suffer from angina (chest pain) or have heart disease, diabetes, or an underactive thyroid.

What is the usual dosage?

Please see general statement regarding dosage on page xii.

Adults and children: Your doctor will prescribe the appropriate dose for you based on your age, weight, and condition.

If you have heart disease, your doctor will adjust your dose appropriately. Also, if you have diabetes, your doctor will determine if the dose of your diabetes medication needs to be adjusted.

How should I take this medication?

- Take Armour Thyroid exactly as prescribed by your doctor, preferably at the same time every day.

What should I avoid while taking this medication?

Do not stop taking Armour Thyroid or change your dose without talking to your doctor.

What are possible food and drug interactions associated with this medication?

If Armour Thyroid is taken with certain other drugs, the effects of either could be increased, decreased, or altered. It is especially important to check with your doctor before combining Armour Thyroid with the following: blood thinners (such as aspirin or warfarin), cholestyramine, colestipol, estrogen preparations (including some birth control pills, such as conjugated estrogens), insulin, or oral diabetes medicine (such as chlorpropamide and glipizide).

What are the possible side effects of this medication?

Please see general statement regarding side effects on page xiii.

> **Side effects may include:** changes in appetite, diarrhea, fever, headache, increased heart rate, irritability, nausea, nervousness, sleeplessness, sweating, weight loss

Can I receive this medication if I am pregnant or breastfeeding?

You can continue to take Armour Thyroid during pregnancy. However, a dose adjustment may be necessary. Small amounts of thyroid hormone are excreted in your breast milk. Tell your doctor immediately if you are pregnant, plan to become pregnant, or are breastfeeding.

What should I do if I miss a dose of this medication?

If you miss a dose of Armour Thyroid, take it as soon as you remember. However, if it is almost time for your next dose, skip the one you missed and return to your regular dosing schedule. Do not take two doses at once.

How should I store this medication?

Store at room temperature in a tightly closed container.

Ascorbic Acid/Polyethylene Glycol 3350/Potassium Chloride/Sodium Ascorbate/Sodium Chloride/Sodium Sulfate: *see Moviprep, page 655*

Aspirin/Dipyridamole: *see Aggrenox, page 43*

Astelin

Generic name: Azelastine HCl

What is this medication?

Astelin is a medicine used to treat nasal symptoms (such as stuffy nose, itching, or sneezing) of seasonal allergies. Astelin is also used to treat non-allergic nasal symptoms (such as runny nose, stuffy nose, or postnasal drip). Astelin is available as a nasal spray.

What is the most important information I should know about this medication?

- Astelin is for use in your nose only.
- Astelin can cause drowsiness and decreased mental alertness. Your risk is higher if you drink alcohol or take other medicines that also decrease alertness (such as alprazolam or oxycodone). Do not drink alcohol or take other medicines that can make you drowsy or decrease your alertness while you are taking Astelin.

Who should not take this medication?

Do not use Astelin if you are allergic to it or any of its ingredients.

What should I tell my doctor before I take the first dose of this medication?

Tell your doctor about all prescription, over-the-counter, and herbal medications you are taking before beginning treatment with Astelin. Also, talk to your doctor about your complete medical history, including all of your allergies, and if you are pregnant, plan to become pregnant, or are breastfeeding.

What is the usual dosage?

Please see general statement regarding dosage on page xii.

Treatment of Seasonal Allergy Symptoms
Adults and adolescents ≥12 years: The recommended dose is 1 or 2 sprays in each nostril twice a day.

Children 5-11 years: The recommended dose is 1 spray in each nostril twice a day.

Treatment of Non-Allergic Nasal Symptoms
Adults and adolescents ≥12 years: The recommended dose is 2 sprays in each nostril twice a day.

How should I take this medication?

- Use Astelin exactly as prescribed by your doctor.
- If you are using the nasal spray unit for the first time, you must prime it (to release into the air the dose that is already in the unit). To do this, press the pump 4 times or until a fine spray

appears. If it has not been used for 3 days or longer, you must prime the pump by pressing 2 times or until you see a fine mist.

• Gently blow your nose to clear your nostrils. Close one nostril and tilt your head downward toward your toes when you spray Astelin into each of your nostrils. Gently breathe in through your nostril and while breathing in press down on the applicator to release a spray. You may feel a brief burning or stinging sensation after using Astelin.

• Please review the instructions that came with your prescription on how to properly use Astelin.

What should I avoid while taking this medication?
Do not spray Astelin into your eyes.

Do not take other antihistamines (such as cetirizine or loratadine) while you are taking Astelin without first talking to your doctor.

Do not drive or operate dangerous machinery until you know how Astelin affects you.

What are possible food and drug interactions associated with this medication?
If Astelin is used with certain other drugs, the effects of either could be increased, decreased, or altered. It is especially important to check with your doctor before combining Astelin with the following: alcohol, cimetidine, ketoconazole, or other medicines that decrease alertness.

What are the possible side effects of this medication?
Please see general statement regarding side effects on page xiii.

Side effects may include: abnormal sensation to touch, bitter taste, drowsiness, headache, inflammation of your sinuses or lining of your nose, nasal burning, nosebleed, sneezing, sore throat

---

Can I receive this medication if I am pregnant or breastfeeding?

The effects of Astelin during pregnancy and breastfeeding are unknown. Tell your doctor immediately if you are pregnant, plan to become pregnant, or are breastfeeding.

What should I do if I miss a dose of this medication?

If you miss a dose of Astelin, apply it as soon as you remember. However, if it is almost time for your next dose, skip the one you missed and return to your regular dosing schedule. Do not apply two doses at once.

How should I store this medication?

Store at room temperature.

Astepro

Generic name: Azelastine HCl

What is this medication?

Astepro is an antihistamine used for the relief of nasal (nose) symptoms of seasonal or year-round allergies (such as itching, runny nose, sneezing, or stuffy nose). Astepro comes in the form of a nasal solution.

What is the most important information I should know about this medication?

• Astepro is for use in your nose only.
• Astepro can cause sleepiness. Do not drive, operate machinery, or engage in dangerous activities after you use Astepro. Also, do not drink alcohol or take other medicines that can cause you to feel sleepy while you are using Astepro.

Who should not take this medication?

Do not use Astepro if you are allergic to it or any of its ingredients.

What should I tell my doctor before I take the first dose of this medication?

Tell your doctor about all prescription, over-the-counter, and herbal medications you are taking before beginning treatment with Astepro. Also, talk to your doctor about your complete medical history, especially if you have allergies, or are pregnant, plan to become pregnant, or are breastfeeding.

What is the usual dosage?

Please see general statement regarding dosage on page xii.

Seasonal Allergies

Adults and adolescents ≥12 years: The recommended dose of Astepro 0.1% and Astepro 0.15% is 1-2 sprays in each nostril twice a day. Astepro 0.15% can also be administered as 2 sprays in each nostril once a day.

Year-Round Allergies

Adults and adolescents ≥12 years: The recommended dose of Astepro 0.15% is 2 sprays in each nostril twice a day.

How should I take this medication?

• Use Astepro exactly as prescribed by your doctor.
• You must prime (to release into the air the dose that is already in the device) the nasal spray unit if you are using it for the first time or if it has been disassembled for cleaning. Press the pump until you see a fine mist; this should happen in 6 sprays or less. Also, you must prime the pump by pressing twice or until you see a fine mist if it has not been used for 3 days or longer.
• Gently blow your nose to clear your nostrils. Keep your head tilted downward toward your toes when you spray Astepro into each of your nostrils. Breathe gently and do not tip your head back after using the spray.
• Please review the instructions that came with your prescription on how to properly use Astepro.

What should I avoid while taking this medication?

Do not spray Astepro in your eyes or mouth.

Do not drive, operate machinery, or engage in dangerous activities after you use Astepro.

Do not drink alcohol or take other medicines that can cause you to feel sleepy while you are using Astepro.

What are possible food and drug interactions associated with this medication?

If Astepro is used with certain other drugs, the effects of either could be increased, decreased, or altered. It is especially important to check with your doctor before combining Astepro with the following: alcohol, cimetidine, or other medicines that can cause sleepiness.

What are the possible side effects of this medication?

Please see general statement regarding side effects on page xiii.

> **Side effects may include:** fatigue, headache, nosebleed, nose discomfort or pain, sleepiness, sneezing, unusual taste (bitter or sweet)

Can I receive this medication if I am pregnant or breastfeeding?

The effects of Astepro during pregnancy and breastfeeding are unknown. Tell your doctor immediately if you are pregnant, plan to become pregnant, or are breastfeeding.

What should I do if I miss a dose of this medication?

If you miss a dose of Astepro, apply it as soon as you remember. However, if it is almost time for your next dose, skip the one you missed and return to your regular dosing schedule. Do not apply two doses at once.

How should I store this medication?

Store upright at room temperature. Do not freeze.

Atenolol: see Tenormin, page 979

Atenolol/Chlorthalidone: see Tenoretic, page 976

Ativan

Generic name: Lorazepam

What is this medication?

Ativan is a medicine used for the management of anxiety disorder and short-term relief of anxiety symptoms (such as insomnia due to anxiety or transient situational stress). It is also used to treat anxiety associated with depressive symptoms.

What is the most important information I should know about this medication?

- Ativan has abuse potential. Mental and physical dependence can occur with the use of Ativan.
- Do not stop taking Ativan without first talking to your doctor. Stopping Ativan suddenly can cause withdrawal symptoms.
- Ativan can cause or worsen depression. Do not take Ativan if you have depression or psychosis.

Who should not take this medication?

Do not take Ativan if you are allergic to it or any of its ingredients.

Do not take Ativan if you have an eye condition called acute narrow-angle glaucoma (high pressure in the eye).

What should I tell my doctor before I take the first dose of this medication?

Tell your doctor about all prescription, over-the-counter, and herbal medications you are taking before beginning treatment with Ativan. Also, talk to your doctor about your complete medical history, especially if you have a history of alcohol or drug abuse; liver, kidney, stomach, heart, or breathing problems; glaucoma; seizure disorders; or depression or psychosis. Also, tell your doctor if you are pregnant, plan to become pregnant, or are breastfeeding.

What is the usual dosage?
Please see general statement regarding dosage on page xii.

Anxiety
Adults and children ≥12 years: The usual starting dose is 2-3 milligrams (mg) twice a day or three times a day.

Insomnia Due to Anxiety or Situational Stress
Adults and children ≥12 years: The usual dose is 2-4 mg once a day at bedtime.

Your doctor will increase your dose as needed until the desired effect is achieved.

If you are elderly or have liver impairment, your doctor will adjust your dose appropriately.

How should I take this medication?
- Take Ativan exactly as prescribed by your doctor.
- Do not change your dose or stop taking Ativan without first talking to your doctor.

What should I avoid while taking this medication?
Do not drive a car or operate dangerous machinery until you known how Ativan affects you.

What are possible food and drug interactions associated with this medication?
If Ativan is taken with certain other drugs, the effects of either could be increased, decreased, or altered. It is especially important to check with your doctor before combining Ativan with the following: alcohol, aminophylline, antidepressants (such as phenelzine or tranylcypromine), antihistamines (such as cetirizine or loratadine), antipsychotics (such as clozapine or olanzapine), barbiturates (such as butalbital or phenobarbital), lorazepam, narcotic painkillers (such as hydrocodone or oxycodone), probenecid, seizure medicines (such as valproate or phenytoin), or theophylline.

What are the possible side effects of this medication?
Please see general statement regarding side effects on page xiii.

> **Side effects may include:** dizziness, sedation, unsteadiness, weakness

Can I receive this medication if I am pregnant or breastfeeding?
Do not take Ativan if you are pregnant or breastfeeding. Tell your doctor immediately if you are pregnant, plan to become pregnant, or are breastfeeding.

What should I do if I miss a dose of this medication?
If you miss a dose of Ativan, take it as soon as you remember. However, if it is almost time for your next dose, skip the one you missed and return to your regular dosing schedule. Do not take two doses at once.

How should I store this medication?
Store at room temperature.

Atomoxetine HCl: *see Strattera, page 948*

Atorvastatin Calcium: *see Lipitor, page 555*

Atropine Sulfate/Diphenoxylate HCl: *see Lomotil, page 569*

Atrovent HFA
Generic name: Ipratropium Bromide

What is this medication?
Atrovent HFA is a medicine used to treat bronchospasm (airway narrowing) associated with chronic obstructive pulmonary disease (COPD), including chronic bronchitis (long-term inflammation of the lungs) and emphysema (lung disease that causes shortness

of breath). Atrovent HFA opens up narrow air passages, allowing more oxygen to reach your lungs.

What is the most important information I should know about this medication?

- Atrovent HFA is not used for the relief of sudden episodes of bronchospasm.
- Tell your doctor immediately if Atrovent HFA is less effective in relieving your symptoms. Also, tell your doctor if your symptoms get worse or if you need to use this inhaler more often.
- Atrovent HFA can cause allergic reactions or anaphylaxis (a serious and rapid allergic reaction that may result in death if not immediately treated). Tell your doctor immediately if you experience symptoms such as rash, itchiness, angioedema (a condition involving swelling of the face, extremities, eyes, lips, and tongue), wheezing, or shortness of breath.
- Tell your doctor if you have any eye problems such as glaucoma (high pressure in the eye) or urinary retention (inability to urinate normally). Atrovent HFA can increase the pressure in your eye or can cause urinary retention.

Who should not take this medication?

Do not use Atrovent HFA if you are allergic to it, any of its components, atropine, or atropine-like medications.

Do not use Atrovent HFA for sudden episodes of bronchospasm.

What should I tell my doctor before I take the first dose of this medication?

Tell your doctor about all prescription, over-the-counter, and herbal medications you are taking before beginning treatment with Atrovent HFA. Also, talk to your doctor about your complete medical history, especially if you have glaucoma, benign prostatic hyperplasia (enlargement of the prostate gland, which may in turn block the flow of urine), or urinary retention.

What is the usual dosage?

Please see general statement regarding dosage on page xii.

Adults: The recommended dose is 2 inhalations four times a day with your inhalation device.

How should I take this medication?

- Use Atrovent HFA exactly as prescribed by your doctor. You do not have to shake the Atrovent HFA canister before use. Prime your Atrovent HFA inhaler before using it for the first time or if you have not used it for 3 days by releasing two sprays into the air. The effects of Atrovent HFA should last up to 2-4 hours. Do not take extra doses or use it more often without asking your doctor.
- Please review the instructions that came with your prescription on how to properly use your inhaler.

What should I avoid while taking this medication?

Do not puncture your Atrovent HFA canister. The contents of the canister are under pressure.

Do not use Atrovent HFA near heat, open flame, or fire. Exposure to high temperatures can cause bursting.

Do not spray Atrovent HFA in your eyes.

What are possible food and drug interactions associated with this medication?

If Atrovent HFA is taken with certain other drugs, the effects of either could be increased, decreased, or altered. It is especially important to check with your doctor before combining Atrovent HFA with anticholinergic agents (such as atropine).

What are the possible side effects of this medication?

Please see general statement regarding side effects on page xiii.

Side effects may include: bitter taste, difficulty breathing, dizziness, dry mouth, "flu-like" symptoms, headache, inflammation of the lungs, nausea, shortness of breath, worsening of COPD

Can I receive this medication if I am pregnant or breastfeeding?

The effects of Atrovent HFA during pregnancy and breastfeeding are unknown. Tell your doctor immediately if you are pregnant, plan to become pregnant, or are breastfeeding.

What should I do if I miss a dose of this medication?

If you miss a dose of Atrovent HFA, take it as soon as you remember. However, if it is almost time for your next dose, skip the one you missed and return to your regular dosing schedule. Do not take two doses at once.

How should I store this medication?

Store at room temperature.

Augmentin

Generic name: Amoxicillin/Clavulanate Potassium

What is this medication?

Augmentin is an antibiotic used to treat bacterial infections of the lower (lung) respiratory tract, ear, sinuses, skin, and urinary tract. Augmentin is available as chewable tablets, oral suspension, and tablets.

What is the most important information I should know about this medication?

- Do not take Augmentin if you are allergic to it or other similar antibiotics (such as penicillin or cephalosporins [such as cephalexin or cefdinir]). Tell your doctor right away if you take Augmentin and you feel signs of an allergic reaction (such as a rash, swelling, or difficulty breathing).
- Diarrhea is a common problem when taking antibiotics; it usually ends when the antibiotic is stopped. Sometimes after starting treatment with antibiotics, people may develop watery and bloody stools (with or without stomach cramps and fever) even as late as two or more months after having taken the last dose of the antibiotic. Contact your doctor right away if this occurs.

- Take Augmentin as prescribed by your doctor for the full course of treatment, even if your symptoms improve earlier. Do not skip doses. Skipping doses or not completing the full course of Augmentin can decrease its effectiveness and can lead to the growth of bacteria that are resistant to the effects of Augmentin.
- If you have a condition known as phenylketonuria (an inability to process phenylalanine, a protein in your body), be aware that Augmentin chewable tablets and oral suspension contain phenylalanine.

Who should not take this medication?
Do not take Augmentin if you are allergic to it, any of its ingredients, or other antibiotics such as penicillin or cephalosporins. Also, do not take Augmentin if you have a history of jaundice (yellowing of your skin or whites of your eyes) or liver impairment associated with previous treatment with Augmentin.

Do not take Augmentin if you have mononucleosis (a viral illness commonly referred to as "mono" that results in weakness and fatigue for weeks or months). This can increase your risk of getting a skin rash.

Do not take Augmentin to treat viral infections, such as the common cold.

What should I tell my doctor before I take the first dose of this medication?
Tell your doctor about all prescription, over-the-counter, and herbal medications you are taking before beginning treatment with Augmentin. Also, talk to your doctor about your complete medical history, especially if you have allergies, blood disorders, kidney or liver problems, "mono," phenylketonuria, or any infections.

What is the usual dosage?
Please see general statement regarding dosage on page xii.

Adults: The usual dose is 500 milligrams (mg) every 12 hours or 250 mg every 8 hours.

Children: Your doctor will prescribe the appropriate dose for your child, based on their weight.

If you have renal impairment or are receiving dialysis, your doctor will adjust your dose appropriately.

How should I take this medication?
- Take Augmentin at the start of a meal.
- Shake the oral suspension well before you or your child take the medicine. Use a dosing spoon or medicine dropper to give your child the oral suspension.
- Throw away any unused amount of the oral suspension after 10 days.

What should I avoid while taking this medication?
Do not stop taking Augmentin, even if you feel better.

What are possible food and drug interactions associated with this medication?
If Augmentin is taken with certain other drugs, the effects of either could be increased, decreased, or altered. It is especially important to check with your doctor before combining Augmentin with the following: allopurinol, birth control pills, blood thinners (such as warfarin), or probenecid.

What are the possible side effects of this medication?
Please see general statement regarding side effects on page xiii.

> **Side effects may include:** diarrhea or loss stools, hives, inflammation of your vagina, nausea, skin rash, vomiting

Can I receive this medication if I am pregnant or breastfeeding?
The effects of Augmentin during pregnancy are unknown. Augmentin can be found in your breast milk if you take it while breastfeeding. Tell your doctor immediately if you are pregnant, plan to become pregnant, or are breastfeeding.

What should I do if I miss a dose of this medication?
If you miss a dose of Augmentin, take it as soon as you remember. However, if it is almost time for your next dose, skip the one you missed and return to your regular dosing schedule. Do not take two doses at once.

How should I store this medication?
Store the oral suspension in the refrigerator. Store all other forms of Augmentin at room temperature.

Augmentin XR
Generic name: Amoxicillin/Clavulanate Potassium

What is this medication?
Augmentin XR is an antibiotic used to treat certain bacterial infections of the lung or sinuses. It may also be used to treat other bacterial infections, as determined by your doctor.

What is the most important information I should know about this medication?
- Do not take Augmentin XR if you are allergic to it or other similar antibiotics (such as penicillin or cephalosporins). Tell your doctor immediately if you take Augmentin XR and you feel signs of an allergic reaction, such as a rash, swelling, or difficulty breathing.
- Augmentin XR can cause diarrhea or colitis (inflammation of the colon). This can occur a couple of months after taking the last dose of Augmentin XR. Tell your doctor immediately if you have diarrhea or colitis.
- Take Augmentin XR as prescribed by your doctor for the full course of treatment, even if symptoms improve earlier. Do not skip doses. Skipping doses or not completing the full course of Augmentin XR can decrease its effectiveness and can lead to the growth of bacteria that are resistant to the effects of Augmentin XR.

Who should not take this medication?

Do not take Augmentin XR if you are allergic to it, any of its ingredients, or other penicillin antibiotics; have a history of jaundice (yellowing of the skin or whites of the eyes) or liver impairment associated with previous treatment with Augmentin; or have severe kidney impairment or are receiving hemodialysis.

Do not take Augmentin XR if you have mononucleosis (a viral illness commonly referred to as "mono" that results in weakness and fatigue for weeks or months). This can increase your risk of getting a skin rash.

Do not take Augmentin XR to treat viral infections, such as the common cold.

What should I tell my doctor before I take the first dose of this medication?

Tell your doctor about all prescription, over-the-counter, and herbal medications you are taking before beginning treatment with Augmentin XR. Also, talk to your doctor about your complete medical history, especially if you have allergies, blood disorders, kidney or liver problems, "mono," or infections.

What is the usual dosage?

Please see general statement regarding dosage on page xii.

Sinus Infection
Adults and children ≥40 kg: The recommended dose is 2 tablets every 12 hours for 10 days.

Lung Infections
Adults and children ≥40 kg: The recommended dose is 2 tablets every 12 hours for 7-10 days.

How should I take this medication?

- Take Augmentin XR exactly as prescribed by your doctor. You can take Augmentin XR at the start of a meal or with a snack to help reduce the possibility of stomach upset.

What should I avoid while taking this medication?
Do not skip or miss any scheduled doses.

What are possible food and drug interactions associated with this medication?
If Augmentin XR is taken with certain other drugs, the effects of either could be increased, decreased, or altered. It is especially important to check with your doctor before combining Augmentin XR with the following: allopurinol, birth control pills, blood thinners (such as warfarin), or probenecid.

What are the possible side effects of this medication?
Please see general statement regarding side effects on page xiii.

> **Side effects may include:** agitation, allergic reactions, anxiety, confusion, diarrhea, dizziness, face edema (swelling), headache, indigestion, itching, loose stools, nausea, rash, tooth discoloration, vaginal infection, vomiting

Can I receive this medication if I am pregnant or breastfeeding?
The effects of Augmentin XR during pregnancy and breastfeeding are unknown. Augmentin XR can be found in your breast milk if you take it during breastfeeding. Tell your doctor immediately if you are pregnant, plan to become pregnant, or are breastfeeding.

What should I do if I miss a dose of this medication?
If you miss a dose of Augmentin XR, take it as soon as you remember. However, if it is almost time for your next dose, skip the one you missed and return to your regular dosing schedule. Do not take two doses at once.

How should I store this medication?
Store at room temperature.

Avanafil: *see Stendra, page 945*

Avapro

Generic name: Irbesartan

What is this medication?

Avapro is a medicine known as an angiotensin receptor blocker, which is used to treat high blood pressure. Avapro is also used to slow damage to the kidneys in patients with diabetes and high blood pressure.

What is the most important information I should know about this medication?

- Do not take Avapro if you are pregnant, think you may be pregnant, plan to become pregnant, or are breastfeeding.
- Avapro can cause low blood pressure, especially if you take diuretics (water pills), are on a low-salt diet, or receive dialysis. If you feel faint or dizzy, lie down and call your doctor.

Who should not take this medication?

Do not take Avapro if you are allergic to it or any of its ingredients.

What should I tell my doctor before I take the first dose of this medication?

Tell your doctor about all prescription, over-the-counter, and herbal medications you are taking, before beginning treatment with Avapro. Also, talk to your doctor about your complete medical history, especially if you have heart failure or kidney problems, or are pregnant, plan to become pregnant, or are breastfeeding.

What is the usual dosage?

Please see general statement regarding dosage on page xii.

<u>High Blood Pressure</u>

Adults and children ≥6 years: The recommended starting dose is 150 milligrams (mg) once a day, either alone or in combination with other blood pressure-lowering medicines. Your doctor will increase your dose as needed until the desired effect is achieved.

Kidney Disease
Adults and children ≥6 years: The usual dose is 300 mg once a day.

How should I take this medication?
• Take Avapro exactly as prescribed by your doctor. Take it with or without food.

What should I avoid while taking this medication?
Do not take Avapro if you are pregnant.

What are possible food and drug interactions associated with this medication?
If Avapro is taken with certain other drugs, the effects of either could be increased, decreased, or altered. It is especially important to check with your doctor before combining Avapro with diuretics (water pills) (such as amiloride or spironolactone), nonsteroidal anti-inflammatory drugs (such as ibuprofen or naproxen), potassium supplements, sulphenazole, or tolbutamide.

What are the possible side effects of this medication?
Please see general statement regarding side effects on page xiii.

> **Side effects may include:** diarrhea, dizziness, fatigue, heartburn, low blood pressure, upset stomach

Can I receive this medication if I am pregnant or breastfeeding?
Do not take Avapro during pregnancy or breastfeeding. Tell your doctor immediately if you are pregnant, plan to become pregnant, or are breastfeeding.

What should I do if I miss a dose of this medication?
If you miss a dose of Avapro, take it as soon as you remember. However, if it is almost time for your next dose, skip the one you missed and return to your regular dosing schedule. Do not take two doses at once.

How should I store this medication?
Store at room temperature.

Avelox
Generic name: Moxifloxacin HCl

What is this medication?
Avelox is an antibiotic used to treat certain bacterial infections of the sinuses, respiratory (lung) tract, skin, and abdomen.

What is the most important information I should know about this medication?
- Avelox can cause tendon problems (such as tendon rupture or swelling). Your risk can increase if you are over 60 years; are taking corticosteroids (such as prednisone); have had a kidney, heart, or lung transplant; engage in physical activity or exercise; have kidney failure; or have past tendon problems (such as rheumatoid arthritis [a type of arthritis that involves inflammation of the joints]). Tell your doctor right away if you experience pain, swelling, tears, or inflammation of tendons in the back of your ankle (Achilles), shoulder, hand, or other tendon sites. Also, tell your doctor right away if you hear or feel a snap or pop in a tendon area, bruise right after an injury in a tendon area, or are unable to move the affected area or bear weight.
- Avelox can cause worsening of myasthenia gravis (a disease characterized by long-lasting fatigue and muscle weakness) symptoms. Tell your doctor right away if you develop muscle weakness or breathing problems.
- Serious or severe allergic reactions that may result in death if not immediately treated can occur while you are taking Avelox. Your doctor will not prescribe Avelox if you are allergic to it, any of its ingredients, or similar antibiotics (such as levofloxacin or ciprofloxacin). Tell your doctor right away if you experience a severe rash or difficulty breathing.
- Do not drive, operate machinery, or engage in other activities that require mental alertness or coordination until you know how Avelox affects you. Tell your doctor right away if you experience

dizziness, lightheadedness, pain, burning, tingling, numbness, weakness, or seizures.

- Avelox can cause diarrhea or colitis (inflammation of the colon). This can occur even a couple of months after receiving the last dose of Avelox. Tell your doctor right away if you have diarrhea or colitis.
- Use Avelox as prescribed by your doctor for the full course of treatment, even if symptoms improve earlier. Do not skip doses. Skipping doses or not completing the full course of Avelox can decrease its effectiveness and can lead to the growth of bacteria that are resistant to the effects of Avelox.

Who should not take this medication?

Do not take Avelox if you are allergic to it, any of its ingredients, or similar antibiotics.

Do not take Avelox to you to treat viral infections, such as the common cold.

What should I tell my doctor before I take the first dose of this medication?

Tell your doctor about all prescription, over-the-counter, and herbal medications you are taking before beginning treatment with Avelox. Also, talk to your doctor about your complete medical history, especially if you have tendon, nerve, or kidney problems; myasthenia gravis; central nervous system (CNS) problems (such as seizures); arrhythmia (life-threatening irregular heartbeat); have a history of joint problems; rheumatoid arthritis; or if you are pregnant, plan to become pregnant, or are breastfeeding.

What is the usual dosage?

Please see general statement regarding dosage on page xii.

Adults: The recommended dose is 400 milligrams once a day. Your doctor will determine the duration of your treatment based on the type of your infection.

How should I take this medication?

- Take Avelox at the same time each day. Take Avelox with or without food.
- Be sure to drink plenty of fluids while you are taking Avelox.

What should I avoid while taking this medication?

Do not drive, operate heavy machinery, or engage in dangerous activities until you know how Avelox affects you. Avelox can make you feel dizzy and lightheaded.

Do not expose your skin to sunlamps, tanning beds, and the sun while you are taking Avelox. Avelox can make your skin more sensitive to light and cause sunburns. Wear sunscreen or protective clothing if you are going to be outside for long periods.

Do not take Avelox within 4 hours before or 8 hours after aluminum-, magnesium-, calcium-, iron-, or zinc-containing products, sucralfate, or didanosine.

What are possible food and drug interactions associated with this medication?

If Avelox is taken with certain other drugs, the effects of either could be increased, decreased, or altered. Avelox may interact with numerous medications. Therefore, it is very important that you tell your doctor about any other medications you are taking.

What are the possible side effects of this medication?

Please see general statement regarding side effects on page xiii.

Side effects may include: allergic reactions, anxiety, burning, changes in your sensation, confusion, depression, diarrhea, dizziness, hallucinations (seeing or hearing things that are really not there), headache, nausea, nervousness, nightmares, paranoia (feel more suspicious), numbness, pain, rash, restlessness, seizures, sensitivity to light, tingling, suicidal thoughts or acts, tremors, trouble sleeping, vomiting, weakness

Can I receive this medication if I am pregnant or breastfeeding?

The effects of Avelox during pregnancy and breastfeeding are unknown. Avelox can be found in your breast milk if you take it while breastfeeding. Tell your doctor immediately if you are pregnant, plan to become pregnant, or are breastfeeding.

What should I do if I miss a dose of this medication?

If you miss a dose of Avelox, take it as soon as you remember. However, if it is almost time for your next dose, skip the one you missed and return to your regular dosing schedule. Do not take two doses at once.

How should I store this medication?

Store at room temperature. Keep away from moisture (humidity).

Aviane

Generic name: Ethinyl Estradiol/Levonorgestrel

What is this medication?

Aviane is a birth control pill used to prevent pregnancy. Aviane contains the hormones levonorgestrel and ethinyl estradiol.

What is the most important information I should know about this medication?

- Cigarette smoking can increase your risk of serious side effects on your heart and blood vessels, including heart attack, blood clots, or stroke. This risk increases with age, especially if you are >35 years and if you smoke ≥15 cigarettes a day. Do not smoke if you are taking Aviane.
- Aviane can increase your risk of heart attack, clotting disorders, stroke, gallbladder disease, or liver tumors. These risks increase if you have high blood pressure, diabetes, high cholesterol, tendency to form blood clots, or obesity. Tell your doctor right away if you experience sharp chest pain, coughing of blood, sudden shortness of breath, pain in your calfs, sudden severe headache or vomiting, dizziness or fainting, disturbances of vision

or speech, weakness or numbness in your arms or legs, loss of vision, abdominal (stomach) pain or tenderness, or jaundice (yellowing of your skin or whites of your eyes) accompanied by fever, fatigue, loss of appetite, dark-colored urine, or light-colored bowel movements.

• Aviane can increase your risk of developing cancer of your breasts or reproductive organs. Ask your doctor to show you how to examine your breasts. Tell your doctor right away if you notice lumps in your breasts.

• You can experience breakthrough bleeding or spotting while you are taking birth control pills, especially during the first 3 months of use. You may also have irregular periods. If you have missed more than two periods in a row, use a pregnancy test to determine if you are pregnant. Do not use Aviane if you are pregnant.

• Aviane is intended to prevent pregnancy. It does not protect against HIV infection (AIDS) and other sexually transmitted diseases.

Who should not take this medication?

Do not take Aviane if you are allergic to it or any of its ingredients.

Do not take Aviane if you have had a heart attack or stroke; blood clots in your legs, lungs, or eyes; known or suspected breast cancer, cancer of the lining of your uterus, cervix or vagina, or certain hormonally sensitive cancers; liver disease, including liver tumors; chest pain; unexplained vaginal bleeding; jaundice during pregnancy or during previous use of the pill; known or suspected pregnancy; heart disorders; diabetes; migraine headaches; uncontrolled high blood pressure; or if you are going to have surgery or will be on bedrest.

What should I tell my doctor before I take the first dose of this medication?

Tell your doctor about all prescription, over-the-counter, and herbal medications you are taking before beginning treatment with Aviane. Also, talk to your doctor about your complete medical history, especially if you or a family member has ever had breast nodules or any disease of the breast; certain hormonally sensitive cancers; diabetes; high triglycerides or cholesterol; high blood pressure; a tendency to form blood clots; migraines or other headaches; depression; gallbladder, heart, liver, or kidney disease; or a history of light or irregular menstrual periods. Also, tell your doctor if you are going to have surgery or will be on bedrest.

What is the usual dosage?

Please see general statement regarding dosage on page xii.

Adults and adolescents ≥16 years: Aviane may be started in one of two ways: on the Sunday after your period begins or during the first 24 hours of your period, as outlined below.

Sunday Start: Take the first orange tablet on the Sunday after your period begins, even if you are still bleeding. Take one orange tablet a day for 21 days, followed by one light green tablet a day for 7 days. After taking all 28 tablets, start a new course the next day (Sunday).

Day 1 Start: Take the first orange tablet during the first 24 hours of your period. Take one orange tablet a day for 21 days, followed by one light green tablet a day for 7 days. After taking all 28 tablets, start a new course the next day.

How should I take this medication?

• Before you start taking Aviane, be sure to read the directions. Take Aviane once a day, at the same time every day in the order directed on the package.

• For the *Sunday Start*, use another method of birth control (such as a condom or spermicide) as a back-up method if you have sex anytime from the Sunday you start your first pack until the next Sunday (7 days). This also applies if you start Aviane after having been pregnant and you have not had a period since your pregnancy.

• You will not need to use a back-up method of birth control for the *Day 1 Start* because you are starting the pill at the beginning of your period. However, if you start Aviane later than the first day of your period, you should use another method of birth control as a back-up method until you have taken 7 orange pills.

• Please follow the instructions on the patient handout that comes with your prescription.

What should I avoid while taking this medication?

Do not smoke cigarettes or become pregnant while you are taking Aviane.

Do not skip pills even if you are spotting or bleeding between monthly periods, feel sick to your stomach (nausea), or if you do not have sex very often.

What are possible food and drug interactions associated with this medication?

If Aviane is taken with certain other drugs, the effects of either could be increased, decreased, or altered. It is especially important to check with your doctor before combining Aviane with the following: certain anti-HIV medications (such as modafinil or ritonavir), certain antibiotics (such as ampicillin, penicillin, rifampin, tetracycline, or troleandomycin), seizure medications (such as carbamazepine, lamotrigine, phenobarbital, phenytoin, primidone, or topiramate), or St. John's wort.

What are the possible side effects of this medication?

Please see general statement regarding side effects on page xiii.

> **Side effects may include:** allergic reactions, breast tenderness, change in your appetite, change in your vision, depression, dizziness, edema (swelling), headache, inability to wear your contact lenses, irregular vaginal bleeding or spotting, loss of scalp hair, nausea, nervousness, rash, spotty darkening of your skin

Can I receive this medication if I am pregnant or breastfeeding?

Do not take Aviane if you are pregnant or breastfeeding. Tell your doctor immediately if you are pregnant, plan to become pregnant, or are breastfeeding.

What should I do if I miss a dose of this medication?

If you miss one orange pill, take it as soon as you remember. Take the next pill at your regular time. This means you can take two pills in one day. You do not need a back-up birth control method if you have sex. If you miss two orange pills or more, consult the patient information that accompanied your prescription, or call your pharmacist or doctor for advice.

How should I store this medication?
Store at room temperature.

Avodart
Generic name: Dutasteride

What is this medication?
Avodart is a medicine used to treat symptoms of benign prostatic hyperplasia (BPH). Avodart is used in men with an enlarged prostate to improve symptoms, to reduce the risk of acute urinary retention (a complete blockage of urine flow), and to reduce the risk of the need for BPH-related surgery. It may also be used in combination with a medicine called Flomax to treat symptoms of BPH in men with an enlarged prostate.

What is the most important information I should know about this medication?
- Women who are pregnant or may become pregnant should not handle Avodart capsules.
- Men treated with Avodart should not donate blood until at least 6 months after their final dose to prevent transmitting the medicine to a pregnant woman through a blood transfusion.
- It may take at least 6 months of treatment with Avodart to determine if it is effective for you, though some men experience fewer problems and symptoms after 3 months.
- Avodart can increase the chance of a more serious form of prostate cancer. Avodart can lower readings of the prostate-specific antigen (PSA) screening test for prostate cancer. If you are scheduled to have your PSA level checked, make sure the doctor knows you are taking Avodart. Also, tell your doctor if you have not been taking Avodart as prescribed because this may affect the PSA test results.

Who should not take this medication?
Do not use Avodart if you are allergic to any of its ingredients.

Women and children should not take Avodart.

A woman who is pregnant or capable of becoming pregnant should not handle Avodart capsules.

What should I tell my doctor before I take the first dose of this medication?
Tell your doctor about all prescription, over-the-counter, and herbal medications you are taking before beginning treatment with Avodart. Also, talk to your doctor about your complete medical history, especially if you have liver problems.

What is the usual dosage?
Please see general statement regarding dosage on page xii.

Adults: The recommended dose of Avodart is 0.5 milligrams (mg) taken orally once a day.

How should I take this medication?
• Take one Avodart capsule once a day. Swallow it whole because the contents of the capsule may irritate your mouth and throat. You can take Avodart with or without food.

What should I avoid while taking this medication?
Avoid giving blood during treatment and for at least 6 months after treatment with Avodart.

Do not allow a pregnant woman to handle Avodart capsules, as they may be absorbed through the skin and pose a danger to the unborn baby, particularly a male. If exposed, wash the exposed area immediately with soap and water.

What are possible food and drug interactions associated with this medication?
If Avodart is taken with certain other drugs, the effects of either could be increased, decreased, or altered. It is especially important

to check with your doctor before combining Avodart with any other medications.

What are the possible side effects of this medication?
Please see general statement regarding side effects on page xiii.

> **Side effects may include:** allergic reactions (such as swelling of your face, tongue, or throat) or serious skin reactions (such as skin peeling), decrease in sex drive, decrease in the amount of semen released during sex or problems with ejaculation, depressed mood, enlarged or painful breasts, impotence
>
> Get medical help right away if you develop any type of a serious allergic reaction and talk to your doctor if you notice any breast lumps or nipple discharge.

Can I receive this medication if I am pregnant or breastfeeding?
Women should not take Avodart. Also, do not touch Avodart capsules if you are pregnant, plan to become pregnant, or are breastfeeding. This medicine can cause severe deformities in your unborn child.

What should I do if I miss a dose of this medication?
If you miss a dose, you may take it later that day. Do not make up the missed dose by taking two doses the next day.

How should I store this medication?
Store at room temperature. Do not use if the capsule is deformed, discolored, or leaking.

Azelastine HCl: see Astelin, page 94

Azelastine HCl: see Astepro, page 97

Azelastine HCl: see Optivar, page 731

Azilsartan Medoxomil: *see Edarbi, page 348*

Azilsartan Medoxomil/Chlorthalidone: *see Edarbyclor, page 350*

Azithromycin: *see Zithromax, page 1138*

Azor
Generic name: Amlodipine/Olmesartan Medoxomil

What is this medication?

Azor is a combination medicine used alone or in combination with other medications to treat high blood pressure and lower the risk of stroke or heart attack. Azor contains two medicines: amlodipine (a calcium channel blocker) and olmesartan (an angiotensin receptor blocker).

What is the most important information I should know about this medication?

- If you become pregnant while you are taking Azor, stop taking it and call your doctor right away. Azor can harm your unborn baby, causing injury or even death.
- Low blood pressure can occur with Azor and cause you to feel faint or dizzy. Lie down if you feel faint or dizzy, and call your doctor right away.
- If you experience chest pain that gets worse, or that does not go away during treatment with Azor, get medical help right away.

Who should not take this medication?

Do not take Azor if you are allergic to it or any of its ingredients.

What should I tell my doctor before I take the first dose of this medication?

Tell your doctor about all prescription, over-the-counter, and herbal medications you are taking before beginning treatment with Azor. Also, talk to your doctor about your complete medical history, especially if you have liver, kidney, or heart problems; or if you are pregnant, plan to become pregnant, or are breastfeeding.

What is the usual dosage?
Please see general statement regarding dosage on page xii.

Adults: The usual starting dose is 5/20 (5 milligrams [mg] of amlodipine and 20 mg of olmesartan) once a day. Your doctor will prescribe the appropriate dose for you and will increase your dose as needed, until the desired effect is achieved.

How should I take this medication?
- Take Azor exactly as prescribed by your doctor.
- Take Azor once a day. Take it with or without food.
- Continue to take Azor even if you feel well.

What should I avoid while taking this medication?
Do not become pregnant or breastfeed while you are taking Azor.

What are possible food and drug interactions associated with this medication?
No significant interactions have been reported with Azor at this time. However, always tell your doctor about any medicines you take, including over-the-counter medications, vitamins, and herbal supplements.

What are the possible side effects of this medication?
Please see general statement regarding side effects on page xiii.

Side effects may include: abnormal heartbeat, diarrhea, dizziness, feeling faint, flushing, frequent urination, hair loss, heart palpitations, itching, lightheadedness, rash, sleepiness, swelling, vomiting, weakness

Can I receive this medication if I am pregnant or breastfeeding?
Do not take Azor if you are pregnant. The effects of Azor during breastfeeding are unknown. Tell your doctor immediately if you are pregnant, plan to become pregnant, or are breastfeeding.

What should I do if I miss a dose of this medication?

If you miss a dose of Azor, take it as soon as you remember. However, if it is almost time for your next dose, skip the one you missed and return to your regular dosing schedule. Do not take two doses at once.

How should I store this medication?

Store at room temperature.

Baclofen

Generic name: Baclofen

What is this medication?

Baclofen is a medicine used to relieve the signs and symptoms of multiple sclerosis, including muscle spasms, pain, certain involuntary muscular contractions (clonus), or muscle stiffness. Also, baclofen can be used in people with spinal cord injuries or diseases. This medicine can reduce muscle contractions, relieve pain, and improve your mobility.

What is the most important information I should know about this medication?

- Do not abruptly stop taking baclofen without talking to your doctor. Abrupt withdrawal can cause hallucinations or seizures.
- Baclofen can cause you to become drowsy and sleepy. Do not drive, operate dangerous machinery, or perform potentially hazardous activities if you experience decreased alertness while you are taking baclofen. Also, do not drink alcohol or take other medications that can cause drowsiness while you are taking baclofen.
- You should take baclofen with caution if you have kidney impairment, stroke, or seizure disorders. Tell your doctor if you have or have had these conditions. Baclofen can form ovarian cysts (fluid-filled sacs or pockets within or on the surface of an ovary), which disappear when treatment is stopped.

Who should not take this medication?

Do not take baclofen if you are allergic to it or any of its ingredients.

What should I tell my doctor before I take the first dose of this medication?

Tell your doctor about all prescription, over-the-counter, and herbal medications you are taking before beginning treatment with baclofen. Also, talk to your doctor about your complete medical history, especially if you have kidney impairment, stroke, seizure disorders, or if you are pregnant, plan to become pregnant, or are breastfeeding.

What is the usual dosage?

Please see general statement regarding dosage on page xii.

Adults and adolescents ≥12 years: Your doctor will prescribe the appropriate dose for you and will increase your dose as needed, until the desired effect is achieved.

How should I take this medication?

• Take baclofen exactly as prescribed by your doctor

What should I avoid while taking this medication?

Do not drive, operate dangerous machinery, or perform potentially hazardous activities if you experience decreased alertness while you are taking baclofen.

Do not drink alcohol or take other medications that can cause drowsiness while you are taking baclofen.

What are possible food and drug interactions associated with this medication?

If baclofen is taken with certain other drugs, the effects of either could be increased, decreased, or altered. It is especially important to check with your doctor before combining baclofen with alcohol or other medications that can cause drowsiness.

What are the possible side effects of this medication?

Please see general statement regarding side effects on page xiii.

> **Side effects may include:** ankle swelling, confusion, constipation, dizziness, drowsiness, excessive sweating, frequent urination, headache, itching, low blood pressure, nausea, rash, sleep disturbances, stuffy nose, tiredness, weakness, weight gain

Can I receive this medication if I am pregnant or breastfeeding?

The effects of baclofen during pregnancy and breastfeeding are unknown. Tell your doctor immediately if you are pregnant, plan to become pregnant, or are breastfeeding.

What should I do if I miss a dose of this medication?

If you miss a dose of baclofen, take it as soon as you remember. However, if it is almost time for your next dose, skip the one you missed and return to your regular dosing schedule. Do not take two doses at once.

How should I store this medication?

Store at room temperature.

Baclofen: *see Baclofen, page 125*

Bactrim

Generic name: Sulfamethoxazole/Trimethoprim

What is this medication?

Bactrim is an antibiotic used to treat certain bacterial infections of the urinary tract, ear, and lining of the intestines. Bactrim is also used to treat sudden attacks of chronic bronchitis, pneumonia, and traveler's diarrhea. In addition, Bactrim is used to prevent pneumonia in people with a decreased immune system. Bactrim is available as Bactrim and Bactrim DS (double strength).

What is the most important information I should know about this medication?

- Bactrim can cause skin toxicity, liver problems, blood disorders, or other severe reactions. Tell your doctor right away if you or your child develops a rash, sore throat, fever, joint pain, paleness or discoloration of your skin, or yellowing of your skin or whites of your eyes.
- Diarrhea is a common problem when taking antibiotics; it usually ends when the antibiotic is stopped. Sometimes after starting treatment with antibiotics, people may develop watery and bloody stools (with or without stomach cramps and fever) even as late as two or more months after having taken the last dose of the antibiotic. Contact your doctor right away if this occurs.
- Take Bactrim as prescribed by your doctor for the full course of treatment, even if your symptoms improve earlier. Do not skip doses. Skipping doses or not completing the full course of Bactrim can decrease its effectiveness and can lead to the growth of bacteria that are resistant to the effects of Bactrim.

Who should not take this medication?

Do not take Bactrim if you are allergic to it or any of its ingredients. Also, do not take Bactrim if you have a history of low platelet levels with previous treatment with Bactrim.

Do not take Bactrim if you have anemia due to folic acid deficiency, severe liver or kidney disease, or if you are pregnant or breast-feeding.

Do not give Bactrim to children <2 months of age.

What should I tell my doctor before I take the first dose of this medication?

Tell your doctor about all prescription, over-the-counter, and herbal medications you are taking before beginning treatment with Bactrim. Also, talk to your doctor about your complete medical history, especially if you have any allergies; liver, kidney, or thyroid problems; asthma; porphyria (a disorder that interferes with how your body produces heme, which is the oxygen-carrying component of your red blood cells); or AIDS. Tell your doctor if you drink excessive amounts of alcohol or if your intestines cannot absorb nutrients from food.

What is the usual dosage?
Please see general statement regarding dosage on page xii.

Urinary Tract Infections
Adults: The usual dose is 1 Bactrim DS tablet every 12 hours for 10-14 days or 2 Bactrim tablets every 12 hours for 10-14 days.

Children ≥2 months: Your doctor will prescribe the appropriate dose for your child, based on their weight.

Intestinal Infections
Adults: The usual dose is 1 Bactrim DS tablet every 12 hours for 5 days or 2 Bactrim tablets every 12 hours for 5 days.

Children ≥2 months: Your doctor will prescribe the appropriate dose for your child, based on their weight.

Ear Infections
Children ≥2 months: Your doctor will prescribe the appropriate dose for your child, based on their weight.

Chronic Bronchitis Attack
Adults: The usual dose is 1 Bactrim DS tablet every 12 hours for 14 days or 2 Bactrim tablets every 12 hours for 14 days.

Treatment of Pneumonia
Adults and children ≥2 months: Your doctor will prescribe the appropriate dose for you or your child, based on your weight.

Prevention of Pneumonia
Adults: The usual dose is 1 Bactrim DS tablet once a day.

Children ≥2 months: Your doctor will prescribe the appropriate dose for your child, based on their weight.

Traveler's Diarrhea
Adults: The usual dose is 1 Bactrim DS tablet every 12 hours for 5 days or 2 Bactrim tablets every 12 hours for 5 days.

If you have kidney impairment, your doctor will adjust your dose appropriately.

How should I take this medication?
- Take Bactrim exactly as prescribed by your doctor.
- Drink adequate amounts of fluids while you are taking Bactrim.

What should I avoid while taking this medication?
Do not stop taking Bactrim, even if you feel better.

What are possible food and drug interactions associated with this medication?
If Bactrim is taken with certain other drugs, the effects of either could be increased, decreased, or altered. It is especially important to check with your doctor before combining Bactrim with the following: amantadine, angiotensin converting enzyme (ACE) inhibitors (such as lisinopril or ramipril), cyclosporine, digoxin, certain diuretics (water pills) (such as furosemide or hydrochlorothiazide), indomethacin, methotrexate, oral diabetes medications, phenytoin, pyrimethamine, certain antidepressants (such as amitrityline or imipramine), or blood thinners (such as warfarin).

What are the possible side effects of this medication?
Please see general statement regarding side effects on page xiii.

> **Side effects may include:** hives, loss of appetite, nausea, rash, vomiting

Can I receive this medication if I am pregnant or breastfeeding?
Do not take Bactrim if you are pregnant or breastfeeding. Tell your doctor immediately if you are pregnant, plan to become pregnant, or are breastfeeding.

What should I do if I miss a dose of this medication?
If you miss a dose of Bactrim, take it as soon as you remember. However, if it is almost time for your next dose, skip the one you missed and return to your regular dosing schedule. Do not take two doses at once.

How should I store this medication?
Store at room temperature.

Bactroban
Generic name: Mupirocin Calcium

What is this medication?
Bactroban is a topical medicine (applied directly on the skin) that is used to treat certain bacterial infections of the skin. Bactroban is available in cream and ointment. Bactroban cream is used to treat certain bacterial infections of skin lesions caused by trauma. Bactroban ointment is used to treat impetigo (a highly contagious bacterial skin infection common among pre-school children).

What is the most important information I should know about this medication?
- Bactroban is for external use only. Do not use it in your eyes, mouth, or nose.
- Do not use Bactroban for any other condition other than that which your doctor has prescribed.
- Contact your doctor if you notice irritation or any skin reactions in the area being treated or if your condition does not improve within 3-5 days of treatment.

Who should not take this medication?
Do not use Bactroban if you are allergic to it or any of its ingredients.

What should I tell my doctor before I take the first dose of this medication?
Tell your doctor about all prescription, over-the-counter, and herbal medications you are taking before beginning treatment with

Bactroban. Also, talk to your doctor about your complete medical history, especially if you have kidney problems.

What is the usual dosage?
Please see general statement regarding dosage on page xii.

Impetigo
Adults and children ≥2 months: Apply a small amount of ointment to the affected area(s) three times a day.

Infected Traumatic Skin Lesions
Adults and children ≥3 months: Apply a small amount of cream to the affected area(s) three times a day for 10 days.

How should I take this medication?
• Apply Bactroban exactly as prescribed by your doctor.
• You can cover the treated skin area with gauze dressing if desired.

What should I avoid while taking this medication?
Do not use Bactroban in your eyes, mouth, or nose.

What are possible food and drug interactions associated with this medication?
No significant interactions have been reported with Bactroban at this time. However, always tell your doctor about any medicines you take, including over-the-counter medications, vitamins, and herbal supplements.

What are the possible side effects of this medication?
Please see general statement regarding side effects on page xiii.

Bactroban cream

> **Side effects may include:** abdominal pain, burning at application site, dizziness, headache, infections, inflammation of your skin, itching, rash, nausea

Bactroban ointment

Side effects may include: burning, dry skin, inflammation of your skin, itching, nausea, pain, rash, skin redness, stinging, swelling

---

Can I receive this medication if I am pregnant or breastfeeding?
The effects of Bactroban during pregnancy and breastfeeding are unknown. Tell your doctor immediately if you are pregnant, plan to become pregnant, or are breastfeeding.

What should I do if I miss a dose of this medication?
If you miss a dose of Bactroban, apply it as soon as you remember. However, if it is almost time for your next dose, skip the one you missed and return to your regular dosing schedule. Do not apply two doses at once.

How should I store this medication?
Store at room temperature. Do not freeze.

Beclomethasone Dipropionate: see Qvar, page 876

Benazepril HCl: see Lotensin, page 578

Benazepril HCl/Hydrochlorothiazide: see Lotensin HCT, page 581

Benicar
Generic name: Olmesartan Medoxomil

What is this medication?
Benicar is a medicine used alone or in combination with other medications to treat high blood pressure.

What is the most important information I should know about this medication?

- Benicar can cause a rare but serious allergic reaction leading to extreme swelling of your face, lips, tongue, throat, or gut (causing severe abdominal pain). If you experience any of these symptoms, seek emergency medical attention right away.
- Benicar may not work as well for you if you are African American.

Who should not take this medication?

Do not take Benicar if you are allergic to it or any of its ingredients. Do not take Benicar if you are pregnant, plan to become pregnant, or are breastfeeding.

What should I tell my doctor before I take the first dose of this medication?

Tell your doctor about all prescription, over-the-counter, and herbal medications you are taking before beginning treatment with Benicar. Also, talk to your doctor about your complete medical history, especially if you have kidney or liver problems.

What is the usual dosage?

Please see general statement regarding dosage on page xii.

Adults: The usual starting dose is 20 milligrams (mg) once a day. Your doctor will prescribe the appropriate dose for you and will increase your dose as needed until the desired effect is achieved.

Children 6-16 years: The usual starting dose is 10 mg once a day. Your doctor will prescribe the appropriate dose for your child, based on their weight.

How should I take this medication?

- Take Benicar exactly as prescribed by your doctor. Do not take extra doses or take more often without asking your doctor.
- You can take Benicar with or without food.

What should I avoid while taking this medication?

Do not become pregnant or breastfeed while you are taking Benicar.

What are possible food and drug interactions associated with this medication?

If Benicar is taken with certain other drugs, the effects of either could be increased, decreased, or altered. It is especially important to check with your doctor before combining Benicar with the following: diuretics (water pills) (such as furosemide, hydrochlorothiazide, spironolactone, or triamterene) or nonsteroidal anti-inflammatory medications (such as ibuprofen or naproxen).

What are the possible side effects of this medication?

Please see general statement regarding side effects on page xiii.

> **Side effects may include:** back pain, chest pain, diarrhea, dizziness, "flu-like" symptoms, headache, high blood sugar levels, infections, muscle pain, swelling of your arms or legs

Can I receive this medication if I am pregnant or breastfeeding?

Do not take Benicar if you are pregnant or breastfeeding. Benicar can harm your unborn baby. Tell your doctor immediately if you are pregnant, plan to become pregnant, or are breastfeeding.

What should I do if I miss a dose of this medication?

If you miss a dose of Benicar, take it as soon as you remember. However, if it is almost time for your next dose, skip the one you missed and return to your regular dosing schedule. Do not take two doses at once.

How should I store this medication?

Store at room temperature.

Benicar HCT

Generic name: Hydrochlorothiazide/Olmesartan Medoxomil

What is this medication?

Benicar HCT is a combination medicine used to treat high blood pressure. Benicar HCT contains two medicines: olmesartan (an angiotensin receptor blocker [ARB]) and hydrochlorothiazide (a diuretic [water pill]).

What is the most important information I should know about this medication?

- When taken during pregnancy, ARBs such as Benicar HCT can cause injury to the unborn baby. If you are pregnant or plan to become pregnant, stop taking Benicar HCT and contact your doctor right away.
- Benicar HCT can cause low blood pressure, especially if you take diuretics or are on a low-salt diet. If you feel faint or dizzy, lie down and call your doctor right away.
- Benicar HCT can cause a rare but serious allergic reaction leading to extreme swelling of your face, lips, tongue, throat, or gut (causing severe stomach pain). If you experience any of these symptoms, seek emergency medical attention.
- Benicar HCT can activate lupus (disease that affects the immune system) or gout (severe and painful inflammation of the joints) and increase cholesterol and triglyceride levels in certain patients.
- Benicar HCT can cause problems seeing objects that are farther away, as well as acute angle-closure glaucoma (high pressure in the eye). Tell your doctor immediately if you experience abnormal visual changes or eye pain.
- Benicar HCT can cause imbalances in fluids and electrolytes (chemicals that are important for the cells in your body to function, such as sodium and potassium). Signs and symptoms of this include dry mouth, thirst, weakness, fatigue, drowsiness, restlessness, confusion, seizures, muscle pain or cramps, low blood pressure, decreased urination, fast heart rate, nausea, and vomiting. Your doctor will monitor your blood electrolyte levels periodically during treatment with Benicar HCT.

• If you have diabetes, Benicar HCT can increase your blood sugar levels. Check your blood sugar frequently.

Who should not take this medication?
Do not take Benicar HCT if you are allergic to it or any of its ingredients, or a sulfonamide-derived medication.

Do not take Benicar HCT if you are unable to produce urine.

What should I tell my doctor before I take the first dose of this medication?
Tell your doctor about all prescription, over-the-counter, and herbal medications you are taking before beginning treatment with Benicar HCT. Also, talk to your doctor if you have diabetes, heart failure, severe immune system problems, lupus, asthma, or liver or kidney disease, or if you have ever had an allergy or sensitivity to an ARB or sulfonamide-derived medication.

What is the usual dosage?
Please see general statement regarding dosage on page xii.

Adults: The usual starting dose is 20/12.5 (20 milligrams [mg] of olmesartan and 12.5 mg of hydrochlorothiazide) once a day. Your doctor may give you a higher dose, depending on your needs.

How should I take this medication?
• You can take Benicar HCT tablets with or without food.

What should I avoid while taking this medication?
Do not become pregnant or breastfeed while you are taking Benicar HCT.

Do not become dehydrated. Drink adequate amounts of fluids while you are taking Benicar HCT.

What are possible food and drug interactions associated with this medication?
If Benicar HCT is taken with certain other drugs, the effects of either could be increased, decreased, or altered. It is especially important

to check with your doctor before combining Benicar HCT with the following: alcohol, barbiturates (such as phenobarbital), cholestyramine, colestipol, diabetes medicines (such as insulin), lithium, narcotic painkillers (such as hydrocodone or oxycodone), nonsteroidal anti-inflammatory drugs (such as ibuprofen or naproxen), norepinephrine, other blood pressure medications, steroids, or tubocurarine.

What are the possible side effects of this medication?
Please see general statement regarding side effects on page xiii.

> **Side effects may include:** dizziness, high blood uric acid levels, nausea, upper respiratory tract infection

Can I receive this medication if I am pregnant or breastfeeding?
Do not take Benicar HCT if you are pregnant or breastfeeding. Benicar HCT can harm your unborn baby. It can be found in your breast milk if you take it while breastfeeding. Tell your doctor immediately if you are pregnant, plan to become pregnant, or are breastfeeding.

What should I do if I miss a dose of this medication?
If you miss a dose of Benicar HCT, take it as soon as you remember. However, if it is almost time for your next dose, skip the one you missed and return to your regular dosing schedule. Do not take two doses at once.

How should I store this medication?
Store at room temperature.

Bentyl
Generic name: Dicyclomine HCl

What is this medication?
Bentyl is a medication used to treat functional bowel or irritable bowel syndrome (abdominal pain accompanied by diarrhea and

constipation associated with stress). Bentyl is available in capsules, tablets, and solution for intramuscular injection (injected into the muscle).

What is the most important information I should know about this medication?

- Bentyl can cause an increase in heart rate. This can worsen your condition if you have rapid, irregular heartbeat, heart failure, high blood pressure, or are having cardiac surgery. Tell your doctor if you have any of these conditions before taking Bentyl.
- Bentyl can cause dry mouth, difficulty swallowing and talking, thirst, dilated pupils, visual disturbances, eye sensitivity to light, flushing, dry skin, changes in heartbeat, difficulty urinating, or constipation. Tell your doctor if you experience any of these symptoms.
- Using Bentyl in hot weather can result in heat prostration (fever and heat stroke due to decreased sweating). If symptoms of heat prostration occur, stop taking Bentyl and tell your doctor right away.
- Bentyl can cause drowsiness, dizziness, or blurred vision. Do not drive or operate machinery until you know how Bentyl affects you.
- Psychotic symptoms have been reported in some individuals who have taken Bentyl. Tell your doctor right away if you experience any psychotic symptoms, confusion, disorientation, memory loss, hallucinations, loss of coordination, coma, feeling high, tiredness, trouble sleeping, or agitation. These symptoms can get better after you stop taking this medication.

Who should not take this medication?

Do not take Bentyl if you are allergic to it or any of its ingredients.

Do not take Bentyl if you have an abnormal blood pressure or heart rate due to any type of gastrointestinal or internal bleeding; myasthenia gravis (a disease characterized by long-lasting fatigue and muscle weakness); glaucoma (high pressure in the eye); blockage of the urinary tract, stomach, or intestines; severe ulcerative colitis (inflammatory disease of the large intestine); or reflux esophagitis (inflammation of the esophagus usually caused by the backflow of acid stomach contents).

What should I tell my doctor before I take the first dose of this medication?

Tell your doctor about all prescription, over-the-counter, and herbal medications you are taking before beginning treatment with Bentyl. Also, talk to your doctor about your complete medical history, especially if you have a nerve disorder; liver or kidney problems; hyperthyroidism (an overactive thyroid gland); high blood pressure; coronary heart disease; congestive heart failure; rapid, irregular heartbeat; myasthenia gravis; blockage of the urinary tract, stomach, or intestines; ulcerative colitis; or enlargement of the prostate gland. Tell your doctor if you are sensitive to anticholinergic drugs or if you have had an ileostomy or colostomy performed.

What is the usual dosage?

Please see general statement regarding dosage on page xii.

Capsules or Tablets

Adults: The recommended starting dose is 20 milligrams (mg) four times a day. Your doctor will prescribe the appropriate dose for you and will increase your dose as needed, until the desired effect is achieved.

Intramuscular Injection

Adults: The recommended starting dose is 10 to 20 mg four times a day.

How should I take this medication?

• Take Bentyl exactly as prescribed by your doctor.
• Your doctor will administer Bentyl intramuscular injection to you.

What should I avoid while taking this medication?

Do not drive or operate machinery until you know how Bentyl affects you.

Do not stay in high temperatures (indoors or outdoors) for a long period of time due to the risk of heat prostration while taking Bentyl.

Do not miss any scheduled follow-up appointments with your doctor.

What are possible food and drug interactions associated with this medication?

If Bentyl is taken with certain other drugs, the effects of either could be increased, decreased, or altered. It is important to check with your doctor before combining Bentyl with any other medication.

What are the possible side effects of this medication?

Please see general statement regarding side effects on page xiii.

Side effects may include: blurred vision, dizziness, drowsiness, dry mouth, nausea, nervousness, weakness

---

Can I receive this medication if I am pregnant or breastfeeding?

The effects of Bentyl during pregnancy are unknown. Bentyl can be found in your breast milk if you take it during breastfeeding. Do not take Bentyl if you are breastfeeding. Tell your doctor immediately if you are pregnant, plan to become pregnant, or are breastfeeding.

What should I do if I miss a dose of this medication?

If you miss a dose of Bentyl, take it as soon as you remember. However, if it is almost time for your next dose, skip the one you missed and return to your regular dosing schedule. Do not take two doses at once.

How should I store this medication?

Store at room temperature. Keep tablets out of direct sunlight.

Benzonatate: *see Tessalon, page 983*

Benztropine

Generic name: Benztropine Mesylate

What is this medication?

Benztropine is a medicine used in combination with other medications to treat parkinsonism. It is also used to control tremors caused by other medications that affect your central nervous system (CNS).

What is the most important information I should know about this medication?

- Benztropine can impair your mental and physical abilities, including weakness, inability to move certain muscles, mental confusion, or excitement, especially with large doses. Contact your doctor immediately if you experience these changes. Do not drive or operate heavy machinery until you know how benztropine affects you.
- Benztropine can cause anhidrosis (not being able to sweat) and increase your body temperature. For this reason, you should take benztropine with caution during hot weather, especially if you have been ill for a long time, are an alcoholic, have CNS disease, or are doing manual labor in a hot environment.
- Benztropine can cause painful urination or urinary retention (inability to urinate normally). Contact your doctor if you experience these problems.
- Benztropine can increase your risk for developing glaucoma (high pressure in the eye). Your doctor will examine your eyes regularly while you are taking benztropine. Tell your doctor immediately if you experience any eye problems or change in your vision.

Who should not take this medication?

Do not take benztropine if you are allergic to it or any of its ingredients.

What should I tell my doctor before I take the first dose of this medication?

Tell your doctor about all prescription, over-the-counter, and herbal medications you are taking before beginning treatment with

benztropine. Also, talk to your doctor about your complete medical history, especially if you have been ill for a long time, are an alcoholic, have CNS disease, have mental disorders, or have glaucoma or vision problems.

What is the usual dosage?
Please see general statement regarding dosage on page xii.

Adults and children ≥3 years: Your doctor will prescribe the appropriate dose for you based on your condition, age, and weight.

How should I take this medication?
- Take benztropine exactly as prescribed by your doctor. Do not stop taking this medication abruptly without first speaking to your doctor.

What should I avoid while taking this medication?
Do not drive or operate heavy machinery until you know how benztropine affects you.

What are possible food and drug interactions associated with this medication?
If benztropine is taken with certain other drugs, the effects of either could be increased, decreased, or altered. It is especially important to check with your doctor before combining benztropine with the following: atropine-like medicines, certain antidepressants (such as amitriptyline), or certain antipsychotics (such as haloperidol).

What are the possible side effects of this medication?
Please see general statement regarding side effects on page xiii.

Side effects may include: abnormal heartbeat, allergic reactions, blurred vision, confusion, constipation, depression, difficulty swallowing or speaking, dilated pupils, disorientation, dry mouth, fever, hallucinations, heat stroke, lethargy, loss of appetite, memory impairment, nausea, nervousness, numbing of fingers, painful urination, skin rash, unable to urinate, vomiting, weight loss

Can I receive this medication if I am pregnant or breastfeeding?

The effects of benztropine during pregnancy and breastfeeding are unknown. Tell your doctor immediately if you are pregnant, plan to become pregnant, or are breastfeeding.

What should I do if I miss a dose of this medication?

If you miss a dose of benztropine, take it as soon as you remember. However, if it is almost time for your next dose, skip the one you missed and return to your regular dosing schedule. Do not take two doses at once.

How should I store this medication?

Store at room temperature.

Benztropine Mesylate: see Benztropine, page 142

Betamethasone Dipropionate/Clotrimazole: see Lotrisone, page 587

Beyaz

Generic name: Drospirenone/Ethinyl Estradiol/Levomefolate Calcium

What is this medication?

Beyaz is a birth control pill used to prevent pregnancy. Beyaz is also used to treat premenstrual dysphoric disorder (PMDD) (a severe condition that consists of physical and emotional symptoms, such as depression and irritability, before menstruation) if you choose to use Beyaz for birth control. Beyaz is also used to treat moderate acne in women who are ≥14 years who are able to and wish to use Beyaz for birth control. Beyaz is also used to provide folic acid supplementation in women who choose to use Beyaz for birth control. The amount of folate contained in Beyaz supplements folate in the diet to lower your risk of having a pregnancy with a rare type of birth defect, in case you become pregnant while taking this medicine or shortly after stopping it.

What is the most important information I should know about this medication?

- Cigarette smoking increases the risk of serious heart-related side effects (such as blood clots, stroke, and heart attack) use of birth control pills, such as Beyaz. The risk increases with age (especially if you are >35 years old and smoke). Do not smoke while you are taking birth control pills.
- Birth control pills increase your risk of serious blood clots, especially if you smoke, are obese, or are over 35 years old. This increased risk is highest when you first start taking birth control pills and when you restart the same or different birth control pills after not using them for a month or more.
- Beyaz contains the progestin (a type of hormone) drospirenone. Women who use birth control pills with drospirenone may have a higher risk of getting a blood clot.
- Drospirenone may increase your potassium levels. During the first month that you take Beyaz, your doctor will order a blood test to check your potassium levels.
- A few woman who take birth control pills may get high blood pressure, gallbaldder problems, and rare liver tumors.
- Tell your doctor if you plan to have a major surgery. Your doctor will tell you when to stop taking Beyaz before the surgery and when to restart it after the surgery.
- Beyaz does not protect against HIV infection (AIDS) and other sexually transmitted diseases.
- Some women miss periods or have light periods when they take birth control pills, even when they are not pregnant. Contact your doctor for advice if you think you are pregnant, miss one period and have not taken your birth control pills on time every day, or if you miss two periods in a row.
- If you have vomiting or diarrhea, your birth control pills may not work as well. Use another birth control method, like condoms or spermicide, until you check with your doctor.

Who should not take this medication?

Do not take Beyaz if you smoke cigarettes and are >35 years old.

Do not take Beyaz if you have a history of blood clots in your legs, lungs, or eyes; stroke; heart attack; certain types of headaches; or breast or cervical cancer.

Also, do not take Beyaz if you have certain heart valve problems or heart rhythm abnormalities that can cause blood clots to form in your heart.

Do not take Beyaz if you have an inherited condition that makes your blood clot more than normal; high blood pressure that medication cannot control; diabetes with kidney, eye, nerve, or blood vessel damage; liver disease, including liver tumors; kidney or adrenal disease.

What should I tell my doctor before I take the first dose of this medication?

Tell your doctor about all prescription, over-the-counter, and herbal medications you are taking before beginning treatment with Beyaz. Also, talk to your doctor about your complete medical history, especially if you have ever had any of the health conditions listed above; depression; diabetes; high triglycerides; history of jaundice (yellowing of your skin or whites of your eyes) caused by pregnancy; you smoke; or if you are pregnant, plan to become pregnant, or are breastfeeding.

What is the usual dosage?

Please see general statement regarding dosage on page xii.

Adults: Beyaz may be started in one of two ways: on the Sunday after your period begins or during the first 24 hours of your period, as outlined below.

Sunday Start: Take the first pink pill on the Sunday after your period begins, even if you are still bleeding. Take one pink pill a day for 24 days, followed by one light orange pill a day for 4 days. After taking all 28 pills , start a new course the next day (Sunday).

Day 1 Start: Take the first pink pill during the first 24 hours of your period. Take one pink pill a day for 24 days, followed by one light orange pill a day for 4 days. After taking all 28 pills, start a new course the next day.

How should I take this medication?

- Before you start taking Beyaz, be sure to read the directions. Take Beyaz once a day, at the same time every day in the order directed on the package. Take the pill after the evening meal or at bedtime, with some liquid, as needed. You can take it without regard to meals.
- For the *Sunday Start*, use another method of birth control (such as a condom or spermicide) as a back-up method if you have sex anytime from the Sunday you start your first pack until the next Sunday (7 days). This also applies if you start Beyaz after having been pregnant and you have not had a period since your pregnancy.
- You will not need to use a back-up method of birth control for the *Day 1 Start* because you are starting the pill at the beginning of your period. However, if you start Beyaz later than the first day of your period, you should use another method of birth control as a back-up method until you have taken 7 pink pills.

What should I avoid while taking this medication?

Do not smoke or become pregnant while you are taking Beyaz. Do not skip pills even if you are spotting or bleeding between monthly periods, feel sick to your stomach (nausea), or if you do not have sex very often.

What are possible food and drug interactions associated with this medication?

If Beyaz is taken with certain other drugs, the effects of either could be increased, decreased, or altered. It is especially important to check with your doctor before combining Beyaz with the following: acetaminophen; antibiotics; blood pressure/heart medications known as angiotensin-converting enzyme (ACE) inhibitors (such as captopril, enalapril, or lisinopril), angiotensin-II receptor antagonists (such as losartan, valsartan, or irbesartan), or aldosterone antagonists (such as eplerenone); bosentan; griseofulvin; heparin; nonsteroidal anti-inflammatory drugs (NSAIDs) (such as ibuprofen and naproxen) when taken long-term and daily; potassium-sparing diuretics (water pills) (such as spironolactone); potassium supplements; rifampin; seizure medications (such as carbamazepine, felbamate, lamotrigine, oxcarbazepine, phenobarbital, topiramate, or phenytoin); St. John's wort; or vitamin C.

What are the possible side effects of this medication?
Please see general statement regarding side effects on page xiii.

Side effects may include: acne (pimples), bloating or fluid retention, blotchy darkening of the skin (especially on your face), breast tenderness, depression, headache, high blood sugar, high cholesterol/triglycerides, less sexual desire, nausea, problems tolerating contact lenses, spotting or bleeding between menstrual periods, weight changes

Can I receive this medication if I am pregnant or breastfeeding?
Do not take Beyaz if you are pregnant or breastfeeding. Tell your doctor immediately if you are pregnant, plan to become pregnant, or are breastfeeding.

What should I do if I miss a dose of this medication?
If you miss one pink pill, take it as soon as you remember. Take the next pill at your regular time. This means you can take two pills in one day. You do not need a back-up birth control method if you have sex. If you miss two pink pills or more, consult the patient information that accompanied your prescription, or call your pharmacist or doctor for advice.

How should I store this medication?
Store at room temperature.

Biaxin
Generic name: Clarithromycin

What is this medication?
Biaxin is an antibiotic used to treat certain bacterial infections, including strep throat, pneumonia, sinusitis (inflammation of the

sinuses), tonsillitis (inflammation of the tonsils), acute middle ear infections, acute flare-ups of chronic bronchitis, and skin infections in adults.

Biaxin can also be combined with other medicines to treat duodenal ulcers caused by *Helicobacter pylori* bacteria in adults.

In children, Biaxin tablets and granules (for oral suspension) are used to treat bacterial infections, including sore throat and tonsillitis, pneumonia, acute middle ear infections, and skin infections.

Biaxin is also used to prevent *Mycobacterium avium* complex (a number of bacterial infections that are usually associated with HIV infection [AIDS]) disease in people with advanced HIV infection.

What is the most important information I should know about this medication?
- Do not use Biaxin if you are pregnant, except in circumstances where no alternative therapy is appropriate as determined by your doctor. Biaxin can cause harm to your unborn baby.
- Diarrhea is a common problem when taking antibiotics; it usually ends when the antibiotic is stopped. Sometimes after starting treatment with antibiotics, people may develop watery and bloody stools (with or without stomach cramps and fever) even as late as two or more months after having taken the last dose of the antibiotic. Contact your doctor right away if this occurs.
- Biaxin does not treat viral infections such as the common cold.
- Take Biaxin as prescribed by your doctor for the full course of treatment, even if your symptoms improve earlier. Do not skip doses. Skipping doses or not completing the full course of Biaxin can decrease its effectiveness and can lead to the growth of bacteria that are resistant to the effects of Biaxin.
- Biaxin can cause myasthenia gravis (a disease characterized by long-lasting fatigue and muscle weakness). If you feel weakness in your muscles, tell your doctor immediately.

Who should not take this medication?
Do not take Biaxin if you are allergic to it or any of its ingredients, or if you are allergic to erythromycin or similar antibiotics.

Do not take Biaxin if you are also taking astemizole, cisapride, di-hydroergotamine, ergotamine, pimozide, or terfenadine. Also, do not take Biaxin if you are taking colchicine and have kidney or liver impairment.

Do not take Biaxin if you have a history of liver problems associated with prior use of Biaxin.

Do not take Biaxin if you have a history of certain heart conditions (such as QT prolongation or ventricular arrhythmia [life-threatening irregular heartbeat]).

What should I tell my doctor before I take the first dose of this medication?

Tell your doctor about all prescription, over-the-counter, and herbal medications you are taking before beginning treatment with Biaxin. Also, talk to your doctor about your complete medical history, especially if you have or had severe kidney disease, diarrhea caused by an organism called *Clostridium difficile*, liver or kidney problems, myasthenia gravis (loss of muscle control), abnormal heart rhythm (such as QT prolongation or increased heart rate), porphyria (a blood disorder), have used antibiotics, or if you are or may be pregnant, plan to become pregnant, are breastfeeding, or plan to breastfeed.

What is the usual dosage?

Please see general statement regarding dosage on page xii.

Duodenal Ulcers

Adults: Your doctor will prescribe the appropriate dose for you depending on the combination of other medicines that will be prescribed to treat your ulcer.

Ear, Sinus, Skin, Respiratory, Throat, and Tonsil Infections

Adults: The usual dose is 250-500 milligrams (mg) every 12 hours for 7-14 days. Your doctor will prescribe the appropriate dose for you based on the type and severity of your infection.

Children ≥6 months: Your doctor will prescribe the appropriate dose for your child, based on their weight.

<u>**Prevention or Treatment of *Mycobacterium Avium* Infection**</u>
Adults: The recommended dose of Biaxin is 500 mg twice a day.

Children ≥20 months: Your doctor will prescribe the appropriate dose for your child, based on their weight.

If you or your child has kidney impairment, your doctor will adjust the dose appropriately.

How should I take this medication?
- Take Biaxin exactly as prescribed by your doctor. Do not take extra doses or take more often without asking your doctor.
- Biaxin tablets and Biaxin granules for oral suspension can be taken with or without food.
- For Biaxin oral suspension, shake well before each use.

What should I avoid while taking this medication?
Do not take astemizole, cisapride, dihydroergotamine, ergotamine, pimozide, or terfenadine if you are taking Biaxin. Taking these medicines with Biaxin can lead to an irregular heart rhythm.

Do not skip doses and complete the full course of Biaxin treatment.

Do not become pregnant while you are taking Biaxin.

What are possible food and drug interactions associated with this medication?
If Biaxin is taken with certain other drugs, the effects of either could be increased, decreased, or altered. Biaxin may interact with numerous medications. Therefore, it is very important that you tell your doctor about any other medications you are taking.

What are the possible side effects of this medication?
Please see general statement regarding side effects on page xiii.

Side effects may include: abdominal (stomach) pain, abnormal taste, allergic reactions, anxiety, diarrhea, headache, low blood sugar levels, nausea, nightmares, tinnitus (ringing in your ears), upset stomach, vomiting

Can I receive this medication if I am pregnant or breastfeeding?

The effects of Biaxin during pregnancy and breastfeeding are unknown. Biaxin may only be used in pregnancy if other therapies are not appropriate. Tell your doctor immediately if you are pregnant, plan to become pregnant, or are breastfeeding.

What should I do if I miss a dose of this medication?

If you miss a dose of Biaxin, take it as soon as you remember. However, if it is almost time for your next dose, skip the one you missed and return to your regular dosing schedule. Do not take two doses at once.

How should I store this medication?

Store at room temperature in a tightly closed container. Store away from light.

Do not refrigerate the suspension.

Bimatoprost: *see Lumigan, page 595*

Bisoprolol Fumarate: *see Zebeta, page 1127*

Bisoprolol Fumarate/Hydrochlorothiazide: *see Ziac, page 1135*

Boceprevir: *see Victrelis, page 1071*

Boniva

Generic name: Ibandronate Sodium

What is this medication?

Boniva is a medicine used to treat or prevent osteoporosis (thin, weak bones) in women after menopause.

What is the most important information I should know about this medication?

- Boniva can cause irritation of your stomach and problems with your esophagus (the tube that connects your mouth and stomach).
- Boniva can lower your blood calcium levels. If you have low blood calcium levels before you start taking Boniva, it can get worse during treatment. Tell your doctor right away if you experience spasms, twitches, or cramps in your muscles; or numbness or tingling in your fingers, toes, or around your mouth as these can be symptoms of low calcium levels. Your doctor may prescribe calcium and vitamin D to help prevent low calcium levels while you are taking Boniva.
- Boniva can cause severe jaw bone problems. Your doctor should examine your mouth before you start Boniva. Your doctor may tell you to see your dentist before you start Boniva. It is important that you practice good mouth care during treatment with Boniva.
- Also, Boniva can cause bone, joint, or muscle pain or unusual fractures in your thigh bone. Tell your doctor right away if you develop pain in your hip, groin, or thigh.

Who should not take this medication?

Do not take Boniva if you are allergic to it or any of its ingredients.

Do not take Boniva if you have problems with your esophagus, low blood calcium levels, cannot stand or sit upright for at least 1 hour.

What should I tell my doctor before I take the first dose of this medication?

Tell your doctor about all prescription, over-the-counter, and herbal medications you are taking before beginning treatment with Boniva.

Also, talk to your doctor about your complete medical history, especially if you have swallowing problems, stomach or digestive problems, low blood calcium levels, plan to have dental surgery or teeth removed, kidney problems, have trouble absorbing minerals in your stomach or intestines, or if you are pregnant, plan to become pregnant, or are breastfeeding.

What is the usual dosage?
Please see general statement regarding dosage on page xii.

Adults: The recommended dose is 2.5 milligram (mg) once a day or 150 mg once a month.

How should I take this medication?
- Take Boniva exactly as prescribed by your doctor.
- Take Boniva in the morning at least 1 hour before eating, drinking, or taking any other medicine. Take Boniva with 6 to 8 ounces (about 1 full cup) of plain water.
- Swallow Boniva whole. Do not chew or suck on the tablet.
- After you take Boniva, wait at least 1 hour before lying down. You can sit, stand, walk, and engage in normal activities like reading.

What should I avoid while taking this medication?
Do not take Boniva with mineral water, coffee, tea, soda, or juice.

Do not eat or drink (except plain water), or take any oral medications within 1 hour of taking Boniva.

Do not lie down within 1 hour after taking Boniva.

What are possible food and drug interactions associated with this medication?
If Boniva is taken with certain other drugs, the effects of either could be increased, decreased, or altered. It is especially important to check with your doctor before combining Boniva with the following: antacids, aspirin, nonsteroidal anti-inflammatory drugs (NSAIDs) (such as ibuprofen), or supplements or vitamins containing aluminum, calcium, iron or magnesium.

What are the possible side effects of this medication?
Please see general statement regarding side effects on page xiii.

> **Side effects may include:** allergic reactions, abdominal (stomach) pain, back pain, diarrhea, "flu-like" symptoms, headache, heartburn, muscle pain, pain in your arms and legs

Can I receive this medication if I am pregnant or breastfeeding?
The effects of Boniva during pregnancy and breastfeeding are unknown. Tell your doctor immediately if you are pregnant, plan to become pregnant, or are breastfeeding.

What should I do if I miss a dose of this medication?
If you are taking 2.5-mg once-daily Boniva, do not take Boniva later in the day if you forget a dose. Return to your normal schedule the next morning. Do not take two tablets on the same day.

If you are taking 150-mg once-monthly Boniva, take the missed dose the morning following the day that you remembered that you missed a dose if your next scheduled Boniva day is more than 7 days away. Then, return to taking one Boniva 150-mg tablet every month in the morning of your chosen day, according to your original schedule.

Do not take two 150-mg tablets within the same week. If your next scheduled Boniva day is less than 7 days away, wait until your next scheduled day to take your tablet. Then, return to taking one Boniva 150-mg tablet every month in the morning of your chosen day, according to your original schedule.

How should I store this medication?
Store at room temperature.

Brilinta

Generic name: Ticagrelor

What is this medication?

Brilinta is a medicine used with aspirin to lower your chance of having a heart attack or dying from a heart attack or stroke. Brilinta prevents blood clots.

What is the most important information I should know about this medication?

- Brilinta can cause bleeding that can be serious and sometimes leads to death. While you take Brilinta, you may bruise and bleed more easily, have nose bleeds, or take longer than usual for any bleeding to stop. Call your doctor immediately if you have bleeding that is severe or that you cannot control; pink, red, or brown urine; vomit with blood or your vomit looks like "coffee grounds;" red or black stools (looks like tar); or if you cough up blood or blood clots.
- Do not stop taking Brilinta without talking to your doctor because your risk of a heart attack or stroke may increase.
- You should not take doses of aspirin higher than 100 mg a day because it can affect how Brilinta works.

Who should not take this medication?

Do not take Brilinta if you are bleeding now, have a history of bleeding in the brain, have bleeding from your stomach or intestines now (an ulcer), or have severe liver problems.

If your doctor tells you, you should stop taking Brilinta 5 days before you have an elective surgery.

Do not take Brilinta if you are allergic to it or any of its ingredients.

What should I tell my doctor before I take the first dose of this medication?

Tell your doctor about all prescription, over-the-counter, and herbal medications you are taking before beginning treatment with Brilinta. Also, talk to your doctor about your complete medical history, especially if you have had bleeding problems in the past, have liver problems, are due to have a surgery or had a recent surgery, plan to have a dental procedure, had a recent injury, have lung problems (such as asthma), have stomach ulcers or colon polyps (non-cancerous growth on the surface of the colon), have a history of stroke, are pregnant, are planning to become pregnant, are breastfeeding, or are planning to breastfeed.

What is the usual dosage?
Please see general statement regarding dosage on page xii.

Adults: The usual initial dose is 180-milligrams (mg) (two 90-mg tablets) a day. Thereafter, the recommended dose is 90 mg twice a day. Brilinta should be given with low-dose aspirin (not more than 100 mg a day); your doctor will prescribe the appropriate dose of aspirin for you.

How should I take this medication?
• Take Brilinta exactly as prescribed by your doctor. Swallow Brilinta tablets whole with some water. Take one in the morning and one in the evening, with or without food, around the same time every day. Take Brilinta with a low-dose aspirin.

What should I avoid while taking this medication?
Do not stop taking Brilinta without talking to your doctor who prescribed it for you.

What are possible food and drug interactions associated with this medication?
If Brilinta is taken with certain other drugs, the effects of either could be increased, decreased, or altered. Brilinta may interact with numerous medications. Therefore, it is very important that you tell your doctor about any other medications you are taking.

What are the possible side effects of this medication?
Please see general statement regarding side effects on page xiii.

Side effects may include: back pain, bleeding, bruising, chest pain, cough, diarrhea, dizziness, fatigue, headache, itching, nausea, shortness of breath

Can I receive this medication if I am pregnant or breastfeeding?

The effects of Brilinta during pregnancy and breastfeeding are unknown. Tell your doctor immediately if you are pregnant, plan to become pregnant, or are breastfeeding.

What should I do if I miss a dose of this medication?

If you miss a dose of Brilinta, take it as soon as you remember. However, if it is almost time for your next dose, skip the one you missed and return to your regular dosing schedule. Do not take two doses at once.

How should I store this medication?

Store at room temperature.

Brimonidine Tartrate: *see Alphagan P, page 52*

Brimonidine Tartrate/Timolol Maleate: *see Combigan, page 253*

Budesonide: *see Rhinocort Aqua, page 893*

Budesonide/Formoterol Fumarate Dihydrate: *see Symbicort, page 954*

Buprenorphine/Naloxone: *see Suboxone, page 951*

Bupropion HCl: *see Wellbutrin, page 1091*

Bupropion HCl: *see Wellbutrin SR, page 1094*

Buspirone

Generic name: Buspirone HCl

What is this medication?

Buspirone is a medicine used for the management of anxiety disorders or for short-term relief of anxiety symptoms.

What is the most important information I should know about this medication?

- Buspirone should not be used with monoamine oxidase inhibitors (MAOIs), a class of medications used to treat depression and other psychiatric conditions. Your blood pressure can increase if you take buspirone with MAOIs.
- Buspirone can impair mental or physical abilities. Do not drive a car or operate complex machinery until you know how buspirone affects you.
- Rarely, buspirone can cause restlessness. Tell your doctor if you experience this symptom.

Who should not take this medication?

Do not take buspirone if you are allergic to it or any of its ingredients.

Do not take buspirone if you have severe kidney or liver impairment.

What should I tell my doctor before I take the first dose of this medication?

Tell your doctor about all prescription, over-the-counter, and herbal medications you are taking before beginning treatment with buspirone. Also, talk to your doctor about your complete medical history, especially if you use alcohol, take MAOIs, have kidney or liver problems, are pregnant, plan to become pregnant, or are breastfeeding.

What is the usual dosage?

Please see general statement regarding dosage on page xii.

Adults and children ≥6 years: The recommended starting dose is 7.5 milligrams twice a day. Your doctor will prescribe the appropriate dose for you and will increase your dose as needed, until the desired effect is achieved.

How should I take this medication?

- Take buspirone at the same time each day. Take buspirone the same way, either always with food or always without food.

What should I avoid while taking this medication?

Do not drink large amounts of grapefruit juice or alcohol while taking buspirone.

Do not drive a car or operate complex machinery until you know how buspirone affects you.

What are possible food and drug interactions associated with this medication?

If buspirone is taken with certain other drugs, the effects of either could be increased, decreased, or altered. Buspirone may interact with numerous medications. Therefore, it is very important that you tell your doctor about any other medications you are taking.

What are the possible side effects of this medication?

Please see general statement regarding side effects on page xiii.

Side effects may include: dizziness, drowsiness, excitement, headache, intestinal or stomach disturbances, lightheadedness, nausea, nervousness, tiredness, trouble sleeping

Can I receive this medication if I am pregnant or breastfeeding?

The effects of buspirone during pregnancy and breastfeeding are unknown. Do not take buspirone during breastfeeding. Tell your doctor immediately if you are pregnant, plan to become pregnant, or are breastfeeding.

What should I do if I miss a dose of this medication?

If you miss a dose of buspirone, take it as soon as you remember. However, if it is almost time for your next dose, skip the one you missed and return to your regular dosing schedule. Do not take two doses at once.

How should I store this medication?

Store at room temperature.

Buspirone HCl: *see Buspirone, page 158*

Bydureon
Generic name: Exenatide

What is this medication?
Bydureon is a medicine used with diet and exercise to improve blood sugar in adults with type 2 diabetes. Bydureon is administered subcutaneously (just below the skin).

What is the most important information I should know about this medication?
- While using Bydureon, tell your doctor if you get a lump or swelling in your neck, hoarseness, trouble swallowing, or shortness of breath. These may be symptoms of thyroid cancer. Do not use Bydureon if you or any of your family members have thyroid cancer or if you have multiple endocrine neoplasia syndrome type 2 (MEN2). This is a disease where you have tumors in more than one gland in your body.
- Bydureon can cause pancreatitis (inflammation of the pancreas). Stop using Bydureon and call your doctor immediately if you have severe pain in your stomach area all the way to your back that will not go away. This may happen with or without vomiting. These may be symptoms of pancreatitis.
- Your risk of getting low blood sugar is higher if you use Bydureon with another medicine that can cause low blood sugar (such as glipizide, glyburide, or glimepiride). Signs and symptoms of low blood sugar include shakiness, sweating, headache, drowsiness, weakness, dizziness, confusion, irritability, hunger, fast heartbeat, or feeling jittery. Talk with your doctor about how to recognize and treat low blood sugar.
- Bydureon can cause a serious allergic reaction, including swelling of your face, lips, tongue, or throat; problems breathing or swallowing; severe rash or itching; fainting or feeling dizzy; or very fast heartbeat. If you have an allergic reaction, stop using Bydureon and call your doctor immediately.

Who should not take this medication?

Do not use Bydureon if you are allergic to it or any of its ingredients.

Do not take Bydureon if you or any of your family members have a history of thyroid cancer, MEN2, or type 1 diabetes.

What should I tell my doctor before I take the first dose of this medication?

Tell your doctor about all prescription, over-the-counter, and herbal medications you are taking before beginning treatment with Bydureon. Also, talk to your doctor about your complete medical history, especially if you have or had thyroid cancer, MEN2, pancreatitis, gallstones (stones in your gallbladder), a history of alcoholism, or high blood triglyceride levels. Also, tell your doctor if you have severe problems with your stomach (such as slow emptying of your stomach or problems digesting food), kidney problems or have had a kidney transplant, or if you are pregnant, plan to become pregnant, or are breastfeeding.

What is the usual dosage?

Please see general statement regarding dosage on page xii.

Adults: The recommended dose is 2 milligrams once every 7 days (weekly).

How should I take this medication?

- Inject Bydureon in your stomach area, upper leg (thigh), or back of your upper arm. You can use the same area of your body each week, but choose a different injection site in that area. Inject Bydureon right after you mix it.
- Your doctor will teach you how to mix and inject Bydureon before you use it for the first time. If you have questions or do not understand the instructions, talk to your doctor or pharmacist.
- Follow your doctor's instructions for diet, exercise, and how often to test your blood sugar during treatment with Bydureon.

What should I avoid while taking this medication?

Do not drink alcohol while you are using Bydureon.

What are possible food and drug interactions associated with this medication?

If Bydureon is used with certain other drugs, the effects of either could be increased, decreased, or altered. It is especially important to check with your doctor before combining Bydureon with the following: other diabetes medicines (such as insulin, glipizide, glyburide, or glimepiride), any medicine you take by mouth, or warfarin.

What are the possible side effects of this medication?

Please see general statement regarding side effects on page xiii.

> **Side effects may include:** constipation, diarrhea, headache, indigestion, itching at the injection site, kidney problems, low blood sugar, nausea, small bump at the injection site, vomiting.

Can I receive this medication if I am pregnant or breastfeeding?

The effects of Bydureon during pregnancy and breastfeeding are unknown. Tell your doctor immediately if you are pregnant, plan to become pregnant, or are breastfeeding.

What should I do if I miss a dose of this medication?

If you miss a dose of Bydureon, inject it as soon as you remember, provided the next regularly scheduled dose is due at least 3 days later. If the next regularly scheduled dose is due 1 or 2 days later, skip the missed dose and inject Bydureon on the next regularly scheduled day. Do not inject two doses of Bydureon less than 3 days apart.

How should I store this medication?

Store in the refrigerator. Do not freeze. Protect from light until you are ready to use Bydureon.

Byetta

Generic name: Exenatide

What is this medication?

Byetta is a medicine used with diet and exercise to improve blood sugar in adults with type 2 diabetes. Byetta is administered subcutaneously (just below the skin).

What is the most important information I should know about this medication?

- Byetta can cause pancreatitis (inflammation of the pancreas). Stop using Byetta and call your doctor immediately if you have severe pain in your stomach area all the way to your back that will not go away. This may happen with or without vomiting. These may be symptoms of pancreatitis.
- Your risk of getting low blood sugar is higher if you use Byetta with another medicine that can cause low blood sugar (such as glipizide, glyburide, or glimepiride). Signs and symptoms of low blood sugar include shakiness, sweating, headache, drowsiness, weakness, dizziness, confusion, irritability, hunger, fast heartbeat, or feeling jittery. Talk to your doctor about how to recognize and treat low blood sugar.
- Byetta can cause new or worsen existing kidney problems, including kidney failure. Tell your doctor right away if you have nausea, vomiting, or diarrhea that will not go away or if you cannot tolerate liquids by mouth while you are taking Byetta.
- Byetta can cause a serious allergic reaction, including swelling of your face, lips, tongue, or throat; problems breathing or swallowing; severe rash or itching; fainting or feeling dizzy; or very fast heartbeat. If you have an allergic reaction, stop using Byetta and call your doctor immediately.

Who should not take this medication?

Do not use Byetta if you are allergic to it or any of its ingredients.

What should I tell my doctor before I take the first dose of this medication?

Tell your doctor about all prescription, over-the-counter, and herbal medications you are taking before beginning treatment with Byetta.

Also, talk to your doctor about your complete medical history, especially if you have or had pancreatitis, gallstones (stones in your gallbladder), a history of alcoholism, or high blood triglyceride levels. Also, tell your doctor if you have severe problems with your stomach (such as slow emptying of your stomach or problems digesting food), kidney problems or have had a kidney transplant, or if you are pregnant, plan to become pregnant, or are breastfeeding.

What is the usual dosage?

Please see general statement regarding dosage on page xii.

Adults: The usual starting dose is 5 micrograms twice a day. Your doctor will increase your dose as needed, until the desired effect is achieved.

How should I take this medication?

- Use Byetta exactly as prescribed by your doctor. Do not change your dose without first talking to your doctor.
- Byetta comes in a prefilled pen. Inject Byetta in your stomach area (abdomen), upper leg (thigh), or your upper arm as instructed by your doctor.
- Inject Byetta twice a day, at any time within 1 hour, before your morning and evening meals.
- Throw away a used Byetta pen after 30 days, even if some medicine remains in the pen.
- Pen needles are not included. You may need a prescription to purchase pen needles. Ask your doctor which needle length and gauge is best for you.
- Follow your doctor's instructions for diet, exercise, and how often to test your blood sugar during treatment with Byetta.

What should I avoid while taking this medication?

Do not inject Byetta into a vein or muscle.

Do not use Byetta after a meal.

What are possible food and drug interactions associated with this medication?

If Byetta is used with certain other drugs, the effects of either could be increased, decreased, or altered. Byetta slows stomach emptying and can affect medicines that need to pass through the stomach quickly. Ask your doctor if the time you take any of your oral medicines should be changed. Also, tell your doctor if you are taking acetaminophen, antibiotics, birth control pills, digoxin, lovastatin, or warfarin.

What are the possible side effects of this medication?

Please see general statement regarding side effects on page xiii.

> **Side effects may include:** acid stomach, constipation, diarrhea, dizziness, headache, jitteriness, nausea, vomiting, weakness

Can I receive this medication if I am pregnant or breastfeeding?

The effects of Byetta during pregnancy and breastfeeding are unknown. Tell your doctor immediately if you are pregnant, plan to become pregnant, or are breastfeeding.

What should I do if I miss a dose of this medication?

If you miss a dose of Byetta, skip that dose and inject your next dose at the next prescribed time. Do not inject an extra dose or increase the amount of your next dose to make up for the one you missed.

How should I store this medication?

Store Byetta in the refrigerator in the original carton. Do not freeze; protect from light.

Do not store the Byetta pen with the needle attached. If the needle is left on, medicine may leak from the Byetta pen or air bubbles may form in the cartridge.

Bystolic
Generic name: Nebivolol

What is this medication?
Bystolic is a medicine known as a beta-blocker, which is used to treat high blood pressure.

What is the most important information I should know about this medication?
- Take Bystolic regularly and continuously. Do not stop taking Bystolic without talking to your doctor. Stopping this medication suddenly can cause harmful effects. Your doctor should gradually reduce your dose when stopping treatment with this medication.
- Bystolic can worsen heart failure, cause breathing problems, or hide symptoms of low blood sugar levels if you have diabetes. Tell your doctor if you experience weight gain or trouble breathing while you are taking Bystolic. If you have diabetes, monitor your blood sugar frequently, especially when you first start taking Bystolic.

Who should not take this medication?
Do not take Bystolic if you are allergic to it or any of its ingredients. In addition, do not take Bystolic if you have a slow heart rate, heart failure, heart block, sick sinus syndrome (abnormal heart rhythm), severe liver disease, or severe blood circulation disorders.

What should I tell my doctor before I take the first dose of this medication?
Tell your doctor about all prescription, over-the-counter, and herbal medications you are taking before beginning treatment with Bystolic. Also, talk to your doctor about your complete medical history, especially if you have allergies; heart problems or heart failure; a history of heart attack; breathing problems (such as asthma, bronchitis [inflammation of the lungs], or emphysema [lung disease that causes shortness of breath]); pheochromocytoma (tumor of the adrenal gland); diabetes; liver, kidney, or thyroid problems; peripheral vascular disease (disease of the blood vessels outside the heart and brain); or are planning to have a major surgery.

Tell your doctor if you have a history of severe allergic reactions to any allergens, because Bystolic may decrease the effectiveness of epinephrine used to treat the reaction.

What is the usual dosage?
Please see general statement regarding dosage on page xii.

Adults: The usual starting dose is 5 milligrams once a day, either alone or in combination with other blood pressure-lowering medicines. Your doctor will increase your dose as needed until the desired effect is achieved.

If you have liver or kidney impairment, your doctor will adjust your dose appropriately.

How should I take this medication?
• Take Bystolic exactly as prescribed by your doctor. Take it with or without food.

What should I avoid while taking this medication?
Do not drive a car, operate machinery, or engage in other tasks requiring alertness until you know how Bystolic affects you.

Do not stop taking Bystolic without first talking to your doctor.

What are possible food and drug interactions associated with this medication?
If Bystolic is taken with certain other drugs, the effects of either could be increased, decreased, or altered. It is especially important to check with your doctor before combining Bystolic with the following: blood pressure medications known as calcium channel blockers (such as diltiazem or verapamil), cimetidine, clonidine, digoxin, disopyramide, fluoxetine, guanethidine, paroxetine, propafenone, reserpine, sildenafil, or quinidine.

What are the possible side effects of this medication?
Please see general statement regarding side effects on page xiii.

> **Side effects may include:** dizziness, headache, leg swelling, low blood pressure, slow heartbeat, tiredness

Can I receive this medication if I am pregnant or breastfeeding?
The effects of Bystolic during pregnancy and breastfeeding are unknown. Tell your doctor immediately if you are pregnant, plan to become pregnant, or are breastfeeding.

What should I do if I miss a dose of this medication?
If you miss a dose of Bystolic, take it as soon as you remember. However, if it is almost time for your next dose, skip the one you missed and return to your regular dosing schedule. Do not take two doses at once.

How should I store this medication?
Store at room temperature.

Calan SR
Generic name: Verapamil HCl

What is this medication?
Calan SR belongs to a class of medications called calcium channel blockers; it is used to treat high blood pressure.

What is the most important information I should know about this medication?
- It is important to let your doctor know before starting this medication if you have any heart conditions or heartbeat irregularities.
- Be sure to follow up with your doctor regularly to monitor your liver function. If you already have liver problems, tell your doctor so he or she may determine if the dose of Calan SR is appropriate for you.

Who should not take this medication?

Do not take Calan SR if you have low blood pressure, sick sinus syndrome (abnormal heart rhythm) or a heart block (unless you have a pacemaker), or other abnormal heart rhythms.

Do not take Calan SR if you are allergic to it or any of its ingredients.

What should I tell my doctor before I take the first dose of this medication?

Tell your doctor about all prescription, over-the-counter, and herbal medications you are taking before beginning treatment with Calan SR. Also, talk to your doctor about your complete medical history, especially if you have low blood pressure, heart problems, kidney disease, liver disease, or Duchenne's muscular dystrophy (inherited disorder that causes muscle weakness).

What is the usual dosage?

Please see general statement regarding dosage on page xii.

Adults: The usual starting dose is 180 milligrams (mg) once a day in the morning. Your doctor will adjust your dose as needed until the desired effect is achieved.

How should I take this medication?

• Take Calan SR exactly as prescribed by your doctor. Take this medicine with food.

What should I avoid while taking this medication?

Do not drink alcohol while you are taking Calan SR. This medicine can increase the effects of alcohol.

Do not breastfeed while you are taking Calan SR.

What are possible food and drug interactions associated with this medication?

If Calan SR is taken with certain other drugs, the effects of either could be increased, decreased, or altered. It is especially important to check with your doctor before combining Calan SR with the following: alcohol, blood pressure medications (such as lisinopril or metoprolol), carbamazepine, cimetidine, clonidine, cyclospo-rine, digoxin, medications for life-threatening irregular heartbeats (such as disopyramide), nitrates (such as nitroglycerin), pheno-barbital, rifampin, telithromycin, or theophylline.

What are the possible side effects of this medication?
Please see general statement regarding side effects on page xiii.

> **Side effects may include:** constipation, difficulty breathing, diz-ziness, headache, heart or liver problems, low blood pressure, nausea, rash, slow heart rate, swelling, tiredness

Can I receive this medication if I am pregnant or breastfeeding?
The effects of Calan SR during pregnancy are unknown. Calan SR may cause harm to your baby if you use it during breastfeeding. Do not breastfeed while you are taking Calan SR. Tell your doctor immediately if you are pregnant, plan to become pregnant, or are breastfeeding.

What should I do if I miss a dose of this medication?
If you miss a dose of Calan SR, take it as soon as you remember. However, if it is almost time for your next dose, skip the one you missed and return to your regular dosing schedule. Do not take two doses at once.

How should I store this medication?
Store at room temperature. Protect from light and moisture.

Captopril
Generic name: Captopril

What is this medication?
Captopril is a medicine known as an angiotensin-converting en-zyme (ACE) inhibitor. Captopril is used alone or in combination with other medications to treat high blood pressure or heart failure.

Captopril is also used to treat kidney disease in people with diabetes. In addition, it is used after a heart attack to improve survival in people with a heart condition called left ventricular dysfunction (damage to the section of the heart that is responsible for pumping blood to the rest of the body).

What is the most important information I should know about this medication?

- Captopril can cause a rare but serious allergic reaction leading to swelling of your face, eyes, lips, tongue, throat, or gut (causing severe abdominal pain), or difficulty swallowing or breathing. If you experience any of these symptoms, seek emergency medical attention immediately.
- Tell your doctor if you experience lightheadedness, especially during the first few weeks of Captopril therapy.
- Vomiting, diarrhea, excessive sweating, and dehydration may lead to an excessive fall in your blood pressure. Tell your doctor if you experience any of these.
- Captopril may decrease your blood neutrophil (type of blood cells that fight infections) levels, especially if you have a collagen vascular disease (such as lupus [disease that affects the immune system]) or kidney disease.
- Promptly report any signs of infection (such as sore throat or fever) to your doctor.
- Captopril can cause liver damage. Stop taking Captopril and call your doctor right away if you develop yellowing of your skin or the whites of your eyes.
- Tell your doctor if you develop a persistent dry cough while you are taking Captopril.

Who should not take this medication?
Do not take Captopril if you are allergic to it or any of its ingredients.

Do not take Captopril if you have a history of angioedema (a condition involving swelling of the face, extremities, eyes, lips, and tongue) related to previous treatment with similar medicines.

What should I tell my doctor before I take the first dose of this medication?

Tell your doctor about all prescription, over-the-counter, and herbal medications you are taking before beginning treatment with Captopril. Also, talk to your doctor about your complete medical history, especially if you have liver problems, kidney disease, or diabetes. Tell your doctor if you have bone marrow problems or any blood disease, any disease that affects the immune system (such as lupus or scleroderma [disease that affects the immune system]), collagen vascular disease, narrowing or hardening of the arteries of your brain or heart, chest pain, or if you have ever had an allergy or sensitivity to ACE inhibitors such as Captopril.

What is the usual dosage?

Please see general statement regarding dosage on page xii.

High Blood Pressure
Adults: The usual starting dose is 25 milligrams (mg) two or three times a day. Your doctor will adjust your dose based on your previous blood pressure medication and will increase your dose as needed until the desired effect is achieved.

Heart Failure
Adults: The usual starting dose is 25 mg three times a day. Your doctor will prescribe the appropriate dose for you based on your condition.

After a Heart Attack
Adults: The usual starting dose is 6.25 mg as a single dose, then 12.5 mg three times a day. Your doctor may increase your dose appropriately.

Kidney Disease
Adults: The usual dose is 25 mg three times a day.

If you have kidney impairment, your doctor will adjust your dose appropriately.

How should I take this medication?
- Take Captopril one hour before meals.

What should I avoid while taking this medication?
Do not change your dose or stop taking Captopril without first talking to your doctor.

What are possible food and drug interactions associated with this medication?
If Captopril is taken with certain other drugs, the effects of either could be increased, decreased, or altered. It is especially important to check with your doctor before combining Captopril with the following: certain diuretics (water pills) (such as amiloride, hydrochlorothiazide, spironolactone, or triamterene), dextran, heart medications known as nitrates (such as nitroglycerin), lithium, nonsteroidal anti-inflammatory drugs (NSAIDs) (such as ibuprofen or naproxen), potassium supplements, or salt substitutes containing potassium.

What are the possible side effects of this medication?
Please see general statement regarding side effects on page xiii.

> **Side effects may include:** anemia, itchy rash, low blood pressure

Can I receive this medication if I am pregnant or breastfeeding?
Do not take Captopril if you are pregnant or breastfeeding. Captopril can harm your unborn baby. Tell your doctor immediately if you are pregnant, plan to become pregnant, or are breastfeeding.

What should I do if I miss a dose of this medication?
If you miss a dose of Captopril, take it as soon as you remember. However, if it is almost time for your next dose, skip the one you missed and return to your regular dosing schedule. Do not take two doses at once.

How should I store this medication?
Store at room temperature.

Captopril: *see Captopril, page 171*

Carafate
Generic name: Sucralfate

What is this medication?
Carafate is a medicine used for short-term (up to 8 weeks) treatment of active duodenal ulcers (ulcer in the upper intestine). Carafate tablets can be used for maintenance therapy after healing of acute ulcers. Carafate is available in tablets and suspension.

What is the most important information I should know about this medication?
- A duodenal ulcer is a recurring illness. Short-term treatment with Carafate can completely heal an ulcer, but it cannot prevent other ulcers from developing nor lessen their severity.
- Tell your doctor if you have kidney impairment. Small amounts of aluminum can be absorbed through your stomach and intestines while taking Carafate. If you have kidney problems, you may have difficulty removing this aluminum from your body and further cause bone or brain problems.
- If you have diabetes, you can experience an increase in your blood sugar levels while taking Carafate suspension. Monitor your blood sugar levels closely. Your doctor may need to adjust the dose of your diabetes medication.

Who should not take this medication?
Do not take Carafate if you are allergic to it or any of its ingredients.

What should I tell my doctor before I take the first dose of this medication?
Tell your doctor about all prescription, over-the-counter, and herbal medications you are taking before beginning treatment with Carafate. Also, talk to your doctor about your complete medical history, especially if you have kidney problems, diabetes, or if you are taking aluminum-containing products.

What is the usual dosage?
Please see general statement regarding dosage on page xii.

Carafate oral suspension may be substituted for Carafate tablets for any of the indications below. Each milliliter (mL) of Carafate oral suspension contains 100 milligrams (mg) of sucralfate.

Active Duodenal Ulcer
Adults: The recommended dose is 1 gram (g) or two teaspoonfuls four times a day.

Maintenance Therapy
Adults: The recommended dose is 1 g twice a day.

How should I take this medication?
- Take Carafate exactly as prescribed by your doctor. Take Carafate on an empty stomach.
- Shake Carafate suspension well before use.

What should I avoid while taking this medication?
Do not take antacids within half an hour before or after Carafate. Also, do not take aluminum-containing antacids or products, especially if you have kidney problems.

What are possible food and drug interactions associated with this medication?
If Carafate is taken with certain other drugs, the effects of either could be increased, decreased, or altered. It is especially important to check with your doctor before combining Carafate with the following: aluminum-containing antacids, certain antibiotics (such as ciprofloxacin, norfloxacin, or ofloxacin), cimetidine, digoxin, ketoconazole, levothyroxine, phenytoin, quinidine, ranitidine, tetracycline, or theophylline.

What are the possible side effects of this medication?
Please see general statement regarding side effects on page xiii.

Side effects may include: back pain, constipation, diarrhea, dizziness, dry mouth, gas, headache, indigestion, itching, nausea, rash, stomach discomfort, trouble sleeping, vomiting

Can I receive this medication if I am pregnant or breastfeeding?

The effects of Carafate during pregnancy and breastfeeding are unknown. Tell your doctor immediately if you are pregnant, plan to become pregnant, or are breastfeeding.

What should I do if I miss a dose of this medication?

If you miss a dose of Carafate, take it as soon as you remember. However, if it is almost time for your next dose, skip the one you missed and return to your regular dosing schedule. Do not take two doses at once.

How should I store this medication?

Store at room temperature. Protect the suspension from freezing.

Carbamazepine: see Carbatrol, page 177

Carbamazepine: see Tegretol, page 970

Carbatrol

Generic name: Carbamazepine

What is this medication?

Carbatrol is a medicine used to treat certain types of seizures and trigeminal neuralgia (facial and head pain).

What is the most important information I should know about this medication?

- Do not stop taking Carbatrol without first talking to your doctor. Stopping Carbatrol suddenly can cause serious health problems.
- Carbatrol can cause rare but serious rashes that may be life-threatening. These serious skin reactions are more likely to

happen within the first four months of Carbatrol treatment but may occur at later times. These reactions can happen in anyone, but are more likely in people of Asian descent. If you are of Asian descent you may need a genetic blood test before you take Carbatrol to see if you are at a higher risk for serious skin reactions with this medicine.

- Carbatrol can cause rare but serious blood problems. Tell your doctor immediately if you experience a fever, sore throat, or other infections that come and go or do not go away; easy bruising, red or purple spots on your body, bleeding gums or nose bleeds, or severe fatigue or weakness.

- Carbatrol can cause suicidal thoughts or actions in a very small number of people. If you develop depression or your depression worsens, suicidal thoughts or behavior occur, or you experience unusual changes in mood or behavior, tell your doctor immediately.

Who should not take this medication?

Do not take Carbatrol if you are allergic to it or any of its ingredients.

Do not take Carbatrol if you have a history of bone marrow depression (a condition of the bone marrow in which it is unable to produce normal amounts of blood cells).

Do not take Carbatrol if you take antidepressant medications known as tricyclics (such as amitriptyline, imipramine, or nortriptyline) or nefazodone.

Do not take Carbatrol if you have taken antidepressant medications known as monoamine oxidase inhibitors (MAOIs) (such as phenelzine, selegiline, or tranylcypromine) in the last 14 days.

What should I tell my doctor before I take the first dose of this medication?

Tell your doctor about all prescription, over-the-counter, and herbal medications you are taking before beginning treatment with Carbatrol. Also, talk to your doctor about your complete medical history, especially if you have or ever had blood disorders; heart, liver, or kidney problems; increased pressure in your eye; suicidal thoughts or actions, depression, or mood problems; or use birth control.

What is the usual dosage?
Please see general statement regarding dosage on page xii.

Seizures
Adults and children >12 years: The usual starting dose is 200 milligrams (mg) twice a day.

Your doctor will prescribe the appropriate dose for you and will increase your dose as needed, until the desired effect is achieved.

Trigeminal Neuralgia
Adults: The usual starting dose is 200 mg on the first day. The dose may be increased by up to 200 mg a day every 12 hours as needed for pain relief.

How should I take this medication?
- Take Carbatrol exactly as prescribed by your doctor. Do not take extra doses or take more often without asking your doctor.
- Take Carbatrol with or without food.
- Carbatrol capsules can be opened and sprinkled over food, such as a teaspoon of applesauce. Tell your doctor if you cannot swallow Carbatrol whole.

What should I avoid while taking this medication?
Do not drink alcohol or take other medicines that may make you sleepy or dizzy while you are taking Carbatrol until you talk to your doctor.

Do not drive, operate heavy machinery, or engage in other dangerous activities until you know how Carbatrol affects you. Carbatrol can slow your thinking and motor skills.

Do not crush, chew, or break Carbatrol capsules or the beads inside of the capsules.

What are possible food and drug interactions associated with this medication?

If Carbatrol is taken with certain other drugs, the effects of either could be increased, decreased, or altered. Carbatrol may interact with numerous medications. Therefore, it is very important that you tell your doctor about any other medications you are taking.

What are the possible side effects of this medication?

Please see general statement regarding side effects on page xiii.

> **Side effects may include:** dizziness, drowsiness, lightheaded-ness, nausea, problems with your walking and coordination, shortness of breath, vomiting

Can I receive this medication if I am pregnant or breastfeeding?

Carbatrol can cause harm to your unborn baby if you use it during pregnancy. Carbatrol can be found in your breast milk if you take it while breastfeeding. Tell your doctor immediately if you are pregnant, plan to become pregnant, or are breastfeeding.

What should I do if I miss a dose of this medication?

If you miss a dose of Carbatrol, take it as soon as you remember. However, if it is almost time for your next dose, skip the one you missed and return to your regular dosing schedule. Do not take two doses at once.

How should I store this medication?

Store at room temperature. Protect from light and moisture.

Carbidopa/Levodopa: *see Sinemet, page 928*

Carbidopa/Levodopa: *see Sinemet CR, page 931*

Cardizem

Generic name: Diltiazem HCl

What is this medication?

Cardizem is a medicine known as a calcium channel blocker, which is used to treat chronic stable angina (long-term chest pain) or angina due to temporary narrowing of an artery in the heart.

What is the most important information I should know about this medication?

- Cardizem can increase your risk of having a very slow heart rate, worsened congestive heart failure (a condition in which the heart cannot pump enough blood throughout the body), very low blood pressure, or liver injury.
- Skin reactions (such as light sensitivity; round red, brown, or purple spots on your skin; itching; or hives) can occur with Cardizem and can disappear. Tell your doctor if the skin reaction gets worse or does not go away.

Who should not take this medication?

Do not take Cardizem if you are allergic to it or any of its ingredients.

Do not take Cardizem if you have low blood pressure.

Do not take Cardizem is you have sick sinus syndrome (abnormal heart rhythm) or a heart block (unless you have a pacemaker).

Do not take Cardizem if you have recently had a heart attack or have lung congestion.

What should I tell my doctor before I take the first dose of this medication?

Tell your doctor about all prescription, over-the-counter, and herbal medications you are taking before beginning treatment with Cardizem. Also, talk to your doctor about your complete medical history, especially if you have low blood pressure, heart failure, heart disease, abnormal heart rhythms, kidney or liver disease, lung problems, have recently had a heart attack, or are pregnant, plan to become pregnant, or are breastfeeding.

What is the usual dosage?
Please see general statement regarding dosage on page xii.

Adults: The usual starting dose is 30 milligrams four times a day. Your doctor will adjust your dose appropriately.

How should I take this medication?
• Take Cardizem exactly as prescribed by your doctor. Take it before meals and at bedtime.

What should I avoid while taking this medication?
Do not breastfeed while you are taking Cardizem.

What are possible food and drug interactions associated with this medication?
If Cardizem is taken with certain other drugs, the effects of either could be increased, decreased, or altered. It is especially important to check with your doctor before combining Cardizem with the following: anesthesia, blood pressure/heart medications known as beta-blockers (such as atenolol or propranolol), buspirone, carbamazepine, cholesterol-lowering medications known as statins (such as lovastatin or simvastatin), cimetidine, clonidine, cyclosporine, digoxin, midazolam, quinidine, rifampin, or triazolam.

What are the possible side effects of this medication?
Please see general statement regarding side effects on page xiii.

> **Side effects may include:** dizziness, headache, nausea, rash, swelling, weakness

Can I receive this medication if I am pregnant or breastfeeding?
The effects of Cardizem during pregnancy are unknown. Cardizem can be found in your breast milk if you take it while breastfeeding. Do not breastfeed while you are taking Cardizem. Tell your doctor immediately if you are pregnant, plan to become pregnant, or are breastfeeding.

What should I do if I miss a dose of this medication?

If you miss a dose of Cardizem, take it as soon as you remember. However, if it is almost time for your next dose, skip the one you missed and return to your regular dosing schedule. Do not take two doses at once.

How should I store this medication?

Store at room temperature. Protect from excessive humidity.

Cardizem CD

Generic name: Diltiazem HCl

What is this medication?

Cardizem CD is a medicine known as a calcium channel blocker, which is used to treat high blood pressure, chronic stable angina (long-term chest pain), or angina due to temporary narrowing of an artery in the heart.

What is the most important information I should know about this medication?

- Cardizem CD can increase your risk of having a very slow heart rate, worsened congestive heart failure (a condition in which the heart cannot pump enough blood throughout the body), very low blood pressure, or liver injury.
- Skin reactions (such as light sensitivity; round red, brown, or purple spots on your skin; itching; or hives) can occur with Cardizem CD and can disappear. Tell your doctor if the skin reaction gets worse or does not go away.

Who should not take this medication?

Do not take Cardizem CD if you are allergic to it or any of its ingredients.

Do not take Cardizem CD if you have low blood pressure.

Do not take Cardizem CD if you have sick sinus syndrome (abnormal heart rhythm) or a heart block (unless you have a pacemaker).

Do not take Cardizem CD if you have recently had a heart attack or have lung congestion.

What should I tell my doctor before I take the first dose of this medication?

Tell your doctor about all prescription, over-the-counter, and herbal medications you are taking before beginning treatment with Cardizem CD. Also, talk to your doctor about your complete medical history, especially if you have low blood pressure, heart failure, heart disease, abnormal heart rhythms, kidney or liver disease, lung problems, have recently had a heart attack, or are pregnant, plan to become pregnant, or are breastfeeding.

What is the usual dosage?

Please see general statement regarding dosage on page xii.

High Blood Pressure
Adults: The usual starting dose is 180-240 milligrams (mg) once a day.

Chest Pain
Adults: The usual starting dose is 120-180 mg once a day.

Your doctor will adjust your dose appropriately.

How should I take this medication?
• Take Cardizem CD exactly as prescribed by your doctor.

What should I avoid while taking this medication?
Do not breastfeed while you are taking Cardizem CD.

What are possible food and drug interactions associated with this medication?

If Cardizem CD is taken with certain other drugs, the effects of either could be increased, decreased, or altered. It is especially important to check with your doctor before combining Cardizem CD with the following: anesthesia, blood pressure/heart medications known as beta-blockers (such as atenolol or propranolol), buspirone, carbamazepine, cholesterol-lowering medications known as statins (such as lovastatin or simvastatin), cimetidine, clonidine, cyclosporine, digoxin, midazolam, quinidine, rifampin, or triazolam.

What are the possible side effects of this medication?

Please see general statement regarding side effects on page xiii.

> **Side effects may include:** abnormal heartbeat, dizziness, headache, slow heartbeat, swelling, weakness

Can I receive this medication if I am pregnant or breastfeeding?

The effects of Cardizem CD during pregnancy are unknown. Cardizem CD can be found in your breast milk if you take it while breastfeeding. Do not breastfeed while you are taking Cardizem CD. Tell your doctor immediately if you are pregnant, plan to become pregnant, or are breastfeeding.

What should I do if I miss a dose of this medication?

If you miss a dose of Cardizem CD, take it as soon as you remember. However, if it is almost time for your next dose, skip the one you missed and return to your regular dosing schedule. Do not take two doses at once.

How should I store this medication?

Store at room temperature. Protect from excessive humidity.

Cardura

Generic name: Doxazosin Mesylate

What is this medication?

Cardura is a medicine used alone or in combination with other medications to treat high blood pressure. Cardura is also used to relieve the signs and symptoms of benign prostatic hyperplasia (enlargement of the prostate gland, which may in turn block the flow of urine).

What is the most important information I should know about this medication?

- Cardura can cause a sudden drop in blood pressure, which may cause fainting, dizziness, or lightheadedness. Do not drive or perform other hazardous activities until you know how Cardura affects you.
- Cardura does not treat high blood pressure.
- Rarely, Cardura can cause painful, prolonged erections (priapism). Tell your doctor right away if this occurs.

Who should not take this medication?

Do not take Cardura if you are allergic to it, any of its ingredients, or similar medications (such as prazosin or terazosin).

What should I tell my doctor before I take the first dose of this medication?

Tell your doctor about all prescription, over-the-counter, and herbal medications you are taking before beginning treatment with Cardura. Also, talk to your doctor about your complete medical history, especially if you have kidney or liver problems, have prostate cancer, plan on having cataract surgery, or are pregnant, plan to become pregnant, or are breastfeeding.

What is the usual dosage?

Please see general statement regarding dosage on page xii.

Adults: The recommended starting dose is 1 milligram once a day, in the morning or at night. Your doctor will prescribe the appropriate dose for you and will increase your dose as needed, until the desired effect is achieved.

How should I take this medication?

- Take Cardura exactly as prescribed by your doctor.
- Take Cardura once a day. Take Cardura with or without food.

What should I avoid while taking this medication?

Do not get up too fast from a sitting or lying position.

Do not drive or perform hazardous tasks for 24 hours after the first dose, after a dosage increase, or if your treatment is interrupted then resumed, until you know how Cardura affects you.

What are possible food and drug interactions associated with this medication?

If Cardura is taken with certain other drugs, the effects of either could be increased, decreased, or altered. It is especially important to check with your doctor before combining Cardura with the following: erectile dysfunction medications (such as sildenafil or tadalafil) or certain other blood pressure/heart medications.

What are the possible side effects of this medication?

Please see general statement regarding side effects on page xiii.

Side effects may include: dizziness, low blood pressure, shortness of breath, swelling, tiredness, weight gain

---

Can I receive this medication if I am pregnant or breastfeeding?

The effects of Cardura during pregnancy and breastfeeding are unknown. Tell your doctor immediately if you are pregnant, plan to become pregnant, or are breastfeeding.

What should I do if I miss a dose of this medication?

If you miss a dose of Cardura, take it as soon as you remember. However, if it is almost time for your next dose, skip the one you missed and return to your regular dosing schedule. Do not take two doses at once.

How should I store this medication?

Store at room temperature.

Carisoprodol: *see Soma, page 940*

Cartia XT
Generic name: Diltiazem HCl

What is this medication?
Cartia XT is a medicine known as a calcium channel blocker, which is used to treat high blood pressure, chronic stable angina (long-term chest pain), or angina due to temporary narrowing of an artery in the heart.

What is the most important information I should know about this medication?
- Cartia XT can increase your risk of having a very slow heart rate, worsened congestive heart failure (a condition in which the heart cannot pump enough blood throughout the body), very low blood pressure, or liver injury.
- Skin reactions (such as light sensitivity; round red, brown, or purple spots on your skin; itching; or hives) can occur with Cartia XT and can disappear. Tell your doctor if the skin reaction gets worse or does not go away.

Who should not take this medication?
Do not take Cartia XT if you are allergic to it or any of its ingredients.

Do not take Cartia XT if you have low blood pressure.

Do not take Cartia XT if you have sick sinus syndrome (abnormal heart rhythm) or a heart block (unless you have a pacemaker).

Do not take Cartia XT if you have recently had a heart attack or have lung congestion.

What should I tell my doctor before I take the first dose of this medication?
Tell your doctor about all prescription, over-the-counter, and herbal medications you are taking before beginning treatment with Cartia XT. Also, talk to your doctor about your complete medical history, especially if you have low blood pressure, heart failure, heart disease, abnormal heart rhythms, kidney or liver disease,

lung problems, have recently had a heart attack, or are pregnant, plan to become pregnant, or are breastfeeding.

What is the usual dosage?
Please see general statement regarding dosage on page xii.

High Blood Pressure
Adults: The usual starting dose is 180-240 milligrams (mg) once a day.

Chest Pain
Adults: The usual starting dose is 120-180 mg once a day.

Your doctor will adjust your dose appropriately.

How should I take this medication?
• Take Cartia XT exactly as prescribed by your doctor.
• Swallow Cartia XT capsules whole. Do not open, crush, or chew them.

What should I avoid while taking this medication?
Do not breastfeed while you are taking Cartia XT.

What are possible food and drug interactions associated with this medication?
If Cartia XT is taken with certain other drugs, the effects of either could be increased, decreased, or altered. It is especially important to check with your doctor before combining Cartia XT with the following: anesthesia, blood pressure/heart medications known as beta-blockers (such as atenolol or propranolol), buspirone, carbamazepine, cholesterol-lowering medications known as statins (such as lovastatin or simvastatin), cimetidine, clonidine, cyclosporine, digoxin, midazolam, quinidine, rifampin, or triazolam.

What are the possible side effects of this medication?
Please see general statement regarding side effects on page xiii.

Side effects may include: abnormal heartbeat, dizziness, headache, slow heartbeat, swelling, weakness

Can I receive this medication if I am pregnant or breastfeeding?

The effects of Cartia XT during pregnancy are unknown. Cartia XT can be found in your breast milk if you take it while breastfeeding. Do not breastfeed while you are taking Cartia XT. Tell your doctor immediately if you are pregnant, plan to become pregnant, or are breastfeeding.

What should I do if I miss a dose of this medication?

If you miss a dose of Cartia XT, take it as soon as you remember. However, if it is almost time for your next dose, skip the one you missed and return to your regular dosing schedule. Do not take two doses at once.

How should I store this medication?

Store at room temperature. Protect from excessive humidity.

Carvedilol: *see Coreg, page 268*

Carvedilol: *see Coreg CR, page 271*

Catapres

Generic name: Clonidine HCl

What is this medication?

Catapres is a medicine used alone or in combination with other medications to treat high blood pressure.

What is the most important information I should know about this medication?

- Do not stop taking Catapres without first talking to your doctor. Stopping Catapres suddenly can cause withdrawal symptoms, including nervousness, agitation, headache, and shaking. These symptoms can occur with or be followed by a sudden rise in your blood pressure.

- If you used Catapres-TTS patches in the past and developed an allergic reaction, Catapres tablets can also cause a reaction. Tell your doctor if you experience rash, hives, or swelling of your face, eyes, lips, or tongue.
- Catapres can cause dry eyes if you wear contact lenses.

Who should not take this medication?

Do not take Catapres if you are allergic to it or any of its ingredients.

What should I tell my doctor before I take the first dose of this medication?

Tell your doctor about all prescription, over-the-counter, and herbal medications you are taking before beginning treatment with Catapres. Also, talk to your doctor about your complete medical history, especially if you have kidney disease, or if you are pregnant, plan to become pregnant, or are breastfeeding.

What is the usual dosage?

Please see general statement regarding dosage on page xii.

Adults: The usual starting dose is 0.1 milligrams twice a day. Your doctor will increase your dose as needed until the desired effect is achieved.

If you are elderly or have kidney impairment, your doctor will adjust your dose appropriately.

How should I take this medication?

- Take Catapres exactly as prescribed by your doctor. Take it in the morning and at bedtime.

What should I avoid while taking this medication?

Do not stop taking Catapres without first talking to your doctor.

Do not drive or operate dangerous machinery until you know how Catapres affects you.

What are possible food and drug interactions associated with this medication?

If Catapres is taken with certain other drugs, the effects of either could be increased, decreased, or altered. It is especially important to check with your doctor before combining Catapres with the following: alcohol, antipsychotic medications (such as clozapine or olanzapine), barbiturates (such as phenobarbital), blood pressure/heart medications known as beta-blockers (such as atenolol or propranolol) or calcium channel blockers (such as diltiazem or verapamil), certain antidepressants (such as amitriptyline or imipramine), digoxin, or sedating medicines (such as alprazolam or diazepam).

What are the possible side effects of this medication?

Please see general statement regarding side effects on page xiii.

> **Side effects may include:** constipation, dizziness, drowsiness, dry mouth, sedation

Can I receive this medication if I am pregnant or breastfeeding?

The effects of Catapres during pregnancy are unknown. Catapres can be found in your breast milk if you take it while breastfeeding. Tell your doctor immediately if you are pregnant, plan to become pregnant, or are breastfeeding.

What should I do if I miss a dose of this medication?

If you miss a dose of Catapres, take it as soon as you remember. However, if it is almost time for your next dose, skip the one you missed and return to your regular dosing schedule. Do not take two doses at once.

How should I store this medication?

Store at room temperature.

Catapres-TTS
Generic name: Clonidine HCl

What is this medication?
Catapres-TTS is a medicine used alone or in combination with other medications to treat high blood pressure. Catapres-TTS is available as a patch.

What is the most important information I should know about this medication?
- Do not stop using Catapres-TTS without first talking to your doctor. Stopping Catapres-TTS suddenly can cause withdrawal symptoms, including nervousness, agitation, headache, shaking, and confusion. These symptoms can occur with or be followed by a sudden rise in your blood pressure.
- Catapres-TTS can cause an allergic reaction. Tell your doctor right away if you experience rash, hives, or swelling of your face, eyes, lips, or tongue.
- Contact your doctor about the possible need to remove Catapres-TTS if you have redness and/or vesicle formation at the application site or skin rash. If you experience mild skin irritation before completing 7 days of use, the patch may be removed and replaced with a new patch applied to a fresh skin site.
- Catapres-TTS can cause skin burns at the patch site if you keep it on during an MRI. Remove the patch before undergoing an MRI.
- Catapres-TTS can cause dry eyes if you wear contact lenses.
- Keep both used and unused patches in a safe place away from children. Accidental use by a child can be harmful.

Who should not take this medication?
Do not use Catapres-TTS if you are allergic to it or any of its ingredients.

What should I tell my doctor before I take the first dose of this medication?
Tell your doctor about all prescription, over-the-counter, and herbal medications you are taking before beginning treatment with Catapres-TTS. Also, talk to your doctor about your complete

medical history, especially if you have kidney disease, or if you are pregnant, plan to become pregnant, or are breastfeeding.

What is the usual dosage?
Please see general statement regarding dosage on page xii.

Adults: Apply 1 patch every 7 days. Your doctor will increase your dose as needed until the desired effect is achieved.

If you have kidney impairment, your doctor will adjust your dose appropriately.

How should I take this medication?
- Use Catapres-TTS exactly as prescribed by your doctor. Apply the patch once a week, on the same day each week.
- Apply the patch to a hairless area of skin on your upper, outer arm or upper chest. The area of skin should not have any cuts, abrasions, irritation, scars, or calluses. Do not shave the skin before applying the patch. Do not apply Catapres-TTS on skin folds or under tight undergarments to avoid the patch becoming loose.
- Wear the patch for 7 days, then take it off and apply a new patch. Use a different skin site on your upper, outer arm or upper chest when you apply a new patch.
- If the patch gets loose during the 7-day wear, apply the adhesive cover directly over it to help keep the patch in place.
- After 7 days, fold the patch in half with the sticky sides together and throw it away, out of reach from children.
- Please review the instructions that came with your prescription on how to properly apply Catapres-TTS.

What should I avoid while taking this medication?
Do not stop taking Catapres-TTS without first talking to your doctor.

Do not drive or operate dangerous machinery until you know how Catapres-TTS affects you.

What are possible food and drug interactions associated with this medication?

If Catapres-TTS is used with certain other drugs, the effects of either could be increased, decreased, or altered. It is especially important to check with your doctor before combining Catapres-TTS with the following: alcohol, antipsychotic medications (such as clozapine or olanzapine), barbiturates (such as phenobarbital), blood pressure/heart medications known as beta-blockers (such as atenolol or propranolol) or calcium channel blockers (such as diltiazem or verapamil), certain antidepressants (such as amitriptyline or imipramine), digoxin, or sedating medicines (such as alprazolam or diazepam).

What are the possible side effects of this medication?

Please see general statement regarding side effects on page xiii.

> **Side effects may include:** change in taste, constipation, dizziness, drowsiness, dry mouth or throat, fatigue, headache, insomnia, nausea, nervousness, sedation, skin reaction (such as itching or redness)

Can I receive this medication if I am pregnant or breastfeeding?

The effects of Catapres-TTS during pregnancy are unknown. Catapres-TTS can be found in your breast milk if you take it while breastfeeding. Tell your doctor immediately if you are pregnant, plan to become pregnant, or are breastfeeding.

What should I do if I miss a dose of this medication?

Catapres-TTS should be used under special circumstances. If you miss your scheduled dose, contact your doctor or pharmacist for advice.

How should I store this medication?

Store at room temperature.

Cefdinir: *see Omnicef, page 726*

Ceftin
Generic name: Cefuroxime Axetil

What is this medication?
Ceftin is an antibiotic used to treat certain bacterial infections. Ceftin is available in tablets or oral suspension. Ceftin tablets are used to treat infections of the throat, tonsils, ear, sinuses, skin, or urinary tract. Also, Ceftin tablets are used to treat bronchitis (inflammation of the air passages within the lungs), gonorrhea (a sexually transmitted disease characterized by itching and burning during urination) or Lyme disease. Ceftin oral suspension is used to treat infections of the throat, tonsils, ear, and skin. Ceftin may also be used to treat other bacterial infections, as determined by your doctor.

What is the most important information I should know about this medication?
- Do not take Ceftin if you are allergic to it, any of its ingredients, or similar antibiotics (such as cefazolin or cefotetan). If you are allergic to penicillin antibiotics, it is possible for you to have an allergic reaction to this medication. Tell your doctor right away if you take Ceftin and feel signs of an allergic reaction (such as a rash, swelling, or difficulty breathing).
- Ceftin can cause diarrhea or colitis (inflammation of the colon). This can occur a couple of months after taking the last dose of Ceftin. Tell your doctor right away if you have diarrhea or colitis.
- Take Ceftin as prescribed by your doctor for the full course of treatment, even if symptoms improve earlier. Do not skip doses. Complete the full course of Ceftin. Skipping doses or not completing the full course of Ceftin can decrease its effectiveness and can lead to the growth of bacteria that are resistant to the effects of Ceftin.
- Ceftin oral suspension contains phenylalanine. Tell your doctor if you have a condition called phenylketonuria (an inability to process phenylalanine).

Who should not take this medication?
Do not take Ceftin if you are allergic to it, any of its ingredients, or similar antibiotics.

Do not take Ceftin to treat viral infections, such as the common cold.

What should I tell my doctor before I take the first dose of this medication?

Tell your doctor about all prescription, over-the-counter, and herbal medications you are taking before beginning treatment with Ceftin. Also, talk to your doctor about your complete medical history, especially if you have allergies, phenylketonuria, a history of colitis, stomach or intestinal problems, or kidney or liver disease.

What is the usual dosage?
Please see general statement regarding dosage on page xii.

Throat, Tonsil, Sinus, or Ear Infections
Adults and adolescents ≥13 years: The recommended dose is 250 milligrams (mg) twice a day for 10 days.

Children 3 months to 12 years: Your doctor will prescribe the appropriate dose for your child, based on their weight and type of infection.

Bronchitis
Adults and adolescents ≥13 years: The recommended dose is 250 mg or 500 mg twice a day for 5-10 days.

Skin Infections
Adults and adolescents ≥13 years: The recommended dose is 250 mg or 500 mg twice a day for 10 days.

Children 3 months to 12 years: Your doctor will prescribe the appropriate dose for your child, based on their weight and type of infection.

Urinary Tract Infections
Adults and adolescents ≥13 years: The recommended dose is 250 mg twice a day for 7-10 days.

Gonorrhea
Adults and adolescents ≥13 years: The recommended dose is 1 gram once.

Early Lyme Disease
Adults and adolescents ≥13 years: The recommended dose is 500 mg twice a day for 20 days.

How should I take this medication?
- Take Ceftin exactly as prescribed by your doctor.
- You can take Ceftin tablets with or without food.
- Take Ceftin oral suspension with food. Shake the suspension well before each use.

What should I avoid while taking this medication?
Do not miss your scheduled follow-up appointments with your doctor.

What are possible food and drug interactions associated with this medication?
If Ceftin is taken with certain other drugs, the effects of either could be increased, decreased, or altered. It is especially important to check with your doctor before combining Ceftin with the following: birth control pills, blood thinners (such as warfarin), certain diuretics (water pills) (such as furosemide), or probenecid.

What are the possible side effects of this medication?
Please see general statement regarding side effects on page xiii.

Side effects may include: abdominal pain, allergic reactions, changes in taste, diaper rash in infants, diarrhea, nausea, rash, stomach or intestinal disturbances, vomiting, yellowing of skin or whites of your eyes

---

Can I receive this medication if I am pregnant or breastfeeding?
The effects of Ceftin during pregnancy are unknown. Ceftin can be found in your breast milk if you take it while breastfeeding. Tell

your doctor immediately if you are pregnant, plan to become pregnant, or are breastfeeding.

What should I do if I miss a dose of this medication?

If you miss a dose of Ceftin, take it as soon as you remember. However, if it is almost time for your next dose, skip the one you missed and return to your regular dosing schedule. Do not take two doses at once.

How should I store this medication?

Store at room temperature.

After mixing, store Ceftin oral suspension in the refrigerator. Discard the unused portion after 10 days.

Cefuroxime Axetil: *see Ceftin, page 196*

Celebrex

Generic name: Celecoxib

What is this medication?

Celebrex is a nonsteroidal anti-inflammatory drug (NSAID) used to treat osteoarthritis, rheumatoid arthritis in adults, juvenile rheumatoid arthritis, ankylosing spondylitis (arthritis of the spine), and sudden pain. In addition, Celebrex is used to treat pain associated with menstrual periods.

What is the most important information I should know about this medication?

- Celebrex can cause serious problems (such as heart attack or stroke). Your risk can increase when this medication is used for long periods of time and if you have heart disease. Tell your doctor if you experience chest pain, shortness of breath, weakness, or slurred speech.

- Celebrex can cause high blood pressure and heart failure or worsen existing high blood pressure. Tell your doctor if you experience weight gain or swelling of your face or throat.
- Celebrex can cause discomfort, ulcers, or bleeding in your stomach or intestines. Your risk can increase with long-term use, smoking, drinking alcohol, older age, or with certain medications. Tell your doctor immediately if you experience stomach pain or if you have bloody vomit or stools.
- Long-term use of Celebrex can cause kidney injury. Your risk can increase if you have kidney impairment; heart failure; liver problems; are taking certain medications, including diuretics (water pills) (such as furosemide or hydrochlorothiazide), blood/heart medications known as angiotensin-converting enzyme (ACE) inhibitors (such as lisinopril), or angiotensin receptor blockers (ARBs) (such as losartan or olmesartan); or are elderly.
- Celebrex can also cause liver injury. Stop taking Celebrex and call your doctor if you experience nausea, tiredness, weakness, itchiness, yellowing of your skin or whites of your eyes, right upper abdominal tenderness, or "flu-like" symptoms.
- Celebrex can cause a serious allergic reaction. Stop taking Celebrex and tell your doctor right away if you experience difficulty breathing or swelling of your face or throat.
- Stop taking Celebrex and tell your doctor right away if you experience serious skin reactions, such as rash, blisters, fever, or itchiness.

Who should not take this medication?

Do not take Celebrex if you are allergic to it or any of its ingredients; or if you have ever had an allergy or sensitivity to sulfonamide medications (such as trimethoprim/sulfamethoxazole or sulfisoxazole).

Do not take Celebrex if you have experienced asthma, hives, or allergic-type reactions after taking aspirin or other NSAIDs (such as ibuprofen or naproxen).

Do not take Celebrex right before or after a heart surgery called a coronary artery bypass graft (CABG).

What should I tell my doctor before I take the first dose of this medication?

Tell your doctor about all prescription, over-the-counter, and herbal medications you are taking before beginning treatment with Celebrex. Also, talk to your doctor about your complete medical history, especially if you have any of the following: allergies to medications, heart problems, history of asthma, high blood pressure, kidney or liver disease, or stomach problems, or are pregnant, plan to become pregnant, or are breastfeeding.

What is the usual dosage?

Please see general statement regarding dosage on page xii.

Osteoarthritis and Ankylosing Spondylitis

Adults: The recommended dose is 200 milligrams (mg) once a day or 100 mg twice a day.

Rheumatoid Arthritis

Adults: The recommended dose is 100-200 mg twice a day.

Sudden and Menstrual Pain

Adults: The recommended starting dose is 400 mg at once, followed by 200 mg if needed on the first day. On the following days, the recommended dose is 200 mg twice a day as needed.

Juvenile Rheumatoid Arthritis

Children ≥2 years: Your doctor will prescribe the appropriate dose for your child, based on their weight.

If you have liver impairment, your doctor will adjust your dose appropriately.

How should I take this medication?

- Take Celebrex exactly as prescribed by your doctor.
- If you or your child have difficulty swallowing the capsule, empty the entire contents of the capsule onto a teaspoon of applesauce. Swallow the medicine and applesauce mixture right away with water.

What should I avoid while taking this medication?
Do not take aspirin or other NSAIDs in combination with Celebrex.

What are possible food and drug interactions associated with this medication?
If Celebrex is taken with certain other drugs, the effects of either could be increased, decreased, or altered. It is especially important to check with your doctor before combining Celebrex with the following: alcohol, ACE inhibitors, ARBs, aspirin, blood thinners (such as warfarin), diuretics, fluconazole, lithium, methotrexate, or steroids.

What are the possible side effects of this medication?
Please see general statement regarding side effects on page xiii.

> **Side effects may include:** constipation, diarrhea, dizziness, gas, heartburn, nausea, stomach pain, vomiting

Can I receive this medication if I am pregnant or breastfeeding?
Do not take Celebrex if you are in the late stage of your pregnancy (≥30 weeks). The effects of Celebrex during early pregnancy are unknown. Tell your doctor immediately if you are pregnant, plan to become pregnant, or are breastfeeding.

What should I do if I miss a dose of this medication?
If you miss a dose of Celebrex, take it as soon as you remember. However, if it is almost time for your next dose, skip the one you missed and return to your regular dosing schedule. Do not take two doses at once.

How should I store this medication?
Store at room temperature.

Celecoxib: *see Celebrex, page 199*

Celexa

Generic name: Citalopram HBr

What is this medication?

Celexa is an antidepressant medicine known as a selective serotonin reuptake inhibitor (SSRI). It is used to treat depression.
Celexa is available in tablets and an oral suspension.

What is the most important information I should know about this medication?

- Celexa can increase the risk of suicidal thoughts and behavior in
  children, adolescents, and young adults. Your doctor will monitor you closely for clinical worsening, suicidal or unusual behavior after you start taking Celexa or start a new dose of Celexa.
  Tell your doctor right away if you experience anxiety, hostility,
  sleeplessness, restlessness, impulsive or dangerous behavior,
  or thoughts about suicide or dying; or if you have new symptoms or seem to be feeling worse.

- Celexa can cause QT prolongation (very fast or abnormal heartbeats) or arrhythmia (life-threatening irregular heartbeat). Call
  your doctor right away if you experience chest pain, fast or slow
  heartbeat, shortness of breath, dizziness, or fainting.

- Celexa can cause serotonin syndrome (a potentially life-threatening drug reaction that causes the body to have too much serotonin, a chemical produced by the nerve cells) or neuroleptic
  malignant syndrome (a brain disorder) when you take it alone or
  in combination with other medicines. You can experience mental
  status changes, an increase in your heart rate and temperature,
  lack of coordination, overactive reflexes, muscle rigidity, nausea, vomiting, or diarrhea. Tell your doctor right away if you
  experience any of these signs or symptoms.

- Celexa can cause severe allergic reactions. Tell your doctor right
  away if you develop a rash, trouble breathing, or swelling of your
  face, tongue, eyes, or mouth.

- Your risk of abnormal bleeding or bruising can increase if you
  take Celexa, especially if you also take blood thinners (such as
  warfarin), nonsteroidal anti-inflammatory drugs (NSAIDs) (such
  as ibuprofen or naproxen), or aspirin.

- You can experience manic episodes while you are taking Celexa. Tell your doctor if you experience greatly increased energy, severe trouble sleeping, racing thoughts, reckless behavior, unusually grand ideas, excessive happiness or irritability, or talking more or faster than usual.
- Celexa can cause seizures or changes in your appetite or weight. Your doctor will monitor you for these effects during treatment.
- Celexa can decrease your blood sodium levels, especially if you are elderly. Tell your doctor if you have a headache, weakness, an unsteady feeling, confusion, problems concentrating or thinking, or memory problems while you are taking Celexa.
- Do not stop taking Celexa without first talking to your doctor. Stopping Celexa suddenly can cause serious symptoms, including anxiety, irritability, changes in your mood, feeling restless, changes in your sleep habits, headache, sweating, nausea, dizziness, electric shock-like sensations, shaking, or confusion.

Who should not take this medication?
Do not take Celexa if you are allergic to it or any of its ingredients.

Do not take Celexa while you are taking other medicines known as monoamine oxidase inhibitors (MAOIs) (such as phenelzine), a class of medications used to treat depression and other conditions. Do not take Celexa if you are taking pimozide.

Do not take Celexa if you are taking a medication called Lexapro, since both medicines contain the same active ingredient.

What should I tell my doctor before I take the first dose of this medication?
Tell your doctor about all prescription, over-the-counter, and herbal medications you are taking before beginning treatment with Celexa. Also, talk to your doctor about your complete medical history, especially if you have high blood pressure; heart, liver, or kidney problems; history of stroke; bleeding problems; seizures; mania or bipolar disorder; or low sodium levels in your blood. Also, tell your doctor if you are pregnant, plan to become pregnant, or are breastfeeding.

What is the usual dosage?
Please see general statement regarding dosage on page xii.

Adults: The usual starting dose is 20 milligrams (mg) once a day. Your doctor will increase your dose as needed until the desired effect is achieved.

If you are older than 60 years or have liver impairment, your doctor will adjust your dose appropriately.

How should I take this medication?
• Take Celexa exactly as prescribed by your doctor. Take Celexa once a day, in the morning or in the evening.
• Take Celexa with or without food.

What should I avoid while taking this medication?
Do not drive, operate heavy machinery, or engage in other dangerous activities until you know how Celexa affects you.

Do not drink alcohol while you are taking Celexa.

Do not stop taking Celexa suddenly without first talking to your doctor, as this can cause serious side effects.

Do not take Celexa and MAOIs together or within 14 days of each other. Combining these medicines with Celexa can cause serious and even life-threatening reactions.

What are possible food and drug interactions associated with this medication?
If Celexa is taken with certain other drugs, the effects of either could be increased, decreased, or altered. Celexa may interact with numerous medications. Therefore, it is very important that you tell your doctor about any other medications you are taking.

What are the possible side effects of this medication?
Please see general statement regarding side effects on page xiii.

> **Side effects may include:** constipation, diarrhea, dizziness, dry mouth, feeling anxious, loss of appetite, nausea, respiratory infections, sexual problems, shaking, sleepiness, sweating, trouble sleeping, weakness, yawning

Can I receive this medication if I am pregnant or breastfeeding?

The effects of Celexa during pregnancy are unknown. Celexa can be found in your breast milk if you take it while breastfeeding. Tell your doctor immediately if you are pregnant, plan to become pregnant, or are breastfeeding.

What should I do if I miss a dose of this medication?

If you miss a dose of Celexa, take it as soon as you remember. However, if it is almost time for your next dose, skip the one you missed and return to your regular dosing schedule. Do not take two doses at once.

How should I store this medication?

Store at room temperature.

Cephalexin

Generic name: Cephalexin

What is this medication?

Cephalexin is an antibiotic used to treat bacterial infections of the respiratory (lung) tract, ear, skin, bone, and genital and urinary tract. Cephalexin capsules can be found as brand name Keflex. Cephalexin is also available as tablets and a suspension.

What is the most important information I should know about this medication?

- Cephalexin only works against bacteria; it does not work against viruses like the common cold.
- Do not take cephalexin if you are allergic to it, any of its ingredients, or similar antibiotics (such as cefazolin, cefaclor, or cefotetan). Tell your doctor right away if you take cephalexin and

feel signs of an allergic reaction (such as a rash, swelling, or difficulty breathing).

- Diarrhea is a common problem caused by antibiotics, and usually ends when the antibiotic is stopped. Sometimes after starting treatment with antibiotics, people may develop watery and bloody stools (with or without stomach cramps and fever) even as late as two or more months after having taken the last dose of the antibiotic. Contact your doctor immediately if this occurs.

- Not taking the complete dose of cephalexin may decrease the effectiveness of the treatment and may increase the possibility that bacteria will develop resistance and will not be treatable by cephalexin or other antibiotics in the future.

Who should not take this medication?

Do not take cephalexin if you are allergic to it, any of its ingredients, or similar antibiotics.

Do not take cephalexin to treat viral infections, such as the common cold.

What should I tell my doctor before I take the first dose of this medication?

Tell your doctor about all prescription, over-the-counter, and herbal medications you are taking before beginning treatment with cephalexin. Also, talk to your doctor about your complete medical history, especially if you have allergies, liver or kidney disease, diarrhea, or stomach problems.

What is the usual dosage?

Please see general statement regarding dosage on page xii.

Adults: The usual dose is 250 milligrams (mg) every 6 hours. Your doctor may prescribe a different dose based on the type and severity of your infection.

Children: Your doctor will prescribe the appropriate dose for your child, based on their weight.

How should I take this medication?

- Take cephalexin exactly as prescribed by your doctor.
- Shake the cephalexin suspension well before you or your child take the medicine.

What should I avoid while taking this medication?

Do not miss your scheduled follow-up appointments with your doctor.

What are possible food and drug interactions associated with this medication?

If cephalexin is taken with certain other drugs, the effects of either could be increased, decreased, or altered. It is especially important to check with your doctor before combining cephalexin with metformin or probenecid.

What are the possible side effects of this medication?

Please see general statement regarding side effects on page xiii.

Side effects may include: allergic reactions, diarrhea, fever, indigestion, inflammation of the stomach lining, rash, stomach pain

---

Can I receive this medication if I am pregnant or breastfeeding?

The effects of cephalexin during pregnancy are unknown. Cephalexin can be found in your breast milk if you take it while breastfeeding. Tell your doctor immediately if you are pregnant, plan to become pregnant, or are breastfeeding.

What should I do if I miss a dose of this medication?

If you miss a dose of cephalexin, take it as soon as you remember. However, if it is almost time for your next dose, skip the one you missed and return to your regular dosing schedule. Do not take two doses at once.

How should I store this medication?

Store cephalexin capsules and tablets at room temperature.

Store cephalexin suspension in the refrigerator for up to 14 days.

Cephalexin: *see Cephalexin, page 206*

Certolizumab Pegol: *see Cimzia, page 218*

Chantix
Generic name: Varenicline

What is this medication?
Chantix is a medicine used to help people stop smoking.

What is the most important information I should know about this medication?
- Your body may undergo changes if you stop smoking (with or without Chantix). If you experience changes in behavior, hostility, agitation, depressed mood, and suicidal thoughts, stop taking Chantix and tell your doctor right away.
- You can have an allergic reaction or serious skin reactions while taking Chantix. Tell your doctor right away if you develop swelling of your face, mouth, or throat; trouble breathing; or rash, redness, or peeling of your skin.

Who should not take this medication?
Do not take Chantix if you are allergic to it or any of its ingredients.

What should I tell my doctor before I take the first dose of this medication?
Tell your doctor about all prescription, over-the-counter, and herbal medications you are taking before beginning treatment with Chantix. Also, talk to your doctor about your complete medical history, especially if you have ever had depression or other mental problems; have kidney, heart, or blood vessel problems; are taking insulin, theophylline, or warfarin; or are pregnant, plan to become pregnant, or are breastfeeding.

What is the usual dosage?
Please see general statement regarding dosage on page xii.

Day 1 to Day 3
Adults: The recommended dose is one white tablet (0.5 milligrams [mg]) once a day.

Day 4 to Day 7
Adults: The recommended dose is two white tablets, one in the morning and one in the evening.

Day 8 to the End of Treatment
Adults: The recommended dose is two blue tablets (1 mg each), one in the morning and one in the evening.

How should I take this medication?
- Take Chantix exactly as prescribed by your doctor. Take Chantix after eating and with a full glass of water.
- Choose a date when you will stop smoking. Start taking Chantix 7 days before your quit date, as this lets Chantix build up in your body. You can keep smoking during this time. Be sure to stop smoking on your quit date, and continue to take Chantix as directed.
- You can also start taking Chantix before you choose a quit date. You can pick a quit date between days 8 to 32 of treatment.

What should I avoid while taking this medication?
Do not smoke after your quit date while taking Chantix. If you slip-up and smoke, try again.

Do not drive or operate machinery until you know how Chantix affects you. Chantix can cause you to feel sleepy, dizzy, or have trouble concentrating.

What are possible food and drug interactions associated with this medication?
If Chantix is taken with certain other drugs, the effects of either could be increased, decreased, or altered. It is especially important to check with your doctor before combining Chantix with the following: insulin, other medications for smoking cessation (such as bupropion or nicotine replacement therapy), theophylline, or warfarin.

What are the possible side effects of this medication?
Please see general statement regarding side effects on page xiii.

> **Side effects may include:** abnormal dreams, back or neck pain, chest discomfort, constipation, gas, jaw pain, lightheadedness, nausea, pain or discomfort in one or both arms, shortness of breath, stomach pain, sweating, trouble sleeping, vomiting

Can I receive this medication if I am pregnant or breastfeeding?
The effects of Chantix during pregnancy and breastfeeding are unknown. Do not take Chantix during breastfeeding. Tell your doctor immediately if you are pregnant, plan to become pregnant, or are breastfeeding.

What should I do if I miss a dose of this medication?
If you miss a dose of Chantix , take it as soon as you remember. However, if it is almost time for your next dose, skip the one you missed and return to your regular dosing schedule. Do not take two doses at once.

How should I store this medication?
Store at room temperature.

Chlorhexidine Gluconate: *see Peridex, page 781*

Chlorpheniramine Polistirex/Hydrocodone Polistirex: *see Tussionex, page 1029*

Chlorthalidone: *see Thalitone, page 986*

Cialis
Generic name: Tadalafil

What is this medication?
Cialis is a medicine used to treat erectile dysfunction in men. It can help men get and keep an erection when they become sexually excited. Cialis is also used to treat the signs and symptoms of benign prostatic hyperplasia (enlargement of the prostate gland, which may in turn block the flow of urine).

What is the most important information I should know about this medication?
- Cialis can help you get an erection only when you are sexually excited. You will not get an erection just by taking this medicine.
- Cialis does not cure erectile dysfunction. It is a treatment for erectile dysfunction.
- Cialis does not protect you or your partner from getting any sexually transmitted diseases.
- Sexual activity can put a strain on your heart, especially if it is already weak from a heart disease. Refrain from further activity and talk to your doctor if you experience chest pain, dizziness, or nausea during sex.
- Cialis can cause a sudden decrease or loss of vision or hearing. Loss of vision can occur in one or both eyes. Loss of hearing can occur with ringing in your ears and dizziness. If you experience these symptoms, stop taking Cialis and call your doctor right away.
- Cialis can cause an erection that lasts many hours. Call your doctor immediately if you ever have an erection that lasts more than 4 hours. If this is not treated right away, permanent damage to your penis can occur.
- Cialis contains the same medicine found in another medicine called Adcirca. Do not use these medicines together.

Who should not take this medication?
Do not take Cialis if you are allergic to it or any of its ingredients.

Do not take Cialis if you take any medicines that contain nitrates (such as nitroglycerin, isosorbide mononitrate, or isosorbide dinitrate). If you take Cialis with these medicines, your blood pressure could suddenly drop to an unsafe or life-threatening level.

Do not take Cialis if your doctor told you not to engage in sexual activity due to a heart disease or other heart problems.

What should I tell my doctor before I take the first dose of this medication?

Tell your doctor about all prescription, over-the-counter, and herbal medications you are taking before beginning treatment with Cialis. Also, talk to your doctor about your complete medical history, especially if you have or ever had any heart problems (such as chest pain, heart failure, irregular heartbeats, or heart attack); stroke; low or high blood pressure; bleeding problems; severe vision loss or retinitis pigmentosa (eye disease that involves damage to the layer of tissue in the back of the eye, called the retina); kidney, liver, or blood problems (such as sickle cell anemia or leukemia); any deformation of your penis; an erection that lasted more than 4 hours; or stomach ulcers.

What is the usual dosage?

Please see general statement regarding dosage on page xii.

Erectile Dysfunction
Adults: There are two ways to take Cialis for erectile dysfunction: either for use as needed or once a day. Your doctor will prescribe the appropriate dose for you.

Benign Prostatic Hyperplasia
Adults: The recommended dose is 5 milligrams once a day.

If you have liver or kidney impairment, your doctor will adjust your dose appropriately.

How should I take this medication?
- Take Cialis exactly as prescribed by your doctor. Take it with or without food.
- Do not split Cialis tablets.
- Do not take Cialis more than once a day.

What should I avoid while taking this medication?

Do not change your dose or the way you take Cialis without talking to your doctor.

Do not use other medicines or treatments for erectile dysfunction while you are taking Cialis.

Do not drink excessive amounts of alcohol while you are taking Cialis.

What are possible food and drug interactions associated with this medication?

If Cialis is taken with certain other drugs, the effects of either could be increased, decreased, or altered. It is especially important to check with your doctor before combining Cialis with the following: alcohol, antacids, anti-HIV medications called protease inhibitors (such as ritonavir or saquinavir), erythromycin, grapefruit juice, itraconazole, ketoconazole, medications called alpha-blockers (such as doxazosin or tamsulosin) used to treat high blood pressure or prostate problems, nitrates, other medicines to treat high blood pressure (such as amlodipine, bendrofluazide, enalapril, losartan, or metoprolol), or rifampin.

What are the possible side effects of this medication?

Please see general statement regarding side effects on page xiii.

> **Side effects may include:** back pain, flushing of your face, headache, muscle aches, stuffy or runny nose, upset stomach

Can I receive this medication if I am pregnant or breastfeeding?

Cialis is not for use in women.

What should I do if I miss a dose of this medication?

If you are taking Cialis as needed, it is not for regular use. Take it only before sexual activity.

If you are taking Cialis once a day and miss a dose, take it as soon as you remember. However, if it is almost time for your next dose, skip the one you missed and return to your regular dosing schedule. Do not take two doses at once.

How should I store this medication?
Store at room temperature.

Cilostazol: see Pletal, page 798

Ciloxan
Generic name: Ciprofloxacin HCl

What is this medication?
Ciloxan is an antibiotic known as a quinolone that is available as eye drops and an eye ointment. Ciloxan eye drops and ointment are used to treat conjunctivitis ("pink eye"). Ciloxan eye drops are also used to treat ulcers of the cornea (clear tissue over the pupil of your eye).

What is the most important information I should know about this medication?
- Ciloxan is for use only in your eyes.
- Ciloxan can cause a serious allergic reaction. Stop using Ciloxan and call your doctor right away if you develop difficulty breathing, hives, itching, rash, or swelling of your face, tongue, or throat.
- If you use Ciloxan for a long period of time, it can cause infections, including fungal infections.

Who should not take this medication?
Do not use Ciloxan if you are allergic to it, any of its ingredients, or other quinolone antibiotics (such as levofloxacin or moxifloxacin).

What should I tell my doctor before I take the first dose of this medication?

Tell your doctor about all prescription, over-the-counter, and herbal medications you are taking before beginning treatment with Ciloxan. Also, talk to your doctor about your complete medical history, especially if you are allergic to quinolone antibiotics, or are pregnant, plan to become pregnant, or are breastfeeding.

What is the usual dosage?

Please see general statement regarding dosage on page xii.

Pink Eye

Ciloxan Eye Drops

Adults and children ≥1 year: Apply 1 or 2 drops into the lower eyelid(s) every 2 hours while awake for 2 days, then apply 1 or 2 drops every 4 hours while awake for the next 5 days.

Ciloxan Ointment

Adults and children ≥2 years: Apply a 1/2 inch ribbon into the lower eyelid(s) three times a day for the first 2 days, then apply a 1/2 inch ribbon twice a day for the next 5 days.

Corneal Ulcers

Ciloxan Eye Drops

Adults and children ≥1 year: Your doctor will prescribe the appropriate dose for you.

How should I take this medication?

- Apply Ciloxan exactly as prescribed by your doctor.
- If you are using Ciloxan eye drops, remove your contact lenses before applying the drops.
- Please review the instructions that came with your prescription on how to properly use your eye drops.

What should I avoid while taking this medication?

Do not touch the applicator tip to your eyes, fingers, or any other surface as this can contaminate Ciloxan.

Do not wear contact lenses if you experience signs and symptoms of pink eye while you are using Ciloxan ointment.

What are possible food and drug interactions associated with this medication?

If Ciloxan is used with certain other drugs, the effects of either could be increased, decreased, or altered. It is especially important to check with your doctor before combining Ciloxan with the following: caffeine, cyclosporine, theophylline, or warfarin.

What are the possible side effects of this medication?

Please see general statement regarding side effects on page xiii.

Side effects may include: change in taste, crusting around your eye, eye burning or discomfort, feeling like something is in your eye, formation of crystals on the surface of your eye (with eye drops only), itching, red eye

---

Can I receive this medication if I am pregnant or breastfeeding?

The effects of Ciloxan during pregnancy and breastfeeding are unknown. Tell your doctor immediately if you are pregnant, plan to become pregnant, or are breastfeeding.

What should I do if I miss a dose of this medication?

If you miss a dose of Ciloxan, apply it as soon as you remember. However, if it is almost time for your next dose, skip the one you missed and return to your regular dosing schedule. Do not apply two doses at once.

How should I store this medication?

Store at room temperature or in the refrigerator.

Protect Ciloxan eye drops from light.

Cimzia

Generic name: Certolizumab Pegol

What is this medication?

Cimzia is a medicine called a Tumor Necrosis Factor (TNF) blocker. Cimzia is a medicine used in adults to lessen the signs and symptoms of moderately to severely active Crohn's disease after usual treatments did not help. It is also used to treat moderately to severely active rheumatoid arthritis.

What is the most important information I should know about this medication?

- Cimzia is a medicine that affects your immune system. Cimzia can lower the ability of the immune system to fight infections. Serious infections have happened in patients taking Cimzia. These infections include tuberculosis (TB) and infections caused by viruses, fungi or bacteria that have spread throughout the body. Some patients have died from these infections.
- Your doctor will test you for TB before starting Cimzia and monitor you closely for signs and symptoms of TB during treatment with Cimzia.
- Cimzia can worsen or cause congestive heart failure (a condition in which the heart cannot pump enough blood throughout the body). Symptoms include shortness of breath, swelling of your ankles or feet, or sudden weight gain. Call your doctor immediately if these symptoms develop.
- Cimzia can cause allergic reactions. Signs include a skin rash, trouble breathing, or swelling of the face, tongue, lips, or throat. Call your doctor immediately if these symptoms develop.
- Cimzia can cause serious nervous system problems, such as multiple sclerosis, seizures, or inflammation of the nerves of the eyes. Symptoms include dizziness, numbness or tingling, problems with your vision, and weakness in your arms or legs. Call your doctor if any of these symptoms develop.
- Cimzia can increase the risk of developing lymphoma (a type of cancer involving cells of the immune system called lymphocytes) or other types of cancer. Contact your doctor immediately if you develop unusual lumps or swelling in your neck, armpit, or

groin, night sweats, recurring fever, unusual tiredness or weakness, persistent unexplained itching, or unexplained weight loss.

Who should not take this medication?

Do not take Cimzia if you are allergic to it or any of its ingredients.

What should I tell my doctor before I take the first dose of this medication?

Tell your doctor about all prescription, over-the-counter, and herbal medications you are taking before beginning treatment with Cimzia. Also, talk to your doctor about your complete medical history, especially if you have diabetes, seizures, heart failure, bleeding problems, HIV, or numbness, tingling, or a disease that affects your nervous system (such as multiple sclerosis); have ever had hepatitis B or cancer; or if you are scheduled to have a vaccination. Tell your doctor if you have an infection, signs of an infection (such as fever, cough, or "flu-like" symptoms) or any open cuts or sores on your body, or ever lived in certain parts of the country (such as the Ohio and Mississippi River valleys) where there is an increased risk for getting certain kinds of fungal infections. Also, tell your doctor if you have TB; were born in, lived in, or traveled to countries where there is more risk for getting TB (ask your doctor if you are not sure); or if you have been in close contact with someone who has had it.

What is the usual dosage?

Please see general statement regarding dosage on page xii.

Crohn's Disease

Adults: The dose is 400 milligrams (mg) given as two injections initially. This same dose is then given again at weeks 2 and 4. The maintenance dose is 400 mg given every 4 weeks.

Rheumatoid Arthritis

Adults: The dose is 400 mg given as two injections initially. This same dose is then given at weeks 2 and 4, followed by 200 mg every other week. The maintenance dose is 400 mg every 4 weeks.

How should I take this medication?

- Your doctor will inject Cimzia in your stomach area or upper thigh. If you would like to self-administer or have a caregiver administer your injection, ask your doctor to explain the proper injection and discarding technique.

What should I avoid while taking this medication?

Do not miss doses or appointments with your doctor. Also avoid contact with people who have contagious infections.

What are possible food and drug interactions associated with this medication?

If Cimzia is taken with certain other drugs, the effects of either could be increased, decreased, or altered. It is especially important to check with your doctor before combining Cimzia with the following: abatacept, adalimumab, anakinra, etanercept, golimumab, infliximab, methotrexate, natalizumab, rituximab, or vaccines.

What are the possible side effects of this medication?

Please see general statement regarding side effects on page xiii.

> **Side effects may include:** back pain, fever, headache, high blood pressure, joint pain, rash, tiredness, upper respiratory infection (such as the flu, a cold), urinary tract infection (bladder infection)

Can I receive this medication if I am pregnant or breastfeeding?

The effects of Cimzia during pregnancy and breastfeeding are unknown. Tell your doctor immediately if you are pregnant, plan to become pregnant, or are breastfeeding.

What should I do if I miss a dose of this medication?

If you forget to take Cimzia, inject a dose as soon as you remember. Then, take your next dose at your regularly scheduled time.

How should I store this medication?

Store in the refrigerator. Do not freeze. Keep in the original carton to protect from light.

Cipro

Generic name: Ciprofloxacin

What is this medication?

Cipro is an antibiotic used to treat certain bacterial infections of the urinary tract, lower respiratory (lung) tract, skin, bone, joint, sinuses, and prostate. Cipro may also be used to treat other bacterial infections and conditions, as determined by your doctor. Cipro is available as tablets and an oral suspension.

What is the most important information I should know about this medication?

- Cipro can cause tendon rupture or swelling. Your risk can increase if you are over 60 years; are taking steroids; have had a kidney, heart, or lung transplant; engage in physical activity or exercise; have kidney failure; or have past tendon problems (such as rheumatoid arthritis). Tell your doctor immediately if you experience pain, swelling, tears, or inflammation of tendons in the back of your ankle, shoulder, hand, or other tendon sites. Also, tell your doctor immediately if you hear or feel a snap or pop in a tendon area, bruise right after an injury in a tendon area, or are unable to move the affected area or bear weight.

- Cipro can cause worsening of myasthenia gravis (a disease characterized by long-lasting fatigue and muscle weakness). Tell your doctor immediately if you develop muscle weakness or trouble breathing.

- Cipro can cause seizures and breathing problems if you take it in combination with a medicine called theophylline. Tell your doctor if you are taking theophylline before beginning treatment with Cipro.

- Cipro can cause central nervous system (CNS) effects. Tell your doctor right away if you experience dizziness, seizures, hallucinations, restlessness, shaking, anxiousness or nervousness, confusion, depression, trouble sleeping, nightmares, suspiciousness, or suicidal thoughts or actions.

- Cipro can cause serious allergic reactions that may be life-threatening. Stop taking Cipro and tell your doctor right away if you experience hives, trouble breathing or swallowing, throat tightness, hoarseness, rapid heartbeat, fainting, skin rash, yellowing of your skin or whites of your eyes, or swelling of your lips, tongue, or face.

- Diarrhea is a common problem when taking antibiotics; it usually ends when the antibiotic is stopped. Sometimes after starting treatment with antibiotics, people may develop watery and bloody stools (with or without stomach cramps and fever) even as late as two or more months after having taken the last dose of the antibiotic. Contact your doctor right away if this occurs.
- Cipro can cause damage to the nerves in your arms, hands, legs, or feet. Tell your doctor right away if you develop pain, burning, tingling, numbness, or weakness in any of these areas of your body.
- Cipro can cause low blood sugar if you take it in combination with a diabetes medicine called glyburide. If you have diabetes, check your blood sugar regularly and tell your doctor if you have low blood sugar while you are taking Cipro.
- Take Cipro as prescribed by your doctor for the full course of treatment, even if your symptoms improve earlier. Do not skip doses. Skipping doses or not completing the full course of Cipro can decrease its effectiveness and can lead to the growth of bacteria that are resistant to the effects of Cipro.

Who should not take this medication?
Do not take Cipro if you are allergic to it or any of its ingredients or similar antibiotics.

Do not take Cipro if you are taking a medicine called tizanidine.

Do not take Cipro to treat viral infections, such as the common cold.

What should I tell my doctor before I take the first dose of this medication?
Tell your doctor about all prescription, over-the-counter, and herbal medications you are taking before beginning treatment with Cipro. Also, talk to your doctor about your complete medical history, especially if you have tendon, nerve, or kidney problems; myasthenia gravis; CNS problems (such as seizures); rheumatoid arthritis or a

history of joint problems; or if you or anyone in your family has an irregular heartbeat, especially a condition called QT prolongation.

What is the usual dosage?
Please see general statement regarding dosage on page xii.

<u>Bone, Joint, Lower Respiratory Tract, Prostate, Sinus, and Skin Infections</u>
Adults: The recommended dose for mild or moderate infection is 500 milligrams (mg) every 12 hours. Your doctor will determine the duration of treatment based on the type and severity of your infection. Your doctor may give you a higher dose for more severe or complicated infections.

<u>Urinary Tract Infection</u>
Adults: The recommended dose for mild or moderate infection is 250 mg every 12 hours. For severe or complicated infection, the recommended dose is 500 mg every 12 hours. Your doctor will determine the duration of treatment based on the severity of your infection.

Children 1-17 years: Your doctor will prescribe the appropriate dose for your child, based on their weight.

If you have kidney impairment, your doctor will adjust your dose appropriately.

How should I take this medication?
- Take Cipro exactly as prescribed by your doctor. Take Cipro in the morning and in the evening, at about the same time each day. Take it with or without food.
- Swallow Cipro tablets whole. Do not split, crush, or chew them.
- Shake the Cipro oral suspension bottle well for about 15 seconds before you take the medicine. Always use the measuring spoon provided to get the exact dose of medicine. Close the bottle completely after you take the medicine.
- Do not take Cipro with dairy products (such as milk or yogurt) or calcium-fortified juices alone, but it may be taken with a meal that contains these products.

- Drink plenty of fluids while you are taking Cipro.
- Take Cipro two hours before or six hours after taking antacids containing magnesium or aluminum, sevelamer, lanthanum carbonate, sucralfate, didanosine, chewable/buffered tablets or pediatric powder, or other products that contain calcium, iron, or zinc.

What should I avoid while taking this medication?

Do not drive, operate machinery, or engage in other activities that require mental alertness or coordination until you know how Cipro affects you.

Do not expose yourself to sunlamps or tanning beds, and try to limit your time in the sun, as Cipro can increase your sensitivity to light. If you need to be outdoors, wear loose-fitting clothes that protect your skin for the sun.

Do not skip any doses, or stop taking Cipro even if you begin to feel better, until you finish your prescribed treatment.

What are possible food and drug interactions associated with this medication?

If Cipro is taken with certain other drugs, the effects of either could be increased, decreased, or altered. Cipro may interact with numerous medications. Therefore, it is very important that you tell your doctor about any other medications you are taking.

What are the possible side effects of this medication?

Please see general statement regarding side effects on page xiii.

> **Side effects may include:** abdominal pain or discomfort, changes in your liver function tests, diarrhea, headache, nausea, rash, vaginal yeast infection, vomiting

Can I receive this medication if I am pregnant or breastfeeding?

The effects of Cipro during pregnancy are unknown. Cipro can be found in breast milk if taken while breastfeeding. Do not breastfeed while you are taking Cipro. Tell your doctor immediately if you are pregnant, plan to become pregnant, or are breastfeeding.

What should I do if I miss a dose of this medication?

If you miss a dose of Cipro, take it as soon as you remember. However, if it is almost time for your next dose, skip the one you missed and return to your regular dosing schedule. Do not take two doses at once.

How should I store this medication?

Store at room temperature.

Ciprodex

Generic name: Ciprofloxacin HCl/Dexamethasone

What is this medication?

Ciprodex is an antibiotic known as a quinolone and is available as ear drops. Ciprodex is used to treat bacterial infections in your ears.

What is the most important information I should know about this medication?

- Ciprodex suspension is for use in your ears only.
- Ciprodex can cause an allergic reaction that may result in death if not immediately treated. Stop using Ciprodex and tell your doctor right away if you develop a skin rash or any other signs of an allergic reaction.
- If you use Ciprodex for a long period of time, it can lead to other infections, including fungal infections, which might not respond to this medication. Tell your doctor if your infection does not improve after one week of therapy.

Who should not take this medication?

Do not use Ciprodex if you are allergic to it or any of its ingredients.

Do not use Ciprodex if you are allergic to other quinolone antibiotics (such as levofloxacin or moxifloxacin).

Do not use Ciprodex if you have viral infections of your outer ear (such as varicella or herpes simplex infections).

What should I tell my doctor before I take the first dose of this medication?

Tell your doctor about all prescription, over-the-counter, and herbal medications you are taking before beginning treatment with Ciprodex. Also, talk to your doctor about your complete medical history, especially if you are allergic to quinolone antibiotics or have viral infections of your outer ear.

What is the usual dosage?

Please see general statement regarding dosage on page xii.

Adults and children ≥6 months: Apply 4 drops into the affected ear(s) twice a day for 7 days.

How should I take this medication?

- Apply Ciprodex exactly as prescribed by your doctor.
- Shake the suspension well immediately before you use it. Warm the suspension by holding the container in your hands for 1-2 minutes to minimize the dizziness that can result from the application of a cold solution into your ear. Lie with your affected ear upward and then apply the drops into your ear. You should maintain this position for 60 seconds. Repeat, if necessary, for your opposite ear. Discard unused portion after therapy is completed.

What should I avoid while taking this medication?

Do not get your affected ears(s) wet when bathing. Do not swim unless your doctor has told you otherwise.

Do not use Ciprodex in your eyes.

Do not touch the applicator tip with material from your ear, fingers, or other sources, as this can contaminate Ciprodex.

What are possible food and drug interactions associated with this medication?

No significant interactions have been reported with Ciprodex at this time. However, always tell your doctor about any medicines you take, including over-the-counter medications, vitamins, and herbal supplements.

What are the possible side effects of this medication?

Please see general statement regarding side effects on page xiii.

> **Side effects may include:** abnormal taste, dizziness if drops are applied cold, ear congestion, ear infection, ear pain, ear residue, irritability

Can I receive this medication if I am pregnant or breastfeeding?

The effects of Ciprodex during pregnancy and breastfeeding are unknown. Ciprodex can be found in your breast milk if you use it while breastfeeding. Tell your doctor immediately if you are pregnant, plan to become pregnant, or are breastfeeding.

What should I do if I miss a dose of this medication?

If you miss a dose of Ciprodex, apply it as soon as you remember. However, if it is almost time for your next dose, skip the one you missed and return to your regular dosing schedule. Do not apply two doses at once.

How should I store this medication?

Store at room temperature. Do not freeze. Protect from light.

Ciprofloxacin: *see Cipro, page 221*

Ciprofloxacin HCl: *see Ciloxan, page 215*

Ciprofloxacin HCl/Dexamethasone: *see Ciprodex, page 225*

Citalopram HBr: *see Celexa, page 203*

Clarinex
Generic name: Desloratadine

What is this medication?
Clarinex is a medicine used to help control the symptoms (such as sneezing, stuffy nose, runny nose, or itching of the nose) of seasonal or year-round allergies. Clarinex is also used to help control the symptoms (such as long-term itching) of chronic hives. Clarinex is available as tablets, an oral solution, and orally disintegrating tablets called Clarinex RediTabs.

What is the most important information I should know about this medication?
- Clarinex can cause serious allergic reactions. Stop taking Clarinex and call your doctor right away if you develop a rash, itching, hives, shortness of breath or trouble breathing, or swelling of your lips, tongue, face, or throat.
- If you have a condition known as phenylketonuria (an inability to process phenylalanine, a protein in your body), be aware that Clarinex RediTabs orally disintegrating tablets contain phenylalanine.

Who should not take this medication?
Do not take Clarinex if you are allergic to it, any of its ingredients, or to loratadine (medicine found in Alavert or Claritin).

What should I tell my doctor before I take the first dose of this medication?
Tell your doctor about all prescription, over-the-counter, and herbal medications you are taking before beginning treatment with Clarinex. Also, talk to your doctor about your complete medical history, especially if you have liver or kidney problems, or if you are pregnant, plan to become pregnant, or are breastfeeding.

What is the usual dosage?
Please see general statement regarding dosage on page xii.

Clarinex Tablets
Adults and children ≥12 years: The recommended dose is one 5-milligram (mg) tablet once a day.

Clarinex RediTabs Tablets
Adults and children ≥12 years: The recommended dose is one 5-mg tablet once a day.

Children 6-11 years: The recommended dose is one 2.5-mg tablet once a day.

Clarinex Oral Solution
Adults and children ≥12 years: The recommended dose is 2 teaspoonfuls (10 milliliters [mL]) once a day.

Children 6-11 years: The recommended dose is 1 teaspoonful (5 mL) once a day.

Children 12 months-5 years: The recommended dose is 1/2 teaspoonful (2.5 mL) once a day.

Children 6-11 months: The recommended dose is 2 mL once a day.

If you have liver or kidney impairment, your doctor will adjust your dose appropriately.

How should I take this medication?
- Take Clarinex exactly as prescribed by your doctor. Take it with or without food.
- To take Clarinex RediTabs, open the blister and remove one tablet. Place the tablet on your tongue right away and allow it to dissolve before swallowing. Take it with or without water.
- Use a measuring dropper or oral syringe to give Clarinex oral solution to your child. Ask your pharmacist for a dropper or syringe if you do not have one.

What should I avoid while taking this medication?
Do not change your dose of Clarinex without first talking to your doctor.

What are possible food and drug interactions associated with this medication?
If Clarinex is taken with certain other drugs, the effects of either could be increased, decreased, or altered. It is especially important to check with your doctor before combining Clarinex with the following: azithromycin, cimetidine, erythromycin, fluoxetine, or ketoconazole.

What are the possible side effects of this medication?
Please see general statement regarding side effects on page xiii.

> **Side effects may include:** dry mouth, menstrual pain, muscle pain, sleepiness, sore throat, tiredness

Can I receive this medication if I am pregnant or breastfeeding?
The effects of Clarinex during pregnancy are unknown. Clarinex can be found in your breast milk if you take it while breastfeeding. Do not breastfeed while you are taking Clarinex. Tell your doctor immediately if you are pregnant, plan to become pregnant, or are breastfeeding.

What should I do if I miss a dose of this medication?
If you miss a dose of Clarinex, take it as soon as you remember. However, if it is almost time for your next dose, skip the one you missed and return to your regular dosing schedule. Do not take two doses at once.

How should I store this medication?
Store at room temperature.

Protect Clarinex oral solution from light.

Clarinex-D 12 Hour

Generic name: Desloratadine/Pseudoephedrine Sulfate

What is this medication?

Clarinex-D 12 Hour is a medicine used to help control the symptoms of seasonal allergic rhinitis (inflammation of the lining of the nose), such as sneezing, stuffy or runny nose, and itching of the nose or eyes.

What is the most important information I should know about this medication?

- Clarinex-D 12 Hour may cause dizziness. This effect may be worse if you take it with alcohol or certain medicines.
- Clarinex-D 12 Hour may interfere with skin allergy tests. If you are scheduled for a skin test, tell your doctor you are taking this medication. You may need to stop taking it for a few days before the tests.

Who should not take this medication?

Do not take Clarinex-D 12 Hour if you are allergic to it or any of its ingredients, or to loratadine. You should not take Clarinex-D 12 Hour if you have narrow-angle glaucoma (high pressure in the eye), urinary problems, severe high blood pressure, or heart disease. Do not take Clarinex-D 12 Hour if you are currently receiving or have received antidepressant medications known as monoamine oxidase inhibitors (MAOIs) within the last 2 weeks. If you are unsure whether your antidepressant medication is an MAOI, ask your doctor or pharmacist.

What should I tell my doctor before I take the first dose of this medication?

Tell your doctor about all prescription, over-the-counter, and herbal medications you are taking before beginning treatment with Clarinex-D 12 Hour. Also, talk to your doctor about your complete medical history, especially if you have a history of high blood pressure, diabetes, glaucoma, seizures, stroke, liver, kidney, prostate, or adrenal gland problems, trouble sleeping, an overactive thyroid, or are currently taking an MAOI (or have taken one within the last 14 days).

What is the usual dosage?
Please see general statement regarding dosage on page xii.

Adults and children ≥12 years: The usual dose is 1 tablet twice a day (every 12 hours).

How should I take this medication?
• You can take Clarinex-D 12 Hour with or without food. Do not crush, split, divide, or chew the tablets. Do not take extra doses or take it more often without asking your doctor.

What should I avoid while taking this medication?
Do not drive or perform other unsafe tasks until you know how Clarinex-D 12 Hour affects you. It may cause dizziness. This effect may be worse if you take it with alcohol or certain medicines.

What are possible food and drug interactions associated with this medication?
If Clarinex-D 12 Hour is taken with certain other drugs, the effects of either could be increased, decreased, or altered. It is especially important to check with your doctor before combining Clarinex-D 12 Hour with the following: azithromycin, digitalis, erythromycin, ketoconazole, MAOIs (such as phenelzine or tranylcypromine), methyldopa, reserpine, or over-the-counter antihistamines and decongestants.

What are the possible side effects of this medication?
Please see general statement regarding side effects on page xiii.

> **Side effects may include:** cough, dizziness, drowsiness, dry mouth, headache, inability to sleep, irregular heart beat, loss of appetite, mild stomach upset, nausea, nervousness, sleepiness, sore throat, tiredness, tremor

Can I receive this medication if I am pregnant or breastfeeding?

The effects of Clarinex-D 12 Hour during pregnancy and breast-feeding are unknown. Tell your doctor immediately if you are pregnant, plan to become pregnant, or are breastfeeding.

What should I do if I miss a dose of this medication?

If you miss a dose of Clarinex-D 12 Hour, take it as soon as you remember. However, if it is almost time for your next dose, skip the one you missed and return to your regular dosing schedule. Do not take two doses at once.

How should I store this medication?

Store at room temperature. Keep dry and away from light.

Clarinex-D 24 Hour

Generic name: Desloratadine/Pseudoephedrine Sulfate

What is this medication?

Clarinex-D 24 Hour is a medicine used to help control the symptoms of seasonal allergic rhinitis (inflammation of the lining of the nose) such as sneezing, stuffy or runny nose, and itching of the nose or eyes.

What is the most important information I should know about this medication?

- Do not drive or perform other unsafe tasks until you know how Clarinex-D 24 Hour affects you. It may cause dizziness. This effect may be worse if you take it with alcohol or certain medicines.
- Clarinex-D 24 Hour may interfere with skin allergy tests. If you are scheduled for a skin test, tell your doctor you are taking this medication. You may need to stop taking it for a few days before the tests.

Who should not take this medication?

Do not take Clarinex-D 24 Hour if you are allergic to it or any of its ingredients, or to loratadine. Do not take Clarinex-D 24 Hour if you have narrow-angle glaucoma (high pressure in the eye), urinary problems, severe high blood pressure, or heart disease. Do not take Clarinex-D 24 Hour if you are currently receiving or have received antidepressant medications known as monoamine oxidase inhibitors (MAOIs) (such as phenelzine or tranylcypromine) within the last 2 weeks.

What should I tell my doctor before I take the first dose of this medication?

Tell your doctor about all prescription, over-the-counter, and herbal medications you are taking before beginning treatment with Clarinex-D 24 Hour. Also, talk to your doctor about your complete medical history, especially if you have a history of high blood pressure, diabetes, glaucoma, seizures, stroke, trouble sleeping, an overactive thyroid, currently taking an MAOI (or have taken one within the last 14 days), or have liver, kidney, prostate, or adrenal gland problems.

What is the usual dosage?

Please see general statement regarding dosage on page xii.

Adults and children ≥ 12 years: The usual dose is 1 tablet once a day (every 24 hours).

How should I take this medication?

• You can take Clarinex-D 24 Hour with or without food. Do not crush, split, divide, or chew the tablets. Do not take extra doses or take it more often without asking your doctor.

What should I avoid while taking this medication?

Do not drive or perform other unsafe tasks until you know how Clarinex-D 24 Hour affects you. It may cause dizziness. This effect may be worse if you take it with alcohol or certain medicines.

What are possible food and drug interactions associated with this medication?

If Clarinex-D 24 Hour is taken with certain other drugs, the effects of either could be increased, decreased, or altered. It is especially important to check with your doctor before combining Clarinex-D

24 Hour with the following: azithromycin, digitalis, erythromycin, ketoconazole, MAOIs, methyldopa, over-the-counter antihistamines and decongestants, or reserpine.

What are the possible side effects of this medication?
Please see general statement regarding side effects on page xiii.

> **Side effects may include:** dizziness, drowsiness, dry mouth, headache, inability to sleep, irregular heart beat, loss of appetite, nausea, nervousness, restlessness, seizures, sleepiness, sore throat, tiredness, tremor

Can I receive this medication if I am pregnant or breastfeeding?
The effects of Clarinex-D 24 Hour during pregnancy and breastfeeding are unknown. Tell your doctor immediately if you are pregnant, plan to become pregnant, or are breastfeeding.

What should I do if I miss a dose of this medication?
If you miss a dose of Clarinex-D 24 Hour, take it as soon as you remember. However, if it is almost time for your next dose, skip the one you missed and return to your regular dosing schedule. Do not take two doses at once.

How should I store this medication?
Store at room temperature. Keep dry and away from light.

Clarithromycin: *see Biaxin, page 148*

Cleocin
Generic name: Clindamycin

What is this medication?
Cleocin is an antibiotic used to treat certain serious bacterial infections of the respiratory (lung) tract, skin, blood, abdomen, pelvis,

or genital tract. It may also be used to treat other bacterial infections, as determined by your doctor. Cleocin is available in capsules or granules for oral solution.

What is the most important information I should know about this medication?

- Cleocin can cause diarrhea or colitis (inflammation of the colon). This can happen a couple of months after receiving the last dose of Cleocin. Tell your doctor immediately if you have diarrhea or colitis.
- Take Cleocin as prescribed by your doctor for the full course of treatment, even if symptoms improve earlier. Do not skip doses. Skipping doses or not completing the full course of Cleocin can decrease its effectiveness, and can lead to growth of bacteria that are resistant to the effects of Cleocin.

Who should not take this medication?

Do not take Cleocin if you are allergic to it, any of its ingredients, or lincomycin.

Do not take Cleocin to treat viral infections, such as the common cold.

What should I tell my doctor before I take the first dose of this medication?

Tell your doctor about all prescription, over-the-counter, and herbal medications you are taking before beginning treatment with Cleocin. Also, talk to your doctor about your complete medical history, especially if you have any allergies, liver or kidney disease, gastrointestinal (stomach and intestines) disease, or colitis.

What is the usual dosage?

Please see general statement regarding dosage on page xii.

Capsules

Adults: The recommended dose for serious infections is 150-300 milligrams (mg) every 6 hours. The recommended dose for more severe infections is 300-450 mg every 6 hours. Your doctor will

prescribe the appropriate dose for you based on the severity of
your infection.

Children: Your doctor will prescribe the appropriate dose for your
child, based on their weight and the severity of their infection.

Granules for Oral Solution
Children: Your doctor will prescribe the appropriate dose for your
child, based on their weight and the severity of their infection.

How should I take this medication?
• Take Cleocin exactly as prescribed by your doctor. Take Cleocin
with a full glass of water to avoid the possibility of esophageal
irritation.

What should I avoid while taking this medication?
Do not skip or miss any scheduled doses.

What are possible food and drug interactions associated
with this medication?
If Cleocin is taken with certain other drugs, the effects of either
could be increased, decreased, or altered. It is especially important to check with your doctor before combining Cleocin with
erythromycin.

What are the possible side effects of this medication?
Please see general statement regarding side effects on page xiii.

Side effects may include: abdominal pain, colitis, diarrhea, inflammation of your skin, itchiness, jaundice (yellowing of the skin
or whites of the eyes), nausea, rash, vomiting

Can I receive this medication if I am pregnant or
breastfeeding?
The effects of Cleocin during pregnancy and breastfeeding are unknown. Cleocin can be found in your breast milk if taken during
breastfeeding. Tell your doctor immediately if you are pregnant,
plan to become pregnant, or are breastfeeding.

What should I do if I miss a dose of this medication?

If you miss a dose of Cleocin, take it as soon as you remember. However, if it is almost time for your next dose, skip the one you missed and return to your regular dosing schedule. Do not take two doses at once.

How should I store this medication?

Store at room temperature. Do not refrigerate the oral solution.

Cleocin T

Generic name: Clindamycin Phosphate

What is this medication?

Cleocin T is a topical medicine (applied directly on the skin) that is used to treat acne. It is available in a solution, lotion, or gel.

What is the most important information I should know about this medication?

- Cleocin T is for external use only. This medication can cause burning and irritation of the eyes. Do not use it in your eyes, broken skin, mouth, nose, or inside your vagina. If contact occurs, rinse your eyes thoroughly with water.
- This medication can cause severe colitis (inflammation of the colon) and diarrhea. If you notice severe diarrhea, stop using this medication and tell your doctor right away.

Who should not take this medication?

Do not use Cleocin T if you are allergic to it, any of its ingredients, or similar medications.

Do not use Cleocin T if you have a history of inflammatory disease of the colon or intestines, or inflammation of the colon with past antibiotic use.

What should I tell my doctor before I take the first dose of this medication?

Tell your doctor about all prescription, over-the-counter, and herbal medications you are taking before beginning treatment with Cleocin T. Also, talk to your doctor about your complete medical history, especially if you have allergies, other skin conditions, or a history of inflammatory disease of the colon or intestines.

What is the usual dosage?

Please see general statement regarding dosage on page xii.

Adults and children ≥12 years: Apply a thin film of the solution, lotion, or gel to the affected area(s) twice a day.

How should I take this medication?

- Apply Cleocin T exactly as prescribed by your doctor.
- Remove the pledget (application pad) from foil just before use of Cleocin T solution. You can use more than 1 pledget. Each pledget should be used only once and then be discarded. Do not use the medication if the seal is broken.
- Shake the lotion well immediately before use.

What should I avoid while taking this medication?

Do not use Cleocin T in your eyes.

Cleocin T has an unpleasant taste. You should be careful when you are applying it around your mouth.

What are possible food and drug interactions associated with this medication?

If Cleocin T is used with certain other drugs, the effects of either could be increased, decreased, or altered. It is important to check with your doctor before combining Cleocin T with any other medication.

What are the possible side effects of this medication?

Please see general statement regarding side effects on page xiii.

Side effects may include: abdominal (stomach) pain, burning, colitis, dryness, itching, oily skin, peeling skin, redness

---

Can I receive this medication if I am pregnant or breastfeeding?

The effects of Cleocin T during pregnancy and breastfeeding are unknown. Tell your doctor immediately if you are pregnant, plan to become pregnant, or are breastfeeding.

What should I do if I miss a dose of this medication?

If you miss a dose of Cleocin T, apply it as soon as you remember. However, if it is almost time for your next dose, skip the one you missed and return to your regular dosing schedule. Do not apply two doses at once.

How should I store this medication?

Store at room temperature. Protect from freezing.

Clindamycin: see Cleocin, page 235

Clindamycin Phosphate: see Cleocin T, page 238

Clobetasol Propionate Cream

Generic name: Clobetasol Propionate

What is this medication?

Clobetasol propionate cream is a topical medicine (applied to the skin surface) that is used for the relief of inflammation and itching of the skin.

What is the most important information I should know about this medication?

- Clobetasol propionate is for external use only. Do not use it in your eyes, face, underarms, vagina, or groin areas.
- Clobetasol propionate can have a greater effect on children because they are more likely to absorb large amounts of the

medicine through the skin. Long-term use can affect the growth and development of children. Talk to your doctor if you think your child is not growing at a normal rate after using this medication for a long period of time.

- Do not use clobetasol propionate for any other condition other than that which your doctor has prescribed.
- Contact your doctor if you notice irritation or any skin reactions in the area being treated or if your condition does not improve within two weeks of treatment.

Who should not take this medication?

Do not use clobetasol propionate if you are allergic to it, any of its ingredients, or to similar products.

What should I tell my doctor before I take the first dose of this medication?

Tell your doctor about all prescription, over-the-counter, and herbal medications you are taking before beginning treatment with clobetasol propionate. Also, talk to your doctor about your complete medical history, especially if you are pregnant, plan to become pregnant, or are breastfeeding.

What is the usual dosage?

Please see general statement regarding dosage on page xii.

Adults and children ≥12 years: Apply a thin film to the affected area(s) twice a day.

Limit the treatment to 2 consecutive weeks, and do not use more than 50 grams (g) a week.

How should I take this medication?

- Apply clobetasol propionate exactly as prescribed by your doctor. Do not apply extra doses or apply more often without asking your doctor.
- Rub the cream into skin gently and completely.

What should I avoid while taking this medication?

Do not use clobetasol propionate in your eyes, face, underarms, or groin areas.

Do not bandage, cover, or wrap the treated skin area as to be occlusive.

What are possible food and drug interactions associated with this medication?

No significant interactions have been reported with clobetasol propionate at this time. However, always tell your doctor about any medicines you take, including over-the-counter medications, vitamins, and herbal supplements.

What are the possible side effects of this medication?

Please see general statement regarding side effects on page xiii.

Side effects may include: acne (pimples), burning, cracking of the skin, dermatitis (inflammation of the skin), infection, irritation, itching, numbness of the fingers, redness, stinging, sweat rash, telangiectasia (widely open blood vessels in the outer layer of the skin)

Can I receive this medication if I am pregnant or breastfeeding?

The effects of clobetasol propionate during pregnancy and breastfeeding are unknown. Tell your doctor immediately if you are pregnant, plan to become pregnant, or are breastfeeding.

What should I do if I miss a dose of this medication?

If you miss a dose of clobetasol propionate, apply it as soon as you remember. However, if it is almost time for your next dose, skip the one you missed and return to your regular dosing schedule. Do not apply two doses at once.

How should I store this medication?

Store at room temperature. Do not refrigerate.

Clobetasol Propionate Gel

Generic name: Clobetasol Propionate

What is this medication?

Clobetasol propionate gel is a topical medicine (applied to the skin surface) that is used for the relief of inflammation and itching of the skin.

What is the most important information I should know about this medication?

- Clobetasol propionate is for external use only. Do not use it in your eyes, face, underarms, vagina, or groin areas.
- Clobetasol propionate can have a greater effect on children because they are more likely to absorb large amounts of the medicine through the skin. Long-term use can affect the growth and development of children. Talk to your doctor if you think your child is not growing at a normal rate after using this medication for a long period of time.
- Do not use clobetasol propionate for any other condition other than that which your doctor has prescribed.
- Contact your doctor if you notice irritation or any skin reactions in the area being treated or if your condition does not improve within two weeks of treatment.

Who should not take this medication?

Do not use clobetasol propionate if you are allergic to it, any of its ingredients, or to similar products.

What should I tell my doctor before I take the first dose of this medication?

Tell your doctor about all prescription, over-the-counter, and herbal medications you are taking before beginning treatment with clobetasol propionate. Also, talk to your doctor about your complete medical history, especially if you are pregnant, plan to become pregnant, or are breastfeeding.

What is the usual dosage?

Please see general statement regarding dosage on page xii.

Adults and children ≥12 years: Apply a thin film to the affected area(s) twice a day.

Limit the treatment to 2 consecutive weeks, and do not use more than 50 grams (g) a week.

How should I take this medication?
- Apply clobetasol propionate exactly as prescribed by your doctor. Do not apply extra doses or apply more often without asking your doctor.
- Rub the gel into skin gently and completely.

What should I avoid while taking this medication?
Do not use clobetasol propionate in your eyes, face, underarms, or groin areas.

Do not bandage, cover, or wrap the treated skin area as to be occlusive

What are possible food and drug interactions associated with this medication?
No significant interactions have been reported with clobetasol propionate at this time. However, always tell your doctor about any medicines you take, including over-the-counter medications, vitamins, and herbal supplements.

What are the possible side effects of this medication?
Please see general statement regarding side effects on page xiii.

Side effects may include: acne (pimples), burning, cracking of the skin, dermatitis (inflammation of the skin), infection, irritation, itching, numbness of the fingers, redness, stinging, sweat rash, telangiectasia (widely open blood vessels in the outer layer of the skin)

Can I receive this medication if I am pregnant or breastfeeding?

The effects of clobetasol propionate during pregnancy and breast-feeding are unknown. Tell your doctor immediately if you are pregnant, plan to become pregnant, or are breastfeeding.

What should I do if I miss a dose of this medication?

If you miss a dose of clobetasol propionate, apply it as soon as you remember. However, if it is almost time for your next dose, skip the one you missed and return to your regular dosing schedule. Do not apply two doses at once.

How should I store this medication?

Store at room temperature. Do not refrigerate.

Clobetasol Propionate Ointment

Generic name: Clobetasol Propionate

What is this medication?

Clobetasol propionate ointment is a topical medicine (applied to the skin surface) that is used for the relief of inflammation and itching of the skin.

What is the most important information I should know about this medication?

- Clobetasol propionate is for external use only. Do not use it in your eyes, face, underarms, vagina, or groin areas.
- Clobetasol propionate can have a greater effect on children because they are more likely to absorb large amounts of the medicine through the skin. Long-term use can affect the growth and development of children. Talk to your doctor if you think your child is not growing at a normal rate after using this medication for a long period of time.
- Do not use clobetasol propionate for any other condition other than that which your doctor has prescribed.

- Contact your doctor if you notice irritation or any skin reactions in the area being treated or if your condition does not improve within 2 weeks of treatment.

Who should not take this medication?

Do not use clobetasol propionate if you are allergic to it, any of its ingredients, or to similar products.

What should I tell my doctor before I take the first dose of this medication?

Tell your doctor about all prescription, over-the-counter, and herbal medications you are taking before beginning treatment with clobetasol propionate. Also, talk to your doctor about your complete medical history, especially if you are pregnant, plan to become pregnant, or are breastfeeding.

What is the usual dosage?

Please see general statement regarding dosage on page xii.

Adults and children ≥12 years: Apply a thin film to the affected area(s) twice a day.

Limit the treatment to 2 consecutive weeks, and do not use more than 50 grams (g) a week.

How should I take this medication?

- Apply clobetasol propionate exactly as prescribed by your doctor. Do not apply extra doses or apply more often without asking your doctor.
- Rub the ointment into your skin gently and completely.

What should I avoid while taking this medication?

Do not use clobetasol propionate in your eyes, face, underarms, vagina, or groin areas.

Do not bandage, cover, or wrap the treated skin area as to be occlusive.

What are possible food and drug interactions associated with this medication?

No significant interactions have been reported with clobetasol propionate at this time. However, always tell your doctor about any medicines you take, including over-the-counter medications, vitamins, and herbal supplements.

What are the possible side effects of this medication?

Please see general statement regarding side effects on page xiii.

Side effects may include: acne (pimples), burning, cracking of the skin, dermatitis (inflammation of the skin), infection, irritation, itching, numbness of the fingers, red spider veins, redness, stinging, sweat rash

---

Can I receive this medication if I am pregnant or breastfeeding?

The effects of clobetasol propionate during pregnancy and breastfeeding are unknown. Tell your doctor immediately if you are pregnant, plan to become pregnant, or are breastfeeding.

What should I do if I miss a dose of this medication?

If you miss a dose of clobetasol propionate, apply it as soon as you remember. However, if it is almost time for your next dose, skip the one you missed and return to your regular dosing schedule. Do not apply two doses at once.

How should I store this medication?

Store at room temperature. Do not refrigerate.

Clobetasol Propionate Scalp Solution

Generic name: Clobetasol Propionate

What is this medication?

Clobetasol propionate scalp solution is a topical medicine (applied to the scalp) that is used for the relief of inflammation and itching of the scalp.

What is the most important information I should know about this medication?

- Clobetasol propionate is for external use only. Do not use it in your eyes, face, underarms, vagina, or groin areas.
- Clobetasol propionate can have a greater effect on children because they are more likely to absorb large amounts of the medicine. Long-term use can affect the growth and development of children. Talk to your doctor if you think your child is not growing at a normal rate after using this medication for a long period of time.
- Do not use clobetasol propionate for any other condition other than that which your doctor has prescribed.
- Contact your doctor if you notice irritation or any reactions in the area being treated or if your condition does not improve within 2 weeks of treatment.

Who should not take this medication?

Do not use clobetasol propionate if you are allergic to it, any of its ingredients, or to similar products.

What should I tell my doctor before I take the first dose of this medication?

Tell your doctor about all prescription, over-the-counter, and herbal medications you are taking before beginning treatment with clobetasol propionate. Also, talk to your doctor about your complete medical history, especially if you are pregnant, plan to become pregnant, or are breastfeeding.

What is the usual dosage?

Please see general statement regarding dosage on page xii.

Adults and children ≥12 years: Apply to the affected scalp area(s) twice a day (morning and night).

Limit the treatment to 2 consecutive weeks, and do not use more than 50 milliliters (mL) a week.

How should I take this medication?
- Apply clobetasol propionate exactly as prescribed by your doctor. Do not apply extra doses or apply more often without asking your doctor.

What should I avoid while taking this medication?
Do not use clobetasol propionate in your eyes, face, underarms, vagina, or groin areas.

Do not bandage, cover, or wrap the treated skin area as to be occlusive.

What are possible food and drug interactions associated with this medication?
No significant interactions have been reported with clobetasol propionate at this time. However, always tell your doctor about any medicines you take, including over-the-counter medications, vitamins, and herbal supplements.

What are the possible side effects of this medication?
Please see general statement regarding side effects on page xiii.

> **Side effects may include:** acne (pimples), burning, cracking of the skin, dermatitis (inflammation of the skin), infection, irritation, itching, numbness of the fingers, red spider veins, redness, stinging, sweat rash

Can I receive this medication if I am pregnant or breastfeeding?
The effects of clobetasol propionate during pregnancy and breastfeeding are unknown. Tell your doctor immediately if you are pregnant, plan to become pregnant, or are breastfeeding.

What should I do if I miss a dose of this medication?

If you miss a dose of clobetasol propionate, apply it as soon as you remember. However, if it is almost time for your next dose, skip the one you missed and return to your regular dosing schedule. Do not apply two doses at once.

How should I store this medication?

Store at room temperature. Do not refrigerate.

Clobetasol Propionate: see Clobetasol Propionate Cream, page 240

Clobetasol Propionate: see Clobetasol Propionate Gel, page 243

Clobetasol Propionate: see Clobetasol Propionate Ointment, page 245

Clobetasol Propionate: see Clobetasol Propionate Scalp Solution, page 248

Clonazepam: see Klonopin, page 504

Clonidine HCl: see Catapres, page 190

Clonidine HCl: see Catapres-TTS, page 193

Clopidogrel Bisulfate: see Plavix, page 796

Codeine Phosphate/Promethazine HCl: see Promethazine with codeine, page 853

Colchicine: see Colcrys, page 251

Colcrys
Generic name: Colchicine

What is this medication?
Colcrys is a medicine used to prevent and treat severe and painful inflammation of the joints (gout flares), and treat familial Mediterranean fever, a hereditary inflammatory disorder.

What is the most important information I should know about this medication?
- Colcrys is not a pain medicine and you should not take it to treat pain related to other conditions, unless it was specifically prescribed by your doctor for those conditions.
- Serious side effects, including death, may occur if levels of Colcrys are too high in your body. Call your doctor immediately if you have muscle weakness or pain; numbness or tingling in your fingers or toes; unusual bleeding or bruising; severe diarrhea or vomiting; increased infections; feel weak or tired; or experience a pale or gray color to your lips, tongue, or palms of your hands, severe diarrhea or vomiting.

Who should not take this medication?
Do not take Colcrys if you are allergic to it, any of its ingredients, or if you have liver or kidney problems and you take certain other medications.

What should I tell my doctor before I take the first dose of this medication?
Tell your doctor about all prescription, over-the-counter, and herbal medications you are taking before beginning treatment with Colcrys. Also, talk to your doctor about your complete medical history, especially if you have kidney or liver problems, are pregnant, plan to become pregnant, or are breastfeeding.

What is the usual dosage?
Please see general statement regarding dosage on page xii.

Adults and children: Your doctor will prescribe the appropriate dose for you based on your condition.

If you have kidney or liver problems, your doctor will adjust your dose appropriately.

How should I take this medication?
• Take Colcrys exactly as prescribed by your doctor. You can take Colcrys with or without food. Do not change the dose or stop taking Colycrys, even if you start to feel better, unless your doctor tells you to do so. If you have a gout flare while you are taking Colcrys, report this to your doctor.

What should I avoid while taking this medication?
Do not eat grapefruit or drink grapefruit juice while you are taking Colcrys.

What are possible food and drug interactions associated with this medication?
If Colcrys is taken with certain other drugs, the effects of either could be increased, decreased, or altered. Colcrys may interact with numerous medications. Therefore, it is very important that you tell your doctor about any other medications you are taking.

What are the possible side effects of this medication?
Please see general statement regarding side effects on page xiii.

> **Side effects may include:** abdominal pain, diarrhea, nausea, vomiting

Can I receive this medication if I am pregnant or breastfeeding?
The effects of Colcrys during pregnancy are unknown. Colcrys can be found in your breast milk if you take it while breastfeeding. Tell your doctor immediately if you are pregnant, plan to become pregnant, or are breastfeeding.

What should I do if I miss a dose of this medication?
If you miss a dose of Colcrys, take it as soon as you remember. However, if it is almost time for your next dose, skip the one you

missed and return to your regular dosing schedule. Do not take two doses at once.

How should I store this medication?
Store at room temperature. Protect from light.

Combigan
Generic name: Brimonidine Tartrate/Timolol Maleate

What is this medication?
Combigan is an eye drop used to lower pressure in the eye in people with glaucoma or ocular hypertension (high pressure in the eye).

What is the most important information I should know about this medication?
- Even though Combigan is applied directly to the eye, the medication can still be absorbed in your bloodstream and worsen heart failure, cause breathing problems, or hide symptoms of low blood sugar levels if you have diabetes. Tell your doctor if you experience weight gain or trouble breathing while you are taking Combigan. If you have diabetes, monitor your blood sugar frequently, especially when you first start taking Combigan.
- Combigan can worsen disorders associated with compromised blood flow. Tell your doctor about all your medical conditions, especially if you have depression, brain or heart problems, circulation problems (such as Raynaud's disease), or sudden falls in your blood pressure.
- Do not allow the tip of the bottle to touch your eye or any other surface, as serious eye infections may occur if your bottle becomes contaminated. Tell your doctor immediately if you experience any eye injury, infection, conjunctivitis ("pink eye"), or eyelid reactions with Combigan.

Who should not take this medication?
Do not use Combigan if you are allergic to it or any of its ingredients.

Do not use Combigan if you have or had asthma or severe chronic obstructive pulmonary disease (COPD) (narrowing of the lungs that makes it hard to breath).

Do not use Combigan if you have a slow heartbeat, heart block, heart failure, or cardiogenic shock (when your heart is too damaged to supply sufficient blood to your body).

What should I tell my doctor before I take the first dose of this medication?

Tell your doctor about all prescription, over-the-counter, and herbal medications you are taking before beginning treatment with Combigan. Also, talk to your doctor about your complete medical history, especially if you have allergies; heart problems or heart failure; asthma, COPD, chronic bronchitis, emphysema, or other breathing problems; diabetes; blood circulation problems; myasthenia gravis (a disease characterized by long-lasting fatigue and muscle weakness); thyroid problems; or if you are planning to have a major surgery, including eye surgery.

Tell your doctor if you have a history of severe allergic reactions to any allergens, because Combigan may decrease the effectiveness of epinephrine used to treat the reaction.

What is the usual dosage?
Please see general statement regarding dosage on page xii.

Adults and children ≥2 years: The recommended dose is 1 drop in the affected eye(s) twice a day, about 12 hours apart.

How should I take this medication?
- Apply Combigan exactly as prescribed by your doctor.
- Combigan contains a preservative that may be absorbed by your contact lenses. Remove your contact lenses prior to the administration of Combigan and reinsert them after 15 minutes.
- If you are using Combigan with another eye drop, the drops should be applied at least 5 minutes apart.

What should I avoid while taking this medication?

Do not allow the tip of the bottle to touch your eye or any other surface, as this can contaminate the medication.

Do not drive or operate heavy machinery until you know how Combigan affects you.

What are possible food and drug interactions associated with this medication?

If Combigan is used with certain other drugs, the effects of either could be increased, decreased, or altered. It is especially important to check with your doctor before combining Combigan with the following: alcohol, anesthesia, barbiturates (such as phenobarbital), blood pressure/heart medications known as beta-blockers (such as atenolol or metoprolol) or calcium-channel blockers (such as amlodipine or diltiazem), certain antidepressants (such as citalopram or sertraline), digoxin, narcotic painkillers (such as hydrocodone or oxycodone), other blood pressure/heart medications, quinidine, reserpine, or sedatives (such as lorazepam).

What are the possible side effects of this medication?

Please see general statement regarding side effects on page xiii.

Side effects may include: burning, stinging, or itching of your eye; pink eye; red eye

---

Can I receive this medication if I am pregnant or breastfeeding?

The effects of Combigan during pregnancy are unknown. Combigan can be found in your breast milk if you use it while breastfeeding. Do not breastfeed while you are using Combigan. Tell your doctor immediately if you are pregnant, plan to become pregnant, or are breastfeeding.

What should I do if I miss a dose of this medication?

If you miss a dose of Combigan, apply it as soon as you remember. However, if it is almost time for your next dose, skip the one you missed and return to your regular dosing schedule. Do not apply two doses at once.

How should I store this medication?
Store at room temperature. Protect from light.

Combivent
Generic name: Albuterol Sulfate/Ipratropium Bromide

What is this medication?
Combivent is an inhaled medicine that combines two medications: ipratropium bromide and albuterol, that work together to help open the airways in your lungs. Combivent is used to treat broncho-spasm (airway narrowing) associated with chronic obstructive pulmonary disease (COPD). This medication is used if you are already using a medication to open your airways and need a second one to control your condition.

What is the most important information I should know about this medication?
- Do not use Combivent more frequently than your doctor recommends. Increasing the number of doses can be dangerous and may actually make symptoms of asthma worse. If the dose your doctor recommends does not provide relief of your symptoms, or if your symptoms become worse, tell your doctor right away.
- You can have an immediate, serious allergic reaction to the first dose of Combivent, with hives, rash, and swelling of your mouth, throat, lips, or tongue. This medication can cause life-threatening breathing problems, especially with the first dose from a new canister.

Who should not take this medication?
Do not use Combivent if you are allergic to it, any of its ingredients, atropine, or soya lecithin or related food products (such as soy-bean and peanut).

What should I tell my doctor before I take the first dose of this medication?

Tell your doctor about all prescription, over-the-counter, and herbal medications you are taking before beginning treatment with Combivent. Also, talk to your doctor about your complete medical history, especially if you have a heart condition, seizure disorder, high blood pressure, arrhythmia (life-threatening irregular heartbeat), overactive thyroid gland, low blood potassium levels, diabetes, liver or kidney disease, glaucoma (high pressure in the eye), an enlarged prostate, or problems urinating due to bladder-neck blockage.

What is the usual dosage?

Please see general statement regarding dosage on page xii.

Adults: The recommended dose is 2 inhalations four times a day. Your doctor may give you a higher dose depending on your needs.

How should I take this medication?

- Use Combivent exactly as prescribed by your doctor. Shake the inhaler well for at least 10 seconds before each use.
- You must test spray the inhaler if you are using it for the first time and when it has not been used for more than 24 hours. To do this, press the pump 3 times into the air, away from your face.
- Breathe out deeply through your mouth, then place the mouthpiece into your mouth and close your lips around it. Keep your eyes closed so that no medicine is sprayed into your eyes. While breathing in slowly through your mouth, press down on the top of the canister. Hold your breath for 10 seconds if possible. Then, wait about two minutes, shake the inhaler well for at least 10 seconds again and repeat.
- Keep the mouthpiece clean. Wash it with hot water and dry thoroughly before use.
- Please review the instructions that came with your prescription on how to properly use Combivent.

What should I avoid while taking this medication?

Do not spray Combivent into your eyes.

Do not drive or operate appliances or machinery until you know how Combivent affects you.

What are possible food and drug interactions associated with this medication?

If Combivent is used with certain other drugs, the effects of either could be increased, decreased, or altered. It is especially important to check with your doctor before combining Combivent with the following: anticholinergic medications (such as atropine), blood pressure/heart medications known as beta-blockers (such as metoprolol or propranolol), certain antidepressant medications (such as amitriptyline or phenelzine), certain diuretics (water pills) (such as furosemide or hydrochlorothiazide), or other medications that can affect your heart (such as amphetamine or epinephrine).

What are the possible side effects of this medication?

Please see general statement regarding side effects on page xiii.

> **Side effects may include:** bronchitis (inflammation of the air passages within your lungs), cough, headache, upper respiratory tract infection

Can I receive this medication if I am pregnant or breastfeeding?

The effects of Combivent during pregnancy and breastfeeding are unknown. Do not breastfeed while you are using Combivent. Tell your doctor immediately if you are pregnant, plan to become pregnant, or are breastfeeding.

What should I do if I miss a dose of this medication?

If you miss a dose of Combivent, take it as soon as you remember. However, if it is almost time for your next dose, skip the one you missed and return to your regular dosing schedule. Do not take two doses at once.

How should I store this medication?

Store at room temperature. Protect from heat, open flame, or excessive humidity.

Complera
Generic name: Emtricitabine/Rilpivirine/Tenofovir Disoproxil Fumarate

What is this medication?
Complera is a medicine used to treat HIV infection (AIDS). Complera contains three medications: emtricitabine, rilpivirine, and tenofovir disoproxil.

What is the most important information I should know about this medication?
- Complera does not cure HIV/AIDS, nor does it reduce the risk of passing HIV/AIDS to others through sexual contact, sharing needles, or being exposed to your blood.
- Complera can cause a serious condition called lactic acidosis (a build-up of an acid in the blood). Lactic acidosis can be a medical emergency and may need to be treated in the hospital.
- Complera can cause serious liver problems, including an enlarged liver and fat deposits in the liver.
- You have a higher chance of getting lactic acidosis or liver problems if you are a woman, are very overweight (obese), or if you have been taking Complera or similar products for a long time.
- If you have hepatitis B virus (HBV) and stop taking Complera, your HBV can worsen.

Who should not take this medication?
Do not take Complera if you are allergic to it or any of its ingredients.

Do not take Complera while you are taking dexamethasone (more than one dose); seizure medications (such as carbamazepine, oxcarbazepine, phenobarbital, or phenytoin); medications for tuberculosis (a bacterial infection that affects the lungs) (such as rifabutin, rifampin, or rifapentine); medications for certain stomach or intestinal problems (such as esomeprazole, lansoprazole, omeprazole, pantoprazole, or rabeprazole); or St. John's wort.

What should I tell my doctor before I take the first dose of this medication?
Tell your doctor about all prescription, over-the-counter, and herbal medications you are taking before beginning treatment with

Complera. Also, talk to your doctor about your complete medical history, especially if you have liver problems (including hepatitis B or C); bone, kidney, or mental health problems; are pregnant, plan to become pregnant, or are breastfeeding.

What is the usual dosage?
Please see general statement regarding dosage on page xii.

Adults: The recommended dose is 1 tablet once a day.

How should I take this medication?
- Take Complera as prescribed by your doctor. Take it with a meal to get the right amount of medicine in your body.
- When your Complera supply runs low, renew your prescription promptly. If you stop the medicine for even a short time, the amount of HIV in your body can increase or it can become resistant to the effects of Complera.

What should I avoid while taking this medication?
Do not become pregnant or breastfeed while you are taking Complera. If you do become pregnant, tell your doctor immediately.

Do not reuse or share needles or other injection equipment. Also, do not share personal items that can have blood or bodily fluids on them, such as toothbrushes or razor blades.

Do not have any unprotected sex.

What are possible food and drug interactions associated with this medication?
If Complera is taken with certain other drugs, the effects of either could be increased, decreased, or altered. Complera may interact with numerous medications. Therefore, it is very important that you tell your doctor about any other medications you are taking.

What are the possible side effects of this medication?
Please see general statement regarding side effects on page xiii.

Side effects may include: abnormal dreams, depression, diarrhea, difficulty sleeping (insomnia), dizziness, headache, nausea, rash, tiredness

Can I receive this medication if I am pregnant or breastfeeding?

The effects of Complera during pregnancy and breastfeeding are unknown. It is recommended that you do not breastfeed your baby if you are infected with HIV. This is because your baby could become infected with HIV through your breast milk. Tell your doctor immediately if you are pregnant, plan to become pregnant, or are breastfeeding.

What should I do if I miss a dose of this medication?

If you miss a dose of Complera within 12 hours of the time you usually take it, take it with a meal as soon as you remember. Then, take your next dose at the regular dosing schedule. If you miss a dose of Complera by more than 12 hours of the time you usually take it, wait, and then take the next dose at the regular dosing schedule. Do not take two doses at once.

How should I store this medication?

Store at room temperature.

Concerta

Generic name: Methylphenidate HCl

What is this medication?

Concerta is a medicine used to treat attention-deficit hyperactivity disorder (ADHD). This medicine can help to increase attention and decrease impulsiveness and hyperactivity in people with ADHD.

What is the most important information I should know about this medication?

- Concerta has a high potential for abuse. Taking Concerta for long periods of time may lead to extreme emotional and physical dependence. Your doctor will monitor your response and make

sure you receive the correct dose. Tell your doctor if you have a history of drug or alcohol abuse.
- Concerta can cause serious heart-related and mental problems, stroke and heart attacks in adults, and increased blood pressure and heart rate. It can also cause new or worsening behavior and thought problems, bipolar illness, and aggressive or hostile behavior.
- In addition, new symptoms (such as hearing voices, believing things that are not true, or manic symptoms) can occur. Call your doctor immediately if you or your child experiences chest pain, shortness of breath, fainting, or new mental problems while taking Concerta.
- The doctor will check your child's height and weight while he/she is taking Concerta. If your child is not growing in height or gaining weight as expected, the doctor may stop this medicine.
- Concerta can cause eyesight changes or blurred vision. If this occurs, tell your doctor.
- Concerta can cause a blockage of the esophagus (the tube that connects your mouth and stomach), stomach, small or large intestine. Tell your doctor if you already have narrowing in any of these organs.

Who should not take this medication?
Do not take Concerta if you are allergic to it or any of its ingredients. Do not take Concerta if you are very anxious, tense, or agitated.

Do not take Concerta if you have glaucoma (high pressure in the eye), tics, or if you have been diagnosed or have a family history of Tourette's syndrome.

Also, do not take Concerta if you are taking antidepressant medications known as monoamine oxidase inhibitors (MAOIs) (such as phenelzine or tranylcypromine) or have taken them within the past 14 days.

What should I tell my doctor before I take the first dose of this medication?
Tell your doctor about all prescription, over-the-counter, and herbal medications you are taking before beginning treatment with

Concerta. Also, talk to your doctor about your complete medical history, including heart problems, heart defects, high blood pressure, or a family history of these problems. Tell your doctor if you have a history of mental problems or a family history of psychosis, mania, bipolar disorder, or depression; tics or Tourette's syndrome; esophagus, stomach, or small or large intestine problems; or seizures or an abnormal brain wave test (EEG).

What is the usual dosage?
Please see general statement regarding dosage on page xii.

Adults 18-65 years: The recommended starting dose is 18 milligrams (mg) or 36 mg once a day.

Children and adolescents 6-17 years: The recommended starting dose is 18 mg once a day.

Your or your child's doctor will prescribe the appropriate dose for you based on your previous ADHD medications and may increase the dose as needed, until the desired effect is achieved.

How should I take this medication?
- Take Concerta exactly as prescribed by your doctor. Take Concerta in the morning. Take it with or without food.
- Swallow Concerta tablets whole with water or other liquids. Do not chew, crush, or divide them.
- When you take Concerta, you may see something in your stool that looks like a tablet. This is the empty shell from the tablet after the medicine has been absorbed in your body.

What should I avoid while taking this medication?
Do not drive or operate dangerous machinery until you know how Concerta affects you.

Do not start any new medicine while you are taking Concerta without first talking to your doctor.

What are possible food and drug interactions associated with this medication?

If Concerta is taken with certain other drugs, the effects of either could be increased, decreased, or altered. It is especially important to check with your doctor before combining Concerta with the following: blood thinners (such as warfarin), certain antidepressants (such as amitriptyline or citalopram), dobutamine, epinephrine, MAOIs, or seizure medications (such as phenobarbital, phenytoin, or primidone).

What are the possible side effects of this medication?

Please see general statement regarding side effects on page xiii.

Side effects may include: anxiety, decreased appetite, dizziness, dry mouth, headache, increased sweating, irritability, nausea, stomach ache, trouble sleeping, weight loss

Can I receive this medication if I am pregnant or breastfeeding?

The effects of Concerta during pregnancy and breastfeeding are unknown Tell your doctor immediately if you are pregnant, plan to become pregnant, or are breastfeeding.

What should I do if I miss a dose of this medication?

If you miss a dose of Concerta, take it as soon as you remember. However, if it is almost time for your next dose, skip the one you missed and return to your regular dosing schedule. Do not take two doses at once.

How should I store this medication?

Store at room temperature. Protect from humidity.

Conjugated Estrogens: *see Premarin, page 813*

Conjugated Estrogens/Medroxyprogesterone Acetate: *see Premphase, page 816*

Conjugated Estrogens/Medroxyprogesterone Acetate: *see*
Prempro, page 820

Cordarone
Generic name: Amiodarone HCl

What is this medication?
Cordarone is a medicine used to treat and prevent frequently recurring ventricular fibrillation or ventricular tachycardia (an irregular,
fast heartbeat) with unstable blood circulation.

What is the most important information I should know about this medication?
- Cordarone can cause very low blood pressure. Your doctor will
  monitor your blood pressure while you take Cordarone.
- Cordarone can cause a different type of abnormal heartbeat that
  can be dangerous and life-threatening. Also, Cordarone can increase your risk of having very slow heartbeat; very low blood
  pressure; liver, lung, vision, or thyroid problems. Because of
  these possible side effects, Cordarone should be used in people
  with life-threatening arrhythmias for which other treatments did
  not work or were not tolerated.

Who should not take this medication?
Do not take Cordarone if you are allergic to it or any of its ingredients, or iodine.

Do not take Cordarone if you have an abnormally slow heartbeat or
heart block (unless you have a pacemaker).

What should I tell my doctor before I take the first dose of this medication?
Tell your doctor about all prescription, over-the-counter, and herbal
medications you are taking before beginning treatment with Cordarone. Also, talk to your doctor about your complete medical history, especially if you have certain heart or blood pressure problems;

lung or breathing problems; liver injury or thyroid abnormalities, or are pregnant, plan to become pregnant, or are breastfeeding.

What is the usual dosage?

Please see general statement regarding dosage on page xii.

Adults: The usual starting doses are 800-1600 milligrams a day, divided in one or two doses. Your doctor will prescribe the appropriate dose for you based on your condition.

How should I take this medication?

- Take Cordarone exactly as prescribed by your doctor.
- You can take Cordarone with or without food. Take it the same way each time. Continue to take Cordarone even if you feel well.
- Do not take extra doses or take more often without asking your doctor.

What should I avoid while taking this medication?

Do not drink grapefruit juice while you are taking Cordarone.

Do not expose your skin to the sun or sun lamps. Cordarone can make your skin more sensitive to light and cause sunburns. Wear sunscreen or protective clothing if you are going to be outside for long periods.

What are possible food and drug interactions associated with this medication?

If Cordarone is taken with certain other drugs, the effects of either could be increased, decreased, or altered. It is especially important to check with your doctor before combining Cordarone with the following: anti-HIV medications called protease inhibitors (such as indinavir), antihistamines (such as loratadine or cimetidine), blood pressure/heart medications known as beta-blockers (such as propranolol) or calcium channel blockers (such as diltiazem or verapamil), blood thinners (such as warfarin), certain antibiotics (such as erythromycin, moxifloxacin, or rifampin), certain antidepressants (such as trazodone), cholesterol medications (such as atorvastatin, cholestyramine, or simvastatin), clopidogrel, cyclosporine, dextromethorphan, digoxin, fentanyl, grapefruit juice, lidocaine, other antiarrhythmics (such as disopyramide, procain-amide, or quinidine), phenytoin, or St. John's wort.

What are the possible side effects of this medication?
Please see general statement regarding side effects on page xiii.

> **Side effects may include:** constipation, decreased concentration, depression, difficulty tolerating cold or heat, dizziness, hair thinning, irritability, loss of appetite, menstruation changes, nausea, nervousness, numbness, "pins and needles" sensations, restlessness, sensitivity to the sun, sweating, swelling, tiredness, tremors, uncontrolled movements, visual disturbances, vomiting, weakness, weight changes

Can I receive this medication if I am pregnant or breastfeeding?
Cordarone can harm your unborn baby if you take it during pregnancy. Cordarone can be found in your breast milk if you take it while breastfeeding. Do not breastfeed while you are taking Cordarone. Tell your doctor immediately if you are pregnant, plan to become pregnant, or are breastfeeding.

What should I do if I miss a dose of this medication?
If you miss a dose of Cordarone, take it as soon as you remember. However, if it is almost time for your next dose, skip the one you missed and return to your regular dosing schedule. Do not take two doses at once.

How should I store this medication?
Store at room temperature. Protect from light.

Coreg

Generic name: Carvedilol

What is this medication?

Coreg is a medicine known as a beta-blocker, which is used to treat high blood pressure and heart failure. Coreg is also used after a heart attack that worsens how well the heart pumps (left ventricular dysfunction).

What is the most important information I should know about this medication?

- Do not stop taking Coreg without talking to your doctor. Stopping this medication suddenly can cause harmful effects. Your doctor should gradually reduce your dose when stopping treatment with this medication.
- Coreg can worsen heart failure, cause breathing problems, or hide symptoms of low blood sugar levels if you have diabetes. Tell your doctor if you experience weight gain or trouble breathing while you are taking Coreg. If you have diabetes, monitor your blood sugar frequently, especially when you first start taking Coreg.
- Coreg can cause low blood pressure, which can lead to dizziness and fainting when you stand up. If this happens, sit or lie down and call your doctor right away.

Who should not take this medication?

Do not take Coreg if you are allergic to it or any of its ingredients. In addition, do not take Coreg if you have asthma or other breathing problems, a slow heart rate, heart failure, heart block, sick sinus syndrome (abnormal heart rhythm), severe liver disease, or severe blood circulation disorders.

What should I tell my doctor before I take the first dose of this medication?

Tell your doctor about all prescription, over-the-counter, and herbal medications you are taking before beginning treatment with Coreg. Also, talk to your doctor about your complete medical history, especially if you have allergies; heart problems or heart failure; a history of heart attack; breathing problems; pheochromocytoma (tumor of the adrenal gland); chest pain; diabetes; liver, kidney, or thyroid problems; low blood pressure; peripheral vascular disease (disease of the blood vessels outside the heart and brain); or are planning to have a major surgery, including eye surgery.

Tell your doctor if you have a history of severe allergic reactions to any allergens, because Coreg may decrease the effectiveness of epinephrine used to treat the reaction.

What is the usual dosage?
Please see general statement regarding dosage on page xii.

High Blood Pressure
Adults: The recommended starting dose is 6.25 milligrams (mg) twice a day, either alone or in combination with other blood pressure-lowering medicines. Full effects should be seen in 1-2 weeks. Your doctor will increase your dose as needed until the desired effect is achieved.

Heart Failure
Adults: The recommended starting dose is 3.125 mg twice a day. Your doctor may increase your dose as appropriate.

Left Ventricular Dysfunction Following a Heart Attack
Adults: The recommended starting dose is 6.25 mg twice a day. Your doctor may increase your dose as appropriate.

How should I take this medication?
• Take Coreg exactly as prescribed by your doctor. Take it with food.

What should I avoid while taking this medication?
Do not drive a car, operate machinery, or engage in other tasks requiring alertness until you know how Coreg affects you.

Do not change your dose or stop taking Coreg without first talking to your doctor.

What are possible food and drug interactions associated with this medication?

If Coreg is taken with certain other drugs, the effects of either could be increased, decreased, or altered. It is especially important to check with your doctor before combining Coreg with any of the following: amiodarone, antidepressant medications known as monoamine oxidase inhibitors (such as phenelzine or tranylcypromine), blood pressure medications known as calcium channel blockers (such as diltiazem or verapamil), cimetidine, clonidine, cyclosporine, diabetes medications (such as insulin), digoxin, fluconazole, fluoxetine, paroxetine, propafenone, quinidine, reserpine, or rifampin.

What are the possible side effects of this medication?

Please see general statement regarding side effects on page xiii.

Side effects may include: diarrhea, dizziness, dry eyes, shortness of breath, tiredness, weight gain

---

Can I receive this medication if I am pregnant or breastfeeding?

The effects of Coreg during pregnancy and breastfeeding are unknown. Tell your doctor immediately if you are pregnant, plan to become pregnant, or are breastfeeding.

What should I do if I miss a dose of this medication?

If you miss a dose of Coreg, take it as soon as you remember. However, if it is almost time for your next dose, skip the one you missed and return to your regular dosing schedule. Do not take two doses at once.

How should I store this medication?

Store at room temperature. Protect from moisture.

Coreg CR
Generic name: Carvedilol

What is this medication?
Coreg CR is a medicine known as a beta-blocker, which is used to treat high blood pressure and heart failure. Coreg CR is also used after a heart attack that worsens how well the heart pumps (left ventricular dysfunction).

What is the most important information I should know about this medication?
- Do not stop taking Coreg CR without talking to your doctor. Stopping this medication suddenly can cause harmful effects. Your doctor should gradually reduce your dose when stopping treatment with this medication.
- Coreg CR can worsen heart failure, cause breathing problems, or hide symptoms of low blood sugar levels if you have diabetes. Tell your doctor if you experience weight gain or trouble breathing while you are taking Coreg CR. If you have diabetes, monitor your blood sugar frequently, especially when you first start taking Coreg CR.
- Coreg CR can cause low blood pressure, which can lead to dizziness and fainting when you stand up. If this happens, sit or lie down and call your doctor right away.

Who should not take this medication?
Do not take Coreg CR if you are allergic to it or any of its ingredients. In addition, do not take Coreg CR if you have asthma or other breathing problems, a slow heart rate, heart failure, heart block, sick sinus syndrome (abnormal heart rhythm), severe liver disease, or severe blood circulation disorders.

What should I tell my doctor before I take the first dose of this medication?
Tell your doctor about all prescription, over-the-counter, and herbal medications you are taking before beginning treatment with Coreg CR. Also, talk to your doctor about your complete medical history, especially if you have allergies; heart problems or heart failure; a history of heart attack; breathing problems; pheochromocytoma

(tumor of the adrenal gland); chest pain; diabetes; liver, kidney, or thyroid problems; low blood pressure; or peripheral vascular disease (disease of the blood vessels outside the heart and brain); or are planning to have a major surgery, including eye surgery.

Tell your doctor if you have a history of severe allergic reactions to any allergens, because Coreg CR may decrease the effectiveness of epinephrine used to treat the reaction.

What is the usual dosage?
Please see general statement regarding dosage on page xii.

High Blood Pressure
Adults: The recommended starting dose is 20 milligrams (mg) once a day, either alone or in combination with other blood pressure-lowering medicines. Full effects should be seen in 1-2 weeks. Your doctor will increase your dose as needed until the desired effect is achieved.

Heart Failure
Adults: The recommended starting dose is 10 mg once a day. Your doctor may increase your dose as appropriate.

Left Ventricular Dysfunction Following a Heart Attack
Adults: The recommended starting dose is 20 mg once a day. Your doctor may increase your dose as appropriate.

How should I take this medication?
- Take Coreg CR exactly as prescribed by your doctor. Take it as a single dose with food.
- Swallow Coreg CR capsules whole. Do not crush or chew them. If you have trouble with this, open the capsules and sprinkle the beads over a spoonful of applesauce. Swallow the applesauce mixture right away. Do not sprinkle the beads on any food other than applesauce.

What should I avoid while taking this medication?
Do not drive a car, operate machinery, or engage in other tasks requiring alertness until you know how Coreg CR affects you.

Do not change your dose or stop taking Coreg CR without first talking to your doctor.

What are possible food and drug interactions associated with this medication?

If Coreg CR is taken with certain other drugs, the effects of either could be increased, decreased, or altered. It is especially important to check with your doctor before combining Coreg CR with any of the following: amiodarone, antidepressant medications known as monoamine oxidase inhibitors (MAOIs) (such as phenelzine or tranylcypromine), blood pressure medications known as calcium channel blockers (such as diltiazem or verapamil), cimetidine, clonidine, cyclosporine, diabetes medications (such as insulin), digoxin, fluconazole, fluoxetine, paroxetine, propafenone, quinidine, reserpine, or rifampin.

What are the possible side effects of this medication?

Please see general statement regarding side effects on page xiii.

> **Side effects may include:** diarrhea, dizziness, dry eyes, shortness of breath, tiredness, weight gain

Can I receive this medication if I am pregnant or breastfeeding?

The effects of Coreg CR during pregnancy and breastfeeding are unknown. Tell your doctor immediately if you are pregnant, plan to become pregnant, or are breastfeeding.

What should I do if I miss a dose of this medication?

If you miss a dose of Coreg CR, take it as soon as you remember. However, if it is almost time for your next dose, skip the one you missed and return to your regular dosing schedule. Do not take two doses at once.

How should I store this medication?

Store at room temperature.

Cosopt
Generic name: Dorzolamide HCl/Timolol Maleate

What is this medication?
Cosopt is an eye drop used to lower pressure in the eye in people with open-angle glaucoma or high pressure in the eye.

What is the most important information I should know about this medication?
- Stop using Cosopt if you experience serious or unusual reactions, including severe skin reactions or signs of hypersensitivity, especially if you are allergic to sulfa-containing medicines (such as sulfamethizole). Contact your doctor right away if you experience any signs and symptoms of an allergic reaction, such as a rash or trouble breathing.
- Even though Cosopt is applied directly to the eye, the medication can still be absorbed in your bloodstream and cause serious adverse reactions, such as breathing difficulties, especially in patients with asthma or heart problems.
- Do not allow the tip of the bottle to touch your eye or any other surface, as serious eye infections may occur if your bottle becomes contaminated. Tell your doctor immediately if you experience any eye injury, infection, conjunctivitis ("pink eye"), or eyelid reactions with Cosopt.
- Do not use other eye medications unless your doctor has prescribed it for you. If you use another eye medication, use it at least 5 minutes before or after using Cosopt.
- Cosopt can cause blurred vision. Use caution if you drive or do anything that requires you to be able to see clearly.

Who should not take this medication?
Do not use Cosopt if you are allergic to it or any of its ingredients.

Do not use Cosopt if you have or had asthma or severe breathing or lung problems.

Do not use Cosopt if you have heart problems, including a slow or irregular heartbeat or heart failure.

What should I tell my doctor before I take the first dose of this medication?

Tell your doctor about all prescription, over-the-counter, and herbal medications you are taking before beginning treatment with Cosopt. Also, talk to your doctor about your complete medical history, especially if you have problems with muscle weakness; diabetes; thyroid, kidney, or liver problems; are planning to have surgery (including eye surgery); are allergic to sulfonamides; have or have had eye problems; or are pregnant, plan to become pregnant, or are breastfeeding.

What is the usual dosage?

Please see general statement regarding dosage on page xii.

Adults and children ≥2 years: Apply 1 drop into the affected eye(s) two times a day.

How should I take this medication?

• Apply Cosopt as prescribed by your doctor. Apply one drop of Cosopt in your eye(s) in the morning and one drop in the evening. Please review the instructions that came with your prescription on how to properly use your eye drops.

What should I avoid while taking this medication?

Do not allow the tip of the single-use container to contact your eye, as this can contaminate Cosopt.

Throw away the opened single-use container with any remaining Cosopt right away.

What are possible food and drug interactions associated with this medication?

If Cosopt is used with certain other drugs, the effects of either could be increased, decreased, or altered. It is especially important to check with your doctor before combining Cosopt with any of the following: blood pressure and heart medications known as beta-blockers (such as propranolol) and calcium channel blockers (such as diltiazem), carbonic anhydrase inhibitors (such as acetazolamide), certain antidepressant medications known as selective serotonin reuptake inhibitors (SSRIs) (such as fluoxetine, paroxetine, or sertraline), clonidine, digitalis, epinephrine, quinidine, or reserpine.

What are the possible side effects of this medication?
Please see general statement regarding side effects on page xiii.

> **Side effects may include:** allergic reactions, bitter or sour taste, blurred vision, breathing problems, burning and stinging of your eye, dizziness, eye redness or swelling, fainting, irregular heartbeat, itching of your eye, muscle weakness, rash, sweating, swelling, watery eyes, weight gain

Can I receive this medication if I am pregnant or breastfeeding?
The effects of Cosopt during pregnancy and breastfeeding are unknown. Cosopt can be found in your breast milk if you use it while breastfeeding. Tell your doctor immediately if you are pregnant, plan to become pregnant, or are breastfeeding.

What should I do If I miss a dose of this medication?
If you miss a dose of Cosopt, apply it as soon as you remember. However, if it is almost time for your next dose, skip the one you missed and return to your regular dosing schedule. Do not apply two doses at once.

How should I store this medication?
Store at room temperature. Do not freeze. Protect from light.

Coumadin
Generic name: Warfarin Sodium

What is this medication?
Coumadin is a blood thinner used to prevent and treat blood clots in the legs and lungs associated with an irregular, fast heartbeat and/or heart-valve replacement. Coumadin is also used after a

heart attack to lower the risk of death, having another heart attack, stroke, or blood clots moving to other parts of the body.

What is the most important information I should know about this medication?

- Coumadin can cause bleeding that can be serious and sometimes life-threatening. You may have a higher risk of bleeding if you take Coumadin and are 65 years or older or have high blood pressure, serious heart disease, low blood counts or cancer, kidney problems, a history of stomach or intestinal bleeding, stroke or mini-stroke, or trauma (such as an accident or surgery).
- Call your doctor right away if you are sick with diarrhea, have an infection, have a fever, or if you fall or injure yourself, especially if you hit your head.
- You may have a higher risk of bleeding if you take Coumadin with other medicines that increase your risk of bleeding (such as heparin, nonsteroidal anti-inflammatory drugs [NSAIDs] [such as ibuprofen], or other medicines to prevent or treat blood clots). Tell your doctor if you take any of these medicines.
- Coumadin can cause destruction of skin tissue cells, or gangrene. Call your doctor right away if you have pain or changes in color or temperature in any area of your body.
- Coumadin can cause "purple toes syndrome." Call your doctor right away if you have pain in your toes or they look purple or dark in color.
- Do not take other medicines that contain warfarin sodium while you are taking Coumadin.
- Some foods and beverages can interact with Coumadin and affect your treatment and dose. Eat a normal, balanced diet. Talk to your doctor before you make any changes to your diet. Do not eat large amounts of leafy, green vegetables, as they contain vitamin K. Certain vegetable oils also contain large amounts of vitamin K. Too much vitamin K can lower the effect of Coumadin.
- Always tell all your doctors that you take Coumadin.
- Wear or carry identification stating that you take Coumadin.

Who should not take this medication?

Do not take Coumadin if you are allergic to it or any of its ingredients. Do not take Coumadin if your chance of having bleeding problems is high. Do not take Coumadin if you are pregnant unless you have a mechanical heart valve.

What should I tell my doctor before I take the first dose of this medication?

Tell your doctor about all prescription, over-the-counter, and herbal medications you are taking before beginning treatment with Coumadin. Also, talk to your doctor about your complete medical history, especially if you have bleeding, liver, or kidney problems; high blood pressure; congestive heart failure (a condition in which the heart cannot pump enough blood throughout the body); diabetes; if you fall often; or if you plan to have any surgery or a dental procedure.

What is the usual dosage?

Please see general statement regarding dosage on page xii.

Adults: Your doctor will prescribe the appropriate dose for you based on your condition and will adjust your dose as needed.

How should I take this medication?

- Take Coumadin exactly as prescribed by your doctor.
- Have regular blood tests and visits with your doctor to monitor your condition and check for your response to Coumadin.

What should I avoid while taking this medication?

Do not change or stop any of your medicines or start any new medicines before talking to your doctor.

Do not do any activity or sport that may cause a serious injury.

What are possible food and drug interactions associated with this medication?

If Coumadin is taken with certain other drugs, the effects of either could be increased, decreased, or altered. Coumadin may interact with numerous medications. Therefore, it is very important that you tell your doctor about any other medications you are taking.

What are the possible side effects of this medication?
Please see general statement regarding side effects on page xiii.

> **Side effects may include:** bleeding from cuts that takes a long time to stop; bleeding gums when brushing your teeth; coughing up blood; dizziness, headache, or weakness; menstrual or vaginal bleeding that is heavier than normal; nosebleeds; pain, swelling, or discomfort; pink or brown urine; red or black stools; unusual bruising; or vomiting blood or material that looks like coffee grounds

Can I receive this medication if I am pregnant or breastfeeding?
Do not take Coumadin during pregnancy unless you have a mechanical heart valve. Tell your doctor immediately if you are pregnant, plan to become pregnant, or are breastfeeding.

What should I do if I miss a dose of this medication?
If you miss a dose of Coumadin, take it as soon as you remember on the same day. Do not take two doses the next day to make up for a missed dose.

How should I store this medication?
Store at room temperature in a tightly closed container. Store away from light and moisture.

Cozaar
Generic name: Losartan Potassium

What is this medication?
Cozaar is a medicine used alone or in combination with other medications to treat high blood pressure. Cozaar is also used to lower the risk of stroke if you have high blood pressure and a heart condition called left ventricular hypertrophy (enlargement of the section of the heart that is responsible for pumping blood to the rest of the

body). In addition, Cozaar is used to treat kidney disease in patients with diabetes and high blood pressure.

What is the most important information I should know about this medication?

- Cozaar can cause low blood pressure, especially if you take diuretics (water pills). If you feel faint or dizzy, lie down and call your doctor.
- Cozaar can cause a serious allergic reaction. If you experience swelling of your face, lips, throat, or tongue, stop taking Cozaar and get emergency medical help right away.
- Cozaar can worsen your kidney function if you already have kidney problems. Tell your doctor if you get swelling in your feet, ankles, or hands, or unexplained weight gain.
- Cozaar may not work as well for you if you are African American.

Who should not take this medication?

Do not take Cozaar if you are allergic to it or any of its ingredients. Do not take Cozaar if you are pregnant, plan to become pregnant, or are breastfeeding.

What should I tell my doctor before I take the first dose of this medication?

Tell your doctor about all prescription, over-the-counter, and herbal medications you are taking before beginning treatment with Cozaar. Also, talk to your doctor about your complete medical history, especially if you have kidney or liver problems, or if you are vomiting a lot or have a lot of diarrhea.

What is the usual dosage?

Please see general statement regarding dosage on page xii.

High Blood Pressure

Adults: The usual starting dose is 50 milligrams (mg) once a day. Your doctor will increase your dose as needed until the desired effect is achieved.

Children 6-16 years: Your doctor will prescribe the appropriate dose for your child, based on their weight.

Left Ventricular Hypertrophy and Kidney Disease
Adults: The usual starting dose is 50 mg once a day. Your doctor will increase your dose as needed until the desired effect is achieved.

How should I take this medication?
• Take Cozaar exactly as prescribed by your doctor. Take it with or without food.

What should I avoid while taking this medication?
Do not become pregnant or breastfeed while you are taking Cozaar.

What are possible food and drug interactions associated with this medication?
If Cozaar is taken with certain other drugs, the effects of either could be increased, decreased, or altered. It is especially important to check with your doctor before combining Cozaar with the following: certain diuretics (water pills) (such as amiloride, spironolactone, or triamterene), fluconazole, lithium, nonsteroidal anti-inflammatory drugs (such as ibuprofen or naproxen), phenobarbital, potassium supplements, rifampin, or salt substitutes that contain potassium.

What are the possible side effects of this medication?
Please see general statement regarding side effects on page xiii.

> **Side effects may include:** back pain, chest pain, diarrhea, dizziness, high blood potassium levels, low blood pressure, low blood sugar levels, stuffy nose, tiredness, upper respiratory infection

Can I receive this medication if I am pregnant or breastfeeding?
Do not take Cozaar if you are pregnant or breastfeeding. Cozaar can harm your unborn baby. Tell your doctor immediately if you are pregnant, plan to become pregnant, or are breastfeeding.

What should I do if I miss a dose of this medication?
If you miss a dose of Cozaar, take it as soon as you remember. However, if it is almost time for your next dose, skip the one you missed and return to your regular dosing schedule. Do not take two doses at once.

How should I store this medication?
Store at room temperature. Protect from light.

Crestor
Generic name: Rosuvastatin Calcium

What is this medication?
Crestor belongs to a class of medicines called "statins," which are used to lower your cholesterol when a low-fat diet is not enough. Crestor lowers your total cholesterol and the "bad" low-density lipoprotein (LDL) cholesterol, thereby helping to slow the hardening of your arteries, lower your risk of a heart attack or stroke, or the need for procedures to restore the blood flow back to the heart or to another part of the body.

What is the most important information I should know about this medication?
- Taking Crestor is not a substitute for following a healthy low-fat and low-cholesterol diet and exercising to lower your cholesterol.
- Do not take Crestor if you are pregnant, think you may be pregnant, plan to become pregnant, or are breastfeeding.
- Crestor can cause muscle pain, tenderness, weakness, fatigue, loss of appetite, right upper abdominal discomfort, dark urine, or yellowing of your skin or whites of your eyes. Call your doctor right away if you notice any of these symptoms.

Who should not take this medication?
Do not take Crestor if you are allergic to it or any of its ingredients, or if you currently have liver disease. Also, do not take Crestor if you are pregnant, plan to become pregnant, or are breastfeeding.

What should I tell my doctor before I take the first dose of this medication?

Tell your doctor about all prescription, over-the-counter, and herbal medications you are taking before beginning treatment with Crestor. Also, talk to your doctor about your complete medical history, especially if you drink excessive amounts of alcohol or you have liver, kidney, thyroid, or heart problems; muscle aches or weakness; or diabetes. Tell your doctor if you are pregnant, plan to become pregnant, or are breastfeeding.

What is the usual dosage?

Please see general statement regarding dosage on page xii.

Adults: The usual starting dose is 10-20 milligrams (mg) once a day. Your doctor will check your blood cholesterol levels during treatment with Crestor and will change your dose based on the results.

Adolescents 10-17 years: The usual dose is 5-20 mg once a day. Your doctor will check your blood cholesterol levels during treatment with Crestor and will change your dose based on the results.

If you have kidney impairment or you are taking other medications, your doctor will adjust your dose appropriately.

How should I take this medication?

- Your doctor will likely start you on a low-cholesterol diet before giving you Crestor. Stay on this diet while you are taking Crestor.
- Swallow Crestor tablets whole. Take the tablets at any time of the day, with or without food.
- Wait at least two hours after taking Crestor to take an antacid that contains a combination of aluminum and magnesium.

What should I avoid while taking this medication?

Do not change your dose or stop taking Crestor without first talking to your doctor.

What are possible food and drug interactions associated with this medication?

If Crestor is taken with certain other drugs, the effects of either could be increased, decreased, or altered. It is especially important to check with your doctor before combining Crestor with the following: alcohol, anti-HIV medications (such as atazanavir, lopinavir, or ritonavir), blood thinners (such as warfarin), cholesterol-lowering medicines known as fibrates (such as fenofibrate or gemfibrozil), cimetidine, cyclosporine, ketoconazole, niacin, or spironolactone.

What are the possible side effects of this medication?

Please see general statement regarding side effects on page xiii.

> **Side effects may include:** abdominal pain, headache, muscle pain, nausea, weakness

Can I receive this medication if I am pregnant or breastfeeding?

Do not take Crestor during pregnancy or breastfeeding. Tell your doctor immediately if you are pregnant, plan to become pregnant, or are breastfeeding.

What should I do if I miss a dose of this medication?

If you miss a dose of Crestor, take it as soon as you remember. However, if it is almost time for your next dose, skip the one you missed and return to your regular dosing schedule. Do not take two doses at once.

How should I store this medication?

Store at room temperature.

Cyclobenzaprine HCl: see Amrix, page 73

Cyclobenzaprine HCl: see Flexeril, page 388

Cyclosporine: see Restasis, page 886

Cymbalta
Generic name: Duloxetine HCl

What is this medication?

Cymbalta is an antidepressant medicine known as serotonin and norepinephrine reuptake inhibitor (SNRI). Cymbalta is used to treat major depressive disorder, generalized anxiety disorder, diabetic neuropathy (a painful nerve disorder associated with diabetes that affects your hands, legs, and feet), fibromyalgia (a condition characterized by weakness and pain in the muscles and tissues surrounding the joints), and chronic muscle pain.

What is the most important information I should know about this medication?

- Cymbalta can increase the risk of suicidal thoughts and behavior in children, adolescents, and young adults. Your doctor will monitor you closely for clinical worsening, suicidal or unusual behavior after you start taking Cymbalta or a new dose of Cymbalta. Tell your doctor right away if you experience anxiety, hostility, sleeplessness, restlessness, impulsive or dangerous behavior, or thoughts about suicide or dying; or if you have new symptoms or seem to be feeling worse.
- Cymbalta can cause liver damage. Contact your doctor right away if you experience abdominal pain or yellowing of your skin or the whites of your eyes. Do not drink alcohol while you are taking Cymbalta as this can contribute to liver damage.
- Cymbalta can cause an increase or decrease in blood pressure. Your doctor will check your blood pressure before starting you on Cymbalta and throughout treatment.
- Cymbalta can cause a severe, possibly life-threatening condition called serotonin syndrome (a drug reaction that causes the body to have too much serotonin, a chemical produced by the nerve cells) or neuroleptic malignant syndrome (a life-threatening brain disorder). Contact your doctor immediately if you experience agitation, hallucinations, fast heartbeat, changes in your blood pressure, increased body temperature, lack of coordination, overactive reflexes, nausea, vomiting, or diarrhea.

- Cymbalta can increase your risk of bleeding. Do not take Cymbalta with aspirin, nonsteroidal anti-inflammatory drugs (NSAIDs) (such as ibuprofen), or blood thinners (such as warfarin).
- Cymbalta can cause severe allergic reactions. Tell your doctor right away if you develop skin blisters, peeling rash, sores in your mouth, hives, or any other allergic reactions.
- Do not stop taking Cymbalta without first talking to your doctor as this can cause serious side effects.
- Cymbalta can cause low blood sodium levels. Contact your doctor immediately if you experience headache, difficulty concentrating, confusion, weakness, unsteadiness, hallucinations, falls, or seizures.
- Cymbalta can affect your blood sugar levels. If you are a diabetic, make sure you check your blood sugar levels regularly.
- Cymbalta can make it difficult to urinate. If you experience this problem, contact your doctor.

Who should not take this medication?

Do not take Cymbalta if you are allergic to it or any of its ingredients.

Do not take Cymbalta if you have untreated narrow-angle glaucoma (high pressure in the eye), severe liver or kidney disease, or if you drink excessive amounts of alcohol.

In addition, never take Cymbalta while you are taking other medicines known as monoamine oxidase inhibitors (MAOIs) (such as phenelzine), a class of medications used to treat depression and other conditions.

What should I tell my doctor before I take the first dose of this medication?

Tell your doctor about all prescription, over-the-counter, and herbal medications you are taking before beginning treatment with Cymbalta. Also, talk to your doctor about your complete medical history, especially if you have liver or kidney problems, glaucoma, diabetes, high blood pressure, bleeding problems, seizures, mania or bipolar disorder, or low blood sodium levels. Also, tell your doctor if you are pregnant, plan to become pregnant, or are breastfeeding.

What is the usual dosage?
Please see general statement regarding dosage on page xii.

Major Depressive Disorder
Adults: The recommended starting dose is 40 milligrams (mg) a day (taken as 20 mg twice a day) to 60 mg a day (taken as 30 mg twice a day or 60 mg once a day).

Generalized Anxiety Disorder and Diabetic Neuropathy
Adults: The recommended starting dose is 60 mg once a day.

Fibromyalgia and Chronic Muscle Pain
Adults: The recommended starting dose is 30 mg once a day.

Your doctor will adjust your dose appropriately.

How should I take this medication?
- Take Cymbalta exactly as prescribed by your doctor. Take it with or without food.
- Swallow Cymbalta capsules whole. Do not crush, chew, or open them.

What should I avoid while taking this medication?
Do not drive a car or operate dangerous machinery until you know how Cymbalta affects you.

Do not stop taking Cymbalta suddenly without talking to your doctor first, as this can cause serious side effects.

Do not take Cymbalta and MAOIs together or within 14 days of each other. Wait at least 5 days after stopping Cymbalta before starting an MAOI. Combining these medicines with Cymbalta can cause serious and even fatal reactions.

What are possible food and drug interactions associated with this medication?
If Cymbalta is taken with certain drugs, the effects of either could be increased, decreased, or altered. It is especially important to check with your doctor before combining Cymbalta with

the following: alcohol, antipsychotic medications (such as thioridazine), aspirin, certain antidepressants (such as desipramine, fluoxetine, fluvoxamine, or paroxetine), certain antibiotics (such as ciprofloxacin or enoxacin), certain migraine products, cimetidine, linezolid, lithium, MAOIs, NSAIDs, other SNRIs, quinidine, St. John's wort, tramadol, tryptophan, or warfarin.

What are the possible side effects of this medication?
Please see general statement regarding side effects on page xiii.

> **Side effects may include:** constipation, decreased appetite, drowsiness, dry mouth, excessive sweating, fatigue, nausea

Can I receive this medication if I am pregnant or breastfeeding?
The effects of Cymbalta during pregnancy are unknown. Cymbalta can be found in your breast milk if you take it while breastfeeding. Do not breastfeed while you are taking Cymbalta. Tell your doctor immediately if you are pregnant, plan to become pregnant, or are breastfeeding.

What should I do if I miss a dose of this medication?
If you miss a dose of Cymbalta, take it as soon as you remember. However, if it is almost time for your next dose, skip the one you missed and return to your regular dosing schedule. Do not take two doses at once.

How should I store this medication?
Store at room temperature.

Cyproheptadine
Generic name: Cyproheptadine HCl

What is this medication?
Cyproheptadine is a medicine used to manage allergic reactions, including seasonal and annual allergies, non-allergic nasal

symptoms (such as runny nose, stuffy nose, or postnasal drip), eye allergies, and skin reactions. Cyproheptadine is available as tablets and an oral solution.

What is the most important information I should know about this medication?

- Give cyproheptadine to your child exactly as prescribed by your doctor. Higher doses than prescribed can cause hallucinations, central nervous system depression, convulsions, breathing problems, or heart problems in infants and young children.
- Cyproheptadine can decrease mental alertness. However, in young children it may occasionally make them excited.

Who should not take this medication?

Do not take cyproheptadine if you are allergic to it or any of its ingredients.

Do not give cyproheptadine to newborn or premature infants.

Do not take cyproheptadine if you have closed-angle glaucoma (high pressure in the eye); a stomach ulcer; an enlarged prostate; bladder, intestine, or stomach obstruction; are elderly; or if you are breastfeeding.

Do not take cyproheptadine if you are taking antidepressant medications known as monoamine oxidase inhibitors (MAOIs) (such as phenelzine or selegiline).

What should I tell my doctor before I take the first dose of this medication?

Tell your doctor about all prescription, over-the-counter, and herbal medications you are taking before beginning treatment with cyproheptadine. Also, talk to your doctor about your complete medical history, especially if you have a history of asthma, glaucoma, thyroid or heart disease, or high blood pressure.

What is the usual dosage?

Please see general statement regarding dosage on page xii.

Adults: The recommended starting dose is 4 milligrams (mg) three times a day.

Children 7-14 years: The usual dose is 4 mg three times a day.

Children 2-6 years: The usual dose is 2 mg two or three times a day.

How should I take this medication?
• Take cyproheptadine exactly as prescribed by your doctor.

What should I avoid while taking this medication?
Do not drive or operate heavy machinery until you know how cyproheptadine affects you.

What are possible food and drug interactions associated with this medication?
If cyproheptadine is taken with certain other drugs, the effects of either could be increased, decreased, or altered. It is especially important to check with your doctor before combining cyproheptadine with the following: alcohol, antianxiety medications (such as alprazolam or lorazepam), MAOIs, sedative-hypnotics (such as butalbital or phenobarbital), or tranquilizers (such as chlorpromazine).

What are the possible side effects of this medication?
Please see general statement regarding side effects on page xiii.

Side effects may include: blood disorders; blurred vision; chills; difficult urination; dry mouth, nose, or throat; fatigue; fluttery or throbbing heartbeat; frequent urination; inflammation of the inner ear; liver problems; low blood pressure; rash; sedation; sleepiness; stomach pain; swelling

Can I receive this medication if I am pregnant or breastfeeding?
Do not breastfeed while you are taking cyproheptadine. Tell your doctor immediately if you are pregnant, plan to become pregnant, or are breastfeeding.

What should I do if I miss a dose of this medication?

If you miss a dose of cyproheptadine, take it as soon as you remember. However, if it is almost time for your next dose, skip the one you missed and return to your regular dosing schedule. Do not take two doses at once.

How should I store this medication?

Store at room temperature.

Cyproheptadine HCI: *see Cyproheptadine, page 288*

Cytomel

Generic name: Liothyronine Sodium

What is this medication?

Cytomel is a medicine used to treat hypothyroidism (an underactive thyroid gland). Cytomel is a synthetic hormone that is intended to replace a hormone that is normally produced by your thyroid gland. It is also used to treat or prevent certain other thyroid conditions such as goiter (an enlarged thyroid gland); inflammation of the thyroid gland; or thyroid hormone deficiency due to surgery, radiation, or certain medications. Also, Cytomel is used for thyroid suppression tests as a diagnostic agent to evaluate your thyroid function.

What is the most important information I should know about this medication?

- Do not use Cytomel to treat obesity or weight loss.
- Cytomel is a replacement therapy, so you need to take it every day for life unless your condition is temporary. Continue taking your medication as directed by your doctor. Tell your doctor immediately if you experience rapid or irregular heartbeats, chest pain, excessive sweating, heat intolerance, nervousness, or any other unusual symptoms.

- If you have heart disease, your doctor may need to start you on a lower dose of Cytomel to see how you respond to this medication.
- Also, if you have diabetes, your doctor will determine if the dose of your diabetes medication needs to be adjusted. Your doctor will monitor your blood sugar levels.
- If you are taking an oral blood thinner (such as warfarin), your doctor will monitor your blood clotting status to determine if the dose of your blood thinner needs to be adjusted.
- Cytomel can cause partial hair loss in children. This is usually temporary and the hair grows back later.

Who should not take this medication?
Do not take Cytomel if you are allergic to it or any of its ingredients.

Do not take Cytomel if you have an overactive thyroid gland or reduced adrenal function.

What should I tell my doctor before I take the first dose of this medication?
Tell your doctor about all prescription, over-the-counter, and herbal medications you are taking before beginning treatment with Cytomel. Also, talk to your doctor about your complete medical history, especially if you have diabetes, heart disease, blood clotting disorders, problems with your adrenal glands, or if you are pregnant, plan to become pregnant, or are breastfeeding.

What is the usual dosage?
Please see general statement regarding dosage on page xii.

   Adults and children: Your doctor will prescribe the appropriate dose for you based on your age, weight, and condition.

How should I take this medication?
- Take Cytomel exactly as prescribed by your doctor.

What should I avoid while taking this medication?
Do not stop taking Cytomel or change the amount or how often you take it without talking to your doctor.

What are possible food and drug interactions associated with this medication?

If Cytomel is taken with certain other drugs, the effects of either could be increased, decreased, or altered. It is especially important to check with your doctor before combining Cytomel with the following: birth control pills, blood thinners, certain antidepressants (such as imipramine), cholestyramine, diabetes medicines (such as insulin), digitalis, epinephrine, estrogen, ketamine, or norepinephrine.

What are the possible side effects of this medication?

Please see general statement regarding side effects on page xiii.

> **Side effects may include:** allergic skin reactions

Can I receive this medication if I am pregnant or breastfeeding?

You can continue to take Cytomel during pregnancy. Small amounts of thyroid hormone are excreted in your breast milk. Tell your doctor immediately if you are pregnant, plan to become pregnant, or are breastfeeding.

What should I do if I miss a dose of this medication?

If you miss a dose of Cytomel, take it as soon as you remember. However, if it is almost time for your next dose, skip the one you missed and return to your regular dosing schedule. Do not take two doses at once.

How should I store this medication?

Store at room temperature.

Dabigatran Etexilate Mesylate: *see Pradaxa, page 800*

Daliresp

Generic name: Roflumilast

What is this medication?

Daliresp is a medicine used in adults with severe chronic obstructive pulmonary disease (COPD) to decrease the number of flare-ups or the worsening of COPD symptoms (such as cough and excessive mucus).

What is the most important information I should know about this medication?

- Do not use Daliresp to treat sudden breathing problems. Your doctor may give you other medications to use for sudden breathing problems.
- Some people taking Daliresp can develop mood or behavior problems including: attempts to commit suicide, trouble sleeping (insomnia), new or worse anxiety or depression, acting on dangerous impulses, and other unusual changes in behavior or mood. Tell your doctor immediately if you have any of these signs or symptoms while you are taking Daliresp.
- Daliresp can cause weight loss. You should check your weight on a regular basis. You will also need to see your doctor regularly to have your weight monitored. If you notice that you are losing weight while taking Daliresp, call your doctor. Your doctor may ask you to stop taking Daliresp if you lose too much weight.

Who should not take this medication?

Do not take Daliresp if you have certain liver problems, are breast-feeding, or if you are allergic to it or any of its ingredients.

What should I tell my doctor before I take the first dose of this medication?

Tell your doctor about all prescription, over-the-counter, and herbal medications you are taking before beginning treatment with Daliresp. Also, talk to your doctor about your complete medical history, especially if you have or have had a history of mental health problems, including depression and suicidal behavior, have liver problems, are pregnant, plan to become pregnant, are breast-feeding, or plan to breastfeed.

What is the usual dosage?

Please see general statement regarding dosage on page xii.

Adults: The recommended dose is 1 tablet once a day.

How should I take this medication?

• Take Daliresp exactly as prescribed by your doctor. You can take Daliresp with or without food.

What should I avoid while taking this medication?

Do not use Daliresp to treat sudden breathing problems.

What are possible food and drug interactions associated with this medication?

If Daliresp is taken with certain other drugs, the effects of either could be increased, decreased, or altered. It is important to check with your doctor before combining Daliresp with any other medication.

What are the possible side effects of this medication?

Please see general statement regarding side effects on page xiii.

Side effects may include: back pain, decreased appetite, diarrhea, dizziness, "flu-like" symptoms, headache, nausea, problems sleeping (insomnia), weight loss

---

Can I receive this medication if I am pregnant or breastfeeding?

The effects of Daliresp during pregnany are unknown. Do not take Daliresp if you are breastfeeding. Tell your doctor immediately if you are pregnant, plan to become pregnant, or are breastfeeding.

What should I do if I miss a dose of this medication?

If you miss a dose of Daliresp, take it as soon as you remember. However, if it is almost time for your next dose, skip the one you missed and return to your regular dosing schedule. Do not take two doses at once.

How should I store this medication?
Store at room temperature.

Darifenacin: *see Enablex, page 363*

Depakote
Generic name: Divalproex Sodium

What is this medication?
Depakote is a medicine used to treat manic episodes associated with bipolar disorder, as well as certain types of seizures and migraines.

What is the most important information I should know about this medication?
- Depakote can cause serious liver damage (usually during the first 6 months of treatment) and pancreatitis (inflammation of the pancreas). Tell your doctor right away if you experience abdominal pain, nausea and vomiting, diarrhea, weakness, loss of appetite, or yellowing of your skin or the whites of your eyes.
- Depakote can cause harm to your unborn baby if you take it during pregnancy. Tell your doctor right away if you are pregnant or plan to become pregnant.
- Depakote can cause low blood platelet (type of blood cells that form clots to help stop bleeding) counts, which can cause you to bleed more easily. Tell your doctor right away if you have any unusual bleeding or bruising.
- Depakote can cause elevated ammonia levels and a drop in your body temperature. Contact your doctor right away if you experience abnormal drowsiness, vomiting, or changes in your behavior or mood.
- If you experience a fever and rash while taking Depakote, contact your doctor right away as this can be a sign of a serious allergic reaction.
- Depakote can cause central nervous system (CNS) depression, especially with alcohol or other CNS depressants. Do not drive

or operate dangerous machinery until you know how Depakote affects you.

Who should not take this medication?
Do not take Depakote if you are allergic to it or any of its ingredients.

Do not take Depakote if you have liver problems or urea cycle disorders (lack of an enzyme responsible for removing ammonia [a toxic substance] from the blood).

What should I tell my doctor before I take the first dose of this medication?
Tell your doctor about all prescription, over-the-counter, and herbal medications you are taking before beginning treatment with Depakote. Also, talk to your doctor about your complete medical history, especially if you have liver or kidney problems, have urea cycle disorders, or are pregnant, plan to become pregnant, or are breastfeeding.

What is the usual dosage?
Please see general statement regarding dosage on page xii.

Adults: Your doctor will prescribe the appropriate dose for you based on your condition and will increase your dose as appropriate.

Children: Your doctor will prescribe the appropriate dose for your child, based on their weight.

Attempts to taper or discontinue the medication should be made at specific intervals, through the guidance of your doctor.

How should I take this medication?
- Take Depakote exactly as prescribed by your doctor. Depakote Sprinkle Capsules can be swallowed whole. The capsule contents can be sprinkled onto soft food, such as applesauce or pudding. Swallow this mixture immediately and do not chew.
- If you experience stomach irritation, you may benefit from taking Depakote with food.

• Do not change your dose or stop taking this medication abruptly without first talking to your doctor.

What should I avoid while taking this medication?

Do not drink alcohol while you are taking Depakote. Drinking alcohol while you are taking Depakote can cause serious problems.

Do not drive, operate heavy machinery, or engage in dangerous activities until you know how Depakote affects you. Depakote can make you drowsy.

What are possible food and drug interactions associated with this medication?

If Depakote is taken with certain other drugs, the effects of either could be increased, decreased, or altered. It is especially important to check with your doctor before combining Depakote with the following: alcohol, aspirin, blood thinners (warfarin), certain antibiotics (such as ertapenem, imipenem, or meropenem), certain antidepressants (such as amitriptyline or nortriptyline), certain seizure medications (such as carbamazepine, clonazepam, diazepam, ethosuximide, felbamate, lamotrigine, nortriptyline, phenobarbital, phenytoin, primidone, or topiramate), rifampin, tolbutamide, or zidovudine.

What are the possible side effects of this medication?

Please see general statement regarding side effects on page xiii.

Side effects may include: abdominal (stomach) pain, blurred vision, bruising, change in your appetite, chest pain, constipation, depression, diarrhea, dizziness, drowsiness, emotional instability, fever, "flu-like" symptoms, hair loss, headache, indigestion, infections, lack of coordination, memory loss, nausea, nervousness, runny nose, shortness of breath, skin rash, sleep problems, sore throat, swelling, tremors, visual abnormalities, vomiting, weakness, weight changes

Can I receive this medication if I am pregnant or breastfeeding?

Depakote can cause harm to your unborn baby if you take it during pregnancy. Depakote can be found in your breast milk if you take it while breastfeeding. Tell your doctor immediately if you are pregnant, plan to become pregnant, or are breastfeeding.

What should I do if I miss a dose of this medication?

If you miss a dose of Depakote, take it dose as soon as you remember. However, if it is almost time for your next dose, skip the one you missed and return to your regular dosing schedule. Do not take two doses at once.

How should I store this medication?

Store at room temperature.

Depakote ER
Generic name: Divalproex Sodium

What is this medication?

Depakote ER is a medicine used to treat manic episodes associated with bipolar disorder, as well as certain types of seizures and migraines.

What is the most important information I should know about this medication?

- Depakote ER can cause serious liver damage (usually during the first 6 months of treatment) and pancreatitis (inflammation of the pancreas). Tell your doctor right away if you experience abdominal pain, nausea and vomiting, diarrhea, weakness, loss of appetite, or yellowing of your skin or the whites of your eyes.
- Depakote ER can cause harm to your unborn baby if you take it during pregnancy. Tell your doctor right away if you are pregnant or plan to become pregnant.
- Depakote ER can cause a low blood platelet (type of blood cells that form clots to help stop bleeding) count, which can cause

you to bleed more easily. Tell your doctor right away if you have any unusual bleeding or bruising.

• Depakote ER can cause elevated ammonia levels and a drop in your body temperature. Contact your doctor right away if you experience abnormal drowsiness, vomiting, or changes in your behavior or mood.

• If you experience a fever and rash while taking Depakote ER, contact your doctor right away as this can be a sign of a serious allergic reaction.

• Depakote ER can cause central nervous system (CNS) depression, especially with alcohol or other CNS depressants. Do not drive or operate dangerous machinery until you know how Depakote ER affects you.

Who should not take this medication?

Do not take Depakote ER if you are allergic to it or any of its ingredients.

Do not take Depakote ER if you have liver problems or urea cycle disorders (lack of an enzyme responsible for removing ammonia [a toxic substance] from the blood).

What should I tell my doctor before I take the first dose of this medication?

Tell your doctor about all prescription, over-the-counter, and herbal medications you are taking before beginning treatment with Depakote ER. Also, talk to your doctor about your complete medical history, especially if you have liver or kidney problems, have urea cycle disorders, or are pregnant, plan to become pregnant, or are breastfeeding.

What is the usual dosage?

Please see general statement regarding dosage on page xii.

Adults: Your doctor will prescribe the appropriate dose for you based on your condition and will increase your dose as appropriate.

Children: Your doctor will prescribe the appropriate dose for your child, based on their weight.

Attempts to taper or discontinue the medication should be made at specific intervals, through the guidance of your doctor.

How should I take this medication?
- Take Depakote ER exactly as prescribed by your doctor. Swallow Depakote ER tablets whole. Do not crush or chew the tablet.
- If you experience stomach irritation, you may benefit from taking Depakote ER with food.
- Do not change your dose or stop taking this medication abruptly without first talking to your doctor.

What should I avoid while taking this medication?
Do not drink alcohol while you are taking Depakote ER. Drinking alcohol while you are taking Depakote ER can cause serious problems.

Do not drive, operate heavy machinery, or engage in dangerous activities until you know how Depakote ER affects you. Depakote ER can make you drowsy.

What are possible food and drug interactions associated with this medication?
If Depakote ER is taken with certain other drugs, the effects of either could be increased, decreased, or altered. It is especially important to check with your doctor before combining Depakote ER with the following: alcohol, aspirin, certain antibiotics (such as ertapenem, imipenem, or meropenem), certain antidepressants (such as amitriptyline or nortriptyline), certain seizure medications (such as carbamazepine, clonazepam, diazepam, ethosuximide, felbamate, lamotrigine, nortriptyline, phenobarbital, phenytoin, primidone, topiramate), rifampin, tolbutamide, warfarin, or zidovudine.

What are the possible side effects of this medication?
Please see general statement regarding side effects on page xiii.

Side effects may include: abdominal pain, blurred vision, bruising, change in your appetite, chest pain, constipation, depression, diarrhea, dizziness, drowsiness, emotional instability, fever, "flu-like" symptoms, hair loss, headache, indigestion, infections, lack of coordination, memory loss, nausea, nervousness, runny nose, shortness of breath, skin rash, sleep problems, sore throat, swelling, thinking abnormally, tremors, visual abnormalities, vomiting, weakness, weight changes

---

Can I receive this medication if I am pregnant or breastfeeding?

Depakote ER can cause harm to your unborn baby if you take it during pregnancy. Depakote ER can be found in your breast milk if you take it while breastfeeding. Tell your doctor immediately if you are pregnant, plan to become pregnant, or are breastfeeding.

What should I do if I miss a dose of this medication?

If you miss a dose of Depakote ER, take it dose as soon as you remember. However, if it is almost time for your next dose, skip the one you missed and return to your regular dosing schedule. Do not take two doses at once.

How should I store this medication?

Store at room temperature.

Desloratadine: *see Clarinex, page 228*

Desloratadine/Pseudoephedrine Sulfate: *see Clarinex-D 12 Hour, page 231*

Desloratadine/Pseudoephedrine Sulfate: *see Clarinex-D 24 Hour, page 233*

Desonate
Generic name: Desonide

What is this medication?
Desonate is a topical gel (applied to the skin surface) that is used for the relief of inflammation and itching of the skin.

What is the most important information I should know about this medication?
- Desonate is for external use only. Do not use it in your eyes.
- Desonate can have a greater effect on children because they are more likely to absorb large amounts of the medicine through the skin. Long-term use can affect the growth and development of children. Talk to your doctor if you think your child is not growing at a normal rate after using this medication for a long period of time.
- Do not use Desonate for any other condition other than that which your doctor has prescribed.
- Contact your doctor if you notice irritation or any skin reactions in the area being treated or if your condition does not improve within four weeks of treatment.

Who should not take this medication?
Do not use Desonate if you are allergic to it or any of its ingredients.

What should I tell my doctor before I take the first dose of this medication?
Tell your doctor about all prescription, over-the-counter, and herbal medications you are taking before beginning treatment with Desonate. Also, talk to your doctor about your complete medical history, especially if you are pregnant, plan to become pregnant, or are breastfeeding.

What is the usual dosage?
Please see general statement regarding dosage on page xii.

Adults and children ≥3 months: Apply a thin layer of gel to the affected area(s) twice a day, for no longer than 4 consecutive weeks.

How should I take this medication?
- Apply Desonate exactly as prescribed by your doctor. Do not apply extra doses or apply more often without asking your doctor.
- Rub the gel into your skin gently.

What should I avoid while taking this medication?
Do not use Desonate in your eyes.

Do not bandage, cover, or wrap the treated skin area.

What are possible food and drug interactions associated with this medication?
No significant interactions have been reported with Desonate at this time. However, always tell your doctor about any medicines you take, including over-the-counter medications, vitamins, and herbal supplements.

What are the possible side effects of this medication?
Please see general statement regarding side effects on page xiii.

> **Side effects may include:** acne (pimples), application-site burning or itching, dermatitis (inflammation of the skin), headache, infection, inflammation of the follicles, rash, telangiectasia (widely open blood vessels in the outer layer of the skin)

Can I receive this medication if I am pregnant or breastfeeding?
The effects of Desonate during pregnancy and breastfeeding are unknown. Tell your doctor immediately if you are pregnant, plan to become pregnant, or are breastfeeding.

What should I do if I miss a dose of this medication?
If you miss a dose of Desonate, apply it as soon as you remember. However, if it is almost time for your next dose, skip the one you missed and return to your regular dosing schedule. Do not apply two doses at once.

How should I store this medication?
Store at room temperature.

Desonide: *see Desonate, page 303*

Desvenlafaxine: *see Pristiq, page 838*

Detrol
Generic name: Tolterodine Tartrate

What is this medication?
Detrol treats symptoms of overactive bladder, including frequent urination, urgency (increased need to urinate), and urge incontinence (inability to control urination).

What is the most important information I should know about this medication?
• In a limited number of people, Detrol causes blurred vision, dizziness, or drowsiness. Do not drive or operate machinery until you know how the drug affects you.

Who should not take this medication?
Do not take Detrol if you suffer from urinary retention (inability to urinate normally), gastric retention (a blockage in the digestive system), or uncontrolled narrow-angle glaucoma (high pressure in the eyes). You should also avoid this drug if it gives you an allergic reaction.

What should I tell my doctor before I take the first dose of this medication?
Tell your doctor about all prescription, over-the-counter, and herbal medications you are taking before beginning treatment with Detrol. Also, talk to your doctor about your complete medical history, especially if you have any of the following: a bladder obstruction or digestive disorder that could lead to a complete blockage,

glaucoma, myasthenia gravis (a disease that results in loss of muscular control), or problems with your heart, liver, or kidneys.

What is the usual dosage?

Please see general statement regarding dosage on page xii.

Adults: The usual starting dose is 2 milligrams (mg) twice a day. Some patients may need a lower dose of 1 mg twice a day.

How should I take this medication?

• Detrol can be taken with or without food. Swallow Detrol capsules whole at the same time each day.

What should I avoid while taking this medication?

Do not operate heavy machinery, drive, or do other dangerous activities until you know how Detrol affects you.

What are possible food and drug interactions associated with this medication?

If you take Detrol with certain other drugs, the effects of either could be increased, decreased, or altered. It is especially important to check with your doctor before combining Detrol with any of the following: clarithromycin, cyclosporine, erythromycin, itraconazole, ketoconazole, miconazole, and vinblastine.

What are the possible side effects of this medication?

Please see general statement regarding side effects on page xiii.

Side effects may include: stomach pain, blurred vision, constipation, diarrhea, dizziness, drowsiness, dry eyes, dry mouth, fatigue, flu-like symptoms, headache, indigestion

Can I receive this medication if I am pregnant or breastfeeding?

The effects of Detrol during pregnancy and breastfeeding are unknown. Tell your doctor immediately if you are pregnant, plan to become pregnant, or are breastfeeding.

What should I do if I miss a dose of this medication?
If you miss a dose of Detrol, skip it. Do not take two doses at once.

How should I store this medication?
Store at room temperature.

Detrol LA
Generic name: Tolterodine Tartrate

What is this medication?
Detrol LA is a medicine used to treat symptoms of overactive bladder, including frequent urination, urgency (increased need to urinate), and urge incontinence (inability to control urination).

What is the most important information I should know about this medication?
• Detrol LA can cause drowsiness or blurred vision. Do not drive, operate machinery, or engage in other dangerous activities until you know how Detrol LA affects you.

Who should not take this medication?
Do not take Detrol LA if you have urinary retention (inability to urinate normally), gastric retention (a blockage in the digestive system), or glaucoma (high pressure in the eye).

Do not take Detrol LA if you are allergic to it, any of its ingredients, or a similar medication called fesoterodine (Toviaz).

What should I tell my doctor before I take the first dose of this medication?
Tell your doctor about all prescription, over-the-counter, and herbal medications you are taking before beginning treatment with Detrol LA. Also, talk to your doctor about your complete medical history, especially if you have stomach or intestinal problems, urinary retention, glaucoma, kidney or liver problems, myasthenia gravis (a disease characterized by long-lasting fatigue and muscle

weakness), or a family history of irregular heartbeat; or if you are
pregnant, plan to become pregnant, or are breastfeeding.

What is the usual dosage?
Please see general statement regarding dosage on page xii.

Adults: The recommended dose is 4 milligrams once a day.

If you have severe kidney or liver impairment, or are taking certain
medications that can interact with Detrol LA, your doctor will adjust
your dose appropriately.

How should I take this medication?
- Take Detrol LA exactly as prescribed by your doctor. You can
  take Detrol LA with or without food at the same time each day.
- Swallow Detrol LA capsules whole. Do not chew, divide, or
  crush tablets.

What should I avoid while taking this medication?
Do not drive, operate machinery, or engage in other dangerous
activities until you know how Detrol LA affects you.

What are possible food and drug interactions associated
with this medication?
If you take Detrol LA with certain other drugs, the effects of either
could be increased, decreased, or altered. It is especially important
to check with your doctor before combining Detrol LA with any
of the following: clarithromycin, certain antibiotics (such as clarithromycin, erythromycin, or rifampin), certain antifungals (such
as itraconazole, ketoconazole, or miconazole), certain medications
for the treatment of HIV infection (such as atazanavir, ritonavir, or
squinavir), cyclosporine, fluoxetine, or vinblastine.

What are the possible side effects of this medication?
Please see general statement regarding side effects on page xiii.

Side effects may include: blurred vision, constipation, dizziness,
drowsiness, dry mouth, headache, stomach pain

Can I receive this medication if I am pregnant or breastfeeding?

The effects of Detrol LA during pregnancy and breastfeeding are unknown. Do not take Detrol LA during breastfeeding. Tell your doctor immediately if you are pregnant, plan to become pregnant, or are breastfeeding.

What should I do if I miss a dose of this medication?

If you miss a dose of Detrol LA, take it as soon as you remember. However, if it is almost time for your next dose, skip the one you missed and return to your regular dosing schedule. Do not take two doses at once.

How should I store this medication?

Store at room temperature. Protect from light. Keep in a dry place.

Dexamethasone/Tobramycin: *see Tobradex, page 994*

Dexilant

Generic name: Dexlansoprazole

What is this medication?

Dexilant is a medicine called a proton pump inhibitor (PPI). It reduces the amount of acid in your stomach. Dexilant is used to treat heartburn related to gastroesophageal reflux disease, to heal erosive esophagitis (inflammation and ulceration of the esophagus [the tube that connects your mouth and stomach]), to continue healing erosive esophagitis, and relieve heartburn.

What is the most important information I should know about this medication?

• Dexilant can cause low magnesium levels in your body. Tell your doctor immediately if you have seizures, dizziness, abnormal or fast heartbeat, jitteriness, jerking movements or shaking, muscle weakness, spasms of your hands and feet, cramps or muscle aches, or spasm of your voice box.

- Tell your doctor if you experience any symptoms of a serious allergic reaction with Dexilant (such as rash, face swelling, throat tightness, or difficulty breathing).
- People who are taking multiple daily doses of Dexilant for a long period of time may have an increased risk of fractures of the hip, wrist, or spine.

Who should not take this medication?

Do not take Dexilant if you are allergic to it or any of its ingredients.

What should I tell my doctor before I take the first dose of this medication?

Tell your doctor about all prescription, over-the-counter, and herbal medications you are taking before beginning treatment with Dexilant. Also, talk to your doctor about your complete medical history, especially if you have low magnesium levels, any allergies, or liver problems. Tell your doctor if you are pregnant, plan to become pregnant, or are breastfeeding.

What is the usual dosage?

Please see general statement regarding dosage on page xii.

Healing of Erosive Esophagitis

Adults: The recommended dose is 60 milligrams (mg) once a day for up to 8 weeks. Your doctor may prescribe a lower dose if you have liver problems.

Maintenance of Healed Erosive Esophagitis or Relief of Heartburn

Adults: The recommended dose is 30 mg once a day for up to 6 months.

Heartburn Associated with Gastroesophageal Reflux Disease

Adults: The recommended dose is 30 mg once a day for 4 weeks.

How should I take this medication?

- Take Dexilant exactly as prescribed by your doctor. You can take Dexilant with or without food.

- Swallow Dexilant capsules whole. If you have trouble with this, open the capsules and sprinkle the contents on a tablespoon of applesauce. Swallow the applesauce mixture immediately. Do not chew the mixture or store for later use.

What should I avoid while taking this medication?

Do not change your dose or stop taking Dexilant without talking to your doctor first.

What are possible food and drug interactions associated with this medication?

If Dexilant is taken with certain other drugs, the effects of either could be increased, decreased, or altered. It is especially important to check with your doctor before combining Dexilant with the following: ampicillin, atazanavir, digoxin, ketoconazole, methotrexate, products that contain iron, tacrolimus, or warfarin.

What are the possible side effects of this medication?

Please see general statement regarding side effects on page xiii.

> **Side effects may include:** common cold, diarrhea, gas, nausea, stomach pain, vomiting

Can I receive this medication if I am pregnant or breastfeeding?

The effects of Dexilant during pregnancy and breastfeeding are unknown. Tell your doctor immediately if you are pregnant, plan to become pregnant, or are breastfeeding.

What should I do if I miss a dose of this medication?

If you miss a dose of Dexilant, take it as soon as you remember. However, if it is almost time for your next dose, skip the one you missed and return to your regular dosing schedule. Do not take two doses at once.

How should I store this medication?

Store at room temperature.

Dexlansoprazole: see Dexilant, page 309

Dexmethylphenidate HCl: see Focalin XR, page 405

Dextromethorphan HBr/Promethazine HCl: see Promethazine DM, page 847

Diazepam: see Valium, page 1044

Diclofenac sodium
Generic name: Diclofenac Sodium

What is this medication?
Diclofenac sodium is a nonsteroidal anti-inflammatory drug (NSAID) used to treat signs and symptoms of rheumatoid arthritis, osteoarthritis, and ankylosing spondylitis (arthritis of the spine).

What is the most important information I should know about this medication?
- Diclofenac sodium can cause serious problems (such as heart attack or stroke). Your risk can increase when this medication is used for long periods of time and in people who have heart disease. Tell your doctor if you experience chest pain, shortness of breath, weakness, or slurred speech. Also, diclofenac sodium can cause high blood pressure or worsening of existing high blood pressure, and heart failure which can lead to weight gain or edema (swelling).
- Diclofenac sodium can cause discomfort, ulcers, or bleeding in your stomach or intestines. Your risk can increase with long-term use, smoking, drinking alcohol, older age, or with certain medications. Tell your doctor immediately if you experience abdominal pain or if you have bloody vomit or stools.
- Long-term use of diclofenac sodium can cause kidney injury. Your risk can increase if you have kidney impairment; heart failure; liver problems; are taking certain medications, including diuretics (water pills) (such as furosemide) or blood/heart medications known as angiotensin-converting enzyme (ACE)

inhibitors (such as lisinopril); are dehydrated; or are elderly. Also, diclofenac sodium can cause liver injury. Tell your doctor if you experience nausea, tiredness, weakness, itchiness, yellowing of your skin or whites of your eyes, right upper abdominal tenderness, or "flu-like" symptoms.

- Diclofenac sodium can cause allergic reactions resembling anaphylaxis (a serious and rapid allergic reaction that may result in death if not immediately treated). Stop taking diclofenac sodium and tell your doctor immediately if you experience difficulty breathing or swelling of your face, mouth, or throat.

- Tell your doctor immediately if you experience serious skin reactions which can be characterized by a severe rash, fever, or itchiness.

Who should not take this medication?

Do not take diclofenac sodium if you are allergic to it, any of its ingredients, or if you experienced asthma, difficulty breathing, rash, or allergic-type reactions after taking aspirin or other NSAIDs.

Do not take diclofenac sodium right before or after a heart surgery called coronary artery bypass graft (CABG).

What should I tell my doctor before I take the first dose of this medication?

Tell your doctor about all prescription, over-the-counter, and herbal medications you are taking before beginning treatment with diclofenac sodium. Also, talk to your doctor about your complete medical history, especially if you have heart disease, stomach problems, kidney or liver impairment, high blood pressure, asthma, or are pregnant or plan to become pregnant.

What is the usual dosage?

Please see general statement regarding dosage on page xii.

Osteoarthritis

Adults: The recommended dose is 100-150 milligrams (mg) a day, divided into smaller doses taken 2-3 times a day. Your doctor will adjust the dose for you based on your response to this medication.

Rheumatoid Arthritis
Adults: The recommended dose is 150-200 mg a day, divided into smaller doses taken 2-4 times a day. Your doctor will adjust the dose for you based on your response to this medication.

Ankylosing Spondylitis
Adults: The recommended dose is 100-125 mg a day, divided into smaller doses taken 4-5 times a day. Your doctor will adjust the dose for you based on your response to this medication.

How should I take this medication?
• Take diclofenac sodium exactly as prescribed by your doctor.

What should I avoid while taking this medication?
Do not take aspirin or other NSAIDs in combination with diclofenac sodium.

What are possible food and drug interactions associated with this medication?
If diclofenac sodium is taken with certain other drugs, the effects of either could be increased, decreased, or altered. It is especially important to check with your doctor before combining diclofenac sodium with the following: ACE inhibitors, aspirin, blood thinners (such as warfarin), cyclosporine, diuretics, lithium, or methotrexate.

What are the possible side effects of this medication?
Please see general statement regarding side effects on page xiii.

> **Side effects may include:** abdominal or stomach pain, bleeding, constipation, diarrhea, dizziness, gas, headache, heartburn, indigestion, itchiness, nausea, rash, ringing in your ear, swelling, vomiting

Can I receive this medication if I am pregnant or breastfeeding?
Do not take diclofenac sodium if you are in the late stage of your pregnancy. The effects of diclofenac sodium during early pregnancy

and breastfeeding are unknown. Tell your doctor immediately if you are pregnant, plan to become pregnant, or are breastfeeding.

What should I do if I miss a dose of this medication?

If you miss a dose of diclofenac sodium, take it as soon as you remember. However, if it is almost time for your next dose, skip the one you missed and return to your regular dosing schedule. Do not take two doses at once.

How should I store this medication?

Store at room temperature. Protect from light and moisture.

Diclofenac Sodium: *see Diclofenac sodium, page 312*

Diclofenac Sodium: *see Voltaren-XR, page 1083*

Dicyclomine HCl: *see Bentyl, page 138*

Dificid

Generic name: Fidaxomicin

What is this medication?

Dificid is a medicine used to treat diarrhea caused by a bacteria called *Clostridium difficile*.

What is the most important information I should know about this medication?

- Take Dificid for the full length of time that your doctor has prescribed. If you skip doses or do not complete the full course of therapy, the effectiveness of Dificid in treating your infection may decrease and there is a risk that the disease will not be treatable with Dificid or other similar medications in the future.
- This medication is for use only to treat diarrhea caused by *Clostridium difficile*. Dificid will not treat viral infections such as the common cold or flu.

Who should not take this medication?
Do not use Dificid if you are allergic to it or any of its ingredients.

What should I tell my doctor before I take the first dose of this medication?
Tell your doctor about all prescription, over-the-counter, and herbal medications you are taking before beginning treatment with Dificid. Also, talk to your doctor about your complete medical history, especially if you are pregnant or plan to become pregnant, or are breastfeeding, or plan to breastfeed.

What is the usual dosage?
Please see general statement regarding dosage on page xii.

Adults: The recommended dose is 200 milligrams (mg) twice a day for 10 days.

How should I take this medication?
• Take Dificid exactly as prescribed by your doctor. You can take it with or without food.

What should I avoid while taking this medication?
Do not miss any doses.

What are possible food and drug interactions associated with this medication?
No significant interactions have been reported with Dificid at this time. However, always tell your doctor about any medicines you take, including over-the-counter medications, vitamins, and herbal supplements.

What are the possible side effects of this medication?
Please see general statement regarding side effects on page xiii.

Side effects may include: bloating, bloody or tarry stools, coughing up blood, difficulty swallowing, gas, itching, nausea, rash, stomach pain/tenderness, vomiting

Can I receive this medication if I am pregnant or breastfeeding?

The effects of Dificid during pregnancy and breastfeeding are un-known. Tell your doctor immediately if you are pregnant, plan to become pregnant, or are breastfeeding.

What should I do if I miss a dose of this medication?

If you miss a dose of Dificid, take it as soon as you remember. However, if it is almost time for your next dose, skip the one you missed and return to your regular dosing schedule. Do not take two doses at once.

How should I store this medication?

Store at room temperature.

Diflucan

Generic name: Fluconazole

What is this medication?

Diflucan is a medicine used to treat vaginal yeast infections. It is also used to treat certain fungal infections in your body. These in-fections are called oropharyngeal candidiasis, esophageal candi-diasis, and cryptococcal meningitis in patients with AIDS. In addi-tion, Diflucan is used to lower the risk of fungal infections in people undergoing bone marrow transplants who are receiving chemo-therapy. Diflucan is available in tablets, an oral suspension, and an intravenous solution (administered through a vein in your arm).

What is the most important information I should know about this medication?

- Diflucan can cause liver damage. Tell your doctor if your skin or eyes become yellow, your urine turns a darker color, your stools are light-colored, if you vomit or feel like vomiting, or if you have severe skin itching.
- Diflucan can cause serious allergic reactions or serious skin re-actions. Tell your doctor right away if you experience shortness of breath; coughing; wheezing; fever; chills; throbbing of your

heart or ears; swelling of your eyelids, face, mouth, neck, or any other part of your body; skin rash; hives, or skin blistering or peeling.
• Diflucan can cause QT prolongation (very fast or abnormal heartbeats) or arrhythmias (life-threatening irregular heartbeats).

Who should not take this medication?

Do not take Diflucan if you are allergic to it or any of its ingredients. Also, do not take Diflucan in combination with astemizole, cisapride, erythromycin, pimozide, or quinidine. Do not take Diflucan with terfenadine if you are taking more than 400 milligrams (mg) of Diflucan.

What should I tell my doctor before I take the first dose of this medication?

Tell your doctor about all prescription, over-the-counter, and herbal medications you are taking before beginning treatment with Diflucan. Also, talk to your doctor about your complete medical history, especially if you have heart, kidney, or liver problems; a serious condition (such as AIDS or cancer); or if you have problems absorbing sugar.

What is the usual dosage?

Please see general statement regarding dosage on page xii.

Vaginal Yeast Infection
Adults: The recommended dose is 150 mg as a single oral dose.

Oropharyngeal and Esophageal Candidiasis
Adults: The recommended dose is 200 mg on the first day, followed by 100 mg once a day.

Children: Your doctor will prescribe the appropriate dose for your child, based on their weight.

Cryptococcal Meningitis
Adults and children: Your doctor will administer the appropriate dose of Diflucan intravenously to you or your child.

Infection Prevention in Bone Marrow Transplant Patients
Adults: The recommended dose is 400 mg once a day.

If you have kidney impairment, your doctor will adjust your dose appropriately.

How should I take this medication?
- Take Diflucan tablets and oral suspension by mouth at any time of the day. You can take them with or without food. If there is no change in your symptoms after a few days, call your doctor.
- Shake the oral suspension well before you take the medicine. Throw away any unused amount of oral suspension after 2 weeks.
- Your doctor will administer Diflucan injection (intravenous solution) to you.

What should I avoid while taking this medication?
Do not start any new medicines within 7 days of taking Diflucan without talking to your doctor.

Do not drive or operate machinery until you know how Diflucan affects you.

What are possible food and drug interactions associated with this medication?
If Diflucan is taken with certain other drugs, the effects of either could be increased, decreased, or altered. Diflucan may interact with numerous medications. Therefore, it is very important that you tell your doctor about any other medications you are taking.

What are the possible side effects of this medication?
Please see general statement regarding side effects on page xiii.

Side effects may include: changes in the way food tastes, diarrhea, dizziness, headache, nausea, stomach pain

Can I receive this medication if I am pregnant or breastfeeding?

The effects of Diflucan during pregnancy are unknown. Diflucan can be found in your breast milk if you take it while breastfeeding. Tell your doctor immediately if you are pregnant, plan to become pregnant, or are breastfeeding.

What should I do if I miss a dose of this medication?

If you miss a dose of Diflucan, take it as soon as you remember. However, if it is almost time for your next dose, skip the one you missed and return to your regular dosing schedule. Do not take two doses at once.

How should I store this medication?

Store tablets and liquid at room temperature. Do not freeze.

Your doctor will store the intravenous solution.

Digoxin: see Lanoxin, page 521

Dilantin

Generic name: Phenytoin Sodium

What is this medication?

Dilantin is a medicine used to treat tonic-clonic (grand mal) and complex partial (psychomotor or temporal lobe) seizures. This medicine can also be used to prevent and treat seizures that happen during or after brain surgery. Dilantin is available as capsules, chewable tablets, and an oral suspension.

What is the most important information I should know about this medication?

- Do not stop taking Dilantin without first talking to your doctor. Stopping Dilantin suddenly can cause serious problems, including seizures that will not stop (status epilepticus).

- Dilantin can cause suicidal thoughts or actions. Tell your doctor immediately if you have thoughts about suicide or dying; attempt to commit suicide; have new or worsening depression, anxiety, or irritability; have panic attacks; have trouble sleeping (insomnia); have an extreme increase in activity and talking (mania); are feeling agitated or restless; acting aggressive; being angry or violent; acting on dangerous impulses; or have other unusual changes in behavior or mood.

- Dilantin can cause swollen lymph nodes (glands found throughout the body that remove bacteria and play an important role in your immune system). Your doctor will monitor you for this problem. Also, Dilantin can cause an overgrowth of your gums. Brushing and flossing your teeth and seeing a dentist regularly while you are taking Dilantin can help prevent this.

- Dilantin can also cause allergic reactions or serious problems, which can affect organs and other parts of your body, including your liver or blood cells. Contact your doctor immediately if you experience swelling of your face, eyes, lips, or tongue; trouble swallowing or breathing; a skin rash; fever; swollen lymph nodes or sore throat that do not go away or come and go; painful sores in your mouth or around your eyes; yellowing of your skin or whites of your eyes; unusual bruising or bleeding; severe tiredness or weakness; severe muscle pain; or frequent infections or an infection that does not go away.

Who should not take this medication?

Do not take Dilantin if you are allergic to it, any of its ingredients, or to other similar medications (such as ethotoin, fosphenytoin, or mephenytoin).

Do not take Dilantin oral suspension if you are taking an anti-HIV medication called delavirdine.

What should I tell my doctor before I take the first dose of this medication?

Tell your doctor about all prescription, over-the-counter, and herbal medications you are taking before beginning treatment with Dilantin. Also, talk to your doctor about your complete medical history, especially if you have or had liver disease, porphyria (a blood disorder that interferes with how your body produces heme, which is the oxygen-carrying component of your red blood cells), diabetes, depression, mood problems, suicidal thoughts or behavior, or if you are pregnant, plan to become pregnant, or are breastfeeding.

What is the usual dosage?
Please see general statement regarding dosage on page xii.

Adults: Your doctor will prescribe the appropriate dose for you based on your condition and will increase your dose as appropriate.

Children: Your doctor will prescribe the appropriate dose for your child, based on their weight.

How should I take this medication?
- Take Dilantin exactly as prescribed by your doctor. Do not change your dose or stop taking Dilantin without first talking to your doctor.
- Chew Dilantin Infatabs thoroughly before swallowing them or swallow them whole.
- Shake Dilantin oral suspension well before taking the medicine or giving it to your child.

What should I avoid while taking this medication?
Do not drink alcohol while you are taking Dilantin.

Do not drive, operate heavy machinery, or engage in other dangerous activities until you know how Dilantin affects you.

What are possible food and drug interactions associated with this medication?
If Dilantin is taken with certain other drugs, the effects of either could be increased, decreased, or altered. Dilantin may interact with numerous medications. Therefore, it is very important that you tell your doctor about any other medications you are taking.

What are the possible side effects of this medication?
Please see general statement regarding side effects on page xiii.

> **Side effects may include:** confusion, constipation, dizziness, headache, nausea, nervousness, problems with walking and coordination, rash, shaking, slurred speech, trouble sleeping, vomiting

Can I receive this medication if I am pregnant or breastfeeding?

Dilantin can harm your unborn baby if you take it during pregnancy. Dilantin can be found in your breast milk if you take it while breastfeeding. Do not breastfeed while you are taking Dilantin. Tell your doctor immediately if you are pregnant, plan to become pregnant, or are breastfeeding.

What should I do if I miss a dose of this medication?

If you miss a dose of Dilantin, take it as soon as you remember. However, if it is almost time for your next dose, skip the one you missed and return to your regular dosing schedule. Do not take two doses at once.

How should I store this medication?

Store at room temperature. Protect from light and moisture.

Dilaudid

Generic name: Hydromorphone HCl

What is this medication?

Dilaudid is a pain medicine that contains the narcotic painkiller hydromorphone. Dilaudid is used to treat pain. Dilaudid is available as tablets and a liquid.

Dilaudid is a federally controlled substance because it has abuse potential.

What is the most important information I should know about this medication?

- Dilaudid has abuse potential. Mental and physical dependence can occur with the use of Dilaudid when it is used improperly.

- Dilaudid can cause serious breathing problems that can become life-threatening, especially when it is used in the wrong way.
- Dilaudid can cause low blood pressure. You can experience dizziness, lightheadedness, or fainting.

Who should not take this medication?
Do not take Dilaudid if you are allergic to it or any of its ingredients.

Do not take Dilaudid if you have asthma or other breathing problems.

Do not take Dilaudid to treat pain associated with childbirth.

What should I tell my doctor before I take the first dose of this medication?
Tell your doctor about all prescription, over-the-counter, and herbal medications you are taking before beginning treatment with Dilaudid. Also, talk to your doctor about your complete medical history, especially if you have ever had liver or kidney problems, breathing problems, an underactive thyroid gland, Addison's disease (adrenal gland failure), an enlarged prostate, urethral stricture (narrowing of the urethra, the tube that connects from the bladder to the genitals to lead urine out of your body), gallbladder disease, kyphoscoliosis (an abnormal curve of the spine), head injury, stomach problems, seizures, a history of alcohol or drug abuse, or if you had stomach or intestinal surgery.

What is the usual dosage?
Please see general statement regarding dosage on page xii.

Dilaudid Liquid
Adults: The usual dose is 1/2 teaspoonful (2.5 milliliters [mL]) to 2 teaspoonfuls (10 mL) every 3-6 hours.

Dilaudid Tablets
Adults: The usual starting dose is 2-4 milligrams every 4-6 hours.

Your doctor will increase your dose as needed, until the desired effect is achieve.

How should I take this medication?
• Take Dilaudid exactly as prescribed by your doctor.

What should I avoid while taking this medication?
Do not drink alcohol while you are taking Dilaudid.

Do not drive or operate machinery until you know how Dilaudid affects you.

Do not change your dose or stop taking Dilaudid without first talking to your doctor. Stopping Dilaudid suddenly can cause side effects.

What are possible food and drug interactions associated with this medication?
If Dilaudid is taken with certain other drugs, the effects of either could be increased, decreased, or altered. It is especially important to check with your doctor before combining Dilaudid with the following: alcohol, buprenorphine, butorphanol, general anesthetics, nalbuphine, pentazocine, phenothiazines (such as chlorpromazine), sedative-hypnotics (such as alprazolam or lorazepam), or tranquilizers (such as thioridazine).

What are the possible side effects of this medication?
Please see general statement regarding side effects on page xiii.

> **Side effects may include:** dizziness, dry mouth, dysphoria (feeling unwell and unhappy), euphoria (a feeling of happiness and well-being), flushing, itching, lightheadedness, nausea, sedation, sweating, vomiting

Can I receive this medication if I am pregnant or breastfeeding?
The effects of Dilaudid during pregnancy are unknown. Dilaudid can be found in your breast milk if you take it while breastfeeding. Do not breastfeed while you are taking Dilaudid. Tell your doctor immediately if you are pregnant, plan to become pregnant, or are breastfeeding.

What should I do if I miss a dose of this medication?

If you miss a dose of Dilaudid, take it as soon as you remember. However, if it is almost time for your next dose, skip the one you missed and return to your regular dosing schedule. Do not take two doses at once.

How should I store this medication?

Store at room temperature. Protect from light.

Diltiazem HCl: *see Cardizem, page 181*

Diltiazem HCl: *see Cardizem CD, page 183*

Diltiazem HCl: *see Cartia XT, page 188*

Diovan

Generic name: Valsartan

What is this medication?

Diovan is a medicine called an angiotensin receptor blocker used in adults to treat high blood pressure, heart failure, and improve the chances of living longer after a heart attack. It is also used in children to treat high blood pressure.

What is the most important information I should know about this medication?

- Diovan should not be taken during pregnancy. If you become pregnant, stop taking Diovan and call your doctor right away.
- Diovan may cause low blood pressure, especially if you take diuretics (water pills), are on a low-salt diet, receive dialysis, have heart problems, or get sick with vomiting or diarrhea. Lie down if you feel faint or dizzy and call your doctor right away.

Who should not take this medication?

Do not take Diovan if you are allergic to any of its ingredients, or if you are pregnant. Diovan is not for children with certain kidney problems.

What should I tell my doctor before I take the first dose of this medication?

Tell your doctor about all prescription, over-the-counter, and herbal medications you are taking, before beginning treatment with Diovan. Also, talk to your doctor about your complete medical history, especially if you are pregnant, plan to become pregnant, or are breastfeeding. Also, tell your doctor if you have heart, liver, or kidney problems.

What is the usual dosage?

Please see general statement regarding dosage on page xii.

Blood Pressure

Adults: The starting dose of Diovan is 80 milligrams (mg) or 160 mg once daily. The usual dose of Diovan can range from 80-320 mg once daily.

Children 6-16 years old: Your doctor will prescribe the appropriate dose for your child.

Heart Attack Survivor

Adults: Diovan may be started as early as 12 hours after a heart attack. The recommended starting dose of Diovan is 20 mg twice daily. The usual dose ranges from 20-160 mg twice daily.

Heart Failure

Adults: The recommended starting dose of Diovan is 40 mg twice daily. The usual dose ranges from 40-160 mg twice daily.

How should I take this medication?

- Diovan may be taken with or without food.
- For children who cannot swallow the tablets, your pharmacist will mix this medicine as a liquid suspension. Shake the bottle

of suspension well for at least 10 seconds before giving it to your child.
• Carefully follow your doctor's instructions about any special diet. For treatment of high blood pressure, take Diovan once daily at the same time each day. For treatment of heart failure or after a heart attack, take Diovan twice a day at the same times each day.

What should I avoid while taking this medication?

Avoid becoming pregnant while taking Diovan. Do not take potassium supplements or salt substitutes containing potassium while on Diovan; doing so may lead to increases in potassium levels in your body and may worsen your condition if you have heart failure.

What are possible food and drug interactions associated with this medication?

If Diovan is taken with certain other drugs, the effects of either could be increased, decreased, or altered. It is especially important to check with your doctor before combining Diovan with the following: diuretics (water pills), potassium supplements, or salt substitutes.

What are the possible side effects of this medication?

Please see general statement regarding side effects on page xiii.

Side effects may include: back pain, cough, diarrhea, dizziness, flu symptoms, headache, high blood potassium, joint pain, low blood pressure, rash, stomach pain, tiredness

Can I receive this medication if I am pregnant or breastfeeding?

If you become pregnant while taking Diovan, stop taking it and call your doctor right away. Diovan can harm an unborn baby, causing injury and even death. If you plan to become pregnant, talk to your doctor about other treatment options before taking Diovan. Diovan may pass through your breast milk and cause harm. Notify your doctor if you are breastfeeding.

What should I do if I miss a dose of this medication?

Take the missed dose as soon as you remember. However, if it is almost time for your next dose, skip the one you missed and return to your regular dosing schedule. Do not take two doses at once.

How should I store this medication?

Store at room temperature. Store the bottle of suspension at room temperature for up to 30 days, or in the refrigerator for up to 75 days.

Diovan HCT

Generic name: Hydrochlorothiazide/Valsartan

What is this medication?

Diovan HCT is a combination medicine used to treat high blood pressure. Diovan HCT contains two medicines: valsartan (an angiotensin receptor blocker [ARB]) and hydrochlorothiazide (a diuretic [water pill]).

What is the most important information I should know about this medication?

- When taken during pregnancy, ARBs such as Diovan HCT can cause injury to the unborn baby. If you are pregnant or plan to become pregnant, stop taking Diovan HCT and contact your doctor right away.
- Diovan HCT can cause low blood pressure, especially if you take diuretics or are on a low-salt diet, receive dialysis, have heart problems, get sick with vomiting or diarrhea, or if you drink alcohol. If you feel faint or dizzy, lie down and call your doctor right away.
- Diovan HCT can cause a serious allergic reaction. Call your doctor right away if you develop an unusual skin rash.
- Diovan HCT can activate lupus (disease that affects the immune system) or gout (severe and painful inflammation of the joints) and increase cholesterol and triglyceride levels in certain patients.

- Diovan HCT can cause problems seeing objects that are farther away, as well as acute angle-closure glaucoma (high pressure in the eye). Tell your doctor immediately if you experience abnormal visual changes or eye pain.
- Diovan HCT can cause imbalances in fluids and electrolytes (chemicals that are important for the cells in your body to function, such as sodium and potassium). Signs and symptoms of this include dry mouth, thirst, weakness, fatigue, drowsiness, restlessness, confusion, seizures, muscle pain or cramps, low blood pressure, decreased urination, fast heart rate, nausea, and vomiting. Your doctor will monitor your blood electrolyte levels periodically during treatment with Diovan HCT.
- Diovan HCT can worsen your kidney function if you already have kidney problems. Tell your doctor if your feet, ankles, or hands become swollen, or unexplained weight gain.
- If you have diabetes, Diovan HCT can increase your blood sugar levels. Check your blood sugar frequently.

Who should not take this medication?
Do not take Diovan HCT if you are allergic to it or any of its ingredients, or to a sulfonamide-derived medication.

Do not take Diovan HCT if you are unable to produce urine.

What should I tell my doctor before I take the first dose of this medication?
Tell your doctor about all prescription, over-the-counter, and herbal medications you are taking before beginning treatment with Diovan HCT. Also, talk to your doctor if you have diabetes, heart failure, severe immune system problems, lupus, asthma, liver or kidney disease, gallstones, or if you have ever had an allergy or sensitivity to an ARB or sulfonamide-derived medication.

What is the usual dosage?
Please see general statement regarding dosage on page xii.

Adults: The usual starting dose is 160/12.5 (160 milligrams [mg] of valsartan and 12.5 mg of hydrochlorothiazide) once a day. Your doctor may give you a higher dose, depending on your needs.

How should I take this medication?
- Take Diovan HCT exactly as prescribed by your doctor. Take Diovan HCT once a day. Take it with or without food.

What should I avoid while taking this medication?
Do not become pregnant or breastfeed while you are taking Diovan HCT.

Do not become dehydrated. Drink adequate amounts of fluids while you are taking Diovan HCT to avoid becoming dehydrated.

What are possible food and drug interactions associated with this medication?
If Diovan HCT is taken with certain other drugs, the effects of either could be increased, decreased, or altered. It is especially important to check with your doctor before combining Diovan HCT with the following: alcohol, barbiturates (such as phenobarbital), carbamazapine, cholestyramine, colestipol, cyclosporine, diabetes medicines (such as insulin), digoxin, lithium, muscle relaxants (such as tubocurarine), narcotic painkillers (such as hydrocodone or oxycodone), nonsteroidal anti-inflammatory drugs (NSAIDs) (such as ibuprofen or naproxen), potassium supplements, rifampin, salt substitutes that contain potassium, or water pill.

What are the possible side effects of this medication?
Please see general statement regarding side effects on page xiii.

> **Side effects may include:** common cold, dizziness, headache

Can I receive this medication if I am pregnant or breastfeeding?
Do not take Diovan HCT if you are pregnant or breastfeeding. Diovan HCT can harm your unborn baby. It can be found in your breast milk if you take it while breastfeeding. Tell your doctor immediately if you are pregnant, plan to become pregnant, or are breastfeeding.

What should I do if I miss a dose of this medication?
If you miss a dose of Diovan HCT, take it as soon as you remember. However, if it is almost time for your next dose, skip the one you missed and return to your regular dosing schedule. Do not take two doses at once.

How should I store this medication?
Store at room temperature. Protect from moisture.

Divalproex Sodium: see Depakote, page 296

Divalproex Sodium: see Depakote ER, page 299

Donepezil HCl: see Aricept, page 87

Dorzolamide HCl/Timolol Maleate: see Cosopt, page 274

Doxazosin Mesylate: see Cardura, page 185

Doxepin
Generic name: Doxepin HCl

What is this medication?
Doxepin is a medicine used to treat depression and anxiety.

What is the most important information I should know about this medication?
- Doxepin can increase suicidal thoughts or actions in some children, teenagers, and young adults within the first few months of treatment.
- Depression and other serious mental illnesses are the most important causes of suicidal thoughts and actions. You may have a particularly high risk of having suicidal thoughts or actions if you have (or have a family history of) bipolar illness (also called manic-depressive illness).

- Pay close attention to any changes, especially sudden changes, in mood, behaviors, thoughts, or feelings. Tell your doctor right away if you develop any changes. This is very important when doxepin is started or when the dose is changed.
- Keep all follow-up visits with your doctor as scheduled. Call your doctor between visits as needed, especially if you have concerns about symptoms.

Who should not take this medication?

Do not take doxepin if you are allergic to it or any of its ingredients.

Do not take doxepin if you have glaucoma (high pressure in the eyes) or difficulty urinating.

Do not take doxepin in combination with monoamine oxidase inhibitors (MAOIs), a class of drugs used to treat depression and other psychiatric conditions. You must wait at least 14 days after stopping an MAOI before starting doxepin.

What should I tell my doctor before I take the first dose of this medication?

Tell your doctor about all prescription, over-the-counter, and herbal medications you are taking before beginning treatment with doxepin. Also, talk to your doctor about your complete medical history, especially if you have a history of bipolar disorder or suicidal thoughts or actions; have liver, kidney, or heart problems; have glaucoma or difficulty urinating; or are pregnant, plan to become pregnant, or are breastfeeding.

What is the usual dosage?

Please see general statement regarding dosage on page xii.

Adults: The recommended starting dose is 75 milligrams (mg) a day. Your doctor may increase your dose as appropriate.

How should I take this medication?

- Take doxepin exactly as prescribed by your doctor. You can take doxepin once a day or in divided doses. If you take doxepin once a day, you can take it at bedtime.

What should I avoid while taking this medication?

Do not drive a car or operate dangerous machinery until you know how doxepin affects you. Doxepin can cause drowsiness.

Do not drink alcohol or take other medications that can make you sleepy while you are taking doxepin.

Do not excessively expose yourself to sunlight while you are taking doxepin.

What are possible food and drug interactions associated with this medication?

If doxepin is taken with certain other drugs, the effects of either could be increased, decreased, or altered. It is especially important to check with your doctor before combining doxepin with the following: alcohol, certain antidepressants (such as fluoxetine, paroxetine, or sertraline), carbamazepine, cimetidine, flecainide, MAOIs, propafenone, quinidine, or tolazamide.

What are the possible side effects of this medication?

Please see general statement regarding side effects on page xiii.

Side effects may include: blurred vision, breathing problems, changes in blood pressure, changes in blood sugar levels, chills, confusion, constipation, diarrhea, dizziness, drowsiness, dry mouth, enlargement of breasts, fever, flushing, hair loss, headache, indigestion, itching, light sensitivity, loss of appetite, loss of muscle coordination, nausea, numbness or tingling in your hands or feet, rapid or irregular heartbeat, rash, seizures, swelling, taste disturbances, tiredness, trouble urinating, vomiting, weakness, weight changes

Can I receive this medication if I am pregnant or breastfeeding?

The effects of doxepin during pregnancy and breastfeeding are unknown. Tell your doctor immediately if you are pregnant, plan to become pregnant, or are breastfeeding.

What should I do if I miss a dose of this medication?

If you miss a dose of doxepin, take it as soon as you remember. However, if it is almost time for your next dose, skip the one you missed and return to your regular dosing schedule. Do not take two doses at once.

How should I store this medication?

Store at room temperature.

Doxepin HCl: *see Doxepin, page 332*

Doxycycline Monohydrate: *see Monodox, page 649*

Dronedarone: *see Multaq, page 662*

Drospirenone/Ethinyl Estradiol: *see Yasmin, page 1114*

Drospirenone/Ethinyl Estradiol: *see Yaz, page 1118*

Drospirenone/Ethinyl Estradiol/Levomefolate Calcium: *see Beyaz, page 144*

Duexis

Generic name: Famotidine/Ibuprofen

What is this medication?

Duexis is a medicine that contains ibuprofen (a nonsteroidal anti-inflammatory drug [NSAID]) and famotidine (a medicine that helps to reduce the acid in your stomach). Duexis is used to relieve the signs and symptoms of rheumatoid arthritis and osteoarthritis. Duexis also decreases the risk of developing ulcers of the stomach and upper intestines in people who are taking ibuprofen for rheumatoid arthritis and osteoarthritis.

What is the most important information I should know about this medication?

- Duexis can cause serious problems (such as heart attack or stroke). Your risk can increase when this medication is used for long periods of time and in people who have heart disease. Tell your doctor if you experience chest pain, shortness of breath, weakness, or slurred speech. Also, Duexis can cause heart failure, which can lead to weight gain or edema (swelling).

- Duexis can cause discomfort, ulcers, or bleeding in your stomach or intestines. Your risk can increase with long-term use, smoking, drinking alcohol, older age, or with certain medications. Tell your doctor immediately if you experience abdominal pain or if you have bloody vomit or stools.

- Long-term use of Duexis can cause kidney injury. Your risk can increase if you have kidney impairment; heart failure; liver problems; are taking certain medications, including diuretics (water pills) (such as furosemide) or blood/heart medications known as angiotensin-converting enzyme (ACE) inhibitors (such as lisinopril); or are elderly. Also, Duexis can cause liver injury. Tell your doctor if you experience nausea, tiredness, weakness, itchiness, yellowing of your skin or whites of your eyes, right upper abdominal tenderness, or "flu-like" symptoms.

- Duexis can cause allergic reactions resembling anaphylaxis (a serious and rapid allergic reaction that may result in death if not immediately treated). Stop taking Duexis and tell your doctor immediately if you experience difficulty breathing or swelling of your face, mouth, or throat.

- Tell your doctor immediately if you experience serious skin reactions which can be characterized by a severe rash, fever, or itchiness.

Who should not take this medication?

Do not take Duexis if you are allergic to it, any of its ingredients, or if you experienced asthma, difficulty breathing, rash, or allergic-type reactions after taking aspirin or other NSAIDs.

Do not take Duexis right before or after a heart surgery called coronary artery bypass graft (CABG) or if you are in the late stages of your pregnancy.

What should I tell my doctor before I take the first dose of this medication?

Tell your doctor about all prescription, over-the-counter, and herbal medications you are taking before beginning treatment with Duexis. Also, talk to your doctor about your complete medical history, especially if you have high blood pressure, heart problems, a history of stomach ulcers, bleeding problems, liver or kidney problems, ulcerative colitis or Crohn's disease (a disease which causes inflammation of the intestine), or are pregnant, plan to become pregnant, or are breastfeeding.

What is the usual dosage?

.*Please see general statement regarding dosage on page xii.*

Adults: The recommended dose is 1 tablet three times a day.

How should I take this medication?

- Take Duexis exactly as prescribed by your doctor. Do not stop Duexis without first talking to your doctor.
- Swallow Duexis tablets whole. Do not cut, chew, divide, or crush the tablets.

What should I avoid while taking this medication?

Do not miss your follow-up appointment with your doctor.

What are possible food and drug interactions associated with this medication?

If Duexis is taken with certain other drugs, the effects of either could be increased, decreased, or altered. It is especially important to check with your doctor before combining Duexis with the following: ACE inhibitors (such as enalapril or lisinopril), aspirin, blood thinners (such as warfarin), cholestyramine, certain antidepressant medications (such as fluoxetine or paroxetine), corticosteroids (such as prednisone), diuretics, lithium, or methotrexate.

What are the possible side effects of this medication?

Please see general statement regarding side effects on page xiii.

> **Side effects may include:** constipation, diarrhea, headache, high
> blood pressure, nausea, stomach pain, upper respiratory tract
> infection

Can I receive this medication if I am pregnant or breastfeeding?

Do not take Duexis if you are in the late stage of your pregnancy.
Duexis can be found in your breast milk if you take it while breastfeeding. Do not take Duexis while you are breastfeeding. Tell your
doctor immediately if you are pregnant, plan to become pregnant,
or are breastfeeding.

What should I do if I miss a dose of this medication?

If you miss a dose of Duexis, take it as soon as you remember.
However, if it is almost time for your next dose, skip the one you
missed and return to your regular dosing schedule. Do not take
two doses at once.

How should I store this medication?

Store in the original container at room temperature. Keep it dry and
keep the bottle tightly closed.

Duloxetine HCl: see Cymbalta, page 285

Duoneb

Generic name: Albuterol Sulfate/Ipratropium Bromide

What is this medication?

Duoneb is a combination of two medicines called bronchodilators.
These medicines work together to help open the airways in your
lungs. Duoneb is used to help treat airway narrowing (bronchospasm) that happens with chronic obstructive pulmonary disease
in adult patients requiring more than one bronchodilator medicine.

What is the most important information I should know about this medication?

- Duoneb is used with a nebulizer.
- Do not exceed the recommended dose or frequency of Duoneb without consulting with your doctor.
- Duoneb can cause the narrowing of the airways to get worse in some patients, which may be life-threatening. Stop taking Duoneb and call your doctor or get emergency help if this happens.
- Duoneb can cause serious allergic reactions. Symptoms include itching; swelling of your face, lips, tongue, or throat (which may cause difficulty in breathing or swallowing); skin rash; hives; airway narrowing; or anaphylaxis (a serious and rapid allergic reaction that may result in death if not immediately treated). Stop taking Duoneb and tell your doctor or get emergency help if you get any of these symptoms.
- Duoneb can cause serious heart-related side effects, such as an increase in pulse or blood pressure.

Who should not take this medication?

Do not use Duoneb if you are allergic to it or any of its ingredients.

Do not use Duoneb if you are allergic to atropine or other similar medicines.

What should I tell my doctor before I take the first dose of this medication?

Tell your doctor about all prescription, over-the-counter, and herbal medications you are taking before beginning treatment with Duoneb. Also, talk to your doctor about your complete medical history, especially if you have high blood pressure or heart problems, diabetes, seizures, an underactive thyroid gland, narrow-angle glaucoma (high pressure in the eye), liver or kidney problems, or problems urinating due to bladder-neck blockage or an enlarged prostate (men), or are pregnant, plan to become pregnant, or are breastfeeding.

What is the usual dosage?

Please see general statement regarding dosage on page xii.

Adults: The usual dose is one 3-milliliter (mL) vial administered four times a day via a nebulizer. An increase of two 3-mL doses may be added after consulting with your doctor.

How should I take this medication?

- Duoneb is administered via a jet nebulizer that is connected to an air compressor with adequate air flow, equipped with a face mask. Your doctor will show you how to use a nebulizer.
- Duoneb may help to open your airways for up to 5 hours after taking this medicine. If Duoneb does not help your airway narrowing or your symptoms get worse, call your doctor right away or get emergency help if needed.
- To use Duoneb, remove one vial from the foil pouch. Twist the cap completely off the vial and squeeze the contents into the nebulizer reservoir. Connect the nebulizer to the mouthpiece or face mask. Connect the nebulizer to the compressor, then sit in a comfortable, upright position and turn it on. Breathe as calmly, deeply, and evenly as possible through your mouth until no more mist is formed. Clean the nebulizer according to the manufacturer's instructions.

What should I avoid while taking this medication?

Do not spray Duoneb into your eyes while you are using your nebulizer as it may lead to enlarged pupils, blurry vision, or eye pain. In addition, do not use more than required without consulting with your doctor.

What are possible food and drug interactions associated with this medication?

If Duoneb is used with certain other drugs, the effects of either could be increased, decreased, or altered. It is especially important to check with your doctor before combining Duoneb with the following: certain antidepressants (such as desipramine or isocarboxazid), diuretics (water pills) (such as furosemide or hydrochlorothiazide), heart pressure/heart medications known as beta-blockers (such as metoprolol), other medicines that contain anticholinergics (such as ipratropium bromide, benztropine, oxybutyn, or scopolamine), or other medicines that contain beta-agonists (such as ephedrine or salmeterol).

What are the possible side effects of this medication?
Please see general statement regarding side effects on page xiii.

> **Side effects may include:** bronchitis, chest pain, constipation, diarrhea, leg cramps, lung disease, nausea, pain, sore throat, upset stomach, urinary tract infection, voice changes

Can I receive this medication if I am pregnant or breastfeeding?
The effects of Duoneb during pregnancy and breastfeeding are unknown. Tell your doctor immediately if you are pregnant, plan to become pregnant, or are breastfeeding.

What should I do if I miss a dose of this medication?
If you miss a dose of Duoneb, apply it as soon as you remember. However, if it is almost time for your next dose, skip the one you missed and return to your regular dosing schedule. Do not apply two doses at once.

How should I store this medication?
Store at room temperature. Keep the vials in the foil pouch to protect from light.

Duragesic
Generic name: Fentanyl

What is this medication?
Duragesic patch is a medicine used to treat persistent, moderate to severe chronic (long-term) pain in patients who are already routinely taking other opioid pain medicines around-the-clock, and have been using the medicine regularly for a week or longer. Duragesic is started only after you have been taking another opioid pain medicine and your body is used to it (opioid-tolerant). Duragesic is a federally controlled substance because it has abuse potential.

What is the most important information I should know about this medication?

- Do not use Duragesic if you are not opioid-tolerant.
- Duragesic can cause life-threatening breathing problems if you are not opioid-tolerant, if you do not use Duragesic exactly as prescribed by your doctor, or if a child applies Duragesic by accident.
- Keep Duragesic in a safe place away from children. Accidental use by a child is a medical emergency. Get emergency help immediately.
- Call your doctor or get emergency medical help immediately if you have breathing problems, drowsiness, slow heartbeat, faintness, dizziness, confusion, or any other unusual symptoms after using Duragesic. These can be signs of an overdose. Your dose of Duragesic may be too high for you. These symptoms may lead to serious problems if not treated right away. Do not apply another Duragesic patch.

Who should not take this medication?

Do not use Duragesic if you are allergic to it or any of its ingredients, or if you have asthma symptoms.

Do not use Duragesic if you are not already taking another opioid pain medicine around-the-clock for your constant pain and are not opioid-tolerant.

Do not use Duragesic if you only have pain for a short time or if your pain is from surgery, medical procedures, or dental work.

What should I tell my doctor before I take the first dose of this medication?

Tell your doctor about all prescription, over-the-counter, and herbal medications you are taking before beginning treatment with Duragesic. Also, talk to your doctor about your complete medical history, especially if you have trouble breathing or lung problems (such as asthma, wheezing, or shortness of breath), liver or kidney problems, seizures, a slow heart rate or other heart problems, low blood pressure, mental health problems, past or present alcohol or drug abuse or a family history of alcohol or drug abuse, or you have or had a head injury or brain problem.

What is the usual dosage?
Please see general statement regarding dosage on page xii.

Adults and children ≥*2 years:* Apply 1 patch continuously for 72 hours. Your doctor will prescribe the appropriate dose for you or your child based on your previous pain medication.

How should I take this medication?
• Use Duragesic exactly as prescribed by your doctor. Do not adjust the dose or use Duragesic more often than prescribed.
• Apply Duragesic to intact, nonirritated skin on a flat surface (such as your chest, back, or upper arm). For children or individuals with cognitive impairment, the patch should be put on the upper back to prevent removal.
• Hair at the application site should be clipped (not shaved). Make sure your skin is dry before applying the patch. Do not use soaps, oils, lotions, alcohol, or any other agents that might irritate or alter your skin.
• Apply Duragesic immediately upon removal from the sealed package. Press the patch firmly in place with the palm of your hand for 30 seconds. If there are problems with the patch not sticking, apply first aid tape to the patch edges or cover the patch with only Bioclusive or Tegaderm, which are special see-through adhesive dressings.

What should I avoid while taking this medication?
Do not drive, operate machinery, or do other dangerous activities until you know how Duragesic affects you. Duragesic can make you sleepy. Ask your doctor when it is safe to do these activities.

Do not drink alcohol while you are using Duragesic. It can increase your chance of having dangerous side effects.

Do not change your dose of Duragesic yourself. Your doctor will change the dose until you and your doctor find the right dose for you.

Do not share Duragesic with anyone else, even if they have the same symptoms you have. It can harm them.

Do not use Duragesic patch if the pouch seal is broken, or the patch is cut, damaged, or changed in any way.

Do not sunbathe or use heat sources (such as heating pads, electric blankets, heat lamps, or hot tubs) while wearing a Duragesic patch.

Do not stop using Duragesic suddenly. Your doctor will slowly reduce this medicine so you don't have withdrawal symptoms.

What are possible food and drug interactions associated with this medication?

If Duragesic is used with certain other drugs, the effects of either could be increased, decreased, or altered. Duragesic may interact with numerous medications. Therefore, it is very important that you tell your doctor about any other medications you are taking.

What are the possible side effects of this medication?

Please see general statement regarding side effects on page xiii.

Side effects may include: confusion, constipation, dry mouth, life-threatening breathing problems, low blood pressure, nausea, pain and redness at the application site, sleepiness, sweating, vomiting, weakness

Can I receive this medication if I am pregnant or breastfeeding?

The effects of Duragesic during pregnancy are unknown. Duragesic can be found in your breast milk if you take it while breastfeeding. Tell your doctor immediately if you are pregnant, plan to become pregnant, or are breastfeeding.

What should I do if I miss a dose of this medication?

Duragesic is intended to be worn as a patch for 72 hours; it is unlikely you will miss your dose. However, if your patch falls off before 72 hours, fold the sticky side together and flush down the toilet. Put a new one on at a different skin site.

How should I store this medication?
Store at room temperature.

Dutasteride: *see Avodart, page 120*

Dyazide
Generic name: Hydrochlorothiazide/Triamterene

What is this medication?
Dyazide is a combination of two diuretics (water pills) used to treat high blood pressure and other conditions that require the elimination of the excess of fluid from the body. It can be used alone or together with other blood pressure lowering medications.

What is the most important information I should know about this medication?
- Dyazide may cause high blood potassium levels. This is more likely to occur if you are elderly, severely ill, or have kidney problems or diabetes. Your doctor will monitor your blood potassium levels.
- Dyazide may cause an imbalance in electrolytes (chemicals that are important for the cells in your body to function, such as sodium and potassium). Contact your doctor immediately if you experience dry mouth, thirst, weakness, fatigue, drowsiness, restlessness, muscle pain or cramps, muscular fatigue, low blood pressure, increased heart rate, low urine output, intestine or stomach problems.
- Dyazide may cause visual disturbances, eye pain, or glaucoma (high pressure in the eye). Contact your doctor immediately if any of these occur.

Who should not take this medication?

Do not take Dyazide if you are allergic to it, any of its ingredients, or to any sulfonamide-derived medications.

Do not take Dyazide if you do not produce urine or have kidney problems, high blood potassium levels, or if you are taking potassium-containing salt substitutes, potassium supplements, or other medications that prevent potassium loss (such as spironolactone or amiloride).

What should I tell my doctor before I take the first dose of this medication?

Tell your doctor about all prescription, over-the-counter, and herbal medications you are taking before beginning treatment with Dyazide. Also, talk to your doctor about your complete medical history, especially if you have diabetes, gout (severe and painful inflammation of the joints), heart failure, kidney disease, kidney stones, liver disease, or cirrhosis (scarring of the liver). Tell your doctor if you are planning to have any kind of surgery before taking Dyazide.

What is the usual dosage?

Please see general statement regarding dosage on page xii.

Adults: The usual dose is one or two capsules once a day.

How should I take this medication?

• Take Dyazide as prescribed by your doctor.

What should I avoid while taking this medication?

Do not take potassium-containing salt substitutes. Do not take potassium supplements unless your doctor specifically directs you to do so. Your doctor will check your blood potassium levels.

What are possible food and drug interactions associated with this medication?

If Dyazide is taken with certain other drugs, the effects of either could be increased, decreased, or altered. It is especially important to check with your doctor before combining Dyazide with the following: amiloride, amphotericin B, blood pressure/heart medications known as angiotensin-converting enzyme (ACE) inhibitors (such as enalapril), blood-thinning medications (such as warfarin), corticosteroids (such as prednisone), diabetes medications (such as chlorpropamide), electrolyte-exchange resin medications (such as sodium polystyrene sulfonate), gout medications (such as allopurinol), insulin, laxatives, lithium, methenamine, nonsteroidal anti-inflammatory drugs (NSAIDs) (such as indomethacin), norepinephrine, other blood pressure medications, potassium-containing salt substitutes, potassium supplements, or spironolactone.

What are the possible side effects of this medication?

Please see general statement regarding side effects on page xiii.

Side effects may include: abdominal pain, anaphylaxis (a serious and rapid allergic reaction that may result in death if not immediately treated), anemia, change in blood potassium levels, constipation, diabetes, diarrhea, dry mouth, fatigue, headache, hives, impotence, irregular heartbeat, jaundice (yellowing of the skin or whites of the eyes), kidney stones, muscle cramps, nausea, rash, sensitivity to light, sudden fall in blood pressure, vomiting, weakness

Can I receive this medication if I am pregnant or breastfeeding?

The effects of Dyazide during pregnancy are unknown. Dyazide appears in your breast milk and can affect your baby. Do not use Dyazide while you are breastfeeding. Tell your doctor immediately if you are pregnant, plan to become pregnant, or are breastfeeding.

What should I do if I miss a dose of this medication?

If you miss a dose of Dyazide, take it as soon as you remember. However, if it is almost time for your next dose, skip the one you missed and return to your regular dosing schedule. Do not take two doses at once.

How should I store this medication?
Store at room temperature and protect from light.

Edarbi
Generic name: Azilsartan Medoxomil

What is this medication?
Edarbi is a medicine called an angiotensin receptor blocker (ARB) used to treat high blood pressure.

What is the most important information I should know about this medication?
- Edarbi can cause harm or death to your unborn baby. If you think you are pregnant, stop taking Edarbi and tell your doctor immediately. If you plan to become pregnant, talk to your doctor about other ways to lower your blood pressure.
- Edarbi can cause low blood pressure, which may make you feel lightheaded or dizzy. If this occurs, lie down and call your doctor immediately.

Who should not take this medication?
Do not take Edarbi if you are allergic to it or any of its ingredients.

What should I tell my doctor before I take the first dose of this medication?
Tell your doctor about all prescription, over-the-counter, and herbal medications you are taking before beginning treatment with Edarbi. Also, talk to your doctor about your complete medical history, especially if you have abnormal electrolyte levels (chemicals that are important for the cells in your body to function, such as sodium and potassium) in your blood, are pregnant or plan to become pregnant, or are breastfeeding.

What is the usual dosage?
Please see general statement regarding dosage on page xii.

Adults: The usual dose is 80 milligrams (mg) once a day. If you were on previous blood pressure medications, your doctor will adjust your dose appropriately.

How should I take this medication?

• Take Edarbi exactly as prescribed by your doctor. You can take it with or without food.

What should I avoid while taking this medication?

Avoid becoming dehydrated while taking Edarbi by drinking enough fluids.

What are possible food and drug interactions associated with this medication?

If Edarbi is taken with certain other drugs, the effects of either could be increased, decreased, or altered. It is important to check with your doctor before combining Edarbi with any other medication.

What are the possible side effects of this medication?

Please see general statement regarding side effects on page xiii.

Side effects may include: cough, diarrhea, dizziness, fainting, low blood pressure, nausea, tiredness

Can I receive this medication if I am pregnant or breastfeeding?

Edarbi can cause harm or death to your unborn baby if you use it during pregnancy. The effects of Edarbi during breastfeeding are unknown. Tell your doctor immediately if you are pregnant, plan to become pregnant, or are breastfeeding.

What should I do if I miss a dose of this medication?

If you miss a dose of Edarbi, take it as soon as you remember. However, if it is almost time for your next dose, skip the one you missed and return to your regular dosing schedule. Do not take two doses at once.

How should I store this medication?
Store at room temperature.

Edarbyclor
Generic name: Azilsartan Medoxomil/Chlorthalidone

What is this medication?
Edarbyclor is a combination medicine used to treat high blood pressure. Edarbyclor contains two medicines: azilsartan medoxomil (an angiotension receptor blocker) and chlorthalidone (a diuretic [water pill]).

What is the most important information I should know about this medication?
- Edarbyclor can cause harm or death to your unborn baby. If you become pregnant while you are taking Edarbyclor, tell your doctor immediately. Your doctor may switch you to a different medicine to treat your high blood pressure. If you plan to become pregnant, talk to your doctor about other ways to lower your blood pressure.
- Edarbyclor can cause low blood pressure and dizziness. If you feel faint or dizzy, lie down and call your doctor immediately. If you faint, have someone call your doctor or get medical help. Stop taking Edarbyclor.
- Edarbyclor can cause or worsen kidney problems. Your doctor will monitor how well your kidneys are working during treatment with Edarbyclor.
- Edarbyclor can increase uric acid levels in your blood, which can cause or worsen gout symptoms. Tell your doctor if you are experiencing gout symptoms.

Who should not take this medication?
Do not take Edarbyclor if you are allergic to it or any of its ingredients.

Do not take Edarbyclor if you urinate less because of kidney problems.

What should I tell my doctor before I take the first dose of this medication?

Tell your doctor about all prescription, over-the-counter, and herbal medications you are taking before beginning treatment with Edarbyclor. Also, talk to your doctor about your complete medical history, especially if you have heart, kidney, or liver problems; stroke; gout; abnormal electrolyte levels (chemicals that are important for the cells in your body to function, such as sodium and potassium) in your blood; diarrhea; vomiting; or are pregnant, plan to become pregnant, or are breastfeeding.

What is the usual dosage?

Please see general statement regarding dosage on page xii.

Adults: The recommended starting dose is 40/12.5 milligrams once a day. Your doctor will adjust your dose as needed until the desired effect is achieved.

How should I take this medication?

• Take Edarbyclor exactly as prescribed by your doctor. You can take it with or without food.

What should I avoid while taking this medication?

Avoid becoming dehydrated while you are taking Edarbyclor by drinking enough fluids.

What are possible food and drug interactions associated with this medication?

If Edarbyclor is taken with certain other drugs, the effects of either could be increased, decreased, or altered. It is especially important to check with your doctor before combining Edarbyclor with the following: digoxin, diuretics, nonsteroidal anti-inflammatory drugs (NSAIDs) (such as ibuprofen), other blood pressure/heart medications, or lithium.

What are the possible side effects of this medication?

Please see general statement regarding side effects on page xiii.

Side effects may include: dizziness, fluid and electrolyte problems, low potassium levels, tiredness

Can I receive this medication if I am pregnant or breastfeeding?

Edarbyclor can cause harm or death to your unborn baby. Do not breastfeed while you are taking Edarbyclor. Tell your doctor immediately if you are pregnant, plan to become pregnant, or are breastfeeding.

What should I do if I miss a dose of this medication?

If you miss a dose of Edarbyclor, take it later in the same day. Do not take more than one dose of Edarbyclor in a day.

How should I store this medication?

Store at room temperature. Protect from light and moisture.

Edurant

Generic name: Rilpivirine

What is this medication?

Edurant is a medicine used to treat HIV (human immunodeficiency virus) infection (AIDS) in combination with other anti-HIV medications. Edurant is a type of HIV medicine called a non-nucleoside reverse transcriptase inhibitor (NNRTI). Edurant is used in adults who have never taken HIV medicines before.

What is the most important information I should know about this medication?

- You have to take Edurant with other HIV medicines.
- Always stay on continuous HIV therapy to control your HIV infection and decrease HIV-related illnesses. Though Edurant can slow the progress of HIV, it is not a cure. You may continue to develop infections and other complications associated with HIV.
- Always practice safe sex to reduce the risk of transmitting HIV to others. Use latex or polyurethane condoms to lower the chance

of sexual contact with any body fluids, such as semen, vaginal secretions, or blood.

- Edurant can cause depression or mood changes. Tell your doctor immediately if you have feelings of sadness or hopelessness, if you are feeling anxious or restless, or if you have thoughts of hurting yourself (suicide) or have tried to hurt yourself.
- Edurant can cause changes in your body fat. These changes may include an increased amount of fat in your upper back and neck ("buffalo hump"), breasts, and around the middle of your body. Loss of fat from your legs, arms, and face may also occur.
- Changes in your immune system can occur when you start taking Edurant. Your immune system may get stronger and begin to fight infections that have been hidden in your body for a long time. Call your doctor immediately if you start having new symptoms after starting Edurant.

Who should not take this medication?

Do not take Edurant if you are allergic to it or any of its ingredients.

Do not take Edurant if you have been previously treated with anti-HIV medications.

Do not take Edurant if you are currently taking carbamazepine, dexamethasone (if you are taking more than one dose), oxcarbazepine, phenobarbital, phenytoin, proton pump inhibitors (such as esomeprazole, lansoprazole, omeprazole, pantoprazole, or rabeprazole), rifabutin, rifampin, rifapentine, or if you are taking St. John's wort.

What should I tell my doctor before I take the first dose of this medication?

Tell your doctor about all prescription, over-the-counter, and herbal medications you are taking before beginning treatment with Edurant. Also, talk to your doctor about your complete medical history, especially if you have had or currently have liver problems, including hepatitis B or C, have ever had a mental health problem, are pregnant, plan to become pregnant, or if you are breastfeeding or plan to breastfeed.

What is the usual dosage?
Please see general statement regarding dosage on page xii.

Adults: The recommended dose is one 25-milligram (mg) tablet taken once a day with a meal.

How should I take this medication?
- Take Edurant every day exactly as prescribed by your doctor. Do not change your dose or stop taking Edurant without first talking with your doctor. You have to see your doctor regularly while taking Edurant.
- Always take Edurant with a meal. Taking Edurant with a meal is important to help get the right amount of medicine in your body. Keep in mind that a protein drink alone does not replace a meal.
- When your supply of Edurant starts to run low, get more from your doctor or pharmacy. It is important that you do not run out of Edurant. The amount of HIV in your blood may increase if the medicine is stopped even for a short time.

What should I avoid while taking this medication?
Do not breastfeed while you are taking Edurant.

Avoid high-risk activities such as unprotected sex and the sharing of needles. Edurant does not cure HIV or AIDS. You can still transmit the virus to others during therapy with this medication.

What are possible food and drug interactions associated with this medication?
If Edurant is taken with certain other drugs, the effects of either could be increased, decreased, or altered. Edurant may interact with numerous medications. Therefore, it is very important that you tell your doctor about any other medications you are taking.

What are the possible side effects of this medication?
Please see general statement regarding side effects on page xiii.

Side effects may include: headache, rash, trouble sleeping

Can I receive this medication if I am pregnant or breastfeeding?

The effects of Edurant during pregnancy and breastfeeding are unknown. It is recommended that you do not breastfeed your baby if you are infected with HIV. This is because your baby could become infected with HIV through your breast milk. Tell your doctor immediately if you are pregnant, plan to become pregnant, or are breastfeeding.

What should I do if I miss a dose of this medication?

If you miss a dose of Edurant within 12 hours of the time you usually take it, take your dose of Edurant with a meal as soon as possible. Then, take your next dose of Edurant at the regularly scheduled time. If you miss a dose of Edurant by more than 12 hours of the time you usually take it, wait, and then take the next dose of Edurant at the regularly scheduled time. Do not take more than your prescribed dose to make up for a missed dose.

How should I store this medication?

Store at room temperature and keep it in the original bottle to protect from light.

Effexor XR

Generic name: Venlafaxine HCl

What is this medication?

Effexor XR belongs to the class of medications called serotonin-norepinephrine reuptake inhibitors (SNRIs). Effexor XR is used to treat major depressive disorder, generalized anxiety disorder, social anxiety disorder, and panic disorder in adults.

What is the most important information I should know about this medication?

- Effexor XR can increase suicidal thoughts or actions in some children, teenagers, and young adults when the medicine is first started.

- Depression and other serious mental illnesses are the most important causes of suicidal thoughts and actions. People with bipolar disorder, or who have a family history of bipolar disorder (also called manic-depressive illness) are at a greater risk. Contact your doctor immediately if you experience any changes in your mood, behavior, thoughts, or feelings. This is very important when an antidepressant medicine is first started or when the dose is changed.

- Effexor XR can cause a severe, possibly life-threatening condition called serotonin syndrome (a drug reaction that causes the body to have too much serotonin, a chemical produced by the nerve cells) or neuroleptic malignant syndrome (a life-threatening brain disorder). Contact your doctor immediately if you experience agitation, hallucinations, coma, fast heartbeat, changes in your blood pressure, increased body temperature, lack of coordination, overactive reflexes, nausea, vomiting, or diarrhea.

- Effexor XR can cause an increase in your blood pressure. Check your blood pressure regularly, especially if you already have high blood pressure.

- Do not suddenly stop taking Effexor XR without talking to your doctor first, as this can cause serious side effects.

- Effexor XR can cause mydriasis (prolonged dilation of the pupils of your eye). Notify your doctor if you have a history of glaucoma (high pressure in your eye).

- Effexor XR can cause low blood sodium levels. Contact your doctor immediately if you experience headache, difficulty concentrating, confusion, weakness, unsteadiness, hallucinations, falls, or seizures.

- Effexor XR can cause seizures to develop, especially if you have a history of seizures. Your doctor will discontinue Effexor XR if seizures occur.

- Effexor XR can increase your risk of bleeding. Do not take Effexor XR with aspirin, nonsteroidal anti-inflammatory drugs (NSAIDs) (such as ibuprofen) or blood thinners (such as warfarin).

- Effexor XR can increase your cholesterol. Your doctor may measure your cholesterol levels if you will be on long-term treatment with Effexor XR.

Who should not take this medication?

Do not take Effexor XR if you are allergic to it or any of its ingredients.

Also, never take Effexor XR while you are taking other medicines known as monoamine oxidase inhibitors (MAOIs) (such as phenelzine), a class of medications used to treat depression and other conditions.

What should I tell my doctor before I take the first dose of this medication?

Tell your doctor about all prescription, over-the-counter, and herbal medications you are taking before beginning treatment with Effexor XR. Also, talk to your doctor about your complete medical history, especially if you have high blood pressure; heart, liver, or kidney disease; a history of seizures, mania, or glaucoma; or a thyroid problem. Also, tell your doctor if you are pregnant, plan to become pregnant, or are breastfeeding.

What is the usual dosage?

Please see general statement regarding dosage on page xii.

Major Depressive Disorder and Generalized Anxiety Disorder

Adults: The recommended starting dose is 75 milligrams (mg) a day. If needed, the doctor may increase your dose up to a maximum of 225 mg a day.

Panic Disorder

Adults: The recommended starting dose is 37.5 mg a day for 7 days. After that, the dose should be increased to 75 mg a day. Your doctor may further increase your dose if needed, up to a maximum of 225 mg a day.

Social Anxiety Disorder

Adults: The recommended starting dose is 75 mg a day, given as a single dose.

How should I take this medication?
- Take Effexor XR as a single dose with food. Take it at about the same time every day, either in the morning or evening.
- Swallow the capsule whole with water. Do not divide, crush, chew, or place it in water.
- You can also open the capsule carefully and sprinkle its contents onto a spoonful of applesauce. Swallow this mixture immediately and follow with a glass of water. Do not chew this mixture before swallowing.

What should I avoid while taking this medication?
Do not drive or operate dangerous machinery or participate in any dangerous activity that requires full mental alertness until you know how Effexor XR affects you.

Effexor XR may cause you to feel drowsy or less alert and may affect your judgment.

Do not drink alcohol while you are taking Effexor XR, as it can worsen these side effects.

Do not stop taking Effexor XR suddenly without talking to your doctor first, as this can cause serious side effects.

Effexor XR can increase your risk of bleeding. Do not take aspirin, NSAIDs, or blood thinners while you are taking Effexor XR.

Do not take Effexor XR and MAOIs together or within 14 days of each other. Wait at least 7 days after stopping Effexor XR before starting an MAOI. Combining these medicines with Effexor XR can cause serious and even fatal reactions.

What are possible food and drug interactions associated with this medication?
If Effexor XR is taken with certain other drugs, the effects of either could be increased, decreased, or altered. It is especially important to check with your doctor before combining Effexor XR with the following: alcohol, antipsychotic medications, aspirin, cimetidine, haloperidol, imipramine, indinavir, ketoconazole, linezolid, lithium,

metoprolol, MAOIs, NSAIDs, phenelzine, other SNRIs, risperidone, tranylcypromine, fluoxetine, paroxetine, St. John's wort, tramadol, certain migraine products, tryptophan,, warfarin, or weight-loss products.

What are the possible side effects of this medication?
Please see general statement regarding side effects on page xiii.

Side effects may include: abnormal ejaculation, changes in vision, constipation, decreased sexual desire, dizziness, drowsiness, dry mouth, increased blood pressure, loss of appetite, nausea, nervousness, sweating, trouble sleeping, weakness, weight loss

Can I receive this medication if I am pregnant or breastfeeding?
The effects of Effexor XR during pregnancy are unknown. Effexor XR can be found in your breast milk if you take it during breastfeeding. Tell your doctor immediately if you are pregnant, plan to become pregnant, or are breastfeeding.

What should I do if I miss a dose of this medication?
If you miss a dose of Effexor XR, take it as soon as you remember. However, if it is almost time for your next dose, skip the one you missed and return to your regular dosing schedule. Do not take two doses at once.

How should I store this medication?
Store at room temperature.

Effient
Generic name: Prasugrel

What is this medication?
Effient is a medicine used to treat people who have had a heart attack or severe chest pain that happens when your heart does not

get enough oxygen, and have been treated with a procedure called "angioplasty" (also called balloon angioplasty).

Effient is used to lower your chance of having another serious problem with your heart or blood vessels, such as another heart attack, a stroke, blood clots in your stent, or death.

Platelets are blood cells that help with normal blood clotting. Effient helps prevent platelets from sticking together and forming a clot that can block an artery or a stent.

What is the most important information I should know about this medication?

- Effient can cause bleeding, which can be serious, and sometimes lead to death. You should not start to take Effient if it is likely that you will have heart bypass surgery (coronary artery bypass graft surgery or CABG) right away. You have a higher risk of bleeding if you take Effient and then have heart bypass surgery.
- When possible, discontinue Effient at least 7 days before any surgery, as instructed by your doctor. Notify your doctor prior to any surgery or dental procedure.
- You may have a higher bleeding risk if you have had trauma or surgery, have stomach or intestinal bleeding, a stomach ulcer, severe liver problems, weigh <132 pounds, or take certain other medications.
- Effient may cause a rare but serious condition called thrombotic thrombocytopenic purpura (TTP) that needs to be treated right away. TTP is a condition in which blood clots form in the blood vessels and can occur all over the body. Get medical help right away if you develop any of these symptoms that cannot otherwise be explained: fever, weakness, extreme skin paleness, purple skin patches, yellowing of your skin or the whites of your eyes, fast heart rate, shortness of breath, or neurological changes (such as confusion, speech changes).
- Serious allergic reactions can happen with Effient. Get medical help right away if you get swelling or hives of your face, lips, in or around your mouth, or throat; if you have trouble breathing or swallowing; if you develop chest pain or pressure; or if you develop dizziness or fainting.

Who should not take this medication?

Do not take Effient if you are allergic to it or any of its ingredients; currently have abnormal bleeding, such as stomach or intestinal bleeding, or bleeding in your head; or if you have had a stroke or "mini-stroke" (also known as transient ischemic attack or TIA).

What should I tell my doctor before I take the first dose of this medication?

Tell your doctor about all prescription, over-the-counter, and herbal medications you are taking before beginning treatment with Effient. Also, talk to your doctor about your complete medical history, especially if you have any bleeding problems; have had a stroke or "mini-stroke" (also known as transient ischemic attack or TIA); are allergic to any medicines, including clopidogrel or ticlopidine; have a history of stomach ulcers, colon polyps (a non-cancerous growth on the surface of the colon), or diverticulosis (a condition in which pockets form in the large intestine); have liver problems; have had any recent severe injury or surgery; plan to have surgery or a dental procedure; are pregnant, planning to become pregnant, or are breastfeeding.

What is the usual dosage?

Please see general statement regarding dosage on page xii.

Adults: The initial dose is a single dose of 60 milligrams (mg). Afterward, the maintenance dose is 10 mg once daily. Underweight people may be instructed to take a lower maintenance dose of 5 mg once daily.

How should I take this medication?

• Take Effient exactly as prescribed by your doctor. Take Effient one time each day. You can take Effient with or without food. Take Effient with aspirin as instructed by your doctor.

What should I avoid while taking this medication?

Avoid stopping Effient without talking to your doctor.

What are possible food and drug interactions associated with this medication?

If Effient is taken with certain other drugs, the effects of either could be increased, decreased, or altered. It is especially important to check with your doctor before combining Effient with the following: heparin, other medicines to prevent or treat blood clots (such as alteplase), pain relievers called nonsteroidal anti-inflammatory drugs (NSAIDs) (such as ibuprofen and naproxen), and warfarin.

What are the possible side effects of this medication?

Please see general statement regarding side effects on page xiii.

> **Side effects may include:** back pain, bleeding, chest pain, cough, dizziness, fatigue, headache, high or low blood pressure, high cholesterol, nausea, shortness of breath

Can I receive this medication if I am pregnant or breastfeeding?

The effects of Effient during pregnancy and breastfeeding are unknown. Tell your doctor immediately if you are pregnant, plan to become pregnant, or are breastfeeding.

What should I do if I miss a dose of this medication?

If you miss a dose, take Effient as soon as you remember. If it is almost time for your next dose, skip the missed dose. Just take the next dose at your regular time. Do not take two doses at the same time unless your doctor tells you to.

How should I store this medication?

Store at room temperature. Keep it in the container it comes in and keep the container closed tightly with the gray cylinder inside. Protect from moisture.

Emtricitabine/Rilpivirine/Tenofovir Disoproxil Fumarate: *see Complera, page 259*

Enablex
Generic name: Darifenacin

What is this medication?
Enablex is a medicine used to treat symptoms of overactive bladder, including frequent urination, urgency (increased need to urinate), and urge incontinence (inability to control urination).

What is the most important information I should know about this medication?
- Enablex can cause blurred vision or dizziness. Do not drive or operate hazardous machinery until you know how Enablex affects you.

Who should not take this medication?
Do not take Enablex if you are allergic to it or any of its ingredients.

Do not take Enablex if you are not able to empty your bladder (urinary retention) or have delayed or slow emptying of your stomach (gastric retention).

Also, do not take Enablex if you have an eye problem called uncontrolled narrow-angle glaucoma (high pressure in the eyes).

What should I tell my doctor before I take the first dose of this medication?
Tell your doctor about all prescription, over-the-counter, and herbal medications you are taking before beginning treatment with Enablex. Also, talk to your doctor about your complete medical history, especially if you have any stomach or intestinal problems, problems with constipation, have trouble emptying your bladder or have a weak urine stream, have liver problems, or if you are pregnant, plan to become pregnant, or are breastfeeding.

What is the usual dosage?
Please see general statement regarding dosage on page xii.

Adults: The recommended starting dose is 7.5 milligrams (mg) once a day. Your doctor may give you a higher dose, depending on your needs.

How should I take this medication?
- Take Enablex once a day with water. Take Enablex with or without food.
- Swallow the Enablex tablet whole. Do not crush, split, or chew it.

What should I avoid while taking this medication?
Do not drive or operate hazardous machinery until you know how Enablex affects you.

Avoid becoming overheated in hot weather or during activity.

What are possible food and drug interactions associated with this medication?
If Enablex is taken with certain other drugs, the effects of either could be increased, decreased, or altered. It is especially important to check with your doctor before combining Enablex with the following: clarithromycin, flecainide, itraconazole, ketoconazole, nefazodone, nelfinavir, ritonavir, thioridazine, or certain antidepressants (such as amitriptyline or imipramine).

What are the possible side effects of this medication?
Please see general statement regarding side effects on page xiii.

> **Side effects may include:** blurred vision, constipation, dry mouth, headache, heartburn, nausea, overheated feeling, urinary tract infection

Can I receive this medication if I am pregnant or breastfeeding?
The effects of Enablex during pregnancy and breastfeeding are unknown. Tell your doctor immediately if you are pregnant, plan to become pregnant, or are breastfeeding.

What should I do if I miss a dose of this medication?
If you miss a dose of Enablex, take it as soon as you remember. However, if it is almost time for your next dose, skip the one you missed and return to your regular dosing schedule. Do not take two doses at once.

How should I store this medication?
Store at room temperature.

Enalapril Maleate: *see Vasotec, page 1055*

Enalapril Maleate/Hydrochlorothiazide: *see Vaseretic, page 1052*

Enoxaparin Sodium: *see Lovenox, page 592*

Epiduo
Generic name: Adapalene/Benzoyl Peroxide

What is this medication?
Epiduo is a topical gel (applied directly on the skin) that is used to treat acne.

What is the most important information I should know about this medication?
- Epiduo is for external use only. Do not use it in your mouth, eyes, lips, vagina, open wounds, or on sunburned skin.
- Epiduo can cause swelling, redness, scaling, dryness, and burning of your skin. This usually happens during the first 4 weeks of treatment and are mostly mild to moderate in severity. Depending upon the severity of these reactions, you may use a moisturizer, reduce the frequency of Epiduo use, or stop using Epiduo. Tell your doctor if these reactions get worse.
- Limit sun exposure while you are using Epiduo. If you have sunburn, wait until it fully recovers before you start this medicine. Use sunscreen products and wear protective clothing over treated areas when you cannot avoid being exposed to the sun.

Weather extremes, such as wind and cold, can irritate your skin and should also be avoided.

Who should not take this medication?
Do not use Epiduo if you are allergic to it or any of its ingredients.

What should I tell my doctor before I take the first dose of this medication?
Tell your doctor about all prescription, over-the-counter, and herbal medications you are taking before beginning treatment with Epiduo. Also, talk to your doctor about your complete medical history, especially if you have other skin problems including cuts, sunburn or eczema (an inflammation or irritation of the skin).

What is the usual dosage?
Please see general statement regarding dosage on page xii.

Adults and children ≥12 years: Apply a pea-sized amount of the gel to the affected area(s) once a day.

How should I take this medication?
• Apply Epiduo as prescribed by your doctor. Use only enough cream to lightly cover the affected area. Wash your face gently with a mild soap and dry your skin gently. Apply a pea-sized amount of Epiduo gel to the affected area(s) and smooth it lightly into your skin.

What should I avoid while taking this medication?
Do not use Epiduo in your mouth, eyes, lips, vagina, open wounds, or on sunburned skin.

Do not excessively expose your skin to the sun, wind, or cold to prevent further irritation.

Do not use skin products that may dry or irritate your skin, such as harsh soaps.

Do not use waxing as a hair removal method on skin treated with Epiduo.

Do not get Epiduo in your hair or on colored fabric. Epiduo may cause bleaching.

What are possible food and drug interactions associated with this medication?

No significant interactions have been reported with Epiduo at this time. However, always tell your doctor about any medicines you take, including over-the-counter medications, vitamins, and herbal supplements.

What are the possible side effects of this medication?

Please see general statement regarding side effects on page xiii.

> **Side effects may include:** local skin reactions such as burning, dryness, redness, scaling, stinging, swelling

Can I receive this medication if I am pregnant or breastfeeding?

The effects of Epiduo during pregnancy and breastfeeding are unknown. Tell your doctor immediately if you are pregnant, plan to become pregnant, or are breastfeeding.

What should I do if I miss a dose of this medication?

If you miss a dose of Epiduo, apply it as soon as you remember. However, if it is almost time for your next dose, skip the one you missed and return to your regular dosing schedule. Do not apply two doses at once.

How should I store this medication?

Store at room temperature.

Epinephrine: see Epipen, page 368

Epipen
Generic name: Epinephrine

What is this medication?
Epipen Auto-Injector is a prefilled injection used in emergency situations to treat severe allergic reactions (anaphylaxis) to insect stings or bites, foods, drugs, and other allergens. Epipen Jr is available for use for children.

What is the most important information I should know about this medication?
- If you have a severe allergic reaction, use Epipen right away and immediately go to your doctor or emergency room for more medical treatment.
- Inject Epipen into your outer thigh. Do not inject Epipen into your hands, fingers, feet, or toes. This can cause a loss of blood flow and result in tissue damage to these areas. If you accidentally inject Epipen into any of these areas, seek immediate emergency medical attention.
- It is important for you not to be afraid to use Epipen for emergency treatment of allergic reactions. Use Epipen early at the start of such allergic reactions to help prevent the reaction from becoming worse.
- It is important that you carry the Epipen Auto-Injector with you at all times since you cannot predict when a life-threatening allergic reaction may occur.
- Keep your Epipen in the carrier tube with the blue safety release on until you need to use it.

Who should not take this medication?
There is absolutely no reason why you should not use Epipen since it is used to treat a life-threatening allergic reaction.

What should I tell my doctor before I take the first dose of this medication?
Tell your doctor about all prescription, over-the-counter, and herbal medications you are taking before beginning treatment with Epipen. Also, talk to your doctor about your complete medical

history, especially if you have heart disease or high blood pressure, thyroid problems, asthma, depression, or diabetes.

What is the usual dosage?
Please see general statement regarding dosage on page xii.

Adults and children: The usual dose is one injection. Your doctor will prescribe the appropriate strength based on your or your child's weight.

How should I take this medication?
• Inject Epipen into the middle of the outer side of your thigh (upper leg).
• In case of emergency, use Epipen exactly as prescribed by your doctor. Please review the instructions that came with your prescription on how to properly use your Epipen Auto-Injector.
• Check your Epipen regularly. If the solution is discolored or contains solid particles, replace the unit. The solution should be clear.
• Do not put your thumb, fingers, or hand over the orange tip of the auto-injector. The needle comes out of the orange tip. If you accidently inject yourself into your thumb, finger, or hand, go immediately to the nearest emergency room.

What should I avoid while taking this medication?
Do not inject Epipen into your buttock or into a vein.

Do not drop the carrier tube or auto-injector. If either is dropped, inspect for damage and leakage. Discard the auto-injector and carrier tube, and replace if damage or leakage is noticed or suspected.

What are possible food and drug interactions associated with this medication?
If Epipen is used with certain other drugs, the effects of either could be increased, decreased, or altered. It is especially important to check with your doctor before combining Epipen with antidepressant medications known as monoamine oxidase inhibitors (MAOIs) (such as phenelzine), antihistamines (such as chlorpheniramine or diphenhydramine), beta-blockers (such as atenolol

or propranolol), ergot alkaloids (such as dihydroergotamine or ergonovine), heart medications known as cardiac glycosides, levothyroxine, tricyclic antidepressants (such as amitriptyline, imipramine, or nortriptyline), water pills (such as hydrochlorothiazide or furosemide).

What are the possible side effects of this medication?
Please see general statement regarding side effects on page xiii.

> **Side effects may include:** abnormal heart beat, anxiety, dizziness, headache, nausea, pale skin, respiratory (lung) difficulties, restlessness, sweating, tremor, vomiting, weakness

Can I receive this medication if I am pregnant or breastfeeding?
The effects of Epipen during pregnancy and breastfeeding are unknown. Tell your doctor if you are pregnant, plan to become pregnant, or are breastfeeding.

What should I do if I miss a dose of this medication?
Epien is only used in emergency situations and is not to be used regularly.

How should I store this medication?
Store at room temperature and protect from light.

Do not store in refrigerator and do not expose to extreme cold or heat.

If your Epipen expires or is about to expire, discard it and replace it with a new one.

Erlotinib: *see Tarceva, page 967*

Escitalopram Oxalate: *see Lexapro, page 549*

Esomeprazole Magnesium: *see Nexium, page 684*

Estrace

Generic name: Estradiol

What is this medication?

Estrace is an estrogen hormone used to treat moderate to severe symptoms of menopause, such as hot flashes or severe dryness, itching, and burning in or around your vagina. Also, Estrace is used to treat certain conditions in which a young woman's ovaries do not produce enough estrogens naturally, certain prostate cancers in men, certain breast cancers in selected women and men, and to reduce your chances of getting postmenopausal osteoporosis (thin, weak bones).

What is the most important information I should know about this medication?

- Estrogens increase your risk of developing cancer of the uterus. Tell your doctor right away if you experience any unusual vaginal bleeding while you are using Estrace.
- Do not take Estrace to prevent heart disease, heart attacks, strokes, or dementia (an illness involving loss of memory, judgment, and confusion.) Using Estrace can increase your chances of getting heart attacks, strokes, breast cancer, or blood clots.
- Estrace can also increase your risk of dementia, gallbladder disease, ovarian cancer, visual abnormalities, high blood pressure, pancreatitis (inflammation of your pancreas), or thyroid problems. Talk regularly with your doctor about whether you still need treatment with Estrace.
- You can lower your chances of serious side effects with Estrace by having a breast exam and mammogram (breast x-ray) every year, unless directed by your doctor to have it more often. See your doctor right away if you get vaginal bleeding while you are taking Estrace. Also, ask your doctor for ways to lower your chances of getting heart disease, especially if you have high blood pressure, high cholesterol, or diabetes, if you are overweight, or if you use tobacco.

Who should not take this medication?

Do not take Estrace if you are allergic to it or any of its ingredients.

Do not take Estrace if you are pregnant or think you may be pregnant.

Do not take Estrace if you have a history of stroke or heart attack, blood clots, liver problems, unusual vaginal bleeding, or certain cancers, including cancer of your breast or uterus.

What should I tell my doctor before I take the first dose of this medication?

Tell your doctor about all prescription, over-the-counter, and herbal medications you are taking before beginning treatment with Estrace. Also, talk to your doctor about your complete medical history, especially if you are pregnant or breastfeeding, or have any unusual vaginal bleeding, asthma, seizures, diabetes, migraine headaches, endometriosis (a common gynecological disorder that may result in sores and pain), porphyria (a blood disorder that interferes with how your body produces heme, which is the oxygen-carrying component of your red blood cells), lupus (disease that affects the immune system), high blood calcium levels, or problems with your heart, liver, thyroid, or kidneys. Also, tell your doctor if you are going to have surgery or will be on bedrest.

What is the usual dosage?

Please see general statement regarding dosage on page xii.

Your doctor might prescribe different doses than those listed below based on your condition and will adjust your dose according to your individual response to the medication.

<u>Treatment of Menopausal Symptoms</u>
Adults: The recommended starting dose is 1-2 milligrams (mg) once a day for 3 weeks, followed by 1 week of no medication, then return to the normal cycle.

Attempts to taper or discontinue the medication should be made at specific intervals, through the guidance of your doctor.

<u>Treatment of Low Estrogen Levels</u>
Adults: The recommended starting dose is 1-2 mg once a day.

Treatment of Breast Cancer
Adults: The recommended dose is 10 mg three times a day for at least 3 months.

Treatment of Androgen-Dependent Prostate Cancer
Adults: The recommended dose is 1-2 mg three times a day.

Prevention of Osteoporosis
Adults: Your doctor will prescribe the appropriate dose for you.

How should I take this medication?
- Take Estrace exactly as prescribed by your doctor.
- Talk to your doctor regularly (every 3-6 months) about the dose you are taking and whether you still need treatment with Estrace.
- Please follow the instructions on the patient handout that comes with your prescription.

What should I avoid while taking this medication?
Do not take Estrace for conditions for which it was not prescribed.

Grapefruit juice can increase your risk of side effects with Estrace. Talk to your doctor before including grapefruit or grapefruit juice in your diet while you are taking Estrace.

What are possible food and drug interactions associated with this medication?
If Estrace is taken with certain other drugs, the effects of either could be increased, decreased, or altered. It is especially important to check with your doctor before combining Estrace with the following: carbamazepine, clarithromycin, erythromycin, grapefruit juice, itraconazole, ketoconazole, phenobarbital, rifampin, ritonavir, or St. John's wort.

What are the possible side effects of this medication?
Please see general statement regarding side effects on page xiii.

Side effects may include: abdominal (stomach) pain, bloating, breast pain, fluid retention, hair loss, headache, high blood pressure, high blood sugar, irregular vaginal bleeding or spotting, liver problems, nausea, spotty darkening of your skin, vaginal yeast infections, vomiting

If you experience symptoms of breast lumps, changes in your speech, changes in your vision, chest pain, dizziness and faintness, pain in your legs, severe headaches, shortness of breath, unusual vaginal bleeding, vomiting, or yellowing of your skin or whites of your eyes, contact your doctor right away.

Can I receive this medication if I am pregnant or breastfeeding?

Do not take Estrace if you are pregnant. Estrace can be found in your breast milk if you take it while breastfeeding. Tell your doctor immediately if you are pregnant, plan to become pregnant, or are breastfeeding.

What should I do if I miss a dose of this medication?

If you miss a dose of Estrace, take it as soon as you remember. However, if it is almost time for your next dose, skip the one you missed and return to your regular dosing schedule. Do not take two doses at once.

How should I store this medication?

Store at room temperature.

Estradiol: *see Estrace, page 371*

Estradiol: *see Vagifem, page 1041*

Estradiol: *see Vivelle-Dot, page 1079*

Eszopiclone: *see Lunesta, page 597*

Ethinyl Estradiol/Etonogestrel: *see Nuvaring, page 711*

Ethinyl Estradiol/Ferrous Fumarate/Norethindrone Acetate: see
Loestrin 24 Fe, page 561

Ethinyl Estradiol/Ferrous Fumarate/Norethindrone Acetate: see
Loestrin Fe, page 565

Ethinyl Estradiol/Levonorgestrel: see Aviane, page 116

Ethinyl Estradiol/Norelgestromin: see Ortho Evra, page 737

Ethinyl Estradiol/Norgestimate: see Ortho-Cyclen, page 733

Ethinyl Estradiol/Norgestimate: see Ortho Tri-Cyclen, page 741

Ethinyl Estradiol/Norgestimate: see Ortho Tri-Cyclen Lo, page 745

Etodolac
Generic name: Etodolac

What is this medication?

Etodolac is a nonsteroidal anti-inflammatory drug (NSAID)
used to treat rheumatoid arthritis, osteoarthritis, and acute pain
(short-term). Etodolac is available as tablets and capsules.

What is the most important information I should know about this medication?

- Etodolac can cause serious problems (such as heart attack or
  stroke). Your risk can increase when this medication is used for
  long periods of time and if you have heart disease. Tell your doctor if you experience chest pain, shortness of breath, weakness,
  or slurred speech.
- Etodolac can cause high blood pressure and heart failure or
  worsen existing high blood pressure. Tell your doctor if you experience weight gain or swelling.
- Etodolac can cause discomfort, ulcers, or bleeding in your
  stomach or intestines. Your risk can increase with long-term
  use, smoking, drinking alcohol, older age, poor health, or with

certain medications. Tell your doctor immediately if you experience stomach pain or if you have bloody vomit or stools.

- Long-term use of etodolac can cause kidney injury. Your risk can increase if you have kidney impairment; heart failure; liver problems; are taking certain medications, including diuretics (water pills) (such as furosemide or hydrochlorothiazide) or blood/heart medications known as angiotensin-converting enzyme (ACE) inhibitors (such as enalapril or lisinopril); or are elderly.

- Etodolac can also cause liver injury. Stop taking etodolac and call your doctor if you experience nausea, tiredness, weakness, itchiness, yellowing of your skin or whites of your eyes, right upper abdominal tenderness, or "flu-like" symptoms.

- Etodolac can cause a serious allergic reaction. Stop taking etodolac and tell your doctor right away if you experience trouble breathing or swelling of your face, mouth, or throat.

- Stop taking etodolac and tell your doctor right away if you experience serious skin reactions, such as rash, blisters, fever, or itchiness.

Who should not take this medication?

Do not take etodolac if you are allergic to it or any of its ingredients, or if you have experienced asthma, rash, or allergic-type reactions after taking aspirin or other NSAIDs (such as ibuprofen).

Do not take etodolac right before or after a heart surgery called a coronary artery bypass graft (CABG).

What should I tell my doctor before I take the first dose of this medication?

Tell your doctor about all prescription, over-the-counter, and herbal medications you are taking before beginning treatment with etodolac. Also, talk to your doctor about your complete medical history, especially if you have any of the following: allergies to medications, heart problems, history of asthma, high blood pressure, kidney or liver disease, or stomach problems, or are pregnant, plan to become pregnant, or are breastfeeding.

What is the usual dosage?

Please see general statement regarding dosage on page xii.

Acute Pain
Adults: The recommended dose is 200-400 milligrams (mg) every 6-8 hours.

Osteoarthritis and Rheumatoid Arthritis
Adults: The recommended starting dose is 300 mg two or three times a day, or 400 mg or 500 mg twice a day.

How should I take this medication?
• Take etodolac exactly as prescribed by your doctor.

What should I avoid while taking this medication?
Do not drink alcohol while you are taking etodolac.

Do not take aspirin or any other anti-inflammatory medications while taking etodolac, unless your doctor tells you to do so.

What are possible food and drug interactions associated with this medication?
If etodolac is taken with certain other drugs, the effects of either could be increased, decreased, or altered. It is especially important to check with your doctor before combining etodolac with the following: aspirin, blood pressure/heart medications known as ACE inhibitors (such as enalapril or lisinopril), cyclosporine, digoxin, lithium, methotrexate, phenylbutazone, warfarin, water pills (such as furosemide or hydrochlorothiazide).

What are the possible side effects of this medication?
Please see general statement regarding side effects on page xiii.

> **Side effects may include:** blurred vision, constipation, depression, dizziness, gas, nausea, nervousness, rash, ringing in your ears, stomach pain, upset stomach, vomiting

Can I receive this medication if I am pregnant or breastfeeding?
Do not take etodolac if you are in the late stage of your pregnancy or if you are breastfeeding. The effects of etodolac during early

pregnancy are unknown. Tell your doctor immediately if you are pregnant, plan to become pregnant, or are breastfeeding.

What should I do if I miss a dose of this medication?

If you miss a dose of etodolac, take it as soon as you remember. However, if it is almost time for your next dose, skip the one you missed and return to your regular dosing schedule. Do not take two doses at once.

How should I store this medication?

Store at room temperature.

Etodolac: *see Etodolac, page 375*

Evista

Generic name: Raloxifene HCl

What is this medication?

Evista is used after menopause to treat or reduce your chances of getting osteoporosis (thin, weak bones). Evista is also used to lower your chance of getting breast cancer.

What is the most important information I should know about this medication?

• Evista can cause serious and life-threatening side effects, such as blood clots. Do not take it 72 hours prior to or during long periods of immobilization, such as recovery from surgery, prolonged bed rest, and long air or car travel. Tell your doctor if you will go through long periods of immobilization, or if you have conditions that increase your risk of getting blood clots, such as previous blood clots, stroke, irregular heartbeat, heart failure, blood vessel problems, or cancer. Stop taking Evista and call your doctor if you have leg pain, feeling of warmth in your lower leg (calf), or swelling of your legs, hands, or feet.

• Evista can increase your risk of dying from a stroke, especially if you have had a heart attack or are at risk for a heart attack. Stop

taking Evista and call your doctor if you have sudden chest pain, shortness of breath, coughing up blood, or sudden change in your vision, such as loss of vision or blurred vision.
- Evista is not for use in women who have not passed menopause.
- If you develop unusual uterine bleeding or breast problems while taking Evista, tell your doctor right away.

Who should not take this medication?
Do not take Evista if you are allergic to it, any of its ingredients, or other similar medications.

Do not take Evista if you have or have had blood clot formation, including blood clots in your legs, lungs, or the retina of your eye.

Do not take Evista if you are pregnant, plan to become pregnant, or are breastfeeding.

What should I tell my doctor before I take the first dose of this medication?
Tell your doctor about all prescription, over-the-counter, and herbal medications you are taking before beginning treatment with Evista. Also, talk to your doctor about your complete medical history, especially if you have or have had clots in your legs, lungs, or eyes; have heart, liver, or kidney problems; are at risk of a stroke; have breast cancer; have high triglyceride levels; or are pregnant, plan to become pregnant, or are breastfeeding.

What is the usual dosage?
Please see general statement regarding dosage on page xii.

Adults: The recommended dose is 60 milligrams (mg) once a day.

How should I take this medication?
- Take Evista exactly as prescribed by your doctor. You can take Evista at any time of the day, with or without food. Take it at about the same time each day to help you remember to take Evista.
- Take calcium and vitamin D with Evista as directed by your doctor to prevent or treat osteoporosis.

What should I avoid while taking this medication?

Do not be still for a long time (such as during long trips or being in bed after surgery) while taking Evista.

Do not smoke or drink alcohol while taking Evista.

What are possible food and drug interactions associated with this medication?

If Evista is taken with certain other drugs, the effects of either could be increased, decreased, or altered. It is especially important to check with your doctor before combining Evista with the following: blood thinners (such as warfarin), cholestyramine, diazepam, diazoxide, estrogens, or lidocaine.

What are the possible side effects of this medication?

Please see general statement regarding side effects on page xiii.

> **Side effects may include:** "flu-like" symptoms, hot flashes, joint pain, leg cramps or swelling, sweating, swelling of your feet or ankles

Can I receive this medication if I am pregnant or breastfeeding?

Evista can harm your baby if you take it during pregnancy or breastfeeding. Do not take Evista if you are pregnant, plan to become pregnant, or are breastfeeding.

What should I do if I miss a dose of this medication?

If you miss a dose of Evista, take it as soon as you remember. However, if it is almost time for your next dose, skip the one you missed and return to your regular dosing schedule. Do not take two doses at once.

How should I store this medication?

Store at room temperature.

Exenatide: *see Byrdureon, page 161*

Exenatide: *see Byetta, page 164*

Exforge
Generic name: Amlodipine/Valsartan

What is this medication?
Exforge is a combination medicine used alone or in combination with other medications to treat high blood pressure and lower the risk of stroke or heart attack. Exforge contains two medicines: amlodipine (a calcium channel blocker) and valsartan (an angiotensin receptor blocker).

What is the most important information I should know about this medication?
- If you become pregnant while you are taking Exforge, stop taking it and call your doctor right away. Exforge can harm your unborn baby, causing injury or even death.
- Low blood pressure can occur with Exforge and cause you to feel faint or dizzy. Lie down if you feel faint or dizzy, and call your doctor right away.
- If you experience chest pain that gets worse, or that does not go away during treatment with Exforge, get medical help right away.

Who should not take this medication?
Do not take Exforge if you are allergic to it or any of its ingredients.

What should I tell my doctor before I take the first dose of this medication?
Tell your doctor about all prescription, over-the-counter, and herbal medications you are taking before beginning treatment with Exforge. Also, talk to your doctor about your complete medical history, especially if you have liver, kidney, or heart problems; if you are vomiting or have a lot of diarrhea; or if you are pregnant, plan to become pregnant, or are breastfeeding.

What is the usual dosage?

Please see general statement regarding dosage on page xii.

Adults: The recommended starting dose is 5/160 (5 milligrams [mg] of amlodipine and 160 mg of valsartan) once a day. Your doctor will prescribe the appropriate dose for you and will increase your dose as needed, until the desired effect is achieved.

How should I take this medication?

- Take Exforge exactly as prescribed by your doctor.
- Take Exforge once a day. Take it with or without food.
- Continue to take Exforge even if you feel well.

What should I avoid while taking this medication?

Do not become pregnant or breastfeed while you are taking Exforge.

What are possible food and drug interactions associated with this medication?

No significant interactions have been reported with Exforge at this time. However, always tell your doctor about any medicines you take, including over-the-counter medications, vitamins, and herbal supplements.

What are the possible side effects of this medication?

Please see general statement regarding side effects on page xiii.

> **Side effects may include:** discomfort when swallowing, dizziness, nasal congestion, sore throat, swelling, upper respiratory infection

Can I receive this medication if I am pregnant or breastfeeding?

Do not take Exforge if you are pregnant. The effects of Exforge during breastfeeding are unknown. Tell your doctor immediately if you are pregnant, plan to become pregnant, or are breastfeeding.

What should I do if I miss a dose of this medication?
If you miss a dose of Exforge, take it as soon as you remember. However, if it is almost time for your next dose, skip the one you missed and return to your regular dosing schedule. Do not take two doses at once.

How should I store this medication?
Store at room temperature.

Ezetimibe: *see Zetia, page 1133*

Ezetimibe/Simvastatin: *see Vytorin, page 1086*

Famotidine: *see Pepcid, page 775*

Famotidine/Ibuprofen: *see Duexis, page 335*

Felodipine ER
Generic name: Felodipine

What is this medication?
Felodipine extended-release (ER) is a medicine known as a calcium channel blocker, which is used alone or in combination with other medications to treat high blood pressure.

What is the most important information I should know about this medication?
- Your blood pressure can become lower than normal during treatment with felodipine ER. Tell your doctor if you experience dizziness, lightheadedness, or fainting while on felodipine ER.
- Although this happens rarely, patients with severe heart disease can experience worsening of chest pain when starting treatment with felodipine ER or if the dose is increased. If this happens, call your doctor right away or go directly to an emergency room.

Who should not take this medication?

Do not take felodipine ER if you are allergic to it or any of its ingredients.

What should I tell my doctor before I take the first dose of this medication?

Tell your doctor about all prescription, over-the-counter, and herbal medications you are taking before beginning treatment with felodipine ER. Also, talk to your doctor about your complete medical history, especially if you have kidney or liver problems, heart disease, or are pregnant, plan to become pregnant, or are breastfeeding.

What is the usual dosage?

Please see general statement regarding dosage on page xii.

Adults: The recommended starting dose is 5 milligrams (mg) once a day. Your doctor may adjust your dose as needed, until the desired effect is achieved.

Adults >65 years: The recommended starting dose is 2.5 mg once a day.

If you have liver impairment, your doctor will adjust your dose appropriately.

How should I take this medication?

• Take felodipine ER once a day, at the same time every day. You can take it without food or with a light meal.

What should I avoid while taking this medication?

Do not stop taking your other prescription medicines, including any other blood pressure medicines while you are taking felodipine ER, without talking to your doctor.

Do not drink grapefruit juice while you are taking felodipine ER.

What are possible food and drug interactions associated with this medication?

If felodipine ER is taken with certain other drugs, the effects of either could be increased, decreased, or altered. It is especially important to check with your doctor before combining felodipine ER with the following: anti-seizure medications (such as carbamazepine, phenobarbital, or phenytoin), blood pressure/heart medications known as beta-blockers (such as atenolol, metoprolol, or propranolol), cimetidine, erythromycin, grapefruit and grapefruit juice, itraconazole, ketoconazole, tacrolimus, or theophylline.

What are the possible side effects of this medication?

Please see general statement regarding side effects on page xiii.

> **Side effects may include:** dizziness, chest pain, flushing, headache, nausea, swelling, upper respiratory (lung) infection, upset stomach, weakness

Can I receive this medication if I am pregnant or breastfeeding?

The effects of felodipine ER during pregnancy and breastfeeding are unknown. Do not take felodipine ER if you are breastfeeding. Tell your doctor immediately if you are pregnant, plan to become pregnant, or are breastfeeding.

What should I do if I miss a dose of this medication?

If you miss a dose of felodipine ER, take it as soon as you remember. However, if it is almost time for your next dose, skip the one you missed and return to your regular dosing schedule. Do not take two doses at once.

How should I store this medication?

Store at room temperature.

Felodipine: *see Felodipine ER, page 383*

Fenofibrate: *see Tricor, page 1017*

Fenofibrate: see Triglide, page 1020

Fenofibric acid: see Trilipix, page 1026

Fentanyl: see Abstral, page 5

Fentanyl: see Duragesic, page 341

Fentanyl: see Lazanda, page 531

Fidaxomicin: see Dificid, page 315

Finasteride: see Propecia, page 856

Fioricet

Generic name: Acetaminophen/Butalbital/Caffeine

What is this medication?

Fioricet is a medicine used to relieve symptoms of tension (or muscle contraction) headaches. Fioricet contains three medications: butalbital, acetaminophen, and caffeine.

What is the most important information I should know about this medication?

- Fioricet contains a medicine called butalbital that is habit-forming and has potential for abuse. Do not take more or use Fioricet longer than your doctor tells you.
- Fioricet contains acetaminophen, which can cause severe liver injury. Do not take more than 4000 milligrams (mg) of acetaminophen a day or take other products containing acetaminophen. The risk of liver injury can be higher if you have underlying liver disease or drink alcohol while you are taking Fioricet.
- Fioricet can cause a severe allergic reaction or anaphylaxis (a serious and rapid allergic reaction that may result in death if not immediately treated). Stop taking this medication and tell your doctor immediately if you experience swelling of your

face, mouth, or throat; difficulty breathing; rash; itchiness; or vomiting.

Who should not take this medication?

Do not take Fioricet if you are allergic to it or any of its ingredients.

Do not take Fioricet or if you have porphyria (a blood disorder that interferes with how your body produces heme, which is the oxygen-carrying component of your red blood cells).

What should I tell my doctor before I take the first dose of this medication?

Tell your doctor about all prescription, over-the-counter, and herbal medications you are taking before beginning treatment with Fioricet. Also, talk to your doctor about your complete medical history, especially if you have porphyria, liver or kidney disease, or abdominal (stomach) problems.

What is the usual dosage?

Please see general statement regarding dosage on page xii.

Adults and children ≥12 years: The recommended dose is 1 or 2 tablets every 4 hours as needed.

How should I take this medication?

- Take Fioricet capsules exactly as prescribed by your doctor. Do not take more than six capsules in one day.

What should I avoid while taking this medication?

Fioricet can cause drowsiness or dizziness. Do not drive or operate machinery until you know how Fioricet affects you.

Do not drink alcohol while you are taking Fioricet.

What are possible food and drug interactions associated with this medication?

If Fioricet is taken with certain other drugs, the effects of either could be increased, decreased, or altered. It is especially important to check with your doctor before combining Fioricet with the following: alcohol, certain painkillers (such as morphine or oxycodone), or monoamine oxidase inhibitors (MAOIs) (such as phenelzine), a class of medications used to treat depression and other psychiatric conditions, or other medications that slow down your brain function (such as alprazolam, chlordiazepoxide, or phenobarbital).

What are the possible side effects of this medication?
Please see general statement regarding side effects on page xiii.

> **Side effects may include:** abdominal pain, drowsiness, intoxicated feeling, lightheadedness, nausea, sedation, shortness of breath, vomiting

Can I receive this medication if I am pregnant or breastfeeding?
The effects of Fioricet during pregnancy and breastfeeding are unknown. Tell your doctor immediately if you are pregnant, plan to become pregnant, or are breastfeeding.

What should I do if I miss a dose of this medication?
Fioricet should be given only as needed.

How should I store this medication?
Store at room temperature. Protect from light and moisture.

Flexeril
Generic name: Cyclobenzaprine HCl

What is this medication?
Flexeril is a muscle relaxant used in combination with rest and physical therapy to relieve symptoms associated with sudden, painful musculoskeletal conditions, such as muscle spasms.

What is the most important information I should know about this medication?

- Do not stop taking Flexeril abruptly; you may develop symptoms such as nausea, headache, or discomfort.

Who should not take this medication?

Do not take Flexeril if you are allergic to it or any of its ingredients.

Do not take Flexeril while you are taking other medicines known as monoamine oxidase inhibitors (MAOIs) (such as phenelzine), a class of medications used to treat depression and other conditions.

Do not take Flexeril if you have an irregular heartbeat, heart failure, heart block, or an overactive thyroid gland, or had a recent heart attack.

What should I tell my doctor before I take the first dose of this medication?

Tell your doctor about all prescription, over-the-counter, and herbal medications you are taking before beginning treatment with Flexeril. Also, talk to your doctor about your complete medical history, especially if you have liver disease, have ever had glaucoma (high pressure in the eye), or have ever been unable to urinate normally.

What is the usual dosage?

Please see general statement regarding dosage on page xii.

Adults and children ≥15 years: The recommended dose is 5 milligrams (mg) three times a day. Your doctor may increase your dose as needed.

If you are elderly or have liver impairment, your doctor will adjust your dose appropriately.

How should I take this medication?

- Take Flexeril exactly as prescribed by your doctor.

What should I avoid while taking this medication?

Do not take Flexeril for a longer period than prescribed by your doctor.

Do not take Flexeril and MAOIs together or within 14 days after stopping treatment with an MAOI.

Do not drive or operate dangerous machinery until you know how Flexeril affects you.

What are possible food and drug interactions associated with this medication?

If Flexeril is taken with certain other drugs, the effects of either could be increased, decreased, or altered. It is especially important to check with your doctor before combining Flexeril with the following: alcohol, barbiturates (such as phenobarbital), guanethidine, ipratropium or tolterodine, MAOIs, naproxen, or tramadol.

What are the possible side effects of this medication?

Please see general statement regarding side effects on page xiii.

> **Side effects may include:** dizziness, drowsiness, dry mouth, fatigue, headache

Can I receive this medication if I am pregnant or breastfeeding?

The effects of Flexeril during pregnancy and breastfeeding are unknown. Tell your doctor immediately if you are pregnant, plan to become pregnant, or are breastfeeding.

What should I do if I miss a dose of this medication?

If you miss a dose of Flexeril, take it as soon as you remember. However, if it is almost time for your next dose, skip the one you missed and return to your regular dosing schedule. Do not take two doses at once.

How should I store this medication?

Store at room temperature.

Flomax

Generic name: Tamsulosin HCl

What is this medication?

Flomax is a medicine used to treat signs and symptoms of benign prostatic hyperplasia (BPH), a condition characterized by an enlargement of the prostate gland, which may in turn block the flow of urine.

What is the most important information I should know about this medication?

- Flomax does not treat high blood pressure.
- Flomax can cause a sudden drop in blood pressure, which may cause fainting, dizziness, or lightheadedness. Until you learn how you react to Flomax, slowly sit or stand up from a lying or sitting position. If you begin to feel dizzy, sit or lie down until you feel better.
- Flomax can cause serious allergic reactions. Tell your doctor right away if you experience rash, itching, hives, difficulty breathing, blistering of your skin, or swelling of your face, tongue, or throat.
- Flomax can cause a painful erection that will not go away. This could happen even when you are not having sex. If this is not treated right away, it could lead to permanent sexual problems (such as impotence). Tell your doctor immediately if this happens.
- Flomax can cause complications in your eyes. Tell your eye doctor that you are taking Flomax before having cataract surgery or other procedures involving the eyes.

Who should not take this medication?

Flomax is not for use in women or children.

Do not take Flomax if you are allergic to it or any of its ingredients.

What should I tell my doctor before I take the first dose of this medication?

Tell your doctor about all prescription, over-the-counter, and herbal medications you are taking before beginning treatment with

Flomax. Also, talk to your doctor about your complete medical history, especially if you have kidney or liver problems, a history of low blood pressure, plan on having cataract surgery, or are allergic to sulfa medications (such as sulfamethoxazole).

What is the usual dosage?
Please see general statement regarding dosage on page xii.

Adults: The recommended dose is 0.4 milligrams once a day. Your doctor will increase your dose as needed.

How should I take this medication?
• Take Flomax exactly as prescribed by your doctor. Take it about 30 minutes after the same meal each day.
• Swallow Flomax capsules whole. Do not crush, chew, or open them.

What should I avoid while taking this medication?
Do not drive, operate machinery, or perform other dangerous activities until you know how Flomax affects you.

What are possible food and drug interactions associated with this medication?
If Flomax is taken with certain other drugs, the effects of either could be increased, decreased, or altered. It is especially important to check with your doctor before combining Flomax with the following: cimetidine, erythromycin, ketoconazole, medications for erectile dysfunction (such as sildenafil or tadalafil); other medications in the same class as Flomax (such as alfuzosin or doxazosin), paroxetine, terbinafine, or warfarin.

What are the possible side effects of this medication?
Please see general statement regarding side effects on page xiii.

> **Side effects may include:** decreased semen, dizziness, runny nose

Can I receive this medication if I am pregnant or breastfeeding?

Flomax is intended for use only by men and must not be used by women.

What should I do if I miss a dose of this medication?

If you miss a dose of Flomax, take it as soon as you remember. However, if it is almost time for your next dose, skip the one you missed and return to your regular dosing schedule. Do not take two doses at once.

How should I store this medication?

Store at room temperature.

Flonase

Generic name: Fluticasone Propionate

What is this medication?

Flonase is a medicine used to treat nasal symptoms (such as stuffy and runny nose, itching, or sneezing) of seasonal or year-round allergies, as well as non-allergic nasal symptoms. Flonase is available as a nasal spray.

What is the most important information I should know about this medication?

- Flonase is for use in your nose only.
- Flonase can cause infections in your nose and throat, form a hole in the wall between your nostrils, or impair wound healing. Do not use Flonase if you have a sore in your nose, have had nasal surgery, or a recent nasal injury until healing has occurred.
- Cataracts (clouding of the eye's lens), glaucoma (high pressure in the eye), or other eye problems can occur while you are using Flonase. Tell your doctor if you experience a change in your vision.
- If you use Flonase, you can have a higher risk of getting an infection. Do not expose yourself to chickenpox or measles while

you are using Flonase. This can be very serious and even fatal in children and adults who have not had chickenpox or measles.

- Use Flonase with caution if you have active or inactive tuberculosis (a bacterial infection that affects the lungs), or untreated fungal, bacterial, or viral infections.
- Flonase can cause slowed or delayed growth in children. Check your child's growth regularly during treatment with Flonase.
- A decrease in nasal symptoms may occur 12 hours after starting treatment with Flonase. The full benefit of Flonase may not be achieved until you have used it for several days. Tell your doctor if your symptoms do not improve within that time, or if your condition worsens.

Who should not take this medication?

Do not use Flonase if you are allergic to it or any of its ingredients.

What should I tell my doctor before I take the first dose of this medication?

Tell your doctor about all prescription, over-the-counter, and herbal medications you are taking before beginning treatment with Flonase. Also, talk to your doctor about your complete medical history, especially if you recently had nasal sores, surgery, or injury; have eye or vision problems; have any infections or had exposure to chickenpox or measles; or if you have asthma or other medical conditions that require long-term steroid treatment.

What is the usual dosage?

Please see general statement regarding dosage on page xii.

Adults: The recommended starting dose is two sprays in each nostril once a day or one spray in each nostril twice a day.

Children ≥4 years and adolescents: The recommended starting dose is one spray in each nostril once a day.

Your doctor may adjust your dose as appropriate.

How should I take this medication?
- Use Flonase exactly as prescribed by your doctor. Shake the bottle gently before each use.
- You must prime the nasal spray unit if you are using it for the first time. To do this, press the pump six times. Also, you must prime the pump by pressing until you see a fine mist if it has not been used for 7 days or longer.
- Gently blow your nose to clear your nostrils. Close one nostril and tilt your head forward slightly when you spray Flonase into each of your nostrils. Gently breathe in through your nostril and while breathing in press down on the applicator to release a spray.
- Please review the instructions that came with your prescription on how to properly use Flonase.

What should I avoid while taking this medication?
Do not spray Flonase into your eyes.

Do not apply extra doses or stop using Flonase without talking to your doctor.

What are possible food and drug interactions associated with this medication?
If Flonase is used with certain other drugs, the effects of either could be increased, decreased, or altered. It is especially important to check with your doctor before combining Flonase with ketoconazole or ritonavir.

What are the possible side effects of this medication?
Please see general statement regarding side effects on page xiii.

Side effects may include: asthma symptoms, cough, headache, nasal burning or irritation, nausea, nosebleed, throat inflammation, vomiting, wheezing

Can I receive this medication if I am pregnant or breastfeeding?

The effects of Flonase during pregnancy and breastfeeding are un-known. Tell your doctor immediately if you are pregnant, plan to become pregnant, or are breastfeeding.

What should I do if I miss a dose of this medication?

If you miss a dose of Flonase, apply it as soon as you remember. However, if it is almost time for your next dose, skip the one you missed and return to your regular dosing schedule. Do not apply two doses at once.

How should I store this medication?

Store in the refrigerator or at room temperature.

Flovent Diskus

Generic name: Fluticasone Propionate

What is this medication?

Flovent Diskus is an inhaled corticosteroid medicine used for the long-term treatment of asthma. It also helps to prevent symptoms of asthma.

What is the most important information I should know about this medication?

- Flovent Diskus does not treat the symptoms of a sudden asthma attack. Always have a short-acting rescue inhaler (such as alb-uterol) to treat sudden symptoms. If you do not have a short-acting inhaler, tell your doctor to have one prescribed for you. Tell your doctor immediately if an asthma attack does not re-spond to the rescue inhaler or if you require more doses than usual.
- Flovent Diskus can cause infections in your mouth and throat. Tell your doctor if you have any redness or white colored patch-es in your mouth.

- Cataracts (clouding of the eye's lens) or glaucoma (high pressure in the eye) can occur while you are using Flovent Diskus. Tell your doctor if you experience a change in your vision.
- If you use Flovent Diskus, you can have a higher risk of getting an infection. Do not expose yourself to chickenpox or measles while you are using Flovent Diskus. Tell your doctor if you experience any signs or symptoms of infection (such as a fever, pain, aches, chills, feeling tired, nausea, or vomiting).
- Flovent Diskus can cause slowed or delayed growth in children. Check your child's growth regularly during treatment with Flovent Diskus.
- Flovent Diskus can cause a serious allergic reaction. Stop using Flovent Diskus and call your doctor right away if you experience breathing problems, hives, rash, or swelling of your face, throat, or tongue.
- Do not stop using Flovent Diskus, even if your symptoms get better. Your doctor will change your medicine as needed.
- You may not feel or taste the medication from your Flovent Diskus when you inhale it. This does not mean that you did not get the medication. Do not repeat your inhalations even if you did not feel the medication when inhaling.

Who should not take this medication?
Do not use Flovent Diskus if you are allergic to it, any of its ingredients, or to milk protein. Also, do not use Flovent Diskus to treat an asthma attack.

What should I tell my doctor before I take the first dose of this medication?
Tell your doctor about all prescription, over-the-counter, and herbal medications you are taking before beginning treatment with Flovent Diskus. Also, talk to your doctor about your complete medical history, especially if you have or had chickenpox or measles, or have recently been near anyone with chickenpox or measles; have tuberculosis (a bacterial infection that affects the lungs), or any type of infection; osteoporosis (thin, weak bones); liver problems; cataracts or glaucoma; or are planning to have surgery. Also, tell your doctor if you take a corticosteroid medicine, seizure medications, or medicines that suppress your immune system.

What is the usual dosage?
Please see general statement regarding dosage on page xii.

Adults and adolescents ≥12 years: Your doctor will prescribe the appropriate dose for you based on your previous asthma medication.

Children 4-11 years: The recommended starting dose is 50 micrograms twice a day.

How should I take this medication?
• Use Flovent Diskus as prescribed by your doctor. Do not use Flovent Diskus more often or use more puffs than you have been prescribed.
• Rinse your mouth with water and spit it out after each dose. Do not swallow the water. This will reduce your chance of getting a fungal infection (thrush) in your mouth.
• Please review the instructions that came with your prescription on how to properly use your inhaler.

What should I avoid while taking this medication?
Do not use Flovent Diskus for a condition for which it was not prescribed.

Do not give Flovent Diskus to other people, even if they have the same symptoms that you have. It may harm them.

What are possible food and drug interactions associated with this medication?
If Flovent Diskus is used with certain other drugs, the effects of either could be increased, decreased, or altered. It is especially important to check with your doctor before combining Flovent Diskus with the following: atazanavir, clarithromycin, indinavir, itraconazole, ketoconazole, nefazodone, nelfinavir, ritonavir, saquinavir, or telithromycin.

What are the possible side effects of this medication?
Please see general statement regarding side effects on page xiii.

> **Side effects may include:** cold, fever, headache, nausea, throat irritation, upper respiratory tract infection, vomiting

Can I receive this medication if I am pregnant or breastfeeding?

The effects of Flovent Diskus during pregnancy and breastfeeding are unknown. Tell your doctor immediately if you are pregnant, plan to become pregnant, or are breastfeeding.

What should I do if I miss a dose of this medication?

If you miss a dose of Flovent Diskus, take it as soon as you remember. However, if it is almost time for your next dose, skip the one you missed and return to your regular dosing schedule. Do not take two doses at once.

How should I store this medication?

Store at room temperature, away from heat or sunlight.

Flovent HFA

Generic name: Fluticasone Propionate

What is this medication?

Flovent HFA is an inhaled corticosteroid medicine for the long-term treatment of asthma. It also helps to prevent symptoms of asthma.

What is the most important information I should know about this medication?

- Flovent HFA does not treat the symptoms of a sudden asthma attack. Always have a short-acting rescue inhaler (such as albuterol) to treat sudden symptoms. If you do not have a short-acting inhaler, tell your doctor to have one prescribed for you. Tell your doctor immediately if an asthma attack does not respond to the rescue inhaler or if you require more doses than usual.
- Flovent HFA can cause infections in your mouth and throat. Tell your doctor if you have any redness or white colored patches in your mouth.

- Cataracts (clouding of the eye's lens) or glaucoma (high pressure in the eye) can occur while you are using Flovent HFA. Tell your doctor if you experience a change in your vision.
- If you use Flovent HFA, you can have a higher risk of getting an infection. Do not expose yourself to chickenpox or measles while you are using Flovent HFA. Tell your doctor if you experience any signs or symptoms of infection (such as a fever, pain, aches, chills, feeling tired, nausea, or vomiting).
- Flovent HFA can cause slowed or delayed growth in children. Check your child's growth regularly during treatment with Flovent HFA.
- Flovent HFA can cause a serious allergic reaction. Stop using Flovent HFA and call your doctor right away if you experience breathing problems, hives, rash, or swelling of your face, throat, or tongue.
- Do not stop using Flovent HFA, even if your symptoms get better. Your doctor will change your medicine as needed.

Who should not take this medication?

Do not use Flovent HFA if you are allergic to it or any of its ingredients.

Do not use Flovent HFA to treat a sudden asthma attack.

What should I tell my doctor before I take the first dose of this medication?

Tell your doctor about all prescription, over-the-counter, and herbal medications you are taking before beginning treatment with Flovent HFA. Also, talk to your doctor about your complete medical history, especially if you have or had chickenpox or measles, or have recently been near anyone with chickenpox or measles; have tuberculosis (a bacterial infection that affects the lungs), or any type of infection; osteoporosis (thin, weak bones); liver problems; cataracts or glaucoma; or are planning to have surgery. Also, tell your doctor if you take a corticosteroid medicine, seizure medications, or medicines that suppress your immune system.

What is the usual dosage?

Please see general statement regarding dosage on page xii.

Adults and adolescents ≥12 years: Your doctor will prescribe the appropriate dose for you based on your previous asthma medication.

Children 4-11 years: The recommended starting dose is 88 micrograms twice a day.

How should I take this medication?
- Use Flovent HFA exactly as prescribed by your doctor. Shake the inhaler well before each use.
- If you are using the inhaler for the first time, you must prime it. To do this, take the cap off the mouthpiece and shake the inhaler well for 5 seconds. Then spray the inhaler into the air, away from your face. Shake and spray the inhaler in this way 3 more times. The counter should now read 120.
- If the inhaler has not been used for 7 days or if you drop it, you must prime it. To do this, take the cap off the mouthpiece and shake the inhaler well for 5 seconds. Then spray the inhaler one time into the air, away from your face.
- Breathe out through your mouth pushing as much air from your lungs as you can, then place the mouthpiece into your mouth and close your lips around it. While breathing in deeply and slowly through your mouth, press down on the top of the metal canister. Hold your breath for 10 seconds if possible.
- Rinse your mouth and spit the water after each dose. Do not swallow the water. This will reduce your chance of getting a fungal infection (thrush) in your mouth.
- Please review the instructions that came with your prescription on how to properly use Flovent HFA.

What should I avoid while taking this medication?
Do not spray Flovent HFA in your eyes.

If you have not had or not been vaccinated against chickenpox, measles, or active tuberculosis, stay away from people who are infected while you are using Flovent HFA.

Do not try to change the numbers or take the counter off the metal canister.

Do not use the plastic actuator with a canister of any other medicine. And do not use the Flovent HFA canister with any other plastic actuator.

What are possible food and drug interactions associated with this medication?

If Flovent HFA is used with certain other drugs, the effects of either could be increased, decreased, or altered. It is especially important to check with your doctor before combining Flovent HFA with the following: atazanavir, clarithromycin, indinavir, itraconazole, ketoconazole, nefazodone, nelfinavir, ritonavir, saquinavir, or telithromycin.

What are the possible side effects of this medication?
Please see general statement regarding side effects on page xiii.

Side effects may include: colds, diarrhea, ear infection, fever, headache, throat irritation, upper respiratory tract infection

Can I receive this medication if I am pregnant or breastfeeding?

The effects of Flovent HFA during pregnancy and breastfeeding are unknown. Tell your doctor immediately if you are pregnant, plan to become pregnant, or are breastfeeding.

What should I do if I miss a dose of this medication?

If you miss a dose of Flovent HFA, take it as soon as you remember. However, if it is almost time for your next dose, skip the one you missed and return to your regular dosing schedule. Do not take two doses at once.

How should I store this medication?

Store at room temperature, away from heat or open flame.

Fluconazole: *see Diflucan, page 317*

Fluocinonide

Generic name: Fluocinonide

What is this medication?

Fluocinonide is a topical medicine (applied to the skin surface) that is used for the relief of inflammation and itching of the skin. It is available in a cream, gel, ointment, and topical solution.

What is the most important information I should know about this medication?

- Fluocinonide is for external use only. Do not use it in your eyes.
- Fluocinonide can have a greater effect on children because they are more likely to absorb large amounts of the medicine through the skin. Long-term use can affect the growth and development of children. Talk to your doctor if you think your child is not growing at a normal rate after using this medication for a long period of time.
- Do not use fluocinonide for any other condition other than that which your doctor has prescribed.
- Fluocinonide should not be applied in the diaper area, as diapers or plastic pants may be occlusive dressings.
- Contact your doctor if you notice irritation or any skin reactions in the area being treated.

Who should not take this medication?

Do not use fluocinonide if you are allergic to it or any of its ingredients.

What should I tell my doctor before I take the first dose of this medication?

Tell your doctor about all prescription, over-the-counter, and herbal medications you are taking before beginning treatment with fluocinonide. Also, talk to your doctor about your complete medical history, especially if you have skin infections, or are pregnant, plan to become pregnant, or are breastfeeding.

What is the usual dosage?

Please see general statement regarding dosage on page xii.

Adults and children: Apply a thin film to the affected area(s) 2-4 times a day depending on the severity of your condition.

How should I take this medication?
- Apply fluocinonide exactly as prescribed by your doctor. Do not apply extra doses or apply more often without asking your doctor.
- You can use occlusive dressings (such as bandages) for the management of psoriasis (immune disorder that affects the skin) or other skin conditions that are difficult to treat.

What should I avoid while taking this medication?
Do not use fluocinonide in your eyes.

Do not bandage, cover, or wrap the treated skin area as to be occlusive unless directed by your doctor to do so.

What are possible food and drug interactions associated with this medication?
No significant interactions have been reported with fluocinonide at this time. However, always tell your doctor about any medicines you take, including over-the-counter medications, vitamins, and herbal supplements.

What are the possible side effects of this medication?
Please see general statement regarding side effects on page xiii.

Side effects may include: acne (pimples), allergic skin reactions, burning, dryness, infections, inflamed hair follicles, irritation, itching, loss of skin color, skin inflammation, stretch marks, sweat rash, thinning of your skin layers

---

Can I receive this medication if I am pregnant or breastfeeding?
The effects of fluocinonide during pregnancy and breastfeeding are unknown. Tell your doctor immediately if you are pregnant, plan to become pregnant, or are breastfeeding.

What should I do if I miss a dose of this medication?

If you miss a dose of fluocinonide, apply it as soon as you remember. However, if it is almost time for your next dose, skip the one you missed and return to your regular dosing schedule. Do not apply two doses at once.

How should I store this medication?

Store at room temperature.

Fluocinonide: see Fluocinonide, page 403

Fluoxetine HCl: see Prozac, page 871

Fluticasone Propionate: see Flonase, page 393

Fluticasone Propionate: see Flovent Diskus, page 396

Fluticasone Propionate: see Flovent HFA, page 399

Fluticasone Propionate/Salmeterol: see Advair Diskus, page 34

Focalin XR

Generic name: Dexmethylphenidate HCl

What is this medication?

Focalin XR is a medicine used to treat attention-deficit hyperactivity disorder (ADHD). This medicine may help increase attention and decrease impulsiveness and hyperactivity in people with ADHD.

What is the most important information I should know about this medication?

• Focalin XR has a high potential for abuse. Taking Focalin XR for long periods of time may lead to extreme emotional and physical dependence. Your doctor will monitor your response and make sure you receive the correct dose. Tell your doctor if you have a history of drug or alcohol abuse.

- Focalin XR can cause serious heart-related and mental problems, stroke and heart attacks in adults, and increased blood pressure and heart rate. It can also cause new or worsening behavior and thought problems, bipolar illness, and aggressive or hostile behavior.
- In addition, new symptoms (such as hearing voices, believing things that are not true, or manic symptoms) can occur. Call your doctor immediately if you or your child experiences chest pain, shortness of breath, fainting, or new mental problems while taking Focalin XR.
- The doctor will check your child's height and weight while he/she is taking Focalin XR. If your child is not growing in height or gaining weight as expected, the doctor may stop this medicine.

Who should not take this medication?
Do not take Focalin XR if you are allergic to it or any of its ingredients. Do not take Focalin XR if you are very anxious, tense, or agitated.

Do not take Focalin XR if you have glaucoma (high pressure in the eye), tics (repeated movements or sounds that cannot be controlled), or Tourette's syndrome or a family history of Tourette's (a brain disorder characterized by involuntary movements and vocalizations called tics). Also, do not use Focalin XR if you are taking antidepressant medications known as MAO inhibitors (such as phenelzine) or have taken them within the past 14 days.

What should I tell my doctor before I take the first dose of this medication?
Tell your doctor about all prescription, over-the-counter, and herbal medications you are taking before beginning treatment with Focalin XR. Also, talk to your doctor about your complete medical history, including heart problems, heart defects, high blood pressure, or a family history of these problems. Tell your doctor if you have a history of mental problems or a family history of suicide, bipolar disorder, or depression; tics or Tourette's syndrome; or seizures or an abnormal brain wave test (EEG).

What is the usual dosage?
Please see general statement regarding dosage on page xii.

People New to Methylphenidate
Adults: The usual starting dose is 10 milligrams (mg) a day. Your doctor may increase your dose as appropriate.

Children ≥6 years: The usual starting dose is 5 mg a day. Your child's doctor may increase the dose as appropriate.

People Currently Using Methylphenidate or Dexmethylphenidate
Adults and Children ≥6 years: Your doctor will prescribe the appropriate dose for you.

How should I take this medication?
- Swallow your Focalin XR capsule whole. Do not crush, chew, or divide it. Take it in the morning with or without food.
- If you cannot swallow the Focalin XR capsule whole, open the capsule carefully and sprinkle the medicine beads over a spoonful of applesauce. Swallow the medicine and applesauce combination whole right away and do not store it for future use.
- Focalin XR is an extended-release capsule, which means it releases medicine into your body throughout the day.

What should I avoid while taking this medication?
Use caution when driving, operating heavy machinery, or performing activities that require alertness.

Focalin XR may cause dizziness, drowsiness, or blurred vision. This medicine may affect your ability to concentrate.

What are possible food and drug interactions associated with this medication?
If Focalin XR is taken with certain other drugs, the effects of either could be increased, decreased, or altered. It is especially important to check with your doctor before combining Focalin XR with the following: antacids, blood thinners (such as warfarin), blood pressure medications, certain antidepressants (such as clomipramine or

desipramine), cold or allergy preparations containing decongestants, MAOIs, or seizure medications (such as phenobarbital, phenytoin, or primidone).

What are the possible side effects of this medication?
Please see general statement regarding side effects on page xiii.

> **Side effects may include:** anxiety, decreased appetite, dizziness, dry mouth, eyesight changes or blurred vision, headache, nervousness, seizures (mainly in patients with history of seizures), trouble sleeping, upset stomach

Can I receive this medication if I am pregnant or breastfeeding?
The effects of Focalin XR during pregnancy and breastfeeding are unknown. Tell your doctor immediately if you are pregnant, plan to become pregnant, or are breastfeeding.

What should I do if I miss a dose of this medication?
If you miss a dose of Focalin XR, take it as soon as you remember. However, if it is almost time for your next dose, skip the one you missed and return to your regular dosing schedule. Do not take two doses at once.

How should I store this medication?
Store at room temperature.

Folic Acid
Generic name: Folic Acid

What is this medication?
Folic acid is a medicine used to treat anemia due to inadequate folic acid levels. Folic acid is also used to treat anemia due to lack of dietary intake, pregnancy, or in infants and children.

What is the most important information I should know about this medication?

- Folic acid should not be used alone to treat anemias caused by low vitamin B$_{12}$ levels.

Who should not take this medication?

Do not take folic acid if you are allergic to it or any of its ingredients.

What should I tell my doctor before I take the first dose of this medication?

Tell your doctor about all prescription, over-the-counter, and herbal medications you are taking before beginning treatment with folic acid. Also, talk to your doctor about your complete medical history especially if you have low vitamin B$_{12}$ levels, liver problems, seizure disorder, drink excessive amounts of alcohol, have an infection, or are receiving dialysis.

What is the usual dosage?

Please see general statement regarding dosage on page xii.

Adults and children: The usual dose is up to 1 milligram a day. Your doctor may adjust your dose as appropriate.

How should I take this medication?

- Take folic acid exactly as prescribed by your doctor.

What should I avoid while taking this medication?

Do not change your dose or stop taking folic acid without first talking to your doctor.

What are possible food and drug interactions associated with this medication?

If folic acid is taken with certain other drugs, the effects of either could be increased, decreased, or altered. It is especially important to check with your doctor before combining folic acid with the following: alcohol, antibiotics (such as tetracycline), methotrexate, nitrofurantoin, pyrimethamine, or seizure medications (such as diphenylhydantoin, phenobarbital, phenytoin, or primidone).

What are the possible side effects of this medication?
Please see general statement regarding side effects on page xiii.

> **Side effects may include:** breathing problems, itching, lack of energy, low vitamin B_{12} levels, rash, skin redness

Can I receive this medication if I am pregnant or breastfeeding?
You can continue to take folic acid during pregnancy and breast-feeding. However, a dose adjustment may be necessary. Folic acid is excreted in your breast milk. Tell your doctor immediately if you are pregnant, plan to become pregnant, or are breastfeeding.

What should I do if I miss a dose of this medication?
If you miss a dose of folic acid, take it as soon as you remember. However, if it is almost time for your next dose, skip the one you missed and return to your regular dosing schedule. Do not take two doses at once.

How should I store this medication?
Store at room temperature.

Folic Acid: see Folic Acid, page 408

Fosamax
Generic name: Alendronate Sodium

What is this medication?
Fosamax is a medicine used to prevent and treat bone loss (osteo-porosis) in postmenopausal women and to increase bone mass in men with this condition. Fosamax is also used to treat osteo-porosis caused by treatment with corticosteroid medicines (such as prednisone), and to treat Paget's disease of bone in men and women. Fosamax is available as tablets and an oral solution.

What is the most important information I should know about this medication?

- Fosamax can cause problems in your esophagus (the tube that connects your mouth and stomach) (such as irritation, swelling, or ulcers), which can sometimes bleed. Stop taking Fosamax and call your doctor right away if you experience chest pain, new or worsening heartburn, or have trouble or pain when you swallow.
- Fosamax can cause or worsen low blood calcium levels. Call your doctor right away if you experience spasms, twitches, or cramps in your muscles, or numbness or tingling in your fingers, toes, or around your mouth.
- Your doctor may prescribe calcium and vitamin D to help prevent low blood calcium levels while you are taking Fosamax.
- Fosamax can cause bone, joint, or muscle pain. Tell your doctor if you experience any of these symptoms.
- Fosamax can cause severe jaw bone problems. Your doctor will examine your mouth or tell you to see your dentist before you start taking Fosamax. Practice good mouth care during treatment with Fosamax.
- Fosamax can cause unusual fractures in the thigh bone. Tell your doctor if you experience new or unusual pain in your hip, groin, or thigh.

Who should not take this medication?

Do not take Fosamax if you are allergic to it or any of its ingredients.

Do not take Fosamax if you have problems with your esophagus, low blood calcium levels, if you cannot stand or sit upright for at least 30 minutes, or if you have severe kidney impairment.

What should I tell my doctor before I take the first dose of this medication?

Tell your doctor about all prescription, over-the-counter, and herbal medications you are taking before beginning treatment with Fosamax. Also, talk to your doctor about your complete medical history, especially if you have problems swallowing, stomach or digestive problems, low blood calcium levels, kidney problems, or if you plan to have dental surgery or teeth removed. Tell your doctor if you have been told you have trouble absorbing minerals in your stomach or intestines.

What is the usual dosage?
Please see general statement regarding dosage on page xii.

Treatment of Postmenopausal Osteoporosis and Osteoporosis in Men
Adults: The recommended dose is one 70-milligram (mg) tablet or one 70-mg bottle of oral solution once a week or one 10-mg tablet once a day.

Prevention of Postmenopausal Osteoporosis
Adults: The recommended dose is one 35-mg tablet once a week or one 5-mg tablet once a day.

Treatment of Corticosteroid-Induced Osteoporosis
Adults: The recommended dose is one 5-mg tablet once a day. In postmenopausal women not receiving estrogen, the recommended dose is one 10-mg tablet once a day.

Paget's Disease
Adults: The recommended dose is 40 mg, once a day, for six months. Your doctor may decide to retreat you based on your condition.

How should I take this medication?
- Take Fosamax exactly as prescribed by your doctor to lower your risk of developing problems in your esophagus.
- Take Fosamax tablets or oral solution as soon as you get up for the day. Take it at least 30 minutes before eating, drinking, or taking any other medicine. Take it while you are sitting or standing.
- Swallow Fosamax tablets whole with a full glass of plain water only. Do not chew or suck the tablets or take it with any other liquids.
- Drink at least a quarter cup of plain water after you take Fosamax oral solution.

- If you are taking Fosamax once a week, take it on the same day each week.
- After you take Fosamax tablets or oral solution, wait at least 30 minutes before you lie down, eat your first meal or drink of the day (except for water), or take any other medicines.

What should I avoid while taking this medication?

Do not lie down for 30 minutes after taking Fosamax.

Do not eat or drink anything (except plain water) before and for at least 30 minutes after you take Fosamax.

Do not take Fosamax at bedtime or if you will stay in bed after waking up.

What are possible food and drug interactions associated with this medication?

If Fosamax is taken with certain other drugs, the effects of either could be increased, decreased, or altered. It is especially important to check with your doctor before combining Fosamax with the following: antacids, aspirin, calcium supplements, or nonsteroidal anti-inflammatory drugs (NSAIDs) (such as ibuprofen or naproxen).

What are the possible side effects of this medication?

Please see general statement regarding side effects on page xiii.

> **Side effects may include:** abdominal (stomach) pain, constipation, diarrhea, heartburn, nausea, upset stomach

Can I receive this medication if I am pregnant or breastfeeding?

The effects of Fosamax during pregnancy and breastfeeding are unknown. Tell your doctor immediately if you are pregnant, plan to become pregnant, or are breastfeeding.

What should I do if I miss a dose of this medication?

Fosamax should be taken under special circumstances. If you miss your scheduled dose, contact your doctor or pharmacist for advice.

How should I store this medication?
Store at room temperature.

Fosinopril
Generic name: Fosinopril Sodium

What is this medication?
Fosinopril is a medicine known as an angiotensin-converting enzyme (ACE) inhibitor. Fosinopril is used alone or in combination with other medications to treat high blood pressure or heart failure.

What is the most important information I should know about this medication?
- Fosinopril can cause a rare but serious allergic reaction leading to extreme swelling of your face, lips, tongue, throat, or gut (causing severe abdominal pain). You may have an increased risk of experiencing these symptoms if you have ever had an allergy to ACE inhibitor-type medicines or if you are African American. If you experience any of these symptoms, seek emergency medical attention immediately.
- Tell your doctor if you experience lightheadedness, especially during the first few days of fosinopril therapy. If you faint, stop taking fosinopril and tell your doctor immediately.
- Vomiting, diarrhea, fever, exercise, hot weather, drinking alcohol, excessive perspiration, and dehydration may lead to an excessive fall in your blood pressure. Tell your doctor if you experience any of these.
- Fosinopril may decrease your blood neutrophil (type of blood cells that fight infections) levels, especially if you have a collagen vascular disease (such as lupus [disease that affects the immune system]) or kidney disease.
- Promptly report any signs of infection (such as sore throat or fever) to your doctor.
- Fosinopril may not work as well in African Americans, who may also have a higher risk of side effects. Contact your doctor if your symptoms do not improve or become worse.

Who should not take this medication?
Do not take fosinopril if you are allergic to it or any of its ingredients.

Do not take fosinopril if you have a history of angioedema (a condition involving swelling of the face, extremities, eyes, lips, and tongue) related to previous treatment with similar medicines. Also, do not take fosinopril if you have a history of certain types of angioedema (such as hereditary or idiopathic).

What should I tell my doctor before I take the first dose of this medication?
Tell your doctor about all prescription, over-the-counter, and herbal medications you are taking before beginning treatment with fosinopril. Also, talk to your doctor about your complete medical history, especially if you have liver problems, kidney disease, or diabetes. Tell your doctor if you have bone marrow problems or any blood disease, any disease that affects the immune system (such as lupus or scleroderma), collagen vascular disease, narrowing or hardening of the arteries of your brain or heart, chest pain, or if you have ever had an allergy or sensitivity to ACE inhibitors such as fosinopril.

What is the usual dosage?
Please see general statement regarding dosage on page xii.

High Blood Pressure
Adults: The usual starting dose is 10 milligrams (mg) once a day. Your doctor will adjust your dose based on your previous blood pressure medication and will increase your dose as needed until the desired effect is achieved.

Children ≥6 years: Your doctor will prescribe the appropriate dose for your child, based on their weight.

Heart Failure
Adults: The usual starting dose is 10 mg once a day. Your doctor may give you a higher dose depending on your needs.

If you have kidney impairment, your doctor will adjust your dose appropriately.

How should I take this medication?
- Take fosinopril at the same time every day. Continue to take fosinopril even if you feel well.
- Do not take extra doses or take more often without asking your doctor.
- Fosinopril can be taken with or without food.

What should I avoid while taking this medication?
Do not become pregnant or breastfeed while you are taking fosinopril.

Do not drive or operate heavy machinery until you know how fosinopril affects you.

Do not take salt substitutes or supplements containing potassium without consulting your doctor.

Do not stand or sit up quickly when you take fosinopril, especially in the morning. Sit or lie down at the first sign of dizziness, light-headedness, or fainting.

What are possible food and drug Interactions associated with this medication?
If fosinopril is taken with certain other drugs, the effects of either could be increased, decreased, or altered. It is especially important to check with your doctor before combining fosinopril with the following: amiloride, antacids, dextran, diuretics (water pills) (such as furosemide, hydrochlorothiazide, spironolactone, or triamterene), lithium, nonsteroidal anti-inflammatory drugs [NSAIDs] (such as ibuprofen or naproxen), potassium supplements, or salt substitutes containing potassium.

What are the possible side effects of this medication?
Please see general statement regarding side effects on page xiii.

> **Side effects may include:** cough, diarrhea, dizziness, fatigue, headache, low blood pressure, muscle pain, upper respiratory infection

Can I receive this medication if I am pregnant or breastfeeding?

Do not take fosinopril if you are pregnant or breastfeeding. Fosinopril can harm your unborn baby. Tell your doctor immediately if you are pregnant, plan to become pregnant, or are breastfeeding.

What should I do if I miss a dose of this medication?

If you miss a dose of fosinopril, take it as soon as you remember. However, if it is almost time for your next dose, skip the one you missed and return to your regular dosing schedule. Do not take two doses at once.

How should I store this medication?

Store at room temperature.

Fosinopril Sodium: see Fosinopril, page 414

Furosemide: see Lasix, page 528

Gabapentin: see Neurontin, page 680

Gabapentin Enacarbil: see Horizant, page 436

Gemfibrozil: see Lopid, page 572

Geodon

Generic name: Ziprasidone HCl

What is this medication?

Geodon is a medicine used to treat schizophrenia. This medication can also be used to treat manic or mixed episodes associated with bipolar disorder alone or in combination with lithium or valproate.

What is the most important information I should know about this medication?

- Geodon can be life-threatening when used in elderly people with mental problems caused by dementia (an illness involving loss of memory, judgment, and confusion). Geodon is not approved to treat mental problems caused by dementia.

- Geodon can cause an abnormal heartbeat that can be dangerous and life-threatening. Do not take Geodon with other medications that can cause this irregular heartbeat (such as chlorpromazine, quinidine, or thioridazine) or certain antibiotics (such as gatifloxacin or moxifloxacin).

- In rare cases, Geodon can cause neuroleptic malignant syndrome (NMS) (a life-threatening brain disorder). NMS is a medical emergency, get medical help right away. Tell your doctor right away if you experience high fever, muscle rigidity, confusion, fast or irregular heartbeat, changes in your blood pressure, or increased sweating.

- Geodon can cause tardive dyskinesia (abnormal muscle movements, including tremor, shuffling and uncontrolled, involuntary movements). Tell your doctor if you experience uncontrollable muscle movements.

- Geodon can cause an increase in your blood sugar levels or diabetes. Tell your doctor if you experience excessive thirst, an increase in urination, an increase in appetite, or weakness. If you have diabetes or are at risk for diabetes, monitor your blood sugar regularly, as determined by your doctor. Also, you can experience an increase in your blood cholesterol levels or weight gain while you are taking Geodon. Monitor your weight regularly.

- Geodon can cause a sudden decrease in your blood pressure with dizziness, rapid heartbeat, and faintness. Geodon can also cause a rash, seizures, problems with your body temperature regulation, difficulty swallowing, or impairment of your judgment, thinking, or motor skills.

- Geodon can also cause hyperprolactinemia (an increase in a hormone called prolactin, which can affect lactation, menstruation, and fertility). Tell your doctor right away if you experience missed menstrual periods, leakage of milk from your breasts, development of the breasts in men, or problems with erections.

- Geodon can lower the ability of your body to fight infections. Tell your doctor if you notice any signs of infection such as a fever, sore throat, rash, or chills.

Who should not take this medication?

Do not take Geodon if you are allergic to it or any of its ingredients.

Geodon is not approved to treat mental problems caused by dementia in the elderly.

Do not take Geodon if you have certain heart diseases, such as an abnormal heart rhythm, a recent heart attack, or severe heart failure.

What should I tell my doctor before I take the first dose of this medication?

Tell your doctor about all prescription, over-the-counter, and herbal medications you are taking before beginning treatment with Geodon. Also, talk to your doctor about your complete medical history, especially if you have or have had any heart or heartbeat problems; any family history of heart disease, including recent heart attack; problems with fainting or dizziness; liver problems; seizures; a history of suicidal thoughts; or are pregnant, plan to become pregnant, or are breastfeeding.

What is the usual dosage?

Please see general statement regarding dosage on page xii.

<u>Schizophrenia</u>

Adults: The recommended starting dose is 20 milligrams (mg) twice a day. Your doctor will increase your dose as needed, until the desired effect is achieved.

<u>Manic or Mixed Episodes of Bipolar Disorder</u>

Adults: The recommended starting dose is 40 mg twice a day with food. Your doctor will increase your dose as needed, until the desired effect is achieved.

How should I take this medication?

- Take Geodon exactly as prescribed by your doctor. Do not take extra doses or take more often without asking your doctor.
- Take Geodon capsules at the same time each day with food. Swallow the Geodon capsule whole.
- If you feel you need to stop Geodon, talk to your doctor first.

What should I avoid while taking this medication?

Do not drink alcohol while you are taking Geodon.

Do not drive or operate machinery until you know how Geodon affects you.

Do not expose yourself to extreme heat or dehydration while you are taking Geodon.

What are possible food and drug interactions associated with this medication?

If Geodon is taken with certain other drugs, the effects of either could be increased, decreased, or altered. It is especially important to check with your doctor before combining Geodon with the following: carbamazepine, ketoconazole, or other medications that can cause irregular heartbeat (such as arsenic trioxide, chlorpromazine, diuretics [water pills] [such as furosemide], dofetilide, dolasetron, droperidol, gatifloxacin, halofantrine, levomethadyl, mefloquine, mesoridazine, moxifloxacin, pentamidine, pimozide, probucol, quinidine, sotalol, sparfloxacin, tacrolimus, or thioridazine).

What are the possible side effects of this medication?

Please see general statement regarding side effects on page xiii.

Side effects may include: abnormal muscle movements, constipation, cough, diarrhea, dizziness, fainting, fluttery or throbbing heartbeat, loss of consciousness, nausea, rash, restlessness, runny nose, shuffling, sleepiness, tiredness, tremor, uncontrolled involuntary movements, upset stomach

---

Can I receive this medication if I am pregnant or breastfeeding?

The effects of Geodon during pregnancy and breastfeeding are unknown. Do not breastfeed while you are taking Geodon. Tell your doctor immediately if you are pregnant, plan to become pregnant, or are breastfeeding.

What should I do if I miss a dose of this medication?

If you miss a dose of Geodon, take it as soon as you remember. However, if it is almost time for your next dose, skip the one you missed and return to your regular dosing schedule. Do not take two doses at once.

How should I store this medication?

Store at room temperature.

Glimepiride: *see Amaryl, page 61*

Glipizide: *see Glucotrol, page 424*

Glucophage

Generic name: Metformin HCl

What is this medication?

Glucophage is a medicine used in addition to diet and exercise to treat type 2 diabetes. It is also available as Glucophage XR, an extended-release form (allows the medicine to be released slowly in your body over 24 hours).

What is the most important information I should know about this medication?

- Glucophage can cause a rare but serious condition called lactic acidosis. Stop using Glucophage and call your doctor right away if you feel very weak, tired or uncomfortable; have unusual muscle pain, trouble breathing, or unusual or unexpected stomach discomfort; feel cold, dizzy, or lightheaded; or if you suddenly have a slow or uneven heartbeat.

- Glucophage rarely causes low blood sugar alone. However, this can happen if you do not eat enough, if you drink alcohol, or if you take other medicines to lower blood sugar.

Who should not take this medication?

Do not take Glucophage if you are allergic to it or any of its ingredients.

Do not take Glucophage if you have kidney or liver problems, heart failure that is treated with medicines such as digoxin or furosemide, or a serious condition (such as heart attack, severe infection, or a stroke).

Do not take Glucophage if you drink a lot of alcohol, are dehydrated, are going to receive an injection of a dye or contrast agent for an imaging procedure (such as x-ray or CT scan), or are going to have surgery.

Do not take Glucophage if you are 80 years or older and have not had your kidney function tested.

What should I tell my doctor before I take the first dose of this medication?

Tell your doctor about all prescription, over-the-counter, and herbal medications you are taking before beginning treatment with Glucophage. Also, talk to your doctor about your complete medical history, especially if you have a history of kidney, liver, or heart problems. Tell your doctor if you drink alcohol frequently or if you are a binge drinker.

Also, tell your doctor if you have an illness that causes severe vomiting, diarrhea, or fever, or if you drink a much lower amount of liquid than normal. These conditions can lead to severe dehydration.

What is the usual dosage?

Please see general statement regarding dosage on page xii.

Glucophage
Adults: The usual starting dose is 500 milligrams (mg) twice a day or 850 mg once a day with meals. Your doctor may adjust your dose as appropriate.

Children 10-16 years: The usual starting dose is 500 mg twice a day with meals. Your doctor may adjust your dose as appropriate.

Glucophage XR
Adults: The usual starting dose is 500 mg once a day with the evening meal. Your doctor may adjust your dose as appropriate.

How should I take this medication?
- Take Glucophage exactly as prescribed by your doctor. Take it with food to lower the chance of an upset stomach.
- Swallow the Glucophage XR tablet whole. Do not crush or chew it.
- Glucophage XR may be eliminated as a soft mass in your stool; it may look like the original tablet. This is not harmful and will not affect the way the medicine works to control your diabetes.

What should I avoid while taking this medication?
Do not drink too much alcohol while you are taking Glucophage.

What are possible food and drug interactions associated with this medication?
If Glucophage is taken with certain other drugs, the effects of either could be increased, decreased, or altered. It is especially important to check with your doctor before combining Glucophage with the following: albuterol, alcohol, birth control pills, blood pressure medications known as calcium channel blockers (such as nifedipine), certain antibiotics (such as trimethoprim or vancomycin), cimetidine, corticosteroids (such as prednisone), digoxin, diuretics (water pills) (such as amiloride, furosemide, hydrochlorothiazide, or triamterene), estrogens, isoniazid, morphine, nicotinic acid, other diabetes medicines (such as chlorpropamide, glyburide, or insulin), phenothiazines (such as chlorpromazine, mesoridazine, or thioridazine), phenytoin, procainamide, pseudoephedrine, quinidine, quinine, ranitidine, or thyroid medicines.

What are the possible side effects of this medication?
Please see general statement regarding side effects on page xiii.

Side effects may include: abdominal discomfort, diarrhea, gas, headache, indigestion, nausea, vomiting, weakness

Can I receive this medication if I am pregnant or breastfeeding?
The effects of Glucophage during pregnancy and breastfeeding are unknown. Tell your doctor immediately if you are pregnant, plan to become pregnant, or are breastfeeding.

What should I do if I miss a dose of this medication?
If you miss a dose of Glucophage, take it as soon as you remember. However, if it is almost time for your next dose, skip the one you missed and return to your regular dosing schedule. Do not take two doses at once.

How should I store this medication?
Store at room temperature.

Glucotrol
Generic name: Glipizide

What is this medication?
Glucotrol is used along with diet and exercise to help lower high blood sugar in type 2 diabetes. Glucotrol also comes in an extended-release form called Glucotrol XL, which allows the medicine to be released slowly in your body over 24 hours. They belong to a class of drugs called sulfonylureas.

What is the most important information I should know about this medication?
• Treatment with sulfonylureas may increase the risk of death from heart and blood vessel problems compared to treatment of

diabetes with diet alone or diet plus insulin. Discuss with your
doctor the risks and benefits of treatment with Glucotrol.

- Low blood sugar may occur. The signs and symptoms include
  headache, drowsiness, weakness, dizziness, fast heartbeat,
  sweating, tremor, and nausea. If you experience any of these
  signs and symptoms, eat or drink something with sugar in it
  right away. If you do not feel better or if your blood sugar does
  not go up, call your doctor immediately.

- Follow diet, medication, and exercise routines closely. Changing
  any of them can affect blood sugar levels. Blood levels should
  be assessed regularly.

Who should not take this medication?

Do not take Glucotrol if you are sensitive to the drug or any of its
components, or have type 1 diabetes.

What should I tell my doctor before I take the first dose of this medication?

Tell your doctor about all prescription, over-the-counter, and
herbal medications you are taking before beginning treatment with
Glucotrol. Also, talk to your doctor about your complete medical
history, especially if you have ever had diabetic ketoacidosis (a life-
threatening medical emergency caused by insufficient insulin and
marked by excessive thirst, nausea, fatigue, pain below the breast
bone, and fruity breath); a history of kidney or liver disease; thyroid
disease; chronic (continuing) diarrhea; or type 1 diabetes; a serious infection, illness, or injury; glucose-6-phosphate dehydrogenase deficiency (lack of an enzyme responsible for the breakdown
of red blood cells); need surgery; or have narrowing of the stomach
or intestines.

What is the usual dosage?

Please see general statement regarding dosage on page xii.

Glucotrol

Adults: The usual starting dose is 5 milligrams (mg) taken before
breakfast. Depending upon your blood sugar response, your doctor may increase your dose as needed.

Elderly or liver impaired: The usual starting dose is 2.5 mg.

Glucotrol XL
Adults: The usual starting dose is 5 mg each day at breakfast. After 3 months, your doctor may increase your dose to 10 mg daily.

Elderly or liver impaired: The usual starting dose is 5 mg.

How should I take this medication?
- Take Glucotrol exactly as prescribed. To achieve the best control of blood sugar levels, Glucotrol should be taken 30 minutes before a meal. However, the exact dosing schedule, as well as the dosage amount, must be determined by your doctor.
- Glucotrol XL should be taken with breakfast. Swallow the tablets whole. Do not chew, crush, or divide them. Do not be alarmed if you notice something that looks like a tablet in your stool; it is only the empty shell that has been eliminated.

What should I avoid while taking this medication?
Avoid alcohol, as it can interfere with your blood sugar levels and your diabetes treatment.

What are possible food and drug interactions associated with this medication?
If Glucotrol is taken with certain other drugs, the effects of either could be increased, decreased, or altered. It is especially important to check with your doctor before combining Glucotrol with the following: alcohol, aspirin, beta-blockers (such as atenolol and metoprolol), calcium channel blockers (such as diltiazem, nifedipine, verapamil), chloramphenicol, cimetidine, clofibrate, corticosteroids (such as dexamethasone and prednisone), diuretics (water pills) (such as hydrochlorothiazide or furosemide), epinephrine, estrogens, fluconazole, gemfibrozil, isoniazid, miconazole, monamine oxidase inhibitors (such as phenelzine and tranylcypromine), nicotinic acid, nonsteroidal anti-inflammatory drugs (such as ibuprofen or naproxen), norepinephrine, birth control pills, phenothiazines, phenytoin, probenecid, pseudoephedrine, rifampin, sulfa drugs (such as sulfamethoxazole), thyroid drugs, or warfarin.

What are the possible side effects of this medication?

Please see general statement regarding side effects on page xiii.

> **Side effects may include:** low blood sugar, weakness, dizziness, nervousness, tremor, diarrhea

Can I receive this medication if I am pregnant or breastfeeding?

The effects of Glucotrol during pregnancy and breastfeeding are unknown. Tell your doctor immediately if you are pregnant, plan to become pregnant, or are breastfeeding.

What should I do if I miss a dose of this medication?

If you miss a dose of Glucotrol, take the missed dose as soon as you remember it. If it is almost time for your next dose, skip the one you missed and return to your regular dosing schedule. Do not take two doses at once.

How should I store this medication?

Store at room temperature.

Glucovance

Generic name: Glyburide/Metformin HCl

What is this medication?

Glucovance, along with diet and exercise, is used to treat type 2 diabetes. This drug combines two glucose-lowering drugs, glyburide and metformin.

What is the most important information I should know about this medication?

• Glucovance can cause a rare, but serious condition called lactic acidosis (a build-up of lactic acid in the blood) that can be potentially fatal. Lactic acidosis is a medical emergency and must be treated in the hospital. Stop taking Glucovance and call your doctor right away if you feel very weak or tired; have muscle pain; have trouble breathing; have stomach pain with nausea, vomiting, and diarrhea; feel cold, especially in your arms and legs; feel dizzy or lightheaded; have a slow or irregular heartbeat; or if a medical condition suddenly changes.

- Glucovance may cause low blood sugar. This can happen if you do not follow your diet, exercise too much, drink alcohol, are under stress, or get sick. It can also happen if you take other glucose-lowering drugs.

- Taking Glucovance may increase your risk of developing heart problems.

Who should not take this medication?
Do not begin treatment with Glucovance if you have kidney disease, congestive heart failure treated with medications, drink alcohol excessively, or are dehydrated.

Do not use Glucovance if you are scheduled to undergo surgery or an x-ray procedure involving special dye or contrast agents.

Do not use Glucovance if you have a serious infection, a history of heart attack or stroke, are ≥80 years of age and have not had your kidney function tested, or are allergic to any of its ingredients.

What should I tell my doctor before I take the first dose of this medication?
Tell your doctor about all prescription, over-the-counter, and herbal medications you are taking before beginning treatment with Glucovance. Also, talk to your doctor about your complete medical history, especially if you have an illness that causes severe diarrhea, vomiting, or fever; heart, kidney, or liver problems; glucose-6-phosphate dehydrogenase deficiency (lack of an enzyme responsible for the breakdown of red blood cells); low levels of vitamin B_{12}; or are pregnant, plan to become pregnant, or are breastfeeding. Your doctor should also know if you are going to have surgery or an x-ray procedure that requires special dye or contrast agents.

What is the usual dosage?
Please see general statement regarding dosage on page xii.

Patients with Inadequate Diabetes Control on Diet and Exercise

Adults: The recommended starting dose is 1.25 milligrams (mg)/250 mg once or twice daily. Your doctor may increase your dose as appropriate.

Patients with Inadequate Diabetes Control on a Sulfonylurea and/or Metformin

Adults: The recommended starting dose is 2.5 mg/500 mg or 5 mg/500 mg twice daily. Your doctor may increase your dose as appropriate.

How should I take this medication?
• Glucovance should be taken with meals.

What should I avoid while taking this medication?
Avoid alcohol. It can interfere with your blood sugar levels and your diabetes treatment.

What are possible food and drug interactions associated with this medication?
If Glucovance is taken with certain other drugs, the effects of either could be increased, decreased, or altered. It is especially important to check with your doctor before combining Glucovance with the following: albuterol, amiloride, beta-blockers (such as atenolol and metoprolol), calcium channel blockers (such as diltiazem and nifedipine), chloramphenicol, chlorpromazine, ciprofloxacin, corticosteroids (such as prednisone), digoxin, estrogens, isoniazid, miconazole, morphine, monoamine oxidase inhibitors (such as tranylcypromine), nicotinic acid, nonsteroidal anti-inflammatory drugs (such as ibuprofen), birth control pills, phenytoin, procainamide, probenecid, quinidine, quinine, ranitidine, salicylates (such as aspirin), sulfonamides (such as sulfamethoxazole), diuretics (water pills such as hydrochlorothiazide, furosemide, and triamterene), thyroid products, trimethoprim, vancomycin, and warfarin.

What are the possible side effects of this medication?
Please see general statement regarding side effects on page xiii.

> **Side effects may include:** low blood sugar, diarrhea, nausea, upper respiratory infection, headache, vomiting, dizziness, abdominal pain

Can I receive this medication if I am pregnant or breastfeeding?

The effects of Glucovance during pregnancy and breastfeeding are unknown. Tell your doctor immediately if you are pregnant, plan to become pregnant, or are breastfeeding.

What should I do if I miss a dose of this medication?

If you miss a dose of Glucovance, take it as soon as you remember. However, if it is almost time for your next dose, skip the missed dose and return to your regular dosing schedule. Do not take two doses at once.

How should I store this medication?

Store at room temperature.

Glyburide: see Glynase Prestab, page 430

Glyburide/Metformin HCl: see Glucovance, page 427

Glynase Prestab
Generic name: Glyburide

What is this medication?

Glynase Prestab is a medicine used in addition to diet and exercise to control blood sugar in people with type 2 diabetes. It belongs to a class of medications known as sulfonylureas.

What is the most important information I should know about this medication?

• Glynase Prestab can lead to heart and blood vessel problems that are life-threatening. Discuss with your doctor the risks and benefits of treatment with Glynase Prestab.

- Glynase Prestab can cause low blood sugar when taken alone and it is not associated with weight gain. If you do not eat enough, if you take other medicines to lower blood sugar, or if you drink alcohol, you can develop low blood sugar.
- The amount and type of diabetes medication you need can change if you undergo any kind of stress (such as a fever), trauma (such as a car accident), infection, or surgery. Tell your doctor immediately if you are under any kind of stress.
- Glynase Prestab can cause hemolytic anemia (a blood disorder in which red blood cells are destroyed), especially in people with glucose-6-phosphate dehydrogenase (G6PD) deficiency (lack of an enzyme responsible for the breakdown of red blood cells).
- Make sure to stay on your diet and exercise program, and check your blood sugar regularly.

Who should not take this medication?

Do not take Glynase Prestab if you are allergic to it, any of its ingredients, if you have diabetic ketoacidosis (a life-threatening medical emergency caused by insufficient insulin), or type 1 diabetes.

What should I tell my doctor before I take the first dose of this medication?

Tell your doctor about all prescription, over-the-counter, and herbal medications you are taking before beginning treatment with Glynase Prestab. Also, talk to your doctor about your complete medical history, especially if you have kidney or liver disease, are exposed to stress, have G6PD deficiency, or are pregnant, plan to become pregnant, or are breastfeeding.

What is the usual dosage?

Please see general statement regarding dosage on page xii.

Adults: The recommended starting dose is 1.5-3 milligrams (mg) once a day. Your doctor may give you a lower or higher dose depending on your needs.

How should I take this medication?

- Take Glynase Prestab exactly as prescribed by your doctor. You can take Glynase Prestab with breakfast or your first main meal if you take it once a day. If you take more than 6 mg a day, you may benefit from taking it twice a day.

What should I avoid while taking this medication?

Do not consume alcohol while you are taking Glynase Prestab. Alcohol can lower your blood sugar levels and interfere with your diabetes treatment.

What are possible food and drug interactions associated with this medication?

If Glynase Prestab is taken with certain other drugs, the effects of either could be increased, decreased, or altered. It is especially important to check with your doctor before combining Glynase Prestab with the following: aspirin, birth control pills, blood pressure/heart medications known as beta-blockers (such as atenolol or propranolol) or calcium channel blockers (such as nifedipine), blood thinners (such as warfarin), certain antidepressant medications known as monoamine oxidase inhibitors (MAOIs) (such as phenelzine), certain antipsychotics (such as chlorpromazine or perphenazine), chloramphenicol, ciprofloxacin, corticosteroids (such as prednisone), diuretics (water pills) (such as hydrochlorothiazide), epinephrine, estrogens, isoniazid, miconazole, niacin, nonsteroidal anti-inflammatory drugs (NSAIDs) (such as ibuprofen), phenytoin, probenecid, salicylates (such as magnesium salicylate or bismuth subsalicylate), sulfonamides (such as sulfamethoxazole), or thyroid medications (such as levothyroxine).

What are the possible side effects of this medication?

Please see general statement regarding side effects on page xiii.

Side effects may include: allergic reactions, blood disorders, blurred or changes in vision, heartburn, hepatitis (inflammation of the liver), itching, low blood sugar levels, nausea, rash, redness, sensitivity to light, stomach fullness

Can I receive this medication if I am pregnant or breastfeeding?

The effects of Glynase Prestab during pregnancy and breastfeeding are unknown. Tell your doctor immediately if you are pregnant, plan to become pregnant, or are breastfeeding.

What should I do if I miss a dose of this medication?

If you miss a dose of Glynase Prestab, take it as soon as you remember. However, if it is almost time for the next dose, skip the one you missed and return to your regular dosing schedule. Do not take two doses at once.

How should I store this medication?

Store at room temperature.

Guanfacine HCl: *see Guanfacine hydrochloride, page 433*

Guanfacine hydrochloride

Generic name: Guanfacine HCl

What is this medication?

Guanfacine is a medicine used alone or in combination with other medications to treat high blood pressure.

What is the most important information I should know about this medication?

- Do not abruptly stop taking guanfacine; a sudden increase in your blood pressure can occur. Abruptly stopping guanfacine can also cause nervousness and anxiety.
- Guanfacine can cause sedation or drowsiness, especially when beginning therapy. Do not drive or operate dangerous machinery until you know that you do not become drowsy or dizzy from this medication.
- Your tolerance to alcohol and other medications that slow down your brain function can be lowered if you take them with guanfacine.

Who should not take this medication?

Do not take guanfacine if you are allergic to it or any of its ingredients.

What should I tell my doctor before I take the first dose of this medication?

Tell your doctor about all prescription, over-the-counter, and herbal medications you are taking before beginning treatment with guanfacine. Also, talk to your doctor about your complete medical history, especially if you have artery disease, heart problems, kidney or liver disease; or have had a recent heart attack or stroke.

What is the usual dosage?

Please see general statement regarding dosage on page xii.

Adults and children ≥12 years: The recommended initial dose is 1 milligram (mg) once a day at bedtime. Your doctor will prescribe the appropriate dose for you and will increase your dose as needed, until the desired effect is achieved.

How should I take this medication?

• Take guanfacine exactly as prescribed by your doctor. Do not take extra doses or take more often without asking your doctor.
• Take guanfacine at bedtime, since it can cause sleepiness.

What should I avoid while taking this medication?

Do not take guanfacine with alcohol, barbiturates (such as butalbital or phenobarbital), phenothiazines (such as chlorpromazine, fluphenazine, or prochlorperazine), benzodiazepines (such as alprazolam, diazepam, or lorazepam), or other medications that slow down your brain function unless under the recommendation and guidance of your doctor.

Do not abruptly stop taking guanfacine, your doctor will slowly decrease your dose to avoid a sudden increase in your blood pressure.

What are possible food and drug interactions associated with this medication?

If guanfacine is taken with certain other drugs, the effects of either could be increased, decreased, or altered. It is especially important to check with your doctor before combining guanfacine with the following: alcohol, barbiturates, benzodiazepines, medications that slow down your brain function, phenothiazines, or phenytoin.

What are the possible side effects of this medication?

Please see general statement regarding side effects on page xiii.

Side effects may include: confusion, conjunctivitis ("pink eye"), constipation, depression, diarrhea, difficulty sleeping, dizziness, dry mouth, fainting, headache, impotence, leg cramps, low blood pressure, nausea, ringing in the ears, sedation, skin reactions/rash, sleepiness, slow heartbeat, tingling or numbness, tiredness, weakness

Can I receive this medication if I am pregnant or breastfeeding?

The effects of guanfacine during pregnancy and breastfeeding are unknown. Tell your doctor immediately if you are pregnant, plan to become pregnant, or are breastfeeding.

What should I do if I miss a dose of this medication?

If you miss a dose of guanfacine, take it as soon as you remember. However, if it is almost time for your next dose, skip the one you missed and return to your regular dosing schedule. Do not take two doses at once.

How should I store this medication?

Store at room temperature.

Guanfacine: *see Intuniv, page 476*

Horizant
Generic name: Gabapentin Enacarbil

What is this medication?
Horizant is a medicine used to treat adults with moderate to severe primary restless legs syndrome (urge to move one's body to stop uncomfortable or odd sensations) and postherpetic neuralgia (pain from damaged nerves).

What is the most important information I should know about this medication?
- Horizant is not for people who need to sleep during the daytime and need to stay awake at night.
- Do not drive (including the morning after you take your dose), operate heavy machinery, or do other dangerous activities until you know how Horizant affects you. Horizant can cause sleepiness, dizziness, or slow thinking, and can affect your coordination. Ask your doctor when it would be ok to do these activities.
- Horizant can cause suicidal thoughts or actions. Call your doctor immediately if you have thoughts about suicide or dying; attempt to commit suicide; new or worsening depression, anxiety, restlessness, trouble sleeping, or irritability; feel agitated; panic attacks; act aggressive; are angry or violent; act on dangerous impulses; an extreme increase in activity and talking; or other unusual changes in your behavior or mood.
- Keep all follow-up visits with your doctor as scheduled. Call your doctor between visits as needed, especially if you are worried about symptoms.
- Do not stop Horizant without first talking to your doctor. If you stop taking Horizant suddenly, you may develop side effects.
- Horizant can cause a serious allergic reaction, including skin rash, hives, fever, swollen glands that do not go away, swelling of your lips or tongue, yellowing of your skin or whites of your eyes, unusual bruising or bleeding, severe fatigue or weakness, unexpected muscle pain, or frequent infections. Call your doctor immediately if you have an allergic reaction.

Who should not take this medication?
Do not take Horizant if you are allergic to it or any of its ingredients.

What should I tell my doctor before I take the first dose of this medication?

Tell your doctor about all prescription, over-the-counter, and herbal medications you are taking before beginning treatment with Horizant. Also, talk to your doctor about your complete medical history, especially if you have kidney problems or are on hemodialysis; have or have had depression, mood problems, suicidal thoughts or behavior, or seizures. Tell your doctor if you have a history of drug abuse, or are pregnant, plan to become pregnant, or are breastfeeding or plan to breastfeed.

What is the usual dosage?

Please see general statement regarding dosage on page xii.

Restless Legs Syndrome
Adults: The recommended dose is 600 milligrams (mg) once a day at 5 PM.

Postherpetic Neuralgia
Adults: The recommended starting dose is 600 mg once a day in the morning for 3 days. Your doctor will increase to 600 mg twice a day beginning on day 4.

If you have kidney impairment, your doctor will adjust your dose appropriately.

How should I take this medication?
• Take Horizant exactly as prescribed by your doctor.
• Take Horizant tablets whole. Do not cut, crush, or chew your tablet.
• Take Horizant with food.

What should I avoid while taking this medication?
Do not take other medicines that make you sleepy or dizzy while you are taking Horizant without first talking with your doctor. Taking Horizant with medicines that cause sleepiness or dizziness may make your sleepiness or dizziness worse.

Do not take Horizant with other gabapentin medications (such as Neurontin or Gralise). Do not use Horizant to replace them.

What are possible food and drug interactions associated with this medication?

No significant interactions have been reported with Horizant at this time. However, always tell your doctor about any medicines you take, including over-the-counter medications, vitamins, and herbal supplements.

What are the possible side effects of this medication?

Please see general statement regarding side effects on page xiii.

> **Side effects may include:** dizziness, headache, sleepiness

Can I receive this medication if I am pregnant or breastfeeding?

The effects of Horizant during pregnancy are unknown. Do not breastfeed while you are taking Horizant. Tell your doctor immediately if you are pregnant, plan to become pregnant, or are breastfeeding.

What should I do if I miss a dose of this medication?

If you miss a dose of Horizant, take it as soon as you remember. However, if it is almost time for your next dose, skip the one you missed and return to your regular dosing schedule. Do not take two doses at once.

How should I store this medication?

Store at room temperature.

Keep Horizant dry and away from moisture. Keep it tightly closed in the bottle provided to you.

Do not remove any moisture control packs that may come in the bottle.

Humalog

Generic name: Insulin Lispro, rDNA origin

What is this medication?

Humalog is a medicine that is a fast-acting insulin. Humalog is used to control high blood sugar in people with diabetes. Humalog comes as a prefilled pen, vial, and a cartridge.

What is the most important information I should know about this medication?

- Do not change the type of insulin you use unless told to do so by your doctor. Your insulin dose and the time you take your dose can change with different types of insulin. Make sure you have the right type and strength of insulin prescribed for you.

- Do not make any changes to your insulin dose unless you have talked to your doctor. Your insulin needs may change because of illness, stress, other medicines, or changes in your diet or activity level.

- Humalog can cause you to experience low blood sugar. Therefore, it is important to use it as prescribed by your doctor. Symptoms of low blood sugar include: hunger, dizziness, feeling shaky or shakiness, lightheadedness, sweating, irritability, headache, fast heartbeat, or confusion. Always carry a quick source of sugar to treat low blood sugar (such as glucose tablets, hard candy, or juice).

- If you forget to take your dose of Humalog, your blood sugar may get too high. If your high blood sugar is not treated, it can lead to serious problems (such as passing out or loss of consciousness, coma, or even death). Follow your doctor's instructions for treating high blood sugar. Symptoms of high blood sugar include: increased thirst, frequent urination, drowsiness, loss of appetite, difficulty breathing, fruity smelling breath, nausea, vomiting, or stomach ache.

- Humalog starts working faster than other insulins. You should inject it 15 minutes or less before a meal. If you do not plan to eat within 15 minutes, delay the injection until the correct time (15 minutes before eating).

Who should not take this medication?

Do not use Humalog if you are allergic to it or any of its ingredients. Also, do not use Humalog if your blood sugar is too low.

What should I tell my doctor before I take the first dose of this medication?

Tell your doctor about all prescription, over-the-counter, and herbal medications you are taking before beginning treatment with Humalog. Also, talk to your doctor about your complete medical history, especially if you have kidney or liver problems, or are pregnant, plan to become pregnant, or are breastfeeding.

What is the usual dosage?

Please see general statement regarding dosage on page xii.

   Adults and children ≥3 years: Your doctor will determine your dose based on your blood sugar levels.

How should I take this medication?

- Inject Humalog exactly as prescribed by your doctor. Use the proper injection technique taught to you by your doctor. Read the User Manual that comes with your Humalog Prefilled Pen for detailed instructions.
- Inject Humalog 15 minutes before you eat. Inject it under the skin of your stomach area, upper arm, upper leg, or buttocks. Never inject Humalog into a muscle or vein. Change your injection site with each dose.
- Only use Humalog that is clear and colorless.
- Your doctor may tell you to mix your Humalog with a longer-acting human insulin. When mixing these two types of insulin, draw Humalog into the syringe first. Do not dilute or mix Humalog with any other insulin in the same external insulin pump.

What should I avoid while taking this medication?

Do not inject Humalog in the same place twice; rotate the injection sites.

Do not use Humalog in the same external pump with other insulin products.

Do not share Humalog with anyone else, even if they have diabetes.
It may harm them.

What are possible food and drug interactions associated with this medication?

If Humalog is used with certain other drugs, the effects of either
could be increased, decreased, or altered. Humalog may interact
with numerous medications. Therefore, it is very important that
you tell your doctor about any other medications you are taking.

What are the possible side effects of this medication?

Please see general statement regarding side effects on page xiii.

> **Side effects may include:** allergic reactions, injection-site reac-
> tions, itching, low blood sugar, rash, skin thickening or pitting at
> the injection site, swelling of your hands and feet, weight gain

Can I receive this medication if I am pregnant or breastfeeding?

The effects of Humalog during pregnancy and breastfeeding are
unknown. Tell your doctor immediately if you are pregnant, plan to
become pregnant, or are breastfeeding.

What should I do if I miss a dose of this medication?

It is very important to follow your insulin regimen exactly as prescribed by your doctor. Do not miss any doses. Ask your doctor
for specific instructions to follow in case you ever miss a dose of
insulin.

How should I store this medication?

Store unopened Humalog in the refrigerator (not the freezer). Protect from extreme heat, cold, or light.

After you open Humalog vials, store them in the refrigerator or at
room temperature for 28 days.

After you start using Humalog cartridges or prefilled pens, do not refrigerate them. Keep them at room temperature, away from direct heat and light for up to 28 days.

Humalog Mix 50/50

Generic name: Insulin Lispro Protamine/Insulin Lispro, rDNA origin

What is this medication?

Humalog Mix 50/50 is a medicine that contains a mixture of fast-acting and longer-acting insulins. Humalog Mix 50/50 is used to control high blood sugar in people with diabetes. Humalog Mix 50/50 comes as a prefilled pen and a vial.

What is the most important information I should know about this medication?

- Do not change the type of insulin you use unless told to do so by your doctor. Your insulin dose and the time you take your dose can change with different types of insulin. Make sure you have the right type and strength of insulin prescribed for you.
- Do not make any changes to your insulin dose unless you have talked to your doctor. Your insulin needs may change because of illness, stress, other medicines, or changes in your diet or activity level.
- Humalog Mix 50/50 can cause you to experience low blood sugar. Therefore, it is important to use it as prescribed by your doctor. Symptoms of low blood sugar include: hunger, dizziness, feeling shaky or shakiness, lightheadedness, sweating, irritability, headache, fast heartbeat, or confusion. Always carry a quick source of sugar to treat low blood sugar (such as glucose tablets, hard candy, or juice).
- Humalog Mix 50/50 starts working faster than other insulins. You should inject it 15 minutes or less before a meal. If you do not plan to eat within 15 minutes, delay the injection until the correct time (15 minutes before eating).

Who should not take this medication?

Do not use Humalog Mix 50/50 if you are allergic to it or any of its ingredients. Also, do not use Humalog Mix 50/50 if your blood sugar is too low.

What should I tell my doctor before I take the first dose of this medication?

Tell your doctor about all prescription, over-the-counter, and herbal medications you are taking before beginning treatment with Humalog Mix 50/50. Also, talk to your doctor about your complete medical history, especially if you have kidney or liver problems, are pregnant, plan to become pregnant, or are breastfeeding.

What is the usual dosage?

Please see general statement regarding dosage on page xii.

Adults: Your doctor will determine your dose based on your blood sugar levels.

How should I take this medication?

- Administer Humalog Mix 50/50 exactly as prescribed by your doctor. Use the proper injection technique taught to you by your doctor. Read the User Manual that comes with your Humalog Mix 50/50 Prefilled Pen for detailed instructions.
- Inject Humalog Mix 50/50 15 minutes before you eat. Inject it under the skin of your stomach area, upper arm, upper leg, or buttocks. Never inject Humalog Mix 50/50 into a muscle or vein. Change your injection site with each dose.
- Mix Humalog Mix 50/50 well before each use. For Humalog Mix 50/50 in a vial, carefully shake or rotate the vial until completely mixed. For prefilled pens, carefully follow the User Manual for instructions on how to mix the pen. Humalog Mix 50/50 should be cloudy or milky after you mix it well. If it is not evenly mixed or has solid particles or clumps in it, return it to the pharmacy for a replacement.

What should I avoid while taking this medication?

Do not inject Humalog Mix 50/50 in the same place twice; rotate the injection sites.

Do not use Humalog Mix 50/50 in the same syringe with other insulin products and do not use it in an insulin pump.

Do not share Humalog Mix 50/50 with anyone else, even if they have diabetes. It may harm them.

What are possible food and drug interactions associated with this medication?

If Humalog Mix 50/50 is used with certain other drugs, the effects of either could be increased, decreased, or altered. Humalog Mix 50/50 may interact with numerous medications. Therefore, it is very important that you tell your doctor about any other medications you are taking.

What are the possible side effects of this medication?

Please see general statement regarding side effects on page xiii.

> **Side effects may include:** allergic reactions, injection-site reactions, itching, low blood sugar, rash, skin thickening or pitting at the injection site

Can I receive this medication if I am pregnant or breastfeeding?

The effects of Humalog Mix 50/50 during pregnancy and breastfeeding are unknown. Tell your doctor immediately if you are pregnant, plan to become pregnant, or are breastfeeding.

What should I do if I miss a dose of this medication?

It is very important to follow your insulin regimen exactly as prescribed by your doctor. Do not miss any doses. Ask your doctor for specific instructions to follow in case you ever miss a dose of insulin.

How should I store this medication?

Store unopened Humalog Mix 50/50 in the refrigerator (not the freezer). Protect from extreme heat, cold, or light.

After you open Humalog Mix 50/50, store the vials in the refrigerator or at room temperature for 28 days. After you start Humalog Mix 50/50 prefilled pens, do not refrigerate them. Keep them at room temperature, away from direct heat and light for up to 10 days.

Humalog Mix 75/25
Generic name: Insulin Lispro Protamine/Insulin Lispro, rDNA origin

What is this medication?
Humalog Mix 75/25 is a medicine that contains a mixture of fast-acting and longer-acting insulins. Humalog Mix 75/25 is used to control high blood sugar in people with diabetes. Humalog Mix 75/25 comes as a prefilled pen and a vial.

What is the most important information I should know about this medication?
- Do not change the type of insulin you use unless told to do so by your doctor. Your insulin dose and the time you take your dose can change with different types of insulin. Make sure you have the right type and strength of insulin prescribed for you. Do not make any changes with your insulin dose unless you have talked to your doctor. Your insulin needs may change because of illness, stress, other medicines, or changes in your diet or activity level.
- Humalog Mix 75/25 can cause you to experience low blood sugar. Therefore, it is important to take it as prescribed by your doctor. Symptoms of low blood sugar include: hunger, dizziness, feeling shaky or shakiness, lightheadedness, sweating, irritability, headache, fast heartbeat, or confusion. Always carry a quick source of sugar to treat low blood sugar (such as glucose tablets, hard candy, or juice).
- Humalog Mix 75/25 starts working faster than other insulins. You should inject it 15 minutes or less before a meal. If you do not plan to eat within 15 minutes, delay the injection until the correct time (15 minutes before eating).

Who should not take this medication?

Do not take Humalog Mix 75/25 if you are allergic to it or any of its ingredients. Also, do not take Humalog Mix 75/25 if your blood sugar is too low.

What should I tell my doctor before I take the first dose of this medication?

Tell your doctor about all prescription, over-the-counter, and herbal medications you are taking before beginning treatment with Humalog Mix 75/25. Also, talk to your doctor about your complete medical history, especially if you have kidney or liver problems, are pregnant, plan to become pregnant, or are breastfeeding.

What is the usual dosage?

Please see general statement regarding dosage on page xii.

Adults: Your doctor will determine your dose based on your blood sugar levels.

How should I take this medication?

- Administer Humalog Mix 75/25 exactly as prescribed by your doctor. Use the proper injection technique taught to you by your doctor. Read the User Manual that comes with your Humalog Mix 75/25 Prefilled Pen for detailed instructions.
- Inject Humalog Mix 75/25 15 minutes before you eat. Inject it under the skin of your stomach area, upper arm, upper leg, or buttocks. Never inject Humalog Mix 75/25 into a muscle or vein. Change your injection site with each dose.
- Mix Humalog Mix 75/25 well before each use. For Humalog Mix 75/25 in a vial, carefully shake or rotate the vial until completely mixed. For prefilled pens, carefully follow the User Manual for instructions on mixing the pen. Humalog Mix 75/25 should be cloudy or milky after you mix it well. If it is not evenly mixed or has solid particles or clumps in it, return it to the pharmacy for a replacement.

What should I avoid while taking this medication?

Do not inject Humalog Mix 75/25 in the same place twice; rotate the injection sites.

Never use Humalog Mix 75/25 in the same syringe with other insulin products and never use it in an insulin pump.

Do not share Humalog Mix 75/25 with anyone else, even if they have diabetes. It may harm them.

What are possible food and drug interactions associated with this medication?

If Humalog Mix 75/25 is used with certain other drugs, the effects of either could be increased, decreased, or altered. Humalog Mix 75/25 may interact with numerous medications. Therefore, it is very important that you tell your doctor about any other medications you are taking.

What are the possible side effects of this medication?

Please see general statement regarding side effects on page xiii.

> **Side effects may include:** allergic reactions, injection-site reactions, itching, low blood sugar, rash, skin thickenning or pitting at the injection site

Can I receive this medication if I am pregnant or breastfeeding?

The effects of Humalog Mix 75/25 during pregnancy and breastfeeding are unknown. Tell your doctor immediately if you are pregnant, plan to become pregnant, or are breastfeeding.

What should I do if I miss a dose of this medication?

It is very important to follow your insulin regimen exactly as prescribed by your doctor. Do not miss any doses. Ask your doctor for specific instructions to follow in case you ever miss a dose of insulin.

How should I store this medication?

Store unopened Humalog Mix 75/25 in the refrigerator (not the freezer). Protect from extreme heat, cold, or light.

After you open Humalog Mix 75/25, store the vials in the refrigerator or at room temperature for 28 days. After you start Humalog Mix 75/25 prefilled pens, do not refrigerate them. Keep them at room temperature, away from direct heat and light for up to 10 days.

Hydralazine
Generic name: Hydralazine HCl

What is this medication?
Hydralazine is a medicine used alone or with other medicines to treat high blood pressure.

What is the most important information I should know about this medication?
- Hydralazine can cause chest pain and other heart problems. It is important for you to tell your doctor about any heart conditions you have.
- You must take hydralazine regularly for it to be effective. Since blood pressure declines gradually, it may be weeks before you get the full benefit of hydralazine. You must continue taking it even if you are feeling well. Hydralazine does not cure high blood pressure; it only keeps it under control.
- Do not abruptly stop taking hydralazine without consulting your doctor.

Who should not take this medication?
Do not take hydralazine if you have coronary artery disease (narrowing of the small blood vessels that supply blood and oxygen to the heart), problems in the valves of your heart, or are allergic to hydralazine or any of its ingredients.

What should I tell my doctor before I take the first dose of this medication?
Tell your doctor about all prescription, over-the-counter, and herbal medications you are taking before beginning treatment with

hydralazine. Also, talk to your doctor about your complete medical history, especially if you have heart or kidney problems.

What is the usual dosage?
Please see general statement regarding dosage on page xii.

Adults: The recommended dose is 10 milligrams (mg) four times a day. Your doctor will adjust your dose according to your individual response to the medication.

How should I take this medication?
• Take hydralazine exactly as prescribed by your doctor, even if you are feeling well. Do not miss any doses. If hydralazine is not taken regularly, your condition may get worse.

What should I avoid while taking this medication?
Do not stop taking hydralazine suddenly.

What are possible food and drug interactions associated with this medication?
If hydralazine is taken with certain other drugs, the effects of either could be increased, decreased, or altered. It is especially important to check with your doctor before combining hydralazine with the following: diazoxide or monoamine oxidase inhibitors (MAOIs), a class of drugs used to treat depression and other psychiatric conditions (such as phenelzine).

What are the possible side effects of this medication?
Please see general statement regarding side effects on page xiii.

Side effects may include: diarrhea, headache, heart problems, increase in heart beats, nausea, vomiting

Can I receive this medication if I am pregnant or breastfeeding?
The effects of hydralazine during pregnancy and breastfeeding are unknown. Tell your doctor immediately if you are pregnant, plan to become pregnant, or are breastfeeding.

What should I do if I miss a dose of this medication?

If you miss a dose of hydralazine, take it as soon as you remember. However, if it is almost time for your next dose, skip the one you missed and return to your regular dosing schedule. Do not take two doses at once.

How should I store this medication?

Store at room temperature.

Hydralazine HCl: see Hydralazine, page 448

Hydrochlorothiazide

Generic name: Hydrochlorothiazide

What is this medication?

Hydrochlorothiazide is a diuretic (water pill) used alone or in combination with other medications to treat high blood pressure. Hydrochlorothiazide is also used to treat edema (swelling) associated with heart, kidney, liver disease, or corticosteroid and estrogen therapy.

What is the most important information I should know about this medication?

- Hydrochlorothiazide can cause nearsightedness and angle-closure glaucoma (high pressure in the eye). Discontinue hydrochlorothiazide and tell your doctor immediately if you experience abnormal visual changes or eye pain.
- Your doctor will perform regular blood tests to check your fluids and electrolytes (chemicals that are important for the cells in your body to function, such as sodium and potassium). Tell your doctor if you experience confusion, decreased urination, drowsiness, dry mouth, fast heart rate, low blood pressure, muscle pain or cramps, nausea, seizures, tiredness, vomiting, or weakness.

- Hydrochlorothiazide can cause gout (severe and painful inflammation of the joints); and an increase in your cholesterol and triglyceride levels.

Who should not take this medication?

Do not take hydrochlorothiazide if you are allergic to, any of its ingredients, or to other sulfonamide medications (such as sulfamethoxazole). Also, do not take hydrochlorothiazide if you are unable to produce urine.

What should I tell my doctor before I take the first dose of this medication?

Tell your doctor about all prescription, over-the-counter, and herbal medications you are taking before beginning treatment with hydrochlorothiazide. Also, talk to your doctor about your complete medical history, especially if you have a history of allergy or asthma; diabetes; gout; kidney, liver, or thyroid disease; or if you have systemic lupus erythematosus (disease that affects the immune system).

What is the usual dosage?

Please see general statement regarding dosage on page xii.

High Blood Pressure

Adults: The usual starting dose is 25 milligrams (mg) once a day.

Children ≤12 years: Your doctor will prescribe the appropriate dose for your child, based on their weight.

Edema

Adults: The usual dose is 25-100 mg given once a day or as divided doses.

Children ≤12 years: Your doctor will prescribe the appropriate dose for your child, based on their weight.

How should I take this medication?

- Take hydrochlorothiazide exactly as prescribed by your doctor. Do not take extra doses or take more often without asking your doctor.

What should I avoid while taking this medication?

Do not drink alcohol while you are taking hydrochlorothiazide; it can increase your risk for low blood pressure.

What are possible food and drug interactions associated with this medication?

If hydrochlorothiazide is taken with certain other drugs, the effects of either could be increased, decreased, or altered. It is especially important to check with your doctor before combining hydrochlorothiazide with the following: alcohol, barbiturates (such as butalbital or phenobarbital), cholestyramine, colestipol, diabetes medications (such as glyburide, insulin, or metformin), lithium, narcotics (such as morphine or methadone), nonsteroidal anti-inflammatory drugs (NSAIDs) (such as ibuprofen or naproxen), norepinephrine, or skeletal muscle relaxants (such as tubocurarine).

What are the possible side effects of this medication?

Please see general statement regarding side effects on page xiii.

Side effects may include: blood disorders, blurred vision, constipation, cramping, diarrhea, dizziness, electrolyte imbalance, fever, headache, increased blood sugar levels, low blood pressure, nausea, rash, restlessness, sexual dysfunction, vomiting

Can I receive this medication if I am pregnant or breastfeeding?

The effects of hydrochlorothiazide during pregnancy and breastfeeding are unknown. Tell your doctor immediately if you are pregnant, plan to become pregnant, or are breastfeeding.

What should I do if I miss a dose of this medication?

If you miss a dose of hydrochlorothiazide, take it as soon as you remember. However, if it is almost time for your next dose, skip the one you missed and return to your regular dosing schedule. Do not take two doses at once.

How should I store this medication?
Store at room temperature.

Hydrochlorothiazide: see Hydrochlorothiazide, page 450

Hydrochlorothiazide/Lisinopril: see Prinzide, page 834

Hydrochlorothiazide/Losartan Potassium: see Hyzaar, page 456

Hydrochlorothiazide/Olmesartan Medoxomil: see Benicar HCT, page 136

Hydrochlorothiazide/Telmisartan: see Micardis HCT, page 632

Hydrochlorothiazide/Triamterene: see Dyazide, page 345

Hydrochlorothiazide/Triamterene: see Maxzide, page 606

Hydrochlorothiazide/Valsartan: see Diovan HCT, page 329

Hydrocodone Bitartrate/Ibuprofen: see Vicoprofen, page 1069

Hydromorphone HCl: see Dilaudid, page 323

Hydroxychloroquine Sulfate: see Plaquenil, page 792

Hydroxyzine Pamoate
Generic name: Hydroxyzine Pamoate

What is this medication?
Hydroxyzine pamoate is used to relieve anxiety and tension associated with certain mental conditions. It is also used as a sedative before medical procedures. In addition, hydroxyzine pamoate is

used to treat itching due to allergic conditions (such as chronic hives or certain skin rashes). Hydroxyzine pamoate capsules can also be found under the brand name Vistaril.

What is the most important information I should know about this medication?

- Hydroxyzine pamoate can increase the effects of alcohol, narcotic painkillers (such as hydrocodone or oxycodone), barbiturates (such as phenobarbital), or other medicines that impair your mental and/or physical abilities. Tell your doctor if you drink alcohol or are taking any of these medicines.
- Hydroxyzine pamoate can cause drowsiness. Do not drive or operate machinery while you are taking this medicine.

Who should not take this medication?

Do not take hydroxyzine pamoate if you are allergic to it or any of its ingredients.

Do not take hydroxyzine pamoate if you are in the early stage of your pregnancy.

What should I tell my doctor before I take the first dose of this medication?

Tell your doctor about all prescription, over-the-counter, and herbal medications you are taking before beginning treatment with hydroxyzine pamoate. Also talk to your doctor about your complete medical history, especially if you are pregnant, planning to become pregnant, or are breastfeeding.

What is the usual dosage?

Please see general statement regarding dosage on page xii.

Relief of Anxiety and Tension
Adults: The recommended dose is 50-100 milligrams (mg) four times a day.

Children >6 years: The recommended dose is 50-100 mg a day in divided doses.

Children <6 years: The recommended dose is 50 mg a day in divided doses.

Relief of Itching Due to Allergic Conditions
Adults: The recommended dose is 25 mg 3 or 4 times a day.

Children >6 years: The recommended dose is 50-100 mg a day in divided doses.

Children <6 years: The recommended dose is 50 mg a day in divided doses.

As Sedation Before Surgery
Adults and children: Your doctor will administer the appropriate dose to you or your child.

If you are elderly, your doctor will adjust your dose appropriately.

How should I take this medication?
• Take hydroxyzine pamoate exactly as prescribed by your doctor.

What should I avoid while taking this medication?
Do not drive or operate machinery while you are taking hydroxyzine pamoate.

What are possible food and drug interactions associated with this medication?
If hydroxyzine pamoate is taken with certain other drugs, the effects of either could be increased, decreased, or altered. It is especially important to check with your doctor before combining hydroxyzine pamoate with the following: alcohol, barbiturates, narcotic painkillers, or other painkillers.

What are the possible side effects of this medication?
Please see general statement regarding side effects on page xiii.

Side effects may include: allergic reaction, drowsiness, dry mouth, hallucinations, headache

Can I receive this medication if I am pregnant or breastfeeding?

Do not take hydroxyzine pamoate if you are in the early stage of your pregnancy or if you are breastfeeding. Tell your doctor immediately if you are pregnant, plan to become pregnant, or are breastfeeding.

What should I do if I miss a dose of this medication?

If you miss a dose of hydroxyzine pamoate, take it as soon as you remember. However, if it is almost time for your next dose, skip the one you missed and return to your regular dosing schedule. Do not take two doses at once.

How should I store this medication?

Store at room temperature.

Hydroxyzine Pamoate: *see Hydroxyzine Pamoate, page 453*

Hyzaar

Generic name: Hydrochlorothiazide/Losartan Potassium

What is this medication?

Hyzaar is a combination medicine used to treat high blood pressure and lower the risk of stroke if you have high blood pressure and a heart condition called left ventricular hypertrophy (enlargement of the section of the heart that is responsible for pumping blood to the rest of the body). Hyzaar contains two medicines: losartan (an angiotensin receptor blocker [ARB]) and hydrochlorothiazide (a diuretic [water pill]).

What is the most important information I should know about this medication?

- When taken during pregnancy, ARBs such as Hyzaar can cause injury to the unborn baby. If you are pregnant or plan to become pregnant, stop taking Hyzaar and contact your doctor right away.

- Hyzaar can cause low blood pressure, especially if you take diuretics. If you feel faint or dizzy, lie down and call your doctor right away.
- Hyzaar can cause a rare but serious allergic reaction leading to extreme swelling of your face, lips, tongue, or throat. If you experience any of these symptoms, seek emergency medical attention.
- Hyzaar can activate lupus (disease that affects the immune system) or gout (severe and painful inflammation of the joints), and increase cholesterol and triglyceride levels in certain patients.
- Hyzaar can worsen your kidney or liver function if you already have kidney or liver problems. Tell your doctor if your feet, ankles, or hands become swollen; unexplained weight gain; nausea; right upper abdominal pain; or yellowing of your skin or the whites of your eyes.
- Hyzaar can cause problems seeing objects that are farther away, as well as acute angle-closure glaucoma (high pressure in the eye). Tell your doctor immediately if you experience abnormal visual changes or eye pain.
- Hyzaar can cause imbalances in fluids and electrolytes (chemicals that are important for the cells in your body to function, such as sodium and potassium). Signs and symptoms of this include dry mouth, thirst, weakness, fatigue, drowsiness, restlessness, confusion, seizures, muscle pain or cramps, low blood pressure, decreased urination, fast heart rate, nausea, and vomiting. Your doctor will monitor your blood electrolyte levels periodically during treatment with Hyzaar.
- If you have diabetes, Hyzaar can increase your blood sugar levels. Check your blood sugar frequently.

Who should not take this medication?
Do not take Hyzaar if you are allergic to it or any of its ingredients, or to a sulfonamide-derived medication.

Do not take Hyzaar if you are unable to produce urine.

What should I tell my doctor before I take the first dose of this medication?

Tell your doctor about all prescription, over-the-counter, and herbal medications you are taking before beginning treatment with Hyzaar. Also, talk to your doctor if you have diabetes, heart failure, severe immune system problems, lupus, asthma, gout, or liver or kidney disease, or if you have ever had an allergy or sensitivity to an ARB or sulfonamide-derived medication.

What is the usual dosage?

Please see general statement regarding dosage on page xii.

High Blood Pressure and Left Ventricular Hypertrophy

Adults: The usual dose is 50/12.5 (50 milligrams [mg] of losartan and 12.5 mg of hydrochlorothiazide) once a day. Your doctor may give you a higher dose, depending on your needs.

If you have liver impairment, your doctor will adjust your dose appropriately.

How should I take this medication?

• Take Hyzaar exactly as prescribed by your doctor. Take it with or without food.

What should I avoid while taking this medication?

Do not become pregnant or breastfeed while you are taking Hyzaar.

Do not become dehydrated. Drink adequate amounts of fluids while you are taking Hyzaar to avoid becoming dehydrated.

What are possible food and drug interactions associated with this medication?

If Hyzaar is taken with certain other drugs, the effects of either could be increased, decreased, or altered. It is especially important to check with your doctor before combining Hyzaar with the following: alcohol, barbiturates (such as phenobarbital), certain diuretics (such as amiloride, spironolactone, or triamterene), cholestyramine, colestipol, diabetes medicines (such as insulin), fluconazole, lithium, narcotic painkillers (such as hydrocodone or oxycodone), nonsteroidal anti-inflammatory drugs (NSAIDs) (such as ibuprofen or naproxen), norepinephrine, other blood pressure medications, potassium supplements, rifampin, salt substitutes that contain potassium, steroids, or tubocurarine.

What are the possible side effects of this medication?
Please see general statement regarding side effects on page xiii.

Side effects may include: back pain, dizziness, fast or irregular heartbeat, rash, stuffy nose, upper respiratory infection

Can I receive this medication if I am pregnant or breastfeeding?
Do not take Hyzaar if you are pregnant or breastfeeding. Hyzaar can harm your unborn baby. It can be found in your breast milk if you take it while breastfeeding. Tell your doctor immediately if you are pregnant, plan to become pregnant, or are breastfeeding.

What should I do if I miss a dose of this medication?
If you miss a dose of Hyzaar, take it as soon as you remember. However, if it Is almost time for your next dose, skip the one you missed and return to your regular dosing schedule. Do not take two doses at once.

How should I store this medication?
Store at room temperature. Protect from light.

Ibandronate Sodium: *see Boniva, page 153*

Imipramine HCI: *see Tofranil, page 997*

Imipramine Pamoate: *see Tofranil-PM, page 1000*

Imitrex

Generic name: Sumatriptan

What is this medication?

Imitrex is a medicine called a triptan. It is used to treat migraine headaches.

What is the most important information I should know about this medication?

- Imitrex is used only to treat migraine headaches. It is not used to prevent or reduce the number of attacks you have.
- Imitrex can increase your chance of getting a heart attack or stroke. This chance is higher in people who have heart disease. Imitrex is not for people with risk factors for heart disease unless a heart exam is done and shows no problems. Risk factors for heart disease include high blood pressure, high cholesterol levels, smoking, obesity, diabetes, family history of heart disease, women who have gone through menopause, and men over the age of 40.
- Imitrex can cause a serious and life-threatening condition called serotonin syndrome. Tell your doctor right away if you experience mental changes (seeing things that are not there, unusual tension and restlessness), fast heartbeat, changes in your blood pressure, high body temperature, tight muscles, trouble walking, nausea, vomiting, or diarrhea.
- Call your doctor right away if you have severe tightness, pain, pressure or heaviness in your chest, throat, neck or jaw; if you have trouble breathing; hives; swelling of your tongue, mouth, or throat; or if you have any problems with your vision.

Who should not take this medication?

Do not take Imitrex if you are allergic to it or any of its ingredients.

Do not take Imitrex if you have heart disease or a history of heart disease, uncontrolled high blood pressure, have had a stroke, transient ischemic attacks (TIAs), problems with your blood circulation, have narrowing of the blood vessels in your legs, arms, stomach or kidneys (peripheral vascular disease), or if you have severe liver problems.

Do not take Imitrex if you have taken medicines known as triptans (such as almotriptan, eletriptan, frovatriptan, naratriptan, or
rizatriptan) within the last 24 hours, any ergotamine-containing
or ergot-type medicines (such as dihydroergotamine) within the
last 24 hours, or monoamine oxidase inhibitors (MAOIs) (such as
phenelzine), a class of medications used to treat depression and
other psychiatric conditions, within the last 2 weeks.

Also, do not take Imitrex if you have migraines that cause short-
term paralysis (you are unable to move) on one side of your body
or basilar migraine (type of migraine with visual symptoms, and
sensory and language difficulties). If you are not sure if you experience this, talk to your doctor.

What should I tell my doctor before I take the first dose of this medication?

Tell your doctor about all prescription, over-the-counter, and herbal
medications you are taking before beginning treatment with Imitrex. Also, talk to your doctor about your complete medical history, especially if you have high cholesterol, diabetes, heart disease
or a family history of heart disease or stroke, smoke, have gone
through menopause, have had epilepsy or seizures, have kidney or
liver problems, or if you are pregnant, plan to become pregnant, or
are breastfeeding.

What is the usual dosage?

Please see general statement regarding dosage on page xii.

Adults: Your doctor will prescribe the appropriate dose for you
based on your condition.

How should I take this medication?

- Take Imitrex exactly as prescribed by your doctor. Swallow
  Imitrex tablets whole with water or other liquids. Do not split
  the tablets.
- If your symptoms come back or if you have a partial response to
  the first dose, you can take a second tablet 2 hours after the first
  tablet, but not sooner.

What should I avoid while taking this medication?

Do not drive, use machines, or engage in activities that require alertness until you know how Imitrex affects you. Imitrex can make you feel drowsy or dizzy.

If you do not feel better after the first dose of Imitrex, do not take a second tablet without first talking to your doctor.

What are possible food and drug interactions associated with this medication?

If Imitrex is taken with certain other drugs, the effects of either could be increased, decreased, or altered. It is especially important to check with your doctor before combining Imitrex with the following: certain migraine products, citalopram, dihydroergotamine, duloxetine, escitalopram, fluoxetine, fluvoxamine, methysergide, MAOIs, olanzapine paroxetine, sertraline, or venlafaxine.

What are the possible side effects of this medication?

Please see general statement regarding side effects on page xiii.

> **Side effects may include:** abdominal (stomach) pain, confusion, diarrhea, difficulty walking, dizziness, drowsiness, facial flushing, fast heartbeat, feeling faint, feel tingling or heat, fever, hallucinations, heart throbbing, muscle spasm, rash, shortness of breath, sweating, swelling, tiredness, wheeziness

Can I receive this medication if I am pregnant or breastfeeding?

The effects of Imitrex during pregnancy are unknown. Imitrex can be found in your breast milk if you take it while breastfeeding. Tell your doctor immediately if you are pregnant, plan to become pregnant, or are breastfeeding.

What should I do if I miss a dose of this medication?

Imitrex should be given only as needed.

How should I store this medication?

Store at room temperature. Keep Imitrex in the container that it comes in until you are ready to take it.

Incivek

Generic name: Telaprevir

What is this medication?

Incivek is a medicine used with peginterferon alfa and ribavirin to treat long-term hepatitis C infection in adults with stable liver problems, who have not been treated before or who have failed previous treatment.

What is the most important information I should know about this medication?

- Do not take Incivek alone to treat long-term hepatitis C infection. Incivek must be used with peginterferon alfa and ribavirin to treat chronic hepatitis C infection.
- Incivek, in combination with peginterferon alfa and ribavirin, can harm your unborn baby. You, or your female sexual partner, should not become pregnant while taking these medications, and for 6 months after treatment is over. You must have a negative pregnancy test before starting treatment, each month during treatment, and for 6 months after your treatment ends. You must use two forms of effective birth control during treatment and for 6 months after treatment is over.
- Mild skin rashes are common with Incivek combination treatment. Sometimes these skin rashes and other skin reactions can become severe and require treatment in a hospital. Tell your doctor immediately if you develop any skin changes with any of the following symptoms: rash, with or without itching; blisters or skin lesions; mouth sores or ulcers; red or inflamed eyes, such as "pink eye" (conjunctivitis); swelling of your face; or fever.
- Your doctor will perform blood tests before you start treatment, and at other times as needed during treatment, to see how well the medicines are working and to check for side effects.
- Do not stop taking Incivek without first talking to your doctor.

Who should not take this medication?

Do not take Incivek if you are allergic to it or any of its ingredients.

Do not take Incivek if you, or your female sexual partner, are pregnant or may become pregnant.

What should I tell my doctor before I take the first dose of this medication?

Tell your doctor about all prescription, over-the-counter, and herbal medications you are taking before beginning treatment with Incivek. Also, talk to your doctor about your complete medical history, especially if you have low red blood cell counts (anemia), liver problems other than hepatitis C infection, hepatitis B infection, human immunodeficiency virus (HIV) infection (AIDS), history of severe and painful inflammation of the joints (gout) or high uric acid levels, had an organ transplant, plan to have surgery, are pregnant, are breastfeeding, or if you or your female sexual partner plan to become pregnant.

What is the usual dosage?

Please see general statement regarding dosage on page xii.

Adults: The usual dose is 750 milligrams (mg), (two 375-mg tablets), 3 times a day taken 7-9 hours apart.

How should I take this medication?

• Take Incivek exactly as prescribed by your doctor.
• Always take Incivek with food. Eat a meal or snack that contains about 20 grams of fat 30 minutes before you take each dose of Incivek.

What should I avoid while taking this medication?

You, or your female sexual partner, should avoid becoming pregnant while taking this medication.

What are possible food and drug interactions associated with this medication?

If Incivek is taken with certain other drugs, the effects of either could be increased, decreased, or altered. It is especially important to check with your doctor before combining Incivek with any other medication.

What are the possible side effects of this medication?
Please see general statement regarding side effects on page xiii.

> **Side effects may include:** anal or rectal problems (such as hemorrhoids or itching, burning, or discomfort near the anus), anemia, dizziness, itching, nausea, shortness of breath, taste changes, tiredness, vomiting, weakness

Can I receive this medication if I am pregnant or breastfeeding?
Do not take Incivek if you are pregnant, plan to become pregnant, or are breastfeeding. Incivek, in combination with peginterferon alfa and ribavirin, can harm your unborn baby. The effects of Incivek during breastfeeding are unknown. Tell your doctor immediately if you are pregnant, plan to become pregnant, or are breastfeeding.

What should I do if I miss a dose of this medication?
If you miss a dose of Incivek within 4 hours of when you usually take it, take your dose with food as soon as possible. If you miss a dose and it is more than 4 hours after the time you usually take it, skip that dose only and take the next dose at your normal dosing schedule.

How should I store this medication?
Store at room temperature.

Indacaterol: *see Arcapta Neohaler, page 84*

Inderal LA

Generic name: Propranolol HCl

What is this medication?

Inderal LA belongs to a class of medications called beta-blockers. It is used to treat high blood pressure or angina (chest pain) or to prevent common migraine headaches. Inderal LA can also be used to improve symptoms associated with hypertrophic subaortic stenosis, which is a heart condition characterized by heart muscle thickening.

What is the most important information I should know about this medication?

- Do not stop taking Inderal LA abruptly without talking to your doctor. Abruptly stopping this medication can cause worsening of your angina or heart attack. Your doctor should gradually reduce your dose to stop this medication.
- If you have high blood pressure, you must take Inderal LA regularly for it to be effective. Because blood pressure declines gradually, it may take several weeks of treatment for you to get the full benefit of this medication.
- Inderal LA can cause allergic reactions that can have serious symptoms. Stop Inderal LA and call your doctor immediately if you develop any skin reactions.
- Inderal LA can worsen heart failure, can cause asthmatic attacks or breathing problems, or can hide symptoms of low blood sugar levels if you have diabetes. Your doctor will monitor your heart, breathing, and blood sugar levels. Be sure to monitor your blood sugar levels on a regular basis.

Who should not take this medication?

Do not take Inderal LA if you are allergic to it, any of its ingredients, or if you have a slow heart rate, a heart block, or asthma.

What should I tell my doctor before I take the first dose of this medication?

Tell your doctor about all prescription, over-the-counter, and herbal medications you are taking before you start treatment with Inderal LA. Also, talk to your doctor about your complete medical history, especially if you have any allergies, breathing problems (such as asthma, chronic bronchitis [long-term inflammation of the lungs], or emphysema [lung disease that causes shortness of breath]), diabetes, glaucoma (high pressure in the eye), heart failure, kidney or liver problems, thyroid problems, Wolff-Parkinson-White syndrome (a type of heart condition), or are planning to have a major surgery.

What is the usual dosage?
Please see general statement regarding dosage on page xii.

Angina, High Blood Pressure, and Migraine
Adults: The usual starting dose is 80 milligrams (mg) once a day. Your doctor will prescribe the appropriate dose for you and will increase your dose as needed, until the desired effect is achieved.

Hypertrophic Subaortic Stenosis
Adults: The usual dose is 80-160 mg once a day.

How should I take this medication?
• Take Inderal LA exactly as prescribed by your doctor.

What should I avoid while taking this medication?
Do not drink alcohol while you are taking Inderal LA.

Do not stop taking Inderal LA abruptly without first talking to your doctor.

What are possible food and drug interactions associated with this medication?
If Inderal LA is taken with certain other drugs, the effects of either could be increased, decreased, or altered. Inderal LA may interact with numerous medications. Therefore, it is very important that you tell your doctor about any other medications you are taking.

What are the possible side effects of this medication?
Please see general statement regarding side effects on page xiii.

Side effects may include: abdominal cramping, allergic reactions, depression, difficulty breathing, fever, hallucinations, lightheadedness, low blood pressure, male impotence, memory loss, nausea, rash, skin reactions, slower heartbeat, sore throat, tiredness, vivid dreams, vomiting, weakness

Can I receive this medication if I am pregnant or breastfeeding?

The effects of Inderal LA during pregnancy and breastfeeding are unknown. Tell your doctor immediately if you are pregnant, plan to become pregnant, or are breastfeeding.

What should I do if I miss a dose of this medication?

If you miss a dose of Inderal LA, take it as soon as you remember. However, if it is almost time for your next dose, skip the one you missed and return to your regular dosing schedule. Do not take two doses at once.

How should I store this medication?

Store at room temperature. Protect from light, moisture, freezing, and excessive heat.

Indomethacin: see Indomethacin, page 469

Influenza Virus Vaccine: see Afluria, page 38

Insulin Aspart Protamine/Insulin Aspart, rDNA origin: see Novolog Mix 70/30, page 708

Insulin Aspart, rDNA origin: see Novolog, page 704

Insulin Detemir, rDNA origin: see Levemir, page 539

Insulin Glargine, rDNA origin: see Lantus, page 525

Insulin Lispro Protamine/Insulin Lispro, rDNA origin: see Humalog Mix 50/50, page 442

Insulin Lispro Protamine/Insulin Lispro, rDNA origin: *see*
Humalog Mix 75/25, page 445

Insulin Lispro, rDNA origin: *see Humalog, page 439*

Indomethacin

Generic name: Indomethacin

What is this medication?

Indomethacin is a nonsteroidal anti-inflammatory drug (NSAID) used to treat rheumatoid arthritis (a type of arthritis that involves inflammation of the joints), osteoarthritis, ankylosing spondylitis (arthritis of the spine), tendinitis, bursitis (inflammation and pain around joints), acute gout, and pain. Indomethacin is available as capsules and as extended-release (ER) tablets (releases medicine into your body throughout the day).

What is the most important information I should know about this medication?

- Indomethacin can cause serious problems (such as heart attack or stroke). Your risk can increase when this medication is used for long periods of time and if you have heart disease. Tell your doctor if you experience chest pain, shortness of breath, weakness, or slurred speech.
- Indomethacin can cause high blood pressure and heart failure or worsen existing high blood pressure. Tell your doctor if you experience weight gain or swelling.
- Indomethacin can cause discomfort, ulcers, or bleeding in your stomach or intestines. Your risk can increase with long-term use, smoking, drinking alcohol, older age, poor health, or with certain medications. Tell your doctor immediately if you experience stomach pain or if you have bloody vomit or stools.
- Long-term use of indomethacin can cause kidney injury. Your risk can increase if you have kidney impairment; heart failure; liver problems; are taking certain medications, including water pills (such as furosemide or hydrochlorothiazide) or blood/heart

medications known as angiotensin-converting enzyme (ACE) inhibitors (such as lisinopril); or are elderly.

• Indomethacin can also cause liver injury. Stop taking indomethacin and call your doctor if you experience nausea, tiredness, weakness, itchiness, yellowing of your skin or whites of your eyes, right upper abdominal tenderness, or "flu-like" symptoms.

• Indomethacin can cause a serious allergic reaction. Stop taking indomethacin and tell your doctor right away if you experience trouble breathing or swelling of your face, mouth, or throat.

• Stop taking indomethacin and tell your doctor right away if you experience serious skin reactions, such as rash, blisters, fever, or itchiness.

Who should not take this medication?

Do not take indomethacin if you are allergic to it or any of its ingredients, or if you have experienced asthma, rash, or allergic-type reactions after taking aspirin or other NSAIDs (such as ibuprofen).

Do not take indomethacin right before or after a heart surgery called a coronary artery bypass graft (CABG).

What should I tell my doctor before I take the first dose of this medication?

Tell your doctor about all prescription, over-the-counter, and herbal medications you are taking before beginning treatment with indomethacin. Also, talk to your doctor about your complete medical history, especially if you have any of the following: allergies to medications, heart problems, history of asthma, high blood pressure, kidney or liver disease, or stomach problems, or are pregnant, plan to become pregnant, or are breastfeeding.

What is the usual dosage?

Please see general statement regarding dosage on page xii.

Rheumatoid Arthritis, Osteoarthritis, and Ankylosing Spondylitis

Indomethacin
Adults and children >14 years: The recommended starting dose is 25 milligrams (mg) two or three times a day. Your doctor will prescribe the appropriate dose for you and will increase your dose as needed, until the desired effect is achieved.

Indomethacin ER
Adults and children >14 years: The recommended starting dose is 75 mg once a day. Your doctor may increase your dose to 75 mg twice a day if needed.

Bursitis and Tendinitis

Indomethacin
Adults and children >14 years: The recommended starting dose is 75-150 mg daily, divided in 3 or 4 doses and taken for 7-14 days.

Indomethacin ER
Adults and children >14 years: The recommended starting dose is 75 mg once or twice a day for 7-14 days.

Acute Gout

Indomethacin
Adults and children >14 years: The usual dose is 50 mg three times a day.

How should I take this medication?
- Take indomethacin exactly as prescribed by your doctor.
- Take indomethacin with food, immediately after a meal, or with an antacid to reduce stomach irritation.

What should I avoid while taking this medication?
Do not drink alcohol while you are taking indomethacin.

Do not take aspirin or any other anti-inflammatory medications while you are taking indomethacin, unless your doctor tells you to do so.

What are possible food and drug interactions associated with this medication?

If indomethacin is taken with certain other drugs, the effects of either could be increased, decreased, or altered. It is especially important to check with your doctor before combining indomethacin with the following: ACE inhibitors (such as enalapril or lisinopril), aspirin, blood pressure/heart medications known as beta-blockers (such as metoprolol or propranolol), blood thinners (such as warfarin), cyclosporine, diflunisal, digoxin, lithium, methotrexate, other NSAIDs, probenecid, and water pills (such as furosemide or hydrochlorothiazide).

What are the possible side effects of this medication?

Please see general statement regarding side effects on page xiii.

> **Side effects may include:** constipation, depression, diarrhea, dizziness, gas, headache, heartburn, nausea, stomach pain, tiredness, vomiting

Can I receive this medication if I am pregnant or breastfeeding?

Do not take indomethacin if you are in the late stage of your pregnancy or if you are breastfeeding. The effects of indomethacin during early pregnancy are unknown. Tell your doctor immediately if you are pregnant, plan to become pregnant, or are breastfeeding.

What should I do if I miss a dose of this medication?

If you miss a dose of indomethacin, take it as soon as you remember. However, if it is almost time for your next dose, skip the one you missed and return to your regular dosing schedule. Do not take two doses at once.

How should I store this medication?

Store at room temperature.

Intermezzo

Generic name: Zolpidem Tartrate

What is this medication?

Intermezzo is a sedative-hypnotic (sleep) medicine that is used to treat those who have a sleep problem called insomnia. Many people have difficulty returning to sleep after awakening in the middle of the night. Intermezzo is used to specifically treat this problem.

Intermezzo is a federally controlled substance because it has abuse potential.

What is the most important information I should know about this medication?

- Intermezzo has abuse potential and can cause dependence. Mental and physical dependence can occur with the use of Intermezzo when it is used improperly for long periods of time. Keep Intermezzo in a safe place to prevent misuse and abuse. Selling or giving away Intermezzo can harm others, and is against the law. Tell your doctor if you have ever abused or have been dependent on alcohol, prescription medicines, or street drugs.
- It is important that you follow the instructions for use when you take Intermezzo to avoid getting drowsy in the morning.
- Intermezzo can cause serious allergic reactions that may result in death if not immediately treated. Stop taking Intermezzo and tell your doctor immediately if you develop swelling of your tongue or throat, difficulty breathing or swallowing, or nausea and vomiting.
- Intermezzo can cause you to get up out of bed while not being fully awake and do an activity that you do not know you are doing (such as driving a car, making and eating food, talking on the phone, having sex, or sleep-walking). Tell your doctor immediately, if you find out that you have done any of these activities after taking Intermezzo.

Who should not take this medication?

Do not take Intermezzo if you are allergic to it, any of its ingredients, or other medications containing zolpidem (such as Ambien, Ambien CR, Edluar, or Zolpimist).

Do not take Intermezzo if you drank alcohol that day or before bed, if you took another medicine to help you sleep, or if you do not have at least 4 hours of bedtime remaining before the planned time of waking.

What should I tell my doctor before I take the first dose of this medication?

Tell your doctor about all prescription, over-the-counter, and herbal medications you are taking before beginning treatment with Intermezzo. Also, talk to your doctor about your complete medical history, especially if you have a history of depression, mental illness, or suicidal thoughts; have a history of drug or alcohol abuse or addiction; have kidney or liver disease; have lung disease or breathing problems; or are pregnant, plan to become pregnant, or are breastfeeding.

What is the usual dosage?

Please see general statement regarding dosage on page xii.

Adults: The recommended dose is 1.75 milligrams (mg) for women and 3.5 mg for men, taken only once a night if needed.

If you have liver impairment, your doctor will adjust your dose appropriately.

How should I take this medication?

• Take Intermezzo exactly as prescribed by your doctor. Only take 1 tablet at night if needed. You should not take Intermezzo with or right after a meal. Intermezzo can help you fall asleep faster when you take it on an empty stomach. While in bed, place the tablet under your tongue and allow it to break apart completely. Do not swallow it whole. Tell your doctor if your insomnia worsens or is not better within 7-10 days.

• Please review the instructions that came with the prescription on how to properly take Intermezzo.

What should I avoid while taking this medication?

Do not drink alcohol or take another medicine to help you sleep while you are taking Intermezzo.

Do not drive or engage in dangerous activities until at least 4 hours after the dosing and until you feel fully awake.

What are possible food and drug interactions associated with this medication?

If Intermezzo is taken with certain other drugs, the effects of either could be increased, decreased, or altered. It is especially important to check with your doctor before combining Intermezzo with the following: alcohol, chlorpromazine, ketoconazole, rifampin, or other medications that slow down your brain function (such as alprazolam, diazepam, or phenobarbital).

What are the possible side effects of this medication?

Please see general statement regarding side effects on page xiii.

> **Side effects may include:** abnormal thoughts and behavior, anxiety, headache, memory loss, nausea, severe allergic reactions (such as swelling of your tongue or throat, trouble breathing, or nausea and vomiting), tiredness

Can I receive this medication if I am pregnant or breastfeeding?

The effects of Intermezzo during pregnancy and breastfeeding are unknown. Tell your doctor immediately if you are pregnant, plan to become pregnant, or are breastfeeding.

What should I do if I miss a dose of this medication?

Intermezzo should be given only as needed. If you miss your scheduled dose, contact your doctor or pharmacist for advice.

How should I store this medication?

Store at room temperature. Protect from moisture.

Intuniv

Generic name: Guanfacine

What is this medication?

Intuniv is a medicine used to treat the symptoms of attention-deficit hyperactivity disorder (ADHD).

What is the most important information I should know about this medication?

- Intuniv can cause low blood pressure, low heart rate, and fainting. Tell your doctor immediately if you have any of these symptoms while you are taking Intuniv.
- Intuniv can cause dizziness and sleepiness. Do not drive, operate heavy machinery, or engage in other dangerous activities until you know how Intuniv affects you. Do not drink alcohol or take other medicines that make you sleepy or dizzy while you are taking Intuniv until you talk with your doctor.

Who should not take this medication?

Do not take Intuniv if you are allergic to it or any of its ingredients.

What should I tell my doctor before I take the first dose of this medication?

Tell your doctor about all prescription, over-the-counter, and herbal medications you are taking before beginning treatment with Intuniv. Also, talk to your doctor about your complete medical history, especially if you have heart problems or a low heart rate, have fainted, have low blood pressure, have liver or kidney problems, are pregnant or plan to become pregnant, or are breastfeeding or plan to breastfeed.

What is the usual dosage?

Please see general statement regarding dosage on page xii.

Adults and children ≥6 years: Your doctor will prescribe the appropriate dose for you, and will increase your dose as needed.

How should I take this medication?

- Take Intuniv exactly as directed by your doctor. Swallow the tablet whole with a small amount of water, milk, or other liquid. Do not crush, chew, or break it. Do not take it with a high-fat meal.

What should I avoid while taking this medication?

Do not stop taking or change your dose of Intuniv without talking to your doctor.

What are possible food and drug interactions associated with this medication?

If Intuniv is taken with certain other drugs, the effects of either could be increased, decreased, or altered. It is important to check with your doctor before combining Intuniv with any other medication.

What are the possible side effects of this medication?

Please see general statement regarding side effects on page xiii.

Side effects may include: dizziness, fainting, low blood pressure, low heart rate, nausea, sleepiness, stomach pain, tiredness, trouble sleeping

---

Can I receive this medication if I am pregnant or breastfeeding?

The effects of Intuniv during pregnancy and breastfeeding are unknown. Tell your doctor immediately if you are pregnant, plan to become pregnant, or are breastfeeding.

What should I do if I miss a dose of this medication?

If you miss a dose of Intuniv, take it as soon as you remember. However, if it is almost time for your next dose, skip the one you missed and return to your regular dosing schedule. Do not take two doses at once.

How should I store this medication?

Store at room temperature.

Invega
Generic name: Paliperidone

What is this medication?
Invega is a medicine used to treat schizophrenia. It is also used alone or in combination with other medications to treat schizoaffective disorder (a mental condition that causes both a loss of contact with reality [psychosis] and mood problems).

What is the most important information I should know about this medication?
- Invega can increase the risk of stroke in elderly patients. Invega is not approved to treat psychosis in the elderly with dementia (an illness involving loss of memory, judgment, and confusion).
- Invega can cause neuroleptic malignant syndrome (NMS) (a life-threatening brain disorder) marked by muscle stiffness or rigidity, fast heartbeat or irregular pulse, increased sweating, high fever, and blood pressure irregularities. Tell your doctor immediately if you experience any of these symptoms.
- Invega can cause tardive dyskinesia (abnormal muscle movements, including tremor, shuffling, and uncontrolled, involuntary movements). Elderly women appear to be at a higher risk for this condition. Tell your doctor immediately if you begin to have any involuntary muscle movements.
- Invega can increase your risk of developing high blood sugar and diabetes. See your doctor immediately if you develop signs of high blood sugar, including dry mouth, unusual thirst, increased urination, or fatigue. If you have diabetes or have a high risk of developing it, see your doctor regularly for blood sugar testing.
- Invega can increase the amount of prolactin in your blood (a hormone which can affect lactation, menstruation, and fertility). If high prolactin levels develop, you can experience enlarged breasts, missed menstrual periods, decreased sexual ability, or nipple discharge. Tell your doctor immediately if you have any of these symptoms.
- Invega can cause dizziness, lightheadedness, or fainting. To prevent this, sit up or stand slowly, especially in the morning. Sit

or lie down at the first sign of any of these effects. These effects may be more prominent when you first start taking Invega.

- Invega can affect the production of disease-fighting white blood cells. Tell your doctor immediately if you have a fever or infection.
- In rare instances, Invega can cause seizures. Tell your doctor if you have a history of seizures.
- Invega can rarely cause a prolonged, painful erection. This could happen even when you are not having sex. If this is not treated right away, it could lead to permanent sexual problems (such as impotence). Tell your doctor immediately if this happens.
- Invega can mask signs and symptoms of medication overdose and of conditions such as intestinal obstruction, brain tumor, and Reye's syndrome (a potentially fatal disease of the brain and liver that most commonly occurs in children after a viral infection, such as chickenpox). Invega can also cause difficulty when swallowing, which in turn can cause a type of pneumonia.

Who should not take this medication?

Do not take Invega if you are allergic to it, any of its ingredients, or a similar medicine called risperidone.

What should I tell my doctor before I take the first dose of this medication?

Tell your doctor about all prescription, over-the-counter, and herbal medications you are taking before beginning treatment with Invega. Also, talk to your doctor about your complete medical history, especially if you have breast cancer; liver, kidney, or heart disease; high or low blood pressure; heart rhythm problems; a history of heart attack or stroke; seizures; alcohol or substance abuse or dependence; diabetes or elevated blood sugar; Alzheimer's disease or dementia; stomach or bowel problems; history of neuroleptic malignant syndrome; a history of suicidal thoughts; Parkinson's disease; trouble swallowing; or a low white blood cell count.

What is the usual dosage?

Please see general statement regarding dosage on page xii.

Schizophrenia
Adults: The recommended dose is 6 milligrams (mg) once a day.

Adolescents 12-17 years: The recommended starting dose is 3 mg once a day.

Schizoaffective Disorder
Adults: The recommended dose is 6 mg once a day.

Your doctor will adjust your dose as needed, until the desired effect is achieved.

If you have kidney impairment, your doctor will adjust your dose appropriately.

How should I take this medication?
- Take Invega exactly as prescribed by your doctor. Take it with or without food.
- Swallow Invega tablets whole with water. Do not chew, crush, or divide them.
- When you take Invega, you may see something in your stool that looks like a tablet. This is the empty shell from the tablet after the medicine has been absorbed in your body.

What should I avoid while taking this medication?
Do not drive or operate dangerous machinery until you know how Invega affects you.

Do not drink alcohol while you are taking Invega.

Do not become overheated or dehydrated. Drink adequate amounts of fluids while you are taking Invega to avoid becoming dehydrated.

What are possible food and drug interactions associated with this medication?
If Invega is taken with certain other drugs, the effects of either could be increased, decreased, or altered. It is especially important to check with your doctor before combining Invega with the following: alcohol, amiodarone, chlorpromazine, gatifloxacin,

levodopa, moxifloxacin, procainamide, quinidine, sotalol, or thioridazine.

What are the possible side effects of this medication?
Please see general statement regarding side effects on page xiii.

> **Side effects may include:** common cold, constipation, drowsiness, fast heartbeat, involuntary movements, restlessness, upset stomach, weight gain

Can I receive this medication if I am pregnant or breastfeeding?
The effects of Invega during pregnancy are unknown. Invega can be found in your breast milk if you take it while breastfeeding. Tell your doctor immediately if you are pregnant, plan to become pregnant, or are breastfeeding.

What should I do if I miss a dose of this medication?
If you miss a dose of Invega, take it as soon as you remember. However, if it is almost time for your next dose, skip the one you missed and return to your regular dosing schedule. Do not take two doses at once.

How should I store this medication?
Store at room temperature. Protect from moisture.

Ipratropium Bromide: *see Atrovent HFA, page 102*

Irbesartan: *see Avapro, page 111*

Isosorbide Dinitrate

Generic name: Isosorbide Dinitrate

What is this medication?

Isosorbide dinitrate is a medicine used to prevent angina (chest pain) caused by coronary artery disease. Isosorbide dinitrate tablets can be found as brand name Isordil Titradose. Isosorbide dinitrate is also available as a sublingual (under the tongue) tablet which is used to prevent and treat angina.

What is the most important information I should know about this medication?

- Isosorbide dinitrate can cause a severe decrease in your blood pressure. This is most likely to occur while rising from a seated position. This effect can occur more frequently if you drink alcohol. Tell your doctor immediately if you experience dizziness or lightheadedness.
- Headache is a common side effect of isosorbide dinitrate. If you get headaches while you are using isosorbide dinitrate, this is a sign that the medicine is working properly. Do not try to avoid headaches by changing the time you take isosorbide dinitrate. Aspirin or acetaminophen (Tylenol) may relieve the pain.

Who should not take this medication?

Do not take isosorbide dinitrate if you are allergic to it, any of its ingredients, or other nitrates (eg, nitroglycerin, isosorbide mononitrate).

What should I tell my doctor before I take the first dose of this medication?

Tell your doctor about all prescription, over-the-counter, and herbal medications you are taking before beginning treatment with isosorbide dinitrate. Also, talk to your doctor about your complete medical history, especially if you have low blood pressure.

What is the usual dosage?

Please see general statement regarding dosage on page xii.

Adults: Your doctor will prescribe the appropriate dose for you.

How should I take this medication?
• Take isosorbide dinitrate exactly as prescribed by your doctor.

What should I avoid while taking this medication?
Do not abruptly stop taking isosorbide dinitrate.

Do not drink alcohol while you are taking isosorbide dinitrate.

What are possible food and drug interactions associated with this medication?
If isosorbide dinitrate is taken with certain other drugs, the effects of either could be increased, decreased, or altered. It is especially important to check with your doctor before combining isosorbide dinitrate with alcohol, other vasodilators (medication that relaxes the blood vessels), or sildenafil.

What are the possible side effects of this medication?
Please see general statement regarding side effects on page xiii.

> **Side effects may include:** dizziness, headache, lightheadedness, low blood pressure

Can I receive this medication if I am pregnant or breastfeeding?
The effects of isosorbide dinitrate during pregnancy and breast-feeding are unknown. Tell your doctor immediately if you are pregnant, plan to become pregnant, or are breastfeeding.

What should I do if I miss a dose of this medication?
If you miss a dose of isosorbide dinitrate, take it as soon as you remember. However, if it is almost time for your next dose, skip the one you missed and return to your regular dosing schedule. Do not take two doses at once.

How should I store this medication?
Store at room temperature.

Isosorbide Dinitrate: see Isosorbide Dinitrate, page 482

Isosorbide Mononitrate

Generic name: Isosorbide Mononitrate

What is this medication?

Isosorbide mononitrate is a medicine used to prevent and treat angina (chest pain) caused by coronary artery disease.

What is the most important information I should know about this medication?

- Isosorbide mononitrate can cause a severe decrease in your blood pressure. This is most likely to occur while rising from a seated position. This effect can occur more frequently if you drink alcohol. Tell your doctor right away if you experience dizziness or lightheadedness.
- Headache is a common side effect of isosorbide mononitrate. If you get headaches while you are using isosorbide mononitrate, this is a sign that the medicine is working properly. You should not try to avoid headaches by changing the time you take isosorbide mononitrate. Aspirin or acetaminophen (Tylenol) may relieve the pain.

Who should not take this medication?

Do not take isosorbide mononitrate if you are allergic to it, any of its ingredients, or other nitrates or nitrites.

What should I tell my doctor before I take the first dose of this medication?

Tell your doctor about all prescription, over-the-counter, and herbal medications you are taking before beginning treatment with isosorbide mononitrate. Also, talk to your doctor about your complete medical history, especially if you are allergic to nitrates, have heart failure or any other heart condition, suffer from migraines, or are pregnant, plan to become pregnant, or are breastfeeding.

What is the usual dosage?
Please see general statement regarding dosage on page xii.

> *Adults:* The recommended starting dose is 30 or 60 milligrams once a day. Your doctor will prescribe the appropriate dose for you and will increase your dose as needed, until the desired effect is achieved.

How should I take this medication?
- Take isosorbide mononitrate exactly as prescribed by your doctor.
- Take isosorbide mononitrate once a day when you wake up in the morning.
- Swallow isosorbide mononitrate tablets whole. Do not chew, crush, or break the extended-release tablets.

What should I avoid while taking this medication?
Do not drink alcohol while you are taking isosorbide mononitrate.

What are possible food and drug interactions associated with this medication?
If isosorbide mononitrate is taken with certain other drugs, the effects of either could be increased, decreased, or altered. It is especially important to check with your doctor before combining isosorbide mononitrate with the following: alcohol, blood pressure/heart medications known as calcium channel blockers (such as amlodipine), or sildenafil.

What are the possible side effects of this medication?
Please see general statement regarding side effects on page xiii.

> **Side effects may include:** abdominal (stomach) pain, allergic reactions, chest pain, cough, decrease in your blood pressure, diarrhea, dizziness, flushing, headache, irregular heartbeat, light-headedness, nausea, rash, tiredness

Can I receive this medication if I am pregnant or breastfeeding?

The effects of isosorbide mononitrate during pregnancy and breastfeeding are unknown. Tell your doctor immediately if you are pregnant, plan to become pregnant, or are breastfeeding.

What should I do if I miss a dose of this medication?

If you miss a dose of isosorbide mononitrate, take it as soon as you remember. However, if it is almost time for your next dose, skip the one you missed and return to your regular dosing schedule. Do not take two doses at once.

How should I store this medication?

Store at room temperature. Protect from light and moisture.

Isosorbide Mononitrate: see Isosorbide Mononitrate, page 484

Jakafi

Generic name: Ruxolitinib

What is this medication?

Jakafi is a medicine used to treat people with certain types of myelo-fibrosis, including primary myelofibrosis, post-polycythemia vera myelofibrosis, and post-essential thrombocythemia myelofibrosis.

What is the most important information I should know about this medication?

- Jakafi can cause low platelet (type of blood cells that form clots to help stop bleeding) counts, low red blood cell counts, or low white blood cell counts. Your doctor will monitor your blood to check your blood cell counts before you start Jakafi and regularly during your treatment. Tell your doctor immediately if you develop unusual bleeding, bruising, fatigue, shortness of breath, or fever.

- You may be at risk for developing a serious infection while you are taking Jakafi. Tell your doctor if you have chills, aches, fever, nausea, vomiting, weakness, or painful skin rash or blisters.

Who should not take this medication?

Do not take Jakafi if you are allergic to it or any of its ingredients.

What should I tell my doctor before I take the first dose of this medication?

Tell your doctor about all prescription, over-the-counter, and herbal medications you are taking before beginning treatment with Jakafi. Also, talk to your doctor about your complete medical history, especially if you have an infection, have or have had liver or kidney problems, are on dialysis, are pregnant, plan to become pregnant, or are breastfeeding.

What is the usual dosage?

Please see general statement regarding dosage on page xii.

Adults: Your doctor will prescribe the appropriate dose for you based on your condition and platelet counts.

If you have kidney or liver impairment, your doctor will adjust your dose appropriately.

How should I take this medication?

- Take Jakafi exactly as prescribed by your doctor. You can take Jakafi with or without food. Do not stop taking Jakafi or change your dose without first consulting your doctor. Signs and symptoms of myelofibrosis are expected to return after stopping the treatment.

What should I avoid while taking this medication?

Do not drink grapefruit juice while you are taking Jakafi. Grapefruit juice can affect the amount of medicine in your blood.

What are possible food and drug interactions associated with this medication?

If Jakafi is taken with certain other drugs, the effects of either could be increased, decreased, or altered. It is especially important to check with your doctor before combining Jakafi with the following: boceprevir, clarithromycin, conivaptan, erythromycin, grapefruit juice, indinavir, itraconazole, ketoconazole, lopinavir/ritonavir, mibefradil, nefazodone, nelfinavir, posaconazole, rifampin, ritonavir, saquinavir, telaprevir, telithromycin, or voriconazole.

What are the possible side effects of this medication?

Please see general statement regarding side effects on page xiii.

> **Side effects may include:** body aches, bruising, chills, dizziness, fever, headache, nausea, painful skin rash or blisters, shortness of breath, tiredness, unusual bleeding, vomiting, weakness

Can I receive this medication if I am pregnant or breastfeeding?

The effects of Jakafi during pregnancy and breastfeeding are unknown. Tell your doctor immediately if you are pregnant, plan to become pregnant, or are breastfeeding.

What should I do if I miss a dose of this medication?

If you miss a dose of Jakafi, take your next dose at your regular time. Do not take two doses at once.

How should I store this medication?

Store at room temperature.

Janumet

Generic name: Metformin HCl/Sitagliptin

What is this medication?

Janumet contains two medicines (sitagliptan and metformin) that are used to treat type 2 diabetes in addition to diet and exercise.

What is the most important information I should know about this medication?

- Janumet can cause lactic acidosis (a condition involving dangerously high levels of lactic acid in the blood). Tell your doctor if you experience any of the following symptoms: feeling very weak or tired; unusual muscle pain; unusual sleepiness; unexplained rapid breathing; unusual or unexpected stomach problems (such as nausea or vomiting); feeling cold, dizzy, or lightheaded; or suddenly having a slow or uneven heartbeat.

- Janumet can cause a serious allergic reaction, including rash, hives, and swelling of your face, lips, tongue, or throat, which may cause difficulty breathing or swallowing. If you have an allergic reaction, stop taking Janumet and call your doctor right away.

- Janumet can cause pancreatitis (inflammation of the pancreas). You can experience severe pain in the stomach all the way to your back that will not go away, and it may happen with or without vomiting. If you experience any of these symptoms, stop taking Janumet and call your doctor immediately.

- Janumet can cause low blood sugar, making you feel lightheaded, dizzy, shaky, and hungry. Call your doctor if this is a continuous problem for you.

Who should not take this medication?

Do not take Janumet if you are allergic to it or any of its ingredients.

Do not take Janumet if you have type 1 diabetes, kidney disease, a history of pancreatitis, or if you are going to receive an injection of a dye or contrast agent for an x-ray procedure.

What should I tell my doctor before I take the first dose of this medication?

Tell your doctor about all prescription, over-the-counter, and herbal medications you are taking before beginning treatment with Janumet. Also, talk to your doctor about your complete medical history, especially if you have a history of liver, kidney, or heart problems. Tell your doctor if you drink alcohol frequently or if you are a binge drinker. Also, tell your doctor if you are pregnant, plan to become pregnant, or are breastfeeding.

What is the usual dosage?
Please see general statement regarding dosage on page xii.

Adults: Janumet is usually taken twice a day with meals. Your doctor will prescribe the appropriate dose for you based on your previous diabetes medication.

How should I take this medication?
• Take Janumet exactly as prescribed by your doctor. You should take it with food to lower the chance of getting an upset stomach.

What should I avoid while taking this medication?
Do not drink excessive amounts of alcohol while you are taking Janumet.

What are possible food and drug interactions associated with this medication?
If Janumet is taken with certain other drugs, the effects of either could be increased, decreased, or altered. It is especially important to check with your doctor before combining Janumet with the following: birth control pills, blood pressure medications known as calcium channel blockers (such as nifedipine), cimetidine, corticosteroids, digoxin, diuretics (such as furosemide), estrogen, isoniazid, nicotinic acid, phenytoin, or thyroid medications.

What are the possible side effects of this medication?
Please see general statement regarding side effects on page xiii.

> **Side effects may include:** diarrhea; gas, indigestion, or upset stomach; headache; nausea and vomiting; sore throat; stuffy or runny nose; weakness
>
> *Symptoms of low blood sugar:* blurred vision, cold sweats, coma, dizziness, fast heartbeat, fatigue, headache, hunger, lightheadedness, nausea, nervousness, pale skin, shallow breathing

Can I receive this medication if I am pregnant or breastfeeding?

The effects of Janumet during pregnancy and breastfeeding are unknown. Tell your doctor immediately if you are pregnant, plan to become pregnant, or are breastfeeding.

What should I do if I miss a dose of this medication?

If you miss a dose of Janumet, take it with food as soon as you remember. However, if it is almost time for your next dose, skip the one you missed and return to your regular dosing schedule. Do not take two doses at once.

How should I store this medication?

Store at room temperature in a tightly closed container.

Janumet XR

Generic name: Metformin HCl/Sitagliptin

What is this medication?

Janumet XR contains two medicines that are used in combination with diet and exercise to treat type 2 diabetes.

What is the most important information I should know about this medication?

- Janumet XR can cause a rare but serious condition called lactic acidosis, which is a build-up of an acid in your blood. Tell your doctor if you experience any of the following symptoms: feeling very weak or tired; unusual muscle pain; difficulty breathing; sudden stomach problems (such as nausea or vomiting); unusual sleepiness; feeling cold, dizzy, or lightheaded; or having a slow or irregular heartbeat.
- Janumet XR can cause pancreatitis (inflammation of the pancreas). You may experience severe pain in the stomach all the way to your back that will not go away. This may happen with or without vomiting. If you experience any of these symptoms, stop taking Janumet XR and call your doctor immediately.

- Janumet XR can cause low blood sugar, making you feel light-headed, dizzy, shaky, and hungry. Call your doctor if this is a continuous problem for you.
- Janumet XR can cause a serious allergic reaction, including rash, hives, and swelling of your face, lips, tongue, or throat, which may cause difficulty breathing or swallowing. If you have an allergic reaction, stop taking Janumet XR and call your doctor immediately.

Who should not take this medication?

Do not take Janumet XR if you are allergic to it or any of its ingredients. Do not take Janumet XR if you have type 1 diabetes, kidney disease, or are going to get an injection of dye or contrast agents for an x-ray procedure.

What should I tell my doctor before I take the first dose of this medication?

Tell your doctor about all prescription, over-the-counter, and herbal medications you are taking before beginning treatment with Janumet XR. Also, talk to your doctor about your complete medical history, especially if you have or had pancreatitis; kidney, liver, or heart problems; gallstones (stones in your gallbladder); or high blood triglyceride levels. Tell your doctor if you drink alcohol frequently or if you are a binge drinker. Also, tell your doctor if you are pregnant, plan to become pregnant, or are breastfeeding.

What is the usual dosage?

Please see general statement regarding dosage on page xii.

Adults: Your doctor will prescribe the appropriate dose for you.

How should I take this medication?

- Take Janumet XR exactly as prescribed by your doctor. Take it with your evening meal to help reduce the chance of an upset stomach.
- Swallow the Janumet XR tablet whole. Do not crush, split, or chew it.

What should I avoid while taking this medication?

Do not drink excessive amounts of alcohol while you are taking Janumet XR.

What are possible food and drug interactions associated with this medication?

If Janumet XR is taken with certain other drugs, the effects of either could be increased, decreased, or altered. It is especially important to check with your doctor before combining Janumet XR with the following: acetazolamide, blood pressure medications known as calcium channel blockers (such as nifedipine or verapamil), cimetidine, digoxin, diuretics (water pills), estrogen, isoniazid, nicotinic acid, birth control pills, phenytoin, thyroid medications, or topiramate.

What are the possible side effects of this medication?

Please see general statement regarding side effects on page xiii.

> **Side effects may include:** diarrhea, gas, headache, indigestion, low blood sugar, nausea, sore throat, stuffy or runny nose, upper respiratory infection, upset stomach, vomiting, weakness

Can I receive this medication if I am pregnant or breastfeeding?

The effects of Janumet XR during pregnancy and breastfeeding are unknown. Tell your doctor immediately if you are pregnant, plan to become pregnant, or are breastfeeding.

What should I do if I miss a dose of this medication?

If you miss a dose of Janumet XR, take it with food as soon as you remember. However, if it is almost time for your next dose, skip the one you missed and return to your regular dosing schedule. Do not take two doses at once.

How should I store this medication?

Store at room temperature in a dry place. Keep cap tightly closed.

Januvia
Generic name: Sitagliptin

What is this medication?
Januvia is a medicine used to treat type 2 diabetes in addition to diet and exercise. Januvia can be taken alone or with certain other diabetes medications.

What is the most important information I should know about this medication?
- Talk to your doctor if you experience excessive thirst or urination. These may be signs of high blood sugar and improper blood sugar control.
- Januvia can cause a serious allergic reaction, including rash, hives, and swelling of your face, lips, tongue, or throat, which may cause difficulty breathing or swallowing. If you have an allergic reaction, stop taking Januvia and call your doctor right away.
- Januvia can cause pancreatitis (inflammation of the pancreas). You can experience severe pain in your stomach all the way to your back that will not go away, and it may happen with or without vomiting. If you experience any of these symptoms, stop taking Januvia and contact your doctor immediately.
- The amount of diabetes medication you need may change if you undergo any kind of stress (such as a fever, trauma [car accident], infection, or surgery). If you are under any kind of stress, you should notify your doctor immediately.
- Make sure to stay on your diet and exercise program and check your blood sugar regularly.

Who should not take this medication?
Do not take Januvia if you are allergic to it or any of its ingredients.

Do not take Januvia if you have type 1 diabetes or a history of pancreatitis.

What should I tell my doctor before I take the first dose of this medication?

Tell your doctor about all prescription, over-the-counter, and herbal medications you are taking before beginning treatment with Januvia. Also, tell your doctor about your complete medical history, especially if you have a history of kidney problems, pancreatitis, stones in your gallbladder, a history of alcoholism, high blood triglyceride (a type of fat found in your blood) levels, or if you are pregnant, plan to become pregnant, or are breastfeeding.

What is the usual dosage?

Please see general statement regarding dosage on page xii.

Adults: The recommended dose is 100 milligrams once a day.

If you have kidney impairment, your doctor will adjust your dose appropriately.

How should I take this medication?

- Take Januvia exactly as prescribed by your doctor.
- Take Januvia with or without food.
- Your doctor may prescribe Januvia along with other medications that lower blood sugar.

What should I avoid while taking this medication?

Do not drink excessive amounts of alcohol while you are taking Januvia.

What are possible food and drug interactions associated with this medication?

If Januvia is taken with certain other drugs, the effects of either could be increased, decreased, or altered. It is especially important to check with your doctor before combining Januvia with digoxin.

What are the possible side effects of this medication?

Please see general statement regarding side effects on page xiii.

Side effects may include: diarrhea, headache, sore throat, stuffy or runny nose, upper respiratory infection, upset stomach

Symptoms of low blood sugar: confusion, dizziness, drowsiness, fast heartbeat, feeling jittery, headache, hunger, irritability, sweating, weakness

Can I receive this medication if I am pregnant or breastfeeding?

The effects of Januvia during pregnancy and breastfeeding are unknown. Tell your doctor immediately if you are pregnant, plan to become pregnant, or are breastfeeding.

What should I do if I miss a dose of this medication?

If you miss a dose of Januvia, take it as soon as you remember. However, if it is almost time for your next dose, skip the one you missed and return to your regular dosing schedule. Do not take two doses at once.

How should I store this medication?

Store at room temperature.

Juvisync

Generic name: Simvastatin/Sitagliptin

What is this medication?

Juvisync is a medicine used in addition to diet and exercise to lower blood sugar and cholesterol in adults with type 2 diabetes. Juvisync contains two medicines, sitagliptin and simvastatin. It lowers triglycerides and "bad" (low density lipoprotein [LDL]) cholesterol, and it raises the "good" (high density lipoprotein [HDL]) cholesterol. Juvisync can reduce your risk of death from heart problems, heart attack, stroke, or the need for certain blood vessel procedures.

What is the most important information I should know about this medication?

- Juvisync can cause a condition known as pancreatitis (inflammation of the pancreas). You can experience severe pain in the stomach all the way to your back that will not go away, and it can happen with or without vomiting. If you experience any of these symptoms, stop taking Juvisync and contact your doctor immediately. Your risk of having these symptoms can be higher if you already have a history of pancreatitis, stones in your gallbladder, alcoholism, high blood triglyceride levels, or kidney problems.

- The amount of diabetes medication you need can change if you undergo any kind of stress (such as a fever), trauma (such as a car accident), infection, or surgery. Tell your doctor immediately if you are under any kind of stress.

- Make sure to stay on your diet and exercise program, and check your blood sugar regularly.

Who should not take this medication?

Do not take Juvisync if you are allergic to it or any of its ingredients.

Do not take Juvisync if you are taking certain antibiotics (such as erythromycin or clarithromycin); certain medications for fungal infections (such as itraconazole, ketoconazole, or posaconazole); cyclosporine; danazol; gemfibrozil; HIV medications in a class called protease inhibitors (such as indinavir, ritonavir, or atazanavir); or nefazodone.

Do not take Juvisync if you have active liver disease or liver problems, type 1 diabetes, if you are pregnant, plan to become pregnant, or are breastfeeding.

What should I tell my doctor before I take the first dose of this medication?

Tell your doctor about all prescription, over-the-counter, and herbal medications you are taking before beginning treatment with Juvisync. Also, talk to your doctor about your complete medical history, especially if you have pancreatitis, kidney or liver problems, stones in your gallbladder, high blood triglycerides levels, or alcoholism. Also, tell your doctor if you are pregnant, plan to become pregnant, or are breastfeeding.

What is the usual dosage?

Please see general statement regarding dosage on page xii.

Adults: The recommended starting dose is 100/40 (100 milligrams [mg] of sitagliptin and 40 mg of simvastatin) once a day. Your doctor will adjust your dose as needed.

How should I take this medication?

• Take Juvisync as prescribed by your doctor. You can take Juvisync once a day in the evening, with or without food. Do not break, cut, crush, dissolve, or chew Juvisync tablets. Swallow the tablets whole. It is important for you to follow any dietary, exercise, and blood sugar monitoring instructions from your doctor while you are taking this medication.

What should I avoid while taking this medication?

Do not drink large amounts of alcohol or grapefruit juice while you are taking Juvisync.

What are possible food and drug interactions associated with this medication?

If Juvisync is taken with certain other drugs, the effects of either could be increased, decreased, or altered. Juvisync may interact with numerous medications. Therefore, it is very important that you tell your doctor about any other medications you are taking.

What are the possible side effects of this medication?

Please see general statement regarding side effects on page xiii.

Side effects may include: constipation, headache, nausea, sore throat, stomach pain, stuffy or runny nose, upper respiratory (lung) infection

---

Can I receive this medication if I am pregnant or breastfeeding?

Do not take Juvisync if you are pregnant or breastfeeding. It can cause harm to your baby. Tell your doctor immediately if you are pregnant, plan to become pregnant, or are breastfeeding.

What should I do if I miss a dose of this medication?

If you miss a dose of Juvisync, take it as soon as you remember. However, if it is almost time for your next dose, skip the one you missed and return to your regular dosing schedule. Do not take two doses at once.

How should I store this medication?

Store at room temperature.

K-Dur

Generic name: Potassium Chloride

What is this medication?

K-Dur is a potassium supplement that helps prevent and treat low blood potassium levels in your body.

What is the most important information I should know about this medication?

- K-Dur can increase your blood potassium to levels higher than normal, which can result in a heart attack. Your risk is higher if you have kidney disease or any other condition that does not allow potassium to be eliminated from your body. Your doctor will perform blood tests regularly to monitor your blood potassium levels.
- K-Dur can cause serious stomach and intestinal problems. Tell your doctor right away if you experience vomiting, abdominal pain, stomach bloating, or tarry stools.

Who should not take this medication?

Do not take K-Dur if you are allergic to it or any of its ingredients.

Do not take K-Dur if you have high blood potassium levels or any condition that stops or slows the passage of tablets through your stomach or intestinal tract.

What should I tell my doctor before I take the first dose of this medication?

Tell your doctor about all prescription, over-the-counter, and herbal medications you are taking before beginning treatment with K-Dur. Also, talk to your doctor about your complete medical history, especially if you have stomach problems, heart disease, kidney problems, or metabolic acidosis (a condition in which there is too much acid in the body).

What is the usual dosage?
Please see general statement regarding dosage on page xii.

Prevention of Low Potassium Levels
Adults: The usual dose is 20 milliequivalents (mEq) once a day.

Treatment of Low Potassium Levels
Adults: The usual dose is 40-100 mEq a day in divided doses.

Your doctor will increase your dose as appropriate.

How should I take this medication?
- Take K-Dur exactly as prescribed by your doctor. Take each dose of K-Dur with meals and with a full glass of water or other liquid. Do not take more than 20 mEq in a single dose.
- Swallow K-Dur tablets whole. Do not crush, chew, or suck on them.
- If you have difficulty swallowing whole tablets, break the tablet in half and take each half separately with a glass of water.
- You can also prepare a mixture with water by placing the whole tablet(s) in about 1/2 a glass of water (4 fluid ounces). Wait about 2 minutes for the tablet(s) to disintegrate. Stir the mixture for about 30 seconds after the tablet(s) has disintegrated. Swirl the mixture and drink the entire amount in the glass (either directly from the cup or using a straw) right away. Add one fluid

ounce of water, swirl it, and drink it right away. Repeat this one more time.
- Do not use any other liquids besides water to mix K-Dur.

What should I avoid while taking this medication?
Do not take K-Dur on an empty stomach.

What are possible food and drug interactions associated with this medication?
If K-Dur is taken with certain other drugs, the effects of either could be increased, decreased, or altered. It is especially important to check with your doctor before combining K-Dur with the following: blood pressure medicines known as angiotensin converting enzyme (ACE) inhibitors (such as captopril or lisinopril) or certain diuretics (water pills) (such as amiloride or triamterene).

What are the possible side effects of this medication?
Please see general statement regarding side effects on page xiii.

Side effects may include: abdominal pain or discomfort, diarrhea, gas, nausea, vomiting

---

Can I receive this medication if I am pregnant or breastfeeding?
The effects of K-Dur during pregnancy are unknown. You can continue to take K-Dur while you are breastfeeding. Tell your doctor immediately if you are pregnant, plan to become pregnant, or are breastfeeding.

What should I do if I miss a dose of this medication?
If you miss a dose of K-Dur, take it as soon as you remember. However, if it is almost time for your next dose, skip the one you missed and return to your regular dosing schedule. Do not take two doses at once.

How should I store this medication?
Store at room temperature.

Keppra

Generic name: Levetiracetam

What is this medication?

Keppra is a medicine used to treat partial-onset, myoclonic, and tonic-clonic (grand mal) seizures. Keppra is available in tablets and an oral solution.

What is the most important information I should know about this medication?

- Do not stop taking Keppra without first talking to your doctor. Stopping Keppra suddenly can cause serious problems, including seizures that will not stop (status epilepticus).
- Keppra can cause suicidal thoughts or actions. Tell your doctor immediately if you have thoughts about suicide or dying; attempts to commit suicide; have new or worse depression, anxiety, or irritability; have panic attacks; have trouble sleeping (insomnia); have an extreme increase in activity and talking (mania); are feeling agitated or restless; acting aggressive; being angry or violent; acting on dangerous impulses; or have other unusual changes in behavior or mood.

Who should not take this medication?

Do not take Keppra if you are allergic to it or any of its ingredients.

What should I tell my doctor before I take the first dose of this medication?

Tell your doctor about all prescription, over-the-counter, and herbal medications you are taking before beginning treatment with Keppra. Also, talk to your doctor about your complete medical history, especially if you have or have had depression, mood problems, suicidal thoughts or behavior, have kidney problems, or are pregnant, plan to become pregnant, or are breastfeeding.

What is the usual dosage?

Please see general statement regarding dosage on page xii.

Adults: Your doctor will prescribe the appropriate dose for you based on your condition and will increase your dose as appropriate.

If you have kidney impairment, your doctor will adjust your dose appropriately.

Children: Your doctor will prescribe the appropriate dose for your child, based on their weight.

Attempts to taper or discontinue the medication should be made at specific intervals, through the guidance of your doctor.

How should I take this medication?
- Take Keppra exactly as prescribed by your doctor.
- Keppra is usually taken twice a day. Take this medication at the same time each day. Take Keppra with or without food.
- Swallow Keppra tablets whole. Do not chew or crush the tablets.
- Do not change your dose or stop taking this medication abruptly without first talking to your doctor.
- If your doctor has prescribed Keppra oral solution, ask your pharmacist for a medicine dropper or medicine cup to help you measure the correct amount of solution. Do not use a household teaspoon.

What should I avoid while taking this medication?
Do not drive, operate machinery, or engage in dangerous activities until you know how Keppra affects you. Keppra can make you dizzy or sleepy.

What are possible food and drug interactions associated with this medication?
If Keppra is taken with certain other drugs, the effects of either could be increased, decreased, or altered. It is important to check with your doctor before combining Keppra with any other medication.

What are the possible side effects of this medication?
Please see general statement regarding side effects on page xiii.

Side effects may include: aggression, agitation, anger, anxiety, delusions (false or strange thoughts or beliefs), depression, dizziness, hallucinations (seeing or hearing things that are really not there), headache, hostility, infections, irritability, lack of interest, loss of appetite, mood swings, nasal congestion, problems with your muscle coordination, skin rash, sleepiness, tiredness, unusual behavior, weakness

Can I receive this medication if I am pregnant or breastfeeding?

The effects of Keppra during pregnancy and breastfeeding are unknown. Keppra can be found in your breast milk if you take it while breastfeeding. Tell your doctor immediately if you are pregnant, plan to become pregnant, or are breastfeeding.

What should I do if I miss a dose of this medication?

If you miss a dose of Keppra, take it as soon as you remember. However, if it is almost time for your next dose, skip the one you missed and return to your regular dosing schedule. Do not take two doses at once.

How should I store this medication?

Store at room temperature. Protect from heat and light.

Ketoconazole: see Nizoral, page 696

Klonopin

Generic name: Clonazepam

What is this medication?

Klonopin is a medicine used to treat panic disorder in adults and certain types of seizure disorders in adults and children. Klonopin is available as a tablet or wafer.

What is the most important information I should know about this medication?

- Klonopin has abuse potential. Mental and physical dependence can occur with the use of Klonopin.
- Do not stop taking Klonopin without first talking to your doctor. Stopping Klonopin suddenly can cause withdrawal symptoms, including seizures.
- Klonopin can cause suicidal thoughts or actions in a small number of people. Tell your doctor right away if you have thoughts about suicide or dying; attempt to commit suicide; have new or worse depression, anxiety, or irritability; have panic attacks, trouble sleeping, an extreme increase in activity and talking; are feeling agitated or restless or acting aggressive; being angry or violent; acting on dangerous impulses; or have other unusual changes in behavior or mood.

Who should not take this medication?

Do not take Klonopin if you are allergic to it or any of its ingredients. In addition, do not take Klonopin if you have severe liver disease or an eye condition called acute narrow-angle glaucoma (high pressure in the eye).

What should I tell my doctor before I take the first dose of this medication?

Tell your doctor about all prescription, over-the-counter, and herbal medications you are taking before beginning treatment with Klonopin. Also, talk to your doctor about your complete medical history, especially if you have a history of alcohol or drug abuse; liver, kidney, or breathing problems; glaucoma; or depression or suicidal tendencies. Also, tell your doctor if you are pregnant, plan to become pregnant, or are breastfeeding.

What is the usual dosage?

Please see general statement regarding dosage on page xii.

Panic Disorder

Adults: The usual starting dose is 0.25 milligrams (mg) twice a day. Your doctor will increase your dose as needed until the desired effect is achieved.

—Seizures

Adults: The usual starting dose is 0.5 mg three times a day. Your doctor will increase your dose as needed until your seizures are controlled.

Children ≤10 years: Your doctor will prescribe the appropriate dose for your child based on their weight.

If you are elderly, your doctor will adjust your dose appropriately.

How should I take this medication?
- Take Klonopin exactly as prescribed by your doctor. Swallow Klonopin tablets whole with water.
- Take Klonopin wafers with or without water. Open the pouch and peel back the foil on the blister pack. Do not push the wafer through the foil. With dry hands, place the wafer in your mouth. It will melt quickly.
- Do not change your dose or stop taking Klonopin without first talking to your doctor.

What should I avoid while taking this medication?
Do not drink alcohol while you are taking Klonopin.

Do not drive, operate heavy machinery, or do other dangerous activities until you know how Klonopin affects you.

What are possible food and drug interactions associated with this medication?
If Klonopin is taken with certain other drugs, the effects of either could be increased, decreased, or altered. It is especially important to check with your doctor before combining Klonopin with the following: alcohol, antifungals (such as fluconazole or itraconazole), barbiturates (such as butalbital or phenobarbital), carbamazepine, certain antidepressants (such as amitriptyline or phenelzine), certain antipsychotics (such as chlorpromazine or haloperidol), narcotic painkillers (such as hydrocodone or oxycodone), propantheline, or seizure medicines (such as valproate or phenytoin).

Labetalol / **507**

What are the possible side effects of this medication?
Please see general statement regarding side effects on page xiii.

Side effects may include: depression, dizziness, drowsiness, fatigue, memory problems, problems with your coordination or walking

Can I receive this medication if I am pregnant or breastfeeding?
Do not take Klonopin if you are pregnant or breastfeeding. Klonopin can harm your unborn baby. Tell your doctor immediately if you are pregnant, plan to become pregnant, or are breastfeeding.

What should I do if I miss a dose of this medication?
If you miss a dose of Klonopin, take it as soon as you remember. However, if it is almost time for your next dose, skip the one you missed and return to your regular dosing schedule. Do not take two doses at once.

How should I store this medication?
Store at room temperature.

Labetalol
Generic name: Labetalol HCl

What is this medication?
Labetalol is a medicine known as a beta-blocker, which is used to treat high blood pressure.

What is the most important information I should know about this medication?
• Do not stop taking labetalol without talking to your doctor. Stopping this medication suddenly can cause harmful effects. Your doctor should gradually reduce your dose when stopping treatment with this medication.

- Labetalol can worsen heart failure, cause breathing problems, or hide symptoms of low blood sugar levels if you have diabetes. Tell your doctor if you experience weight gain or trouble breathing while you are taking labetalol. If you have diabetes, monitor your blood sugar frequently, especially when you first start taking labetalol.
- Labetalol can cause liver impairment. Tell your doctor if you experience itching, dark urine, loss of appetite, yellowing of your skin or whites of your eyes, right upper abdominal pain, or "flu-like" symptoms.

Who should not take this medication?

Do not take labetalol if you are allergic to it or any of its ingredients. In addition, do not take labetalol if you have asthma, a slow heart rate, heart failure, heart block, or severe blood circulation disorders.

What should I tell my doctor before I take the first dose of this medication?

Tell your doctor about all prescription, over-the-counter, and herbal medications you are taking before beginning treatment with labetalol. Also, talk to your doctor about your complete medical history, especially if you have allergies, heart problems or heart failure, a history of heart attack, breathing problems (such as bronchitis [inflammation of the air passages within the lungs] or emphysema [lung disease that causes shortness of breath]), pheochromocytoma (tumor of the adrenal gland), diabetes, liver problems, or are planning to have a major surgery, including eye surgery.

Tell your doctor if you have a history of severe allergic reactions to any allergens, because labetalol may decrease the effectiveness of epinephrine used to treat the reaction.

What is the usual dosage?

Please see general statement regarding dosage on page xii.

Adults: The usual starting dose is 100 milligrams twice a day, either alone or in combination with other blood pressure-lowering medicines. Your doctor will increase your dose as needed until the desired effect is achieved.

How should I take this medication?
- Take labetalol exactly as prescribed by your doctor.

What should I avoid while taking this medication?
Do not stop taking labetalol without first talking to your doctor.

What are possible food and drug interactions associated with this medication?
If labetalol is taken with certain other drugs, the effects of either could be increased, decreased, or altered. It is especially important to check with your doctor before combining labetalol with the following: asthma inhalers (such as albuterol or salmeterol), blood pressure medications known as calcium channel blockers (such as diltiazem or verapamil), certain antidepressants (such as amitriptyline or imipramine), cimetidine, diabetes medicines (such as insulin), digoxin, or nitroglycerin.

What are the possible side effects of this medication?
Please see general statement regarding side effects on page xiii.

> **Side effects may include:** dizziness, ejaculation problems, fatigue, impotence, nausea, stuffy nose, temporary scalp tingling, upset stomach

Can I receive this medication if I am pregnant or breastfeeding?
The effects of labetalol during pregnancy are unknown. Labetalol can be found in your breast milk if you take it while breastfeeding. Tell your doctor immediately if you are pregnant, plan to become pregnant, or are breastfeeding.

What should I do if I miss a dose of this medication?
If you miss a dose of labetalol, take it as soon as you remember. However, if it is almost time for your next dose, skip the one you

missed and return to your regular dosing schedule. Do not take two doses at once.

How should I store this medication?
Store at room temperature.

Labetalol HCl: see Labetalol, page 507

Lactulose
Generic name: Lactulose

What is this medication?
Lactulose is a liquid medicine used to treat constipation.

What is the most important information I should know about this medication?
- Lactulose can take 24-48 hours to produce a normal bowel movement. Tell your doctor if you experience unusual diarrhea.
- Tell your doctor if you will be undorgoing any procedures that require bowel cleansing while on lactulose. Your doctor may prescribe you a different solution.
- If you are elderly and have been taking lactulose for more than 6 months, your doctor will order blood tests regularly to check your electrolytes (chemicals that are important for the cells in your body to function, such as potassium, chloride, and carbon dioxide).

Who should not take this medication?
Do not take lactulose if you are allergic to it or any of its ingredients.

Lactulose contains galactose (a simple sugar). Do not take lactulose if you are required to maintain a low galactose diet.

What should I tell my doctor before I take the first dose of this medication?

Tell your doctor about all prescription, over-the-counter, and herbal medications you are taking before beginning treatment with lactulose. Also, talk to your doctor about your complete medical history, especially if you have diabetes, are required to maintain a low galactose diet, are pregnant, plan to become pregnant, or are breastfeeding.

What is the usual dosage?

Please see general statement regarding dosage on page xii.

Adults: The usual dose is 1-2 tablespoonfuls (15-30 milliliters [mL]) once a day. Your doctor may increase the dose to 60 mL once a day, if necessary.

How should I take this medication?

• Take lactulose exactly as prescribed by your doctor. Do not take extra doses or take more often without asking your doctor. If you find the taste of lactulose to be unpleasant, you can mix it with water, fruit juice, or milk.

What should I avoid while taking this medication?

Do not skip or miss any scheduled doses.

What are possible food and drug interactions associated with this medication?

If lactulose is taken with certain other drugs, the effects of either could be increased, decreased, or altered. It is especially important to check with your doctor before combining lactulose with antacids.

What are the possible side effects of this medication?

Please see general statement regarding side effects on page xiii.

Side effects may include: diarrhea, electrolyte imbalance, gas, high blood sodium levels, low blood potassium levels, nausea, stomach cramps, vomiting

Can I receive this medication if I am pregnant or breastfeeding?

The effects of lactulose during pregnancy and breastfeeding are unknown. Tell your doctor immediately if you are pregnant, plan to become pregnant, or are breastfeeding.

What should I do if I miss a dose of this medication?

If you miss a dose of lactulose, take it as soon as you remember. However, if it is almost time for your next dose, skip the one you missed and return to your regular dosing schedule. Do not take two doses at once.

How should I store this medication?

Store at room temperature.

Lactulose: *see Lactulose, page 510*

Lamictal

Generic name: Lamotrigine

What is this medication?

Lamictal is a medicine used alone or with other medicines to treat certain types of seizures. It is also used for long-term treatment of bipolar disorder. Lamictal is available as chewable dispersible tablets, orally disintegrating tablets, and tablets.

What is the most important information I should know about this medication?

- Lamictal can cause a serious skin rash that can be life-threatening. Your risk of getting this rash is higher if you take Lamictal with another medicine called valproate or if you take more Lamictal than your doctor prescribed. Tell your doctor right away if you experience blistering or peeling of your skin, hives, or painful sores in your mouth or around your eyes.
- Lamictal can cause serious blood or liver problems. Call your doctor right away if you experience a fever, frequent infections,

severe muscle pain, unusual bruising or bleeding, weakness, fatigue, yellowing of your skin or the whites of your eyes, or swelling of your face, eyes, lips, or tongue.

- Lamictal can cause suicidal thoughts or actions in a small number of people. Tell your doctor right away if you have thoughts about suicide or dying; attempt to commit suicide; have new or worse depression, anxiety, or irritability; have panic attacks, trouble sleeping, an extreme increase in activity and talking; are feeling agitated or restless or acting aggressive; being angry or violent; acting on dangerous impulses; or have other unusual changes in your behavior or mood.

- Lamictal can rarely cause meningitis (brain or spinal cord inflammation). Tell your doctor right away if you develop a headache, fever, nausea, vomiting, stiff neck, rash, unusual sensitivity to light, muscle pain, chills, confusion, or drowsiness.

- Tell your doctor if you plan to start or stop taking birth control pills as this can affect the amount of Lamictal in your body and may require dose adjustments.

- Do not stop taking Lamictal without first talking to your doctor. Stopping Lamictal suddenly can cause withdrawal symptoms, including seizures.

Who should not take this medication?

Do not take Lamictal if you are allergic to it or any of its ingredients.

What should I tell my doctor before I take the first dose of this medication?

Tell your doctor about all prescription, over-the-counter, and herbal medications you are taking before beginning treatment with Lamictal. Also, talk to your doctor about your complete medical history, especially if you have kidney problems; are taking birth control pills or other hormone medicines for women; have or had depression, mood problems, or suicidal thought or behavior; or have had meningitis after taking Lamictal or a rash or allergic reaction to another anti-seizure medicine.

What is the usual dosage?

Please see general statement regarding dosage on page xii.

Adults and children: Your doctor will prescribe the appropriate dose for you or your child, based on your condition.

How should I take this medication?
- Take Lamictal exactly as prescribed by your doctor. Swallow Lamictal tablets whole.
- Place Lamictal orally disintegrating tablets on your tongue and move it around your mouth. The tablet will rapidly disintegrate. Swallow it with or without water and take it with or without food.
- If you are taking Lamictal chewable dispersible tablets, swallow it whole, chew it, or mix it in water or diluted fruit juice. If you are chewing them, drink a small amount of water or diluted fruit juice to help you swallow.
- To mix the chewable dispersible tablets in liquid, add the tablets to a small amount of water or diluted juice (1 teaspoon or enough amount to cover the tablets) in a glass or spoon. Wait at least 1 minute or until the tablets are completely broken up, then mix the solution together. Take the entire amount right away.

What should I avoid while taking this medication?
Do not change your dose or stop taking Lamictal without first talking to your doctor. Stopping Lamictal suddenly may cause serious side effects.

Do not start or stop taking birth control pills or other hormone medicines for women without first talking to your doctor.

Do not drive or operate dangerous machinery until you know how Lamictal affects you.

What are possible food and drug interactions associated with this medication?
If Lamictal is taken with certain other drugs, the effects of either could be increased, decreased, or altered. It is especially important to check with your doctor before combining Lamictal with the following: birth control pills, carbamazepine, phenobarbital, phenytoin, primidone, rifampin, topiramate, or valproate.

What are the possible side effects of this medication?
Please see general statement regarding side effects on page xiii.

Side effects may include: abdominal pain, back pain, blurred or double vision, dizziness, dry mouth, fever, headache, lack of co-ordination, nausea, rash, shaking, sleepiness, tiredness, trouble sleeping, vomiting

---

Can I receive this medication if I am pregnant or breastfeeding?
The effects of Lamictal during pregnancy are unknown. Lamictal can be found in your breast milk if you take it while breastfeeding. Tell your doctor immediately if you are pregnant, plan to become pregnant, or are breastfeeding.

What should I do if I miss a dose of this medication?
If you miss a dose of Lamictal, take it as soon as you remember. However, if it is almost time for your next dose, skip the one you missed and return to your regular dosing schedule. Do not take two doses at once.

How should I store this medication?
Store at room temperature. Protect from light.

Lamictal XR
Generic name: Lamotrigine

What is this medication?
Lamictal XR is a medicine used alone or with other medicines to treat certain types of seizures.

What is the most important information I should know about this medication?
- Lamictal XR can cause a serious skin rash that can be life-threatening. Your risk of getting this rash is higher if you take Lamictal XR with another medicine called valproate or if

you take more Lamictal XR than your doctor prescribed you. Tell your doctor right away if you experience a skin rash, blistering or peeling of your skin, hives, or painful sores in your mouth or around your eyes.

- Lamictal XR can cause serious blood or liver problems. Call your doctor right away if you experience a fever, frequent infections, severe muscle pain, unusual bruising or bleeding, weakness, fatigue, yellowing of your skin or the whites of your eyes, or swelling of your face, eyes, lips, or tongue.
- Lamictal XR can cause suicidal thoughts or actions in a small number of people. Tell your doctor right away if you have thoughts about suicide or dying; attempt to commit suicide; have new or worse depression, anxiety, or irritability; have panic attacks, trouble sleeping, an extreme increase in activity and talking; are feeling agitated or restless or acting aggressive; become angry or violent; acting on dangerous impulses; or have other unusual changes in your behavior or mood.
- Lamictal XR can rarely cause meningitis (brain or spinal cord inflammation). Tell your doctor right away if you develop a headache, fever, nausea, vomiting, stiff neck, rash, unusual sensitivity to light, muscle pain, chills, confusion, or drowsiness.
- Tell your doctor if you plan to start or stop taking birth control pills as this can affect the amount of Lamictal XR in your body, that may require dose adjustments.
- Do not stop taking Lamictal XR without first talking to your doctor. Stopping Lamictal XR suddenly can cause withdrawal symptoms, including seizures.

Who should not take this medication?

Do not take Lamictal XR if you are allergic to it or any of its ingredients.

What should I tell my doctor before I take the first dose of this medication?

Tell your doctor about all prescription, over-the-counter, and herbal medications you are taking before beginning treatment with Lamictal XR. Also, talk to your doctor about your complete medical history, especially if you have kidney problems; are taking birth control pills or other hormone medicines for women; have or had depression, mood problems, or suicidal thoughts or behavior; or have had meningitis after taking Lamictal or Lamictal XR or a rash or allergic reaction to another anti-seizure medicine.

What is the usual dosage?
Please see general statement regarding dosage on page xii.

Adults and children ≥13 years: Your doctor will prescribe the appropriate dose for you or your child, based on your condition.

How should I take this medication?
• Take Lamictal XR exactly as prescribed by your doctor. Take it with or without food.
• Swallow Lamictal XR tablets whole. Do not chew, crush, or divide them.

What should I avoid while taking this medication?
Do not change your dose or stop taking Lamictal XR without first talking to your doctor. Stopping Lamictal XR suddenly may cause serious side effects.

Do not start or stop taking birth control pills or other hormone medicines for women without first talking to your doctor.

Do not drive or operate dangerous machinery until you know how Lamictal XR affects you.

What are possible food and drug interactions associated with this medication?
If Lamictal XR is taken with certain other drugs, the effects of either could be increased, decreased, or altered. It is especially important to check with your doctor before combining Lamictal XR with the following: birth control pills, carbamazepine, phenobarbital, phenytoin, primidone, rifampin, topiramate, or valproate.

What are the possible side effects of this medication?
Please see general statement regarding side effects on page xiii.

> **Side effects may include:** anxiety, dizziness, double vision, lack of coordination, nausea, shaking, vomiting

Can I receive this medication if I am pregnant or breastfeeding?

The effects of Lamictal XR during pregnancy are unknown. Lamictal XR can be found in your breast milk if you take it while breast-feeding. Tell your doctor immediately if you are pregnant, plan to become pregnant, or are breastfeeding.

What should I do if I miss a dose of this medication?

If you miss a dose of Lamictal XR, take it as soon as you remember. However, if it is almost time for your next dose, skip the one you missed and return to your regular dosing schedule. Do not take two doses at once.

How should I store this medication?

Store at room temperature.

Lamisil

Generic name: Terbinafine HCl

What is this medication?

Lamisil is an antifungal medicine used to treat certain fungal infections. It is available in tablets or oral granules. Lamisil tablets are used to treat tinea unguium or onychomycosis (ringworm of the nails). Lamisil oral granules are used for the treatment of tinea capitis (ringworm of the scalp).

What is the most important information I should know about this medication?

• Lamisil can cause liver damage. Tell your doctor right away if you experience persistent nausea, loss of appetite, fatigue, vomiting, right upper abdominal pain, yellowing of your skin or whites of your eyes, dark urine, or pale stools.

- Lamisil can cause taste or smell disturbances, including loss of taste or smell. Tell your doctor if you experience these changes while taking Lamisil.
- Lamisil can cause lupus (disease that affects the immune system). If you develop a progressive skin rash that is scaly, red, shows scarring, loss of pigment, or unusual sensitivity to the sun that can lead to a rash, stop taking Lamisil and tell your doctor right away.
- Lamisil can cause severe skin reactions. Stop taking Lamisil and tell your doctor right away if you develop a rash.
- Also, Lamisil can cause symptoms of depression. Tell your doctor right away if you feel sad or worthless, or if you have changes in sleep pattern, loss of energy or interest in daily activities, restlessness, or mood changes.

Who should not take this medication?
Do not take Lamisil if you are allergic to it or any of its ingredients.

What should I tell my doctor before I take the first dose of this medication?
Tell your doctor about all prescription, over-the-counter, and herbal medications you are taking before beginning treatment with Lamisil. Also, talk to your doctor about your complete medical history, especially if you have kidney or liver problems, a weak immune system, lupus, are pregnant, plan to become pregnant, or are breastfeeding.

What is the usual dosage?
Please see general statement regarding dosage on page xii.

Lamisil Tablets

Tinea Unguium or Onychomycosis
Adults: The usual dose is 250 milligrams (mg) once a day. Your doctor will determine the duration of treatment based on the type of your infection.

Lamisil Oral Granules

Tinea Capitis
Adults and children >4 years: Your doctor will prescribe the appropriate dose for you, based on your weight.

How should I take this medication?
- Take Lamisil exactly as prescribed by your doctor.
- You can take Lamisil tablets with or without food.
- Sprinkle Lamisil oral granules on food and take it by mouth. Shake the packet of Lamisil oral granules. Carefully pour the entire contents of the packet onto a spoonful of a soft, non-acidic food (such as pudding or mashed potatoes). Make sure that no granules remain in the packet. Swallow the combination of food and granules without chewing.
- Please review the instructions that came with your prescription on how to properly take your Lamisil.

What should I avoid while taking this medication?
Do not take Lamisil oral granules with applesauce or a fruit-based food.

Do not chew Lamisil oral granules.

Do not breastfeed while taking Lamisil.

What are possible food and drug interactions associated with this medication?
If Lamisil is taken with certain other drugs, the effects of either could be increased, decreased, or altered. It is especially important to check with your doctor before combining Lamisil with the following: blood pressure/heart medications known as beta-blockers (such as atenolol or propranolol), caffeine, certain antidepressants (such as desipramine, fluoxetine, imipramine, rasagiline, sertraline, selegiline, or tranylcypromine), certain medications used to treat arrhythmias (life-threatening irregular heartbeat) (such as amiodarone, flecainide, or propafenone), cimetidine, cyclosporine, fluconazole, rifampin, or warfarin.

What are the possible side effects of this medication?
Please see general statement regarding side effects on page xiii.

Side effects may include: abdominal pain, allergic reactions, change in taste or smell, cough, dark urine, depression, fever, headache, nausea, pale or light colored stools, poor appetite, rash, tiredness, vomiting, yellowing of your skin or whites of your eyes

Can I receive this medication if I am pregnant or breastfeeding?
The effects of Lamisil during pregnancy and breastfeeding are unknown. Do not take Lamisil while breastfeeding. Tell your doctor immediately if you are pregnant, plan to become pregnant, or are breastfeeding.

What should I do if I miss a dose of this medication?
If you miss a dose of Lamisil, take it as soon as you remember. However, if it is almost time for your next dose, skip the one you missed and return to your regular dosing schedule. Do not take two doses at once.

How should I store this medication?
Store at room temperature. Protect from light.

Lamotrigine: *see Lamictal, page 512*

Lamotrigine: *see Lamictal XR, page 515*

Lanoxin
Generic name: Digoxin

What is this medication?
Lanoxin is a medicine used to treat heart failure or atrial fibrillation (an irregular, fast heartbeat). Lanoxin is available in tablets and oral

solution, or it can be administered intravenously (through a vein in your arm).

What is the most important information I should know about this medication?

- Lanoxin can cause a different type of abnormal heartbeat, heart block, or other heart problems; which can be dangerous and life-threatening. Your doctor will monitor you while you take Lanoxin. Tell your doctor if you have had any other heart problems before you start this medication.

- Do not stop taking Lanoxin without first speaking to your doctor. If you suddenly stop taking Lanoxin, you can experience serious changes in your heart. Even if you feel better, keep taking this medication to help your heart work properly.

- You can experience serious side effects if you use Lanoxin and have low blood potassium or magnesium levels, high blood calcium levels, or other electrolyte (chemicals that are important for the cells in your body to function, such as sodium and potassium) abnormalities. Your doctor will perform regular blood tests to check your fluids and electrolytes. Tell your doctor if you are malnourished or experienced diarrhea or vomiting.

- Your doctor may schedule certain lab tests periodically while you use Lanoxin. These tests will help to monitor your condition or check for side effects. Do not miss your scheduled follow-up appointments with your doctor.

Who should not take this medication?

Do not take Lanoxin if you are allergic to it, any of its ingredients, or similar medications.

Do not take Lanoxin if you have a type of irregular heartbeat known as ventricular fibrillation.

What should I tell my doctor before I take the first dose of this medication?

Tell your doctor about all prescription, over-the-counter, and herbal medications you are taking before beginning treatment with Lanoxin. Also, talk to your doctor about your complete medical history, especially if you have calcium, potassium, or magnesium imbalances; any heart problems or a history of heart attack; kidney, liver, or lung problems; underactive or overactive thyroid gland; or are pregnant, plan to become pregnant, or are breastfeeding.

What is the usual dosage?
Please see general statement regarding dosage on page xii.

Adults: Your doctor will prescribe or administer the appropriate dose for you based on your weight and condition.

Children: Your doctor will prescribe the appropriate dose for your child, based on their weight.

If you are elderly or have kidney impairment, your doctor will adjust your dose appropriately.

How should I take this medication?
- Take Lanoxin exactly as prescribed by your doctor. Lanoxin is usually taken once a day. You can take Lanoxin on an empty stomach. You can take it with food if it upsets your stomach.
- If you are taking the Lanoxin solution, use the specially marked dropper that comes with it.
- Your doctor will administer Lanoxin injection to you.

What should I avoid while taking this medication?
Do not take Lanoxin with meals high in bran or fiber. Doing so can decrease the amount of absorbed Lanoxin.

Do not miss your scheduled follow-up appointments with your doctor.

What are possible food and drug interactions associated with this medication?
If Lanoxin is taken with certain other drugs, the effects of either could be increased, decreased, or altered. It is especially important to check with your doctor before combining Lanoxin with the following: albuterol; alprazolam; antacids; anticancer medications (such as cyclophosphamide); blood pressure/heart medications known as beta-blockers (such as atenolol or propranolol) or

calcium channel blockers (such as diltiazem, nifedipine, or vera-pamil); certain antibiotics (such as clarithromycin, erythromycin, neomycin, rifampin, or tetracycline); certain antifungals (such as amphotericin B, itraconazole, or ketoconazole); cholestyramine; cough, cold, and allergy medications; diphenoxylate; diuretics (water pills) (such as spironolactone); indomethacin; kaolin-pectin; medications used to treat irregular heartbeat (such as amiodarone, propafenone, or quinidine); metoclopramide; propantheline; suc-cinylcholine; sulfasalazine; or thyroid medications.

What are the possible side effects of this medication?
Please see general statement regarding side effects on page xiii.

> **Side effects may include:** confusion, diarrhea, dizziness, enlargement of breasts, headache, irregular heartbeat, lack of emotion, loss of appetite, mental disturbances (such as anxiety, depression, delirium, or hallucinations), nausea, rash, visual disturbances (blurred or yellow vision), vomiting, weakness

Can I receive this medication if I am pregnant or breastfeeding?
The effects of Lanoxin during pregnancy and breastfeeding are unknown. Lanoxin can be found in your breast milk if you take it while breastfeeding. Tell your doctor immediately if you are pregnant, plan to become pregnant, or are breastfeeding.

What should I do if I miss a dose of this medication?
If you miss a dose of Lanoxin, take it as soon as you remember. However, if it is almost time for your next dose, skip the one you missed and return to your regular dosing schedule. Do not take two doses at once. Lanoxin injection should be given under special circumstances determined by your doctor.

How should I store this medication?
Store at room temperature. Store in a dry place and protect from light.

Your doctor will store Lanoxin injection for you.

Lansoprazole: see Prevacid, page 823

Lantus

Generic name: Insulin Glargine, rDNA origin

What is this medication?

Lantus is a medicine that is a long-acting insulin. Lantus is used to control high blood sugar in people with diabetes. Lantus is available as a prefilled pen, vial, and a cartridge.

What is the most important information I should know about this medication?

- Do not change the type of insulin you use unless told to do so by your doctor. Your insulin dose and the time you take your dose can change with different types of insulin. Make sure you have the right type and strength of insulin prescribed for you.
- Do not make any changes to your insulin dose unless you have talked to your doctor. Your insulin needs may change because of illness, stress, other medicines, or changes in your diet or activity level.
- Lantus can cause you to experience low blood sugar. Therefore, it is important to use it as prescribed by your doctor. Symptoms of low blood sugar include: anxiety, restlessness, trouble concentrating, changes in your personality or mood, blurred vision, dizziness, shakiness, lightheadedness, drowsiness, nightmares or trouble sleeping, sweating, irritability, headache, slurred speech, fast heartbeat, unsteady walking, or tingling in your hands, feet, lips, or tongue. Always carry a quick source of sugar to treat low blood sugar (such as glucose tablets, hard candy, or juice).
- If you forget to take your dose of Lantus, your blood sugar may get too high. If your high blood sugar is not treated, it can lead to serious problems (such as passing out or loss of consciousness, coma, or even death). Follow your doctor's instructions for treating high blood sugar. Symptoms of high blood sugar include: confusion, increased thirst, frequent urination,

drowsiness, loss of appetite, difficulty breathing, fruity smelling breath, nausea, vomiting, or stomach ache.
• Lantus can cause serious and possibly life-threatening allergic reactions. Get medical help right away if you experience shortness of breath, wheezing, a fast heartbeat, sweating, low blood pressure, or develop a rash all over your body.

Who should not take this medication?
Do not use Lantus if you are allergic to it or any of its ingredients.

What should I tell my doctor before I take the first dose of this medication?
Tell your doctor about all prescription, over-the-counter, and herbal medications you are taking before beginning treatment with Lantus. Also, talk to your doctor about your complete medical history, especially if you have kidney or liver problems, or are pregnant, plan to become pregnant, or are breastfeeding.

What is the usual dosage?
Please see general statement regarding dosage on page xii.

Type 1 Diabetes
Adults and children ≥6 years: Your doctor will prescribe the appropriate dose for you.

Type 2 Diabetes
Adults: The recommended starting dose is 10 units once a day.

Your doctor will adjust your dose based on your blood sugar levels.

If you have liver or kidney impairment, your doctor will adjust your dose appropriately.

How should I take this medication?
• Inject Lantus exactly as prescribed by your doctor. Use the proper injection technique taught to you by your doctor. Read the User Manual that comes with your medicine for detailed instructions.

- Inject Lantus at any time during the day, but you must inject it at the same time every day. Inject it under the skin of your stomach area, upper arm, or upper leg. Never inject Lantus into a muscle or vein. Change your injection site with each dose.
- Only use Lantus that is clear and colorless.

What should I avoid while taking this medication?

Do not inject Lantus in the same place twice; rotate the injection sites.

Do not mix Lantus with any other insulin or solution.

Do not share Lantus with anyone else, even if they have diabetes. It may harm them.

What are possible food and drug interactions associated with this medication?

If Lantus is used with certain other drugs, the effects of either could be increased, decreased, or altered. Lantus may interact with numerous medications. Therefore, it is very important that you tell your doctor about any other medications you are taking.

What are the possible side effects of this medication?

Please see general statement regarding side effects on page xiii.

Side effects may include: allergic reactions, eye problems, injection-site reactions, itching, low blood sugar, rash, skin thickening or pitting at the injection site, swelling of your hands and feet, upper respiratory tract infection, weight gain

---

Can I receive this medication if I am pregnant or breastfeeding?

The effects of Lantus during pregnancy and breastfeeding are unknown. Tell your doctor immediately if you are pregnant, plan to become pregnant, or are breastfeeding.

What should I do if I miss a dose of this medication?
It is very important to follow your insulin regimen exactly as prescribed by your doctor. Do not miss any doses. Ask your doctor for specific instructions to follow in case you ever miss a dose of insulin.

How should I store this medication?
Store unopened Lantus vials in the refrigerator (not the freezer). Protect from extreme heat, cold, or light.

After you open Lantus vials, store them in the refrigerator or at room temperature for 28 days. After you start Lantus cartridges or prefilled pens, do not refrigerate them. Keep them at room temperature, away from direct heat and light for up to 28 days.

Lasix
Generic name: Furosemide

What is this medication?
Lasix is a diuretic (water pill) used alone or in combination with other medications to treat high blood pressure. Lasix is also used to treat edema (swelling) associated with heart, liver, or kidney disease.

What is the most important information I should know about this medication?
- Lasix can cause ringing in your ears, other hearing problems, or deafness. Your risk is higher if you have severe kidney disease, hyperproteinemia (high blood protein levels), take a higher dose than prescribed by your doctor, or if you take Lasix with certain medications. Tell your doctor if you experience any changes in your hearing while you are taking Lasix.
- Your doctor will perform regular blood tests to check your fluids and electrolytes (chemicals that are important for the cells in your body to function, such as sodium and potassium). Tell your doctor if you experience dry mouth, thirst, weakness, fatigue, drowsiness, restlessness, muscle pains or cramps, low blood pressure, decreased urination, fast or irregular heartbeat,

nausea, or vomiting. If you experience a sudden drop in your blood pressure, get up slowly.

- Lasix can cause an increase in your blood sugar levels or diabetes. If you have diabetes or are at risk for diabetes, monitor your blood sugar regularly, as determined by your doctor.
- Lasix can cause gout (severe and painful inflammation of the joints).

Who should not take this medication?

Do not take Lasix if you are allergic to it or any of its ingredients.

Do not take Lasix if you are unable to produce urine.

What should I tell my doctor before I take the first dose of this medication?

Tell your doctor about all prescription, over-the-counter, and herbal medications you are taking before beginning treatment with Lasix. Also, talk to your doctor about your complete medical history, especially if you have diabetes, gout, problems emptying your bladder, an enlarged prostate, narrowing of the urethra (the tube that connects from the bladder to the genitals to lead urine out of your body), or if you have systemic lupus erythematosus (disease that affects the immune system).

What is the usual dosage?

Please see general statement regarding dosage on page xii.

High Blood Pressure
Adults: The usual starting dose is 40 milligrams (mg) twice a day.

Edema
Adults: The usual starting dose is 20-80 mg once a day.

Children: Your doctor will prescribe the appropriate dose for your child, based on their weight.

Your doctor will increase your dose as needed, until the desired effect is achieved.

If you are elderly, your doctor will adjust your dose appropriately.

How should I take this medication?
• Take Lasix exactly as prescribed by your doctor.

What should I avoid while taking this medication?
Do not expose yourself to excessive amounts of sunlight while you are taking Lasix, as the medicine can increase your sensitivity to sunlight.

If you have high blood pressure, do not take any medicines that can increase your blood pressure (such as over-the-counter appetite suppressants or cold medicines).

What are possible food and drug interactions associated with this medication?
If Lasix is taken with certain other drugs, the effects of either could be increased, decreased, or altered. It is especially important to check with your doctor before combining Lasix with the following: alcohol, aspirin, barbiturates (such as phenobarbital), blood pressure/heart medications known as angiotensin-converting enzyme (ACE) inhibitors (such as captopril or lisinopril) or angiotensin receptor blockers (ARBs) (such as losartan or valsartan), certain antibiotics (such as cephalexin or tobramycin), chloral hydrate, cisplatin, corticosteroids (such as prednisone), cyclosporine, ethacrynic acid, laxatives (long-term use), licorice (large amounts), lithium, methotrexate, narcotic painkillers (such as hydrocodone or oxycodone), nonsteroidal anti-inflammatory drugs (NSAIDs) (such as ibuprofen or indomethacin), norepinephrine, phenytoin, succinylcholine, sucralfate, or tubocurarine.

What are the possible side effects of this medication?
Please see general statement regarding side effects on page xiii.

Side effects may include: allergic reactions; anemia; increased cholesterol, triglyceride, or blood sugar levels; liver problems; low blood platelet counts; pancreatitis (inflammation of the pancreas); skin reactions; sudden fall in your blood pressure; ringing in your ears or hearing loss; skin tingling and numbness

Can I receive this medication if I am pregnant or breastfeeding?

The effects of Lasix during pregnancy are unknown. Lasix can be found in your breast milk if you take it while breastfeeding. Tell your doctor immediately if you are pregnant, plan to become pregnant, or are breastfeeding.

What should I do if I miss a dose of this medication?

If you miss a dose of Lasix, take it as soon as you remember. However, if it is almost time for your next dose, skip the one you missed and return to your regular dosing schedule. Do not take two doses at once.

How should I store this medication?

Store at room temperature.

Latanoprost: *see Xalatan, page 1098*

Lazanda

Generic name: Fentanyl

What is this medication?

Lazanda is a medicine used to treat breakthrough pain in adults with cancer who are already routinely taking other opioid pain medicines around-the-clock for their constant cancer pain. Lazanda is started only after you have been taking another opioid pain medicine and your body is used to it (opioid-tolerant). Lazanda is a federally controlled substance because it has abuse potential. Lazanda is available as a nasal spray.

What is the most important information I should know about this medication?

- Do not use Lazanda if you are not opioid-tolerant.
- Lazanda can cause life-threatening breathing problems if you are not opioid-tolerant, if you do not use Lazanda exactly as prescribed by your doctor, or if a child takes Lazanda by accident.

- Keep Lazanda in a safe place away from children. Accidental use by a child is a medical emergency. Get emergency help immediately.
- Lazanda is available only through a restricted distribution program called the TIRF REMS Access Program.
- Call your doctor or get emergency medical help immediately if you have breathing problems, drowsiness, faintness, dizziness, confusion, or any other unusual symptoms after taking Lazanda. These can be signs of an overdose. Your dose of Lazanda may be too high for you. These symptoms may lead to serious problems if not treated right away. Do not take another dose of Lazanda.
- If you stop taking your around-the-clock pain medicine for your constant cancer pain, you must stop using Lazanda. You may no longer be opioid-tolerant. Talk to your doctor about how to treat your pain.

Who should not take this medication?

Do not use Lazanda if you are allergic to it or any of its ingredients.

Do not use Lazanda if you are not already taking another opioid pain medicine around-the-clock for your constant cancer pain.

Do not use Lazanda if you only have pain for a short time or if your pain is from surgery, headache or migraine, or dental work.

What should I tell my doctor before I take the first dose of this medication?

Tell your doctor about all prescription, over-the-counter, and herbal medications you are taking before beginning treatment with Lazanda. Also, talk to your doctor about your complete medical history, especially if you have trouble breathing or lung problems (such as asthma, wheezing, or shortness of breath), liver or kidney problems, seizures, a slow heart rate or other heart problems, low blood pressure, mental health problems, past or present alcohol or drug abuse or a family history of alcohol or drug abuse, or you have or had a head injury or brain problem.

What is the usual dosage?

Please see general statement regarding dosage on page xii.

Adults: The starting dose is one 100-micrograms spray into one nostril.

Your doctor will prescribe the appropriate dose for you and will increase your dose as needed, until the desired effect is achieved.

How should I take this medication?
- Use Lazanda exactly as prescribed by your doctor. Do not use Lazanda more often than prescribed by your doctor.
- Use only one dose of Lazanda for each episode of breakthrough cancer pain. As your dose is adjusted, your doctor will tell you whether your dose of Lazanda is one spray or two sprays. Separate doses by at least 2 hours.
- Do not use Lazanda for more than four episodes of breakthrough cancer pain in 1 day. If you have more than four episodes each day, talk to your doctor. The dose of the opioid pain medicine for your constant pain may need to be changed. Also, if the dose of Lazanda does not relieve your breakthrough cancer pain, talk to your doctor. The dose of Lazanda may need to be changed.
- Please review the instructions that came with your prescription on how to properly use Lazanda.

What should I avoid while taking this medication?
Do not drive, operate machinery, or do other dangerous activities until you know how Lazanda affects you. Lazanda can make you sleepy. Ask your doctor when it is ok to do these activities.

Do not drink alcohol or grapefruit juice while you are using Lazanda. It can increase your chance of having dangerous side effects.

Do not change your dose of Lazanda yourself. Your doctor will change the dose until you and your doctor find the right dose for you.

Do not share Lazanda with anyone else, even if they have the same symptoms you have. It can harm them.

What are possible food and drug interactions associated with this medication?

If Lazanda is used with certain other drugs, the effects of either could be increased, decreased, or altered. Lazanda may interact with numerous medications. Therefore, it is very important that you tell your doctor about any other medications you are taking.

What are the possible side effects of this medication?

Please see general statement regarding side effects on page xiii.

> **Side effects may include:** constipation, dizziness, fever, nausea, vomiting

Can I receive this medication if I am pregnant or breastfeeding?

The effects of Lazanda during pregnancy are unknown. Lazanda can be found in your breast milk if you use it while breastfeeding. Tell your doctor immediately if you are pregnant, plan to become pregnant, or are breastfeeding.

What should I do if I miss a dose of this medication?

Lazanda should be used under special circumstances determined by your doctor (or given only as needed). You should use Lazanda only when you experience breakthrough cancer pain.

How should I store this medication?

Store at room temperature. Do not freeze. Protect from light.

To dispose of Lazanda and its bottle when no longer needed, empty all the remaining medicine into the pouch, seal the pouch, and put the sealed pouch into the child-resistant container with the empty bottle. Throw the child-resistant container with the empty bottle and sealed pouch inside it into the trash.

Levalbuterol Tartrate: *see Xopenex HFA, page 1108*

Levaquin

Generic name: Levofloxacin

What is this medication?

Levaquin is an antibiotic used to treat certain bacterial infections of the urinary tract, skin, sinuses, kidneys, and prostate. Levaquin may also be used to treat sudden worsening of chronic bronchitis, inhalation anthrax, plague, and certain types of pneumonia. Levaquin is available as tablets and an oral solution.

What is the most important information I should know about this medication?

- Levaquin can cause tendon rupture or swelling. Your risk can increase if you are over 60 years; are taking steroids; have had a kidney, heart, or lung transplant; engage in physical activity or exercise; have kidney failure; or have past tendon problems (such as rheumatoid arthritis). Tell your doctor immediately if you experience pain, swelling, tears, or inflammation of tendons in the back of your ankle, shoulder, hand, or other tendon sites. Also, tell your doctor immediately if you hear or feel a snap or pop in a tendon area, bruise right after an injury in a tendon area, or are unable to move the affected area or bear weight.

- Levaquin can cause worsening of myasthenia gravis (a disease characterized by long-lasting fatigue and muscle weakness). Tell your doctor immediately if you develop muscle weakness or trouble breathing.

- Levaquin can cause serious allergic reactions that may be life-threatening. Stop taking Levaquin and tell your doctor right away if you experience hives, trouble breathing or swallowing, throat tightness, hoarseness, rapid heartbeat, fainting, skin rash, or swelling of your lips, tongue, or face.

- Levaquin can cause liver damage. Call your doctor right away if you develop unexplained nausea or vomiting, stomach pain, fever, weakness, abdominal pain or tenderness, itching, unusual tiredness, loss of appetite, light color bowel movements, dark colored urine, or yellowing of your skin or whites of your eyes.

- Levaquin can cause central nervous system (CNS) effects. Tell your doctor right away if you experience seizures, hallucinations, restlessness, shaking, anxiousness or nervousness, confusion, depression, trouble sleeping, nightmares, lightheadedness, suspiciousness, headaches that will not go away, or suicidal thoughts or actions.

- Diarrhea is a common problem when taking antibiotics; it usually ends when the antibiotic is stopped. Sometimes after starting treatment with antibiotics, people may develop watery and bloody stools (with or without stomach cramps and fever) even as late as two or more months after having taken the last dose of the antibiotic. Contact your doctor right away if this occurs.

- Levaquin can cause damage to the nerves in your arms, hands, legs, or feet. Tell your doctor right away if you develop pain, burning, tingling, numbness, or weakness in any of these areas of your body.

- Levaquin can cause serious heart rhythm changes. Your risk of this happening is higher if you are elderly, have low blood potassium levels, take certain medicines to control your heart rhythm, or have a family history of prolonged QT interval (very fast or abnormal heartbeats). Tell your doctor right away if you develop a fast or irregular heartbeat, or if you feel faint.

- Levaquin can increase the risk of problems with joints or tissue around joints in children. Tell your child's doctor if your child has any joint problems during or after treatment with Levaquin.

- Levaquin can cause changes in blood sugar if you take it in combination with diabetes medicines. If you have diabetes, check your blood sugar regularly and tell your doctor right away if you have low blood sugar while you are taking Levaquin.

- Take Levaquin as prescribed by your doctor for the full course of treatment, even if your symptoms improve earlier. Do not skip doses. Skipping doses or not completing the full course of Levaquin can decrease its effectiveness and can lead to the growth of bacteria that are resistant to the effects of Levaquin.

Who should not take this medication?
Do not take Levaquin if you are allergic to it, any of its ingredients, or similar antibiotics.

Do not take Levaquin to treat viral infections, such as the common cold.

What should I tell my doctor before I take the first dose of this medication?

Tell your doctor about all prescription, over-the-counter, and herbal medications you are taking before beginning treatment with Levaquin. Also, talk to your doctor about your complete medical history, especially if you have tendon, nerve, bone, kidney, or liver problems; myasthenia gravis; CNS problems (such as seizures); rheumatoid arthritis or a history of joint problems; low blood potassium levels; diabetes or problems with low blood sugar; or if you or anyone in your family has an irregular heartbeat, especially QT prolongation.

What is the usual dosage?

Please see general statement regarding dosage on page xii.

Adults: The usual dose is 250 milligrams (mg), 500 mg, or 750 mg once a day. Your doctor will prescribe the appropriate dose for you based on the type and severity of your infection.

Children: Your doctor will prescribe the appropriate dose for your child, based on their weight.

If you have kidney impairment, your doctor will adjust your dose appropriately.

How should I take this medication?

- Take Levaquin exactly as prescribed by your doctor. Take Levaquin at about the same time each day. Take it with or without food.
- Drink plenty of fluids while you are taking Levaquin.
- Take antacids containing magnesium or aluminum, sucralfate, didanosine, multivitamins that contain zinc, or other products that contain iron at least two hours before or two hours after you take Levaquin.
- Take Levaquin oral solution 1 hour before or 2 hours after eating.

What should I avoid while taking this medication?

Do not drive, operate machinery, or engage in other activities that require mental alertness or coordination until you know how Levaquin affects you.

Do not expose yourself to sunlamps or tanning beds, and try to limit your time in the sun, as Levaquin can increase your sensitivity to light. If you need to be outdoors, wear sunscreen and loose-fitting clothes that protect your skin for the sun.

Do not skip any doses, or stop taking Levaquin even if you begin to feel better, until you finish your prescribed treatment.

What are possible food and drug interactions associated with this medication?

If Levaquin is taken with certain other drugs, the effects of either could be increased, decreased, or altered. It is especially important to check with your doctor before combining Levaquin with the following: diabetes medicines, nonsteroidal anti-inflammatory drugs (NSAIDs) (such as ibuprofen or naproxen), theophylline, or warfarin.

What are the possible side effects of this medication?

Please see general statement regarding side effects on page xiii.

> **Side effects may include:** constipation, diarrhea, dizziness, headache, nausea, trouble sleeping

Can I receive this medication if I am pregnant or breastfeeding?

The effects of Levaquin during pregnancy and breastfeeding are unknown. Do not breastfeed while you are taking Levaquin. Tell your doctor immediately if you are pregnant, plan to become pregnant, or are breastfeeding.

What should I do if I miss a dose of this medication?

If you miss a dose of Levaquin, take it as soon as you remember. However, if it is almost time for your next dose, skip the one you

missed and return to your regular dosing schedule. Do not take two doses at once.

How should I store this medication?
Store at room temperature.

Levemir
Generic name: Insulin Detemir, rDNA origin

What is this medication?
Levemir is a long-acting insulin used to treat adults or children with type 1 diabetes. It is also used in adults with type 2 diabetes who require long-acting insulin to control their high blood sugar levels. Levemir is administered subcutaneously (just below the skin).

What is the most important information I should know about this medication?
- Do not make any changes to your insulin dose unless you have talked to your doctor. Your insulin needs may change because of illness, stress, other medicines, or changes in your diet or activity level.
- If you forget to take your dose of Levemir, your blood sugar may go too high. If high blood sugar is not treated it can lead to serious problems, such as passing out, coma, or even death.
- Tell your doctor if you experience symptoms of high blood sugar such as increased thirst, frequent urination, drowsiness, loss of appetite, difficulty breathing, and fruity smelling breath.
- Levemir can cause low blood sugar, loss or redistribution of your fat, weight gain, or allergic reactions.
- Talk to your doctor about what your blood sugar should be and when you should check your blood sugar levels.
- Do not use Levemir with an insulin infusion pump. Do not dilute or mix Levemir with any other insulin or solution.
- Be careful when you drive a car or operate machinery until you know how you respond to Levemir. Your ability to concentrate or react may be reduced if you have low blood sugar.

- If you use too much Levemir, your blood sugar may fall low. You can treat mild low blood sugar by drinking or eating something sugary immediately (such as fruit juice, sugar candies, or glucose tablets). It is important to treat low blood sugar right away because it could get worse and you could pass out (lose consciousness).
- Your doctor may perform tests, including fasting blood glucose levels or A1C, while you use Levemir. Be sure to keep all doctor and lab appointments.

Who should not take this medication?

Do not use Levemir if you are allergic to it or any of its ingredients.

What should I tell my doctor before I take the first dose of this medication?

Tell your doctor about all prescription, over-the-counter, and herbal medications you are taking before beginning treatment with Levemir. Also, talk to your doctor about your complete medical history, especially if you have thyroid, adrenal gland, or pituitary problems; are fasting; have high blood sodium levels; are on a low-salt diet; or have kidney or liver disease.

What is the usual dosage?

Please see general statement regarding dosage on page xii.

Type 1 Diabetes
Adults and children ≥2 years: Your doctor will prescribe the appropriate dose for you or your child.

Type 2 Diabetes
Adults: The recommended starting dose is 10 units (U) once a day or divided doses twice a day.

Your doctor will prescribe the appropriate dose for you based on your weight and your previous insulin medication.

If you have kidney or liver impairment, your doctor will adjust your dose appropriately.

How should I take this medication?

- Use Levemir exactly as prescribed by your doctor. Do not inject extra doses or use more often without asking your doctor.
- Inspect Levemir visually prior to administration and only use it if the solution appears clear, odorless, and colorless.
- Use the proper injection technique taught to you by your doctor. Refer to the package insert that accompanies Levemir for detailed instructions.
- Inject Levemir subcutaneously, and not into a vein or muscle.
- Rotate the injection areas (abdomen, thigh, or upper arm) from one injection to the next. Check with your doctor if you notice a depression in your skin or skin thickening at the injection site. You may need to change your injection technique.
- Use a new needle for each injection. After each injection, remove the needle without recapping and dispose of it in a puncture-resistant container.

What should I avoid while taking this medication?

Do not inject Levemir in the same place twice. Rotate your injection sites.

Do not mix Levemir with any other insulin.

Do not miss a Levemir dose.

Do not share needles, insulin pens, or syringes with others.

Do not drink alcohol. Alcohol may affect your blood sugar when you use Levemir.

What are possible food and drug interactions associated with this medication?

If Levemir is used with certain other drugs, the effects of either could be increased, decreased, or altered. It is especially important to check with your doctor before combining Levemir with the following: albuterol, antidepressants known as MAO inhibitors (phenelzine, selegiline, or tranylcypromine), antidiabetes medications, birth control pills, blood pressure medications known as ACE inhibitors and beta-blockers, certain cholesterol medications (fibrates), clonidine, corticosteroids, danazol, disopyramide, diuretics (water pills), epinephrine, estrogens, fluoxetine, guanethidine, isoniazid, octreotide, propoxyphene, reserpine, salicylates, somatropin, sulfonamide antibiotics, terbutaline, or thyroid hormones.

What are the possible side effects of this medication?
Please see general statement regarding side effects on page xiii.

> **Side effects may include:** allergic reactions, injection-site reactions, low blood sugar, rash, weight gain
>
> *Signs of low blood sugar:* blurred vision, dizziness, fast heartbeat, headache, hunger, shakiness, sweating, trouble concentrating. If these symptoms occur, tell your doctor immediately.

Can I receive this medication if I am pregnant or breastfeeding?
The effects of Levemir during pregnancy and breastfeeding are unknown. Tell your doctor immediately if you are pregnant, plan to become pregnant, or are breastfeeding.

What should I do if I miss a dose of this medication?
It is very important to follow your insulin regimen exactly. Do not miss any doses. Ask your doctor for specific instructions to follow in case you ever miss a dose of insulin.

How should I store this medication?
Store in the refrigerator. Do not freeze.

Levetiracetam: *see Keppra, page 502*

Levitra

Generic name: Vardenafil HCl

What is this medication?

Levitra is a medicine used to treat erectile dysfunction in men. It can help men get and keep an erection when they become sexually excited.

What is the most important information I should know about this medication?

- Levitra can help you get an erection only when you are sexually excited. You will not get an erection just by taking this medicine.
- Levitra does not cure erectile dysfunction. It is a treatment for erectile dysfunction.
- Levitra does not protect you or your partner from getting any sexually transmitted diseases.
- Sexual activity can put a strain on your heart, especially if it is already weak from a heart disease. Refrain from further activity and talk to your doctor if you experience chest pain, dizziness, or nausea during sex.
- Levitra can cause a sudden decrease or loss of vision or hearing. Loss of vision can occur in one or both eyes. Loss of hearing can occur with ringing in your ears and dizziness. If you experience these symptoms, stop taking Levitra and call your doctor right away.
- Levitra can cause an erection that lasts many hours. Call your doctor immediately if you ever have an erection that lasts more than 4 hours. If this is not treated right away, permanent damage to your penis can occur.

Who should not take this medication?

Do not take Levitra if you are allergic to it, any of its ingredients, or if you are receiving dialysis.

Do not take Levitra if you take any medicines that contain nitrates (such as nitroglycerin, isosorbide mononitrate, or isosorbide dinitrate). If you take Levitra with these medicines, your blood pressure could suddenly drop to an unsafe or life-threatening level.

Do not take Levitra if your doctor told you not to engage in sexual activity due to a heart disease or other heart problems.

What should I tell my doctor before I take the first dose of this medication?

Tell your doctor about all prescription, over-the-counter, and herbal medications you are taking before beginning treatment with Levitra. Also, talk to your doctor about your complete medical history, especially if you have or ever had any heart problems (such as chest pain, heart failure, irregular heartbeats, long QT syndrome, or heart attack); stroke; low or high blood pressure; bleeding problems; seizure(s); hearing problems; severe vision loss or retinitis pigmentosa (eye disease that involves damage to the layer of tissue in the back of the eye, called the retina); kidney, liver, or blood problems (such as sickle cell anemia or leukemia); any deformation of your penis; an erection that lasted more than 4 hours; or stomach ulcers.

What is the usual dosage?

Please see general statement regarding dosage on page xii.

Adults: The recommended starting dose is 10 milligrams as needed about 1 hour before you plan to have sex. Your doctor will increase or decrease your dose as needed.

If you are older than 65 years or have liver impairment, your doctor will adjust your dose appropriately.

How should I take this medication?
- Take Levitra exactly as prescribed by your doctor. Take it with or without food.
- Do not take Levitra more than once a day.

What should I avoid while taking this medication?

Do not change your dose of Levitra without talking to your doctor.

Do not use other medicines or treatments for erectile dysfunction while you are taking Levitra.

What are possible food and drug interactions associated with this medication?

If Levitra is taken with certain other drugs, the effects of either could be increased, decreased, or altered. It is especially important to check with your doctor before combining Levitra with the following: alcohol, anti-HIV medications called protease inhibitors (such as atazanavir, indinavir, ritonavir or saquinavir), clarithromycin, erythromycin, grapefruit juice, itraconazole, ketoconazole, medications called alpha-blockers (such as tamsulosin or terazosin) used to treat high blood pressure, medicines that treat abnormal heartbeat (such as amiodarone, procainamide, quinidine, or sotalol), or nitrates.

What are the possible side effects of this medication?

Please see general statement regarding side effects on page xiii.

> **Side effects may include:** back pain, dizziness, flushing of your face, headache, stuffy or runny nose, upset stomach

Can I receive this medication if I am pregnant or breastfeeding?

Levitra is not for use in women.

What should I do if I miss a dose of this medication?

Levitra is not for regular use. Take it only before sexual activity.

How should I store this medication?

Store at room temperature.

Levocetirizine Dihydrochloride: see Xyzal, page 1111

Levofloxacin: see Levaquin, page 535

Levothyroxine Sodium: see Levoxyl, page 546

Levothyroxine Sodium: see Synthroid, page 958

Levoxyl

Generic name: Levothyroxine Sodium

What is this medication?

Levoxyl is a medicine used to treat hypothyroidism (an underactive thyroid gland). Levoxyl is a synthetic hormone that is intended to replace a hormone that is normally produced by your thyroid gland. It is also used to treat or prevent certain other thyroid conditions such as goiter (an enlarged thyroid gland); inflammation of the thyroid gland; thyroid hormone deficiency due to surgery, radiation, or certain medications; or for the management of certain thyroid cancers.

What is the most important information I should know about this medication?

- Do not use Levoxyl to treat obesity or weight loss.
- Levoxyl is a replacement therapy, so you need to take it every day for life unless your condition is temporary. You will notice improvement in your symptoms several weeks after you start Levoxyl. Continue taking your medication as directed by your doctor. Tell your doctor right away if you experience rapid or irregular heartbeats, chest pain, shortness of breath, leg cramps, headache, nervousness, irritability, sleeplessness, or tremors. Also, tell your doctor if you experience changes in your appetite, weight gain or loss, vomiting, diarrhea, excessive sweating, heat intolerance, fever, changes in your menstrual periods, hives, or skin rash.
- Long-term Levoxyl use can weaken bones, especially in women after menopause.
- If you have a heart disease, your doctor may need to start you on a lower dose of Levoxyl to see how you respond to this medication.
- Also, if you have diabetes, your doctor will determine if the dose of your diabetes medication needs to be adjusted. Your doctor will monitor your blood sugar levels.
- If you are taking an oral blood thinner (such as warfarin), your doctor will monitor your blood clotting status to determine if the dose of your blood thinner needs to be adjusted.

- Tell your doctor or dentist that you are taking Levoxyl before having any surgery.
- Levoxyl can cause partial hair loss during the first few months of treatment. This is usually temporary.

Who should not take this medication?

Do not take Levoxyl if you are allergic to it or any of its ingredients.

Do not take Levoxyl if you have an overactive thyroid gland, reduced adrenal function, or had a recent heart attack.

What should I tell my doctor before I take the first dose of this medication?

Tell your doctor about all prescription, over-the-counter, and herbal medications you are taking before beginning treatment with Levoxyl. Also, talk to your doctor about your complete medical history, especially if you have anemia, diabetes, heart disease, blood clotting disorders, or problems with your pituitary or adrenal glands, or if you are pregnant, plan to become pregnant, or are breastfeeding.

What is the usual dosage?

Please see general statement regarding dosage on page xii.

Adults and children: Your doctor will prescribe the appropriate dose for you based on your age, weight, and condition.

How should I take this medication?

- Take Levoxyl exactly as prescribed by your doctor. Take it in the morning on an empty stomach, at least 30 minutes before eating any food. Take Levoxyl with a full glass of water.
- Certain foods and supplements can decrease the amount of Levoxyl in your body. Do not take Levoxyl within 4 hours of taking antacids and iron or calcium supplements.
- If an infant or child cannot swallow whole tablets, crush the tablet and mix it into 1-2 teaspoonfuls of water. Have the child drink the mixture right away. Do not store it for later use. Soybean infant formula can decrease the amount of Levoxyl in your baby's

body and should not be used for administering the crushed tablets.

What should I avoid while taking this medication?

Do not stop taking Levoxyl or change the amount or how often you take it without talking to your doctor.

What are possible food and drug interactions associated with this medication?

If Levoxyl is taken with certain other drugs, the effects of either could be increased, decreased, or altered. Levoxyl may interact with numerous medications. Therefore, it is very important that you tell your doctor about any other medications you are taking.

What are the possible side effects of this medication?

Please see general statement regarding side effects on page xiii.

> **Side effects may include:** change in your appetite or menstrual periods, chest pain, diarrhea, excessive sweating, fever, headache, heat intolerance, hives, irritability, leg cramps, nervousness, rapid or irregular heartbeats, shortness of breath, skin rash, sleeplessness, tremors, vomiting, weight gain or loss

Can I receive this medication if I am pregnant or breastfeeding?

You can continue to take Levoxyl during pregnancy. However, a dose adjustment may be necessary. Small amounts of thyroid hormone are excreted in your breast milk. Tell your doctor immediately if you are pregnant, plan to become pregnant, or are breastfeeding.

What should I do if I miss a dose of this medication?

If you miss a dose of Levoxyl, take it as soon as you remember. However, if it is almost time for your next dose, skip the one you missed and return to your regular dosing schedule. Do not take two doses at once.

How should I store this medication?

Store at room temperature, away from heat, light, and moisture.

Lexapro

Generic name: Escitalopram Oxalate

What is this medication?

Lexapro is an antidepressant medicine known as a selective serotonin reuptake inhibitor (SSRI). It is used to treat major depressive
disorder and generalized anxiety disorder. Lexapro is available in
tablets and an oral solution.

What is the most important information I should know about this medication?

- Lexapro can increase the risk of suicidal thoughts and behavior in children, adolescents, and young adults. Your doctor will
  monitor you closely for clinical worsening, suicidal or unusual
  behavior after you start taking Lexapro or start a new dose of
  Lexapro.
- Tell your doctor right away if you experience anxiety, hostility,
  sleeplessness, restlessness, impulsive or dangerous behavior,
  or thoughts about suicide or dying; or if you have new symptoms or seem to be feeling worse.
- Lexapro can cause serotonin syndrome (a potentially
  life-threatening drug reaction that causes the body to have too
  much serotonin, a chemical produced by the nerve cells) or neuroleptic malignant syndrome (a brain disorder) when you take it
  alone or in combination with other medicines. You can experience mental status changes, an increase in your heart rate and
  temperature, lack of coordination, overactive reflexes, muscle rigidity, nausea, vomiting, or diarrhea. Tell your doctor right away
  if you experience any of these signs or symptoms.
- Lexapro can cause severe allergic reactions. Tell your doctor
  right away if you develop a rash, trouble breathing, or swelling
  of your face, tongue, eyes, or mouth.
- Your risk of abnormal bleeding or bruising can increase if you
  take Lexapro, especially if you also take blood thinners (such as
  warfarin), nonsteroidal anti-inflammatory drugs (NSAIDs) (such
  as ibuprofen or naproxen), or aspirin.
- You can experience manic episodes while you are taking
  Lexapro. Tell your doctor if you experience greatly increased
  energy, severe trouble sleeping, racing thoughts, reckless

behavior, unusually grand ideas, excessive happiness or irritability, or talking more or faster than usual.
- Lexapro can cause seizures or changes in your appetite or weight. Your doctor will monitor you for these effects during treatment.
- Lexapro can decrease your blood sodium levels, especially if you are elderly. Tell your doctor if you have a headache, weakness, an unsteady feeling, confusion, problems concentrating or thinking, or memory problems while you are taking Lexapro.
- Do not stop taking Lexapro without first talking to your doctor. Stopping Lexapro suddenly can cause serious symptoms, including anxiety, irritability, changes in your mood, feeling restless, changes in your sleep habits, headache, sweating, nausea, dizziness, electric shock-like sensations, shaking, or confusion.

Who should not take this medication?
Do not take Lexapro if you are allergic to it or any of its ingredients.

Do not take Lexapro while you are taking other medicines known as monoamine oxidase inhibitors (MAOIs) (such as phenelzine), a class of medications used to treat depression and other conditions.

Do not take Lexapro if you are taking pimozide.

Do not take Lexapro if you are taking a medication called Celexa, since both medicines contain the same active ingredient.

What should I tell my doctor before I take the first dose of this medication?
Tell your doctor about all prescription, over-the-counter, and herbal medications you are taking before beginning treatment with Lexapro. Also, talk to your doctor about your complete medical history, especially if you have high blood pressure; heart, liver, or kidney problems; history of stroke; bleeding problems; seizures; mania or bipolar disorder; or low sodium levels in your blood. Also, tell your doctor if you are pregnant, plan to become pregnant, or are breastfeeding.

What is the usual dosage?
Please see general statement regarding dosage on page xii.

Major Depressive Disorder
Adults and adolescents 12-17 years: The recommended starting dose is 10 milligrams (mg) once a day.

Generalized Anxiety Disorder
Adults: The recommended starting dose is 10 mg once a day.

Your doctor will increase your dose as needed until the desired effect is achieved.

If you are elderly or have liver impairment, your doctor will adjust your dose appropriately.

How should I take this medication?
- Take Lexapro exactly as prescribed by your doctor. Take Lexapro once a day, in the morning or in the evening.
- Take Lexapro with or without food.

What should I avoid while taking this medication?
Do not drive, operate heavy machinery, or engage in other dangerous activities until you know how Lexapro affects you.

Do not drink alcohol while you are taking Lexapro.

Do not stop taking Lexapro suddenly without first talking to your doctor, as this can cause serious side effects.

Do not take Lexapro and MAOIs together or within 14 days of each other. Combining these medicines with Lexapro can cause serious and even life-threatening reactions.

What are possible food and drug interactions associated with this medication?
If Lexapro is taken with certain other drugs, the effects of either could be increased, decreased, or altered. Lexapro may interact

with numerous medications. Therefore, it is very important that you tell your doctor about any other medications you are taking.

What are the possible side effects of this medication?
Please see general statement regarding side effects on page xiii.

Side effects may include: constipation, dizziness, dry mouth, feeling anxious, infections, loss of appetite, nausea, sexual problems, shaking, sleepiness, sweating, trouble sleeping, weakness, yawning

Can I receive this medication if I am pregnant or breastfeeding?
The effects of Lexapro during pregnancy are unknown. Lexapro can be found in your breast milk if you take it while breastfeeding. Tell your doctor immediately if you are pregnant, plan to become pregnant, or are breastfeeding.

What should I do if I miss a dose of this medication?
If you miss a dose of Lexapro, take it as soon as you remember. However, if it is almost time for your next dose, skip the one you missed and return to your regular dosing schedule. Do not take two doses at once.

How should I store this medication?
Store at room temperature.

Lidocaine: *see Lidoderm, page 553*

Lidoderm
Generic name: Lidocaine

What is this medication?
Lidoderm is a topical patch (applied to the skin surface) used to relieve local nerve pain following an episode of shingles (painful rash caused by chickenpox virus).

What is the most important information I should know about this medication?
- Lidoderm is for external use only, on intact skin. Do not apply Lidoderm to broken or inflamed skin or your eyes. If eye contact occurs, immediately wash out your eye with water or saline and protect your eye until sensation returns.
- After you use a Lidoderm patch, it still contains a large amount of lidocaine. A small child or pet can suffer serious adverse effects from chewing or ingesting a new or used Lidoderm patch. Store and dispose of Lidoderm patches out of reach of children, pets, and others.
- If you apply Lidoderm to larger areas, apply more patches, or apply for longer periods than prescribed by your doctor, you may absorb larger amounts of lidocaine and experience serious side effects. Tell your doctor if you develop blurred or double vision, breathing or lung problems, confusion, dizziness, drowsiness, lightheadedness, nervousness, numbness, seizures, sensations of heat, twitching, unconsciousness, or vomiting.

Who should not take this medication?
Do not use Lidoderm if you are allergic to it, any of its ingredients, or similar medications.

What should I tell my doctor before I take the first dose of this medication?
Tell your doctor about all prescription, over-the-counter, and herbal medications you are taking before beginning treatment with Lidoderm. Also, talk to your doctor about your complete medical history, especially if you have liver disease, irregular heart beat, are pregnant, plan to become pregnant, or are breastfeeding.

What is the usual dosage?
Please see general statement regarding dosage on page xii.

Adults: Apply up to three patches to cover the most painful area. Use only once for up to 12 hours within a 24-hour period.

How should I take this medication?
- Apply Lidoderm exactly as prescribed by your doctor. You can cut Lidoderm patches into smaller sizes with scissors before you remove the release liner.
- Apply Lidoderm right after removal from the protective envelope. Wash your hands after handling Lidoderm patches.
- You can wear clothing over the area of application.
- To safely discard used patches, fold the patches so that the adhesive side sticks to itself.

What should I avoid while taking this medication?
Do not apply external heat sources, such as heating pads or electric blankets, over Lidoderm patches.

Do not apply Lidoderm to broken or inflamed skin or your eyes.

What are possible food and drug interactions associated with this medication?
If Lidoderm is taken with certain other drugs, the effects of either could be increased, decreased, or altered. It is especially important to check with your doctor before combining Lidoderm with other local anesthetics or medications used for arrhythmias (life-threatening irregular heartbeat) (such as mexiletine or tocainide).

What are the possible side effects of this medication?
Please see general statement regarding side effects on page xiii.

Side effects may include: allergic reactions (such as difficulty breathing, itching, rash, or swelling), application-site reactions (such as burning, bruising, discoloration, irritation, itching, redness, or swelling), confusion, disorientation, dizziness, headache, lightheadedness, metallic taste, sleepiness, visual disturbances, vomiting, weakness

Can I receive this medication if I am pregnant or breastfeeding?

The effects of Lidoderm during pregnancy and breastfeeding are unknown. Tell your doctor immediately if you are pregnant, plan to become pregnant, or are breastfeeding.

What should I do if I miss a dose of this medication?

Lidoderm should be given under special circumstances determined by your doctor.

How should I store this medication?

Store at room temperature.

Linagliptin: see Tradjenta, page 1009

Liothyronine Sodium: see Cytomel, page 291

Lipitor

Generic name: Atorvastatin Calcium

What is this medication?

Lipitor belongs to a class of medicines called "statins," which are used to lower your cholesterol when a low-fat diet is not enough. Lipitor lowers your total cholesterol and the "bad" low-density lipoprotein (LDL) cholesterol, thereby helping to lower your risk of a heart attack, stroke, or chest pain; hospitalization for heart failure; or the need for procedures to restore the blood flow back to the heart or to another part of the body.

What is the most important information I should know about this medication?

- Taking Lipitor is not a substitute for following a healthy low-fat and low-cholesterol diet and exercising to lower your cholesterol.
- Do not take Lipitor if you are pregnant, think you may be pregnant, plan to become pregnant, or are breastfeeding.

- Lipitor can cause muscle pain, tenderness, weakness, fatigue, loss of appetite, right upper abdominal discomfort, dark urine, or yellowing of your skin or whites of your eyes. Call your doctor right away if you notice any of these symptoms.
- Lipitor can cause serious allergic reactions. Call your doctor right away if you experience swelling of your face, lips, tongue, or throat or if you have trouble breathing or swallowing.

Who should not take this medication?

Do not take Lipitor if you are allergic to it or any of its ingredients or if you currently have liver disease. Also, do not take Lipitor if you are pregnant, plan to become pregnant, or are breastfeeding.

What should I tell my doctor before I take the first dose of this medication?

Tell your doctor about all prescription, over-the-counter, and herbal medications you are taking before beginning treatment with Lipitor. Also, talk to your doctor about your complete medical history, especially if you drink excessive amounts of alcohol or you have liver, kidney, thyroid, or heart problems; muscle aches or weakness; or diabetes. Tell your doctor if you are pregnant, plan to become pregnant, or are breastfeeding.

What is the usual dosage?

Please see general statement regarding dosage on page xii.

Adults: The recommended starting dose is 10-20 milligrams (mg) once a day. Your doctor will check your blood cholesterol levels during treatment with Lipitor and will change your dose based on the results.

Adolescents 10-17 years: The recommended starting dose is 10 mg once a day. Your doctor will check your child's blood cholesterol levels during treatment with Lipitor and will change his/her dose based on the results.

If you have kidney impairment or you are taking other medications, your doctor will adjust your dose appropriately.

How should I take this medication?

- Your doctor will likely start you on a low-cholesterol diet before prescribing Lipitor. Stay on this diet while you are taking Lipitor.
- Take Lipitor exactly as prescribed by your doctor. Take it at about the same time every day, with or without food. Do not break Lipitor tablets.

What should I avoid while taking this medication?

Do not change your dose or stop taking Lipitor without first talking to your doctor.

What are possible food and drug interactions associated with this medication?

If Lipitor is taken with certain other drugs, the effects of either could be increased, decreased, or altered. It is especially important to check with your doctor before combining Lipitor with the following: alcohol, anti-HIV medications (such as darunavir, fosamprenavir, lopinavir, ritonavir, saquinavir, or tipranavir), birth control pills, blood thinners (such as warfarin), cholesterol-lowering medicines known as fibrates (such as fenofibrate or gemfibrozil), cimetidine, clarithromycin, colchicine, cyclosporine, digoxin, efavirenz, grapefruit juice (>1 liter), itraconazole, ketoconazole, niacin, rifampin, spironolactone, or telaprevir.

What are the possible side effects of this medication?

Please see general statement regarding side effects on page xiii.

> **Side effects may include:** common cold, diarrhea, joint pain, pain in arms and legs, urinary tract infection

Can I receive this medication if I am pregnant or breastfeeding?

Do not take Lipitor during pregnancy or breastfeeding. Tell your doctor immediately if you are pregnant, plan to become pregnant, or are breastfeeding.

What should I do if I miss a dose of this medication?

If you miss a dose of Lipitor, take it as soon as you remember. However, if it is almost time for your next dose, skip the one you missed and return to your regular dosing schedule. Do not take two doses at once.

How should I store this medication?

Store at room temperature.

Lisdexamfetamine Dimesylate: *see Vyvanse, page 1088*

Lisinopril: *see Prinivil, page 831*

Lisinopril: *see Zestril, page 1130*

Lithium

Generic name: Lithium Carbonate

What is this medication?

Lithium is a medicine used to treat manic episodes of bipolar disorder. A manic episode is a time of elevated, unreserved, or irritable mood. Lithium is also used in the maintenance treatment of bipolar disorder. Lithium is available in capsules, a solution, and tablets.

What is the most important information I should know about this medication?

- It may take up to three weeks before you see any improvement in your symptoms.
- While taking lithium, it is very important that you follow your doctor's recommendations and make sure you do not miss any appointments or laboratory tests.
- Toxic levels of this medication can occur at any dose and frequent blood tests will be required. You should stop taking lithium and tell your doctor immediately if you develop signs of lithium toxicity, such as diarrhea, drowsiness, mild lack of coordination, muscular weakness, tremor, or vomiting.

Who should not take this medication?

Do not take lithium if you are allergic to it or any of its ingredients. Also, do not take lithium if you are allergic to Lithobid, Eskalith, Eskalith CR, or any of their components.

What should I tell my doctor before I take the first dose of this medication?

Tell your doctor about all prescription, over-the-counter, and herbal medications you are taking before beginning treatment with lithium. Also, talk to your doctor about your complete medical history, especially if you have a history of kidney or heart disease, thyroid problems, severe debilitation, dehydration, low sodium levels, or are receiving diuretics (water pills).

What is the usual dosage?

Please see general statement regarding dosage on page xii.

Acute Mania in Bipolar Disorder

Adults: **Capsules and tablets:** The optimal dose is 600 milligrams (mg) three times a day. **Solution:** The optimal dose is 10 milliliters (mL) taken as 2 full teaspoons three times a day.

Long-Term Therapy for Bipolar Disorder

Adults: **Capsules and tablets:** The usual dose is 300 mg three or four times a day. **Solution:** The usual dose is 1 full teaspoon three or four times a day.

If you have kidney impairment, your doctor will adjust your dose appropriately.

How should I take this medication?

• Take lithium exactly as prescribed by your doctor. Do not take extra doses or take more often without asking your doctor. Do not chew or crush lithium tablets or capsules; swallow them whole.

What should I avoid while taking this medication?

Do not stop taking lithium without consulting your doctor first.

Do not drive or operate dangerous machinery or participate in activities that require full mental alertness until you know how lithium affects you.

What are possible food and drug interactions associated with this medication?

If lithium is taken with certain other drugs, the effects of either could be increased, decreased, or altered. It is especially important to check with your doctor before combining lithium with the following: blood pressure/heart medications in a class known as angiotensin-converting enzyme (ACE) inhibitors (such as enalapril or fosinopril), diuretics (such as furosemide or hydrochlorothiazide), haloperidol, neuromuscular blocking agents (such as atracurium or succinylcholine), or nonsteroidal anti-inflammatory drugs (NSAIDs) (such as celecoxib, ibuprofen, or naproxen).

What are the possible side effects of this medication?

Please see general statement regarding side effects on page xiii.

> **Side effects may include:** blurred vision, confusion, decreased appetite, diarrhea, dry mouth, frequent urination, general discomfort, sleepiness, slurred speech, temporary and mild nausea, tiredness, tremor, vomiting

Can I receive this medication if I am pregnant or breastfeeding?

Lithium may cause harm to your unborn baby if you take it during pregnancy. Do not breastfeed while you are taking lithium. Tell your doctor immediately if you are pregnant, plan to become pregnant, or are breastfeeding.

What should I do if I miss a dose of this medication?

If you miss a dose of lithium, take it as soon as you remember. However, if it is almost time for your next dose, skip the one you missed and return to your regular dosing schedule. Do not take two doses at once.

How should I store this medication?
Store at room temperature, in a dry place, and away from light.

Lithium Carbonate: see Lithium, page 558

Loestrin 24 Fe
Generic name: Ethinyl Estradiol/Ferrous Fumarate/Norethindrone Acetate

What is this medication?
Loestrin 24 Fe is a birth control pill used to prevent pregnancy.

What is the most important information I should know about this medication?
- Cigarette smoking increases the risk of serious heart-related side effects (such as blood clots, stroke, and heart attack) from use of birth control pills, such as Loestrin 24 Fe. The risk increases with age (especially if you are >35 years old and smoke).
- Use of birth control pills is associated with increased risk of heart attack, clotting disorders, stroke, liver tumors, and gall-bladder disease. These risks increase in people with a history of high blood pressure, high cholesterol, obesity, diabetes, clotting disorders, heart attack, stroke, chest pain, cancer of the breast or sex organs, or liver tumors.
- Birth control pills can increase your cholesterol levels. Women with high cholesterol should be monitored closely.
- Loestrin 24 Fe does not protect against HIV infection (AIDS) and other sexually transmitted diseases.
- You can experience breakthrough bleeding or spotting while you are taking birth control pills, especially during the first 3 months of use. You can also have irregular periods. If you have missed more than two periods in a row, take a pregnancy test to determine if you are pregnant. Do not use Loestrin 24 Fe if you are pregnant.

Who should not take this medication?

Do not take Loestrin 24 Fe if you are allergic to it or any of its ingredients.

Do not take Loestrin 24 Fe if you are >35 years old and smoke cigarettes.

Do not take Loestrin 24 Fe if you have problems with your heart (such as a prior heart attack, stroke, or an abnormal rhythm) or liver; blood clots in your eyes, legs, lungs, or deep veins of your legs; chest pain; unexplained vaginal bleeding; cancer of the breast, lining of the uterus, cervix, or vagina; jaundice (yellowing of the skin or whites of the eyes) during pregnancy or during previous use of birth control pills; a liver tumor; very high blood pressure; diabetes with complications; severe headaches or migraines; or if you plan to have surgery with prolonged bed rest.

Do not take Loestrin 24 Fe if you may be pregnant or if you have not had your first period.

What should I tell my doctor before I take the first dose of this medication?

Tell your doctor about all prescription, over-the-counter, and herbal medications you are taking before beginning treatment with Loestrin 24 Fe. Also, talk to your doctor about your complete medical history, especially if you have or have had breast nodules; fibrocystic disease of the breast (lumpy and painful breasts); an abnormal breast x-ray or mammogram; high cholesterol or triglycerides; water retention; depression; migraines or other headaches; seizures; problems with your gallbladder, kidney, or liver; irregular menstrual bleeding or periods; wear contact lenses; smoke; plan to have surgery with prolonged bed rest; or if you are pregnant, plan to become pregnant, or are breastfeeding.

What is the usual dosage?

Please see general statement regarding dosage on page xii.

Adults: Each white "active" pill of Loestrin 24 Fe contains 1 milligram (mg) of norethindrone acetate and 20 micrograms (mcg) of ethinyl estradiol. Each brown "reminder" pill contains ferrous fumarate (iron) and inactive ingredients.

Sunday Start: Take the first white "active" pill on the Sunday after your period begins, even if you are still bleeding. Take one white "active" pill a day for 24 days followed by one brown "reminder" pill a day for 4 days. After all 28 pills have been taken, start a new course the next day (Sunday).

Day 1 Start: Take the first white "active" pill of the first pack during the first 24 hours of your period. Take one white "active" pill a day from the 1st day through the 24th day of the menstrual cycle (counting the day your period starts as Day 1) followed by one brown "reminder" pill a day for 4 days. Take the pills without interruption for 28 days. After all 28 pills have been taken, start a new course the next day.

How should I take this medication?

- Before you start taking Loestrin 24 Fe, be sure to read the directions. Take Loestrin 24 Fe once a day at the same time every day until the pack is empty.
- When you finish a pack or switch from another birth control pill, start the next pack on the day after your brown "reminder" pill. Do not wait any days between packs.
- For the first cycle of a Sunday Start regimen, use another method of birth control (such as condoms or spermicide) as a backup method if you have sex any time from the Sunday you start your first pack until you have been taking the pills for 7 days. You will not need to use a back-up method of birth control for the first cycle of a Day 1 regimen, since you are starting the pill at the beginning of your period.

What should I avoid while taking this medication?

Do not smoke or become pregnant while you are taking Loestrin 24 Fe.

Do not skip pills, even if you are spotting or bleeding between monthly periods, feel sick to your stomach (nausea), or if you do not have sex very often.

What are possible food and drug interactions associated with this medication?

If Loestrin 24 Fe is taken with certain other drugs, the effects of either could be increased, decreased, or altered. It is especially important to check with your doctor before combining Loestrin 24 Fe with the following: acetaminophen, antibiotics (such as ampicillin), atorvastatin, clofibric acid, cyclosporine, felbamate, griseofulvin, certain medicines used to treat HIV and AIDS, itraconazole, ketoconazole, modafinil, morphine, oxcarbazepine, phenylbutazone, prednisolone, rifampin, salicylic acid, seizure medications (such as carbamazepine, lamotrigine, phenobarbital, phenytoin, primidone, or topiramate), St. John's wort, temazepam, theophylline, troleandomycin, or vitamin C.

What are the possible side effects of this medication?

Please see general statement regarding side effects on page xiii.

> **Side effects may include:** abdominal (stomach area) cramps and bloating, absence of a period, allergic reactions, breakthrough bleeding or spotting, breast tenderness, change in your appetite, change in your vision or inability to wear your contact lenses, dizziness, headache, increase In your blood pressure, irregular vaginal bleeding, loss of scalp hair, mood changes, nausea, nervousness, rash, spotty darkening of the skin (especially on your face), vaginal infections, vomiting, water retention causing swelling of your fingers or ankles, weight change

Can I receive this medication if I am pregnant or breastfeeding?

Do not take Loestrin 24 Fe if you are pregnant or breastfeeding. The effects of Loestrin 24 Fe during pregnancy are unknown. Loestrin 24 Fe can be found in your breast-milk if you take it while breastfeeding. Tell your doctor immediately if you are pregnant, plan to become pregnant, or are breastfeeding.

What should I do if I miss a dose of this medication?

If you miss one white "active" pill, take it as soon as you remember. Take the next pill at your regular time. This means you can take two pills in the same day. You do not need a back-up birth control method if you have sex.

If you miss two pills or more, consult the patient information that accompanied your prescription or call your doctor or pharmacist for advice.

How should I store this medication?
Store at room temperature.

Loestrin Fe
Generic name: Ethinyl Estradiol/Ferrous Fumarate/Norethindrone Acetate

What is this medication?
Loestrin Fe is a birth control pill used to prevent pregnancy.

What is the most important information I should know about this medication?
- Cigarette smoking increases the risk of serious heart-related side effects (such as blood clots, stroke, and heart attack) from use of birth control pills, such as Loestrin Fe. The risk increases with age (especially if you are >35 years old and smoke cigarettes). Do not smoke cigarettes while you are taking birth control pills.
- Use of birth control pills is associated with increased risk of heart attack, clotting disorders, stroke, liver tumors, and gall-bladder disease. These risks increase in people with a history of high blood pressure, high cholesterol, obesity, diabetes, clotting disorders, heart attack, stroke, chest pain, cancer of the breast or sex organs, or liver tumors.
- Birth control pills can increase your cholesterol levels. Women with high cholesterol should be monitored closely.
- Loestrin Fe does not protect against HIV infection (AIDS) and other sexually transmitted diseases.
- You can experience breakthrough bleeding or spotting while you are taking birth control pills, especially during the first 3 months of use. You can also have irregular periods. If you have missed more than two periods in a row, you may be pregnant. Tell your

doctor right away to determine if you are pregnant. Do not take Loestrin Fe if you are pregnant.

Who should not take this medication?
Do not take Loestrin Fe if you are >35 years old and smoke cigarettes.

Do not take Loestrin Fe if you have a history of heart attack or stroke; blood clots in your legs, lungs, or eyes; chest pain (angina); cancer of the breast, lining of the uterus, cervix, or vagina; unexplained vaginal bleeding; yellowing of your skin or the whites of your eyes during pregnancy or previous use of oral birth control pills; liver tumors; or if you are allergic to any of the ingredients in Loestrin Fe. Do not take Loestrin Fe if you think you may be pregnant or if you have not had your first period.

What should I tell my doctor before I take the first dose of this medication?
Tell your doctor about all prescription, over-the-counter, and herbal medications you are taking before beginning treatment with Loestrin Fe. Tell your doctor if you have ever had any of the health conditions listed above. Also, talk to your doctor about your complete medical history, especially if you have breast nodules; fibrocystic disease of the breast (lumpy or painful breasts); an abnormal breast x-ray or mammogram; diabetes; high cholesterol or triglycerides; high blood pressure; migraines or other headaches; seizures; depression; gallbladder, heart, or kidney disease; a history of irregular menstrual bleeding or periods; wear contact lenses; smoke cigarettes; plan to have surgery with prolonged bed rest; or if you are pregnant, plan to become pregnant, or are breastfeeding.

What is the usual dosage?
Please see general statement regarding dosage on page xii.

Loestrin Fe is available as Loestrin Fe 1/20 and Loestrin Fe 1.5/30. Your doctor will prescribe the appropriate birth control for you.

Loestrin Fe 1/20

Women who have reached puberty: Each light yellow "active" pill contains 1 milligram (mg) of norethindrone acetate and 20 micrograms (mcg) of ethinyl estradiol. Each brown "reminder" pill contains 75 mg of ferrous fumarate.

Sunday Start: Take the first light yellow "active" pill of the first pack on the Sunday after your period begins, even if you are still bleeding. If your period begins on Sunday, start the pack that same day. Take one light yellow "active" pill for 21 days followed by one brown "reminder" pill a day for 7 days. After all 28 pills have been taken, start a new course the next day (Sunday).

Day 1 Start: Take the first light yellow "active" pill of the first pack during the first 24 hours of your period. Take one light yellow "active" pill from the 1st day through the 21st day of the menstrual cycle (counting the day your period starts as Day 1) followed by one brown "reminder" pill a day for 7 days. Take the pills without interruption for 28 days. After all 28 pills have been taken, start a new course the next day.

Loestrin Fe 1.5/30

Women who have reached puberty: Each pink "active" pill contains 1.5 mg of norethindrone acetate and 30 mcg of ethinyl estradiol. Each brown "reminder" pill contains 75 mg of ferrous fumarate.

Sunday Start: Take the first pink "active" pill of the first pack on the Sunday after your period begins, even if you are still bleeding. If your period begins on Sunday, start the pack that same day. Take one pink "active" pill for 21 days followed by one brown "reminder" pill a day for 7 days. After all 28 pills have been taken, start a new course the next day (Sunday).

Day 1 Start: Take the first pink "active" pill of the first pack during the first 24 hours of your period. Take one pink "active" pill from the 1st day through the 21st day of the menstrual cycle (counting the day your period starts as Day 1) followed by one brown "reminder" pill a day for 7 days. Take the pills without interruption for 28 days. After all 28 pills have been taken, start a new course the next day.

How should I take this medication?

- Before you start taking Loestrin Fe, be sure to read the directions. Take Loestrin Fe at the same time every day until the pack is empty. When you finish a pack, start the next pack on the day after your last brown "reminder" pill. Do not wait any days between packs. If you are switching from another birth control pill, start Loestrin Fe on the same day that a new pack of the previous pills should have been started.

- For the first cycle of a *Sunday Start* regimen, use another method of birth control (such as condoms or sperimicide) as a backup method if you have sex any time from the Sunday you start your first pack until you have been taking the pills for 7 days. You will not need to use a back-up method of birth control for the first cycle of a *Day 1* regimen, since you are starting the pill at the beginning of your period.

What should I avoid while taking this medication?

Do not smoke cigarettes or become pregnant while you are taking Loestrin Fe.

Do not skip pills, even if you are spotting or bleeding between monthly periods, feel sick to your stomach (nausea), or if you do not have sex very often.

What are possible food and drug interactions associated with this medication?

If Loestrin Fe is taken with certain other drugs, the effects of either could be increased, decreased, or altered. It is especially important to check with your doctor before combining Loestrin Fe with the following: acetaminophen, antibiotics (such as ampicillin, griseofluvin, or tetracycline), atorvastatin, clofibric acid, cyclosporine, morphine, phenylbutazone, prednisolone, rifampin, salicylic acid, seizure medications (such as carbamazepine, phenobarbital, or phenytoin), temazepam, theophylline, troglitazone, or vitamin C.

What are the possible side effects of this medication?

Please see general statement regarding side effects on page xiii.

Side effects may include: abdominal cramps and bloating, absence of a period, blotchy darkening of the skin (especially on your face), breakthrough bleeding or spotting, breast tenderness, change in your appetite, change in your vision or inability to wear your contact lenses, depression, dizziness, gallbladder disease, headache, high blood pressure, irregular vaginal bleeding, nausea, nervousness, rash, vaginal infections, vomiting, water retention causing swelling of your fingers or ankles, weight changes

Can I receive this medication if I am pregnant or breastfeeding?

Do not take Loestrin Fe if you are pregnant or breastfeeding. Tell your doctor immediately if you are pregnant, plan to become pregnant, or are breastfeeding.

What should I do if I miss a dose of this medication?

If you miss one light yellow or pink "active" pill, take it as soon as you remember. Take the next pill at your regular time. This means you can take two pills in one day. You do not need a back-up birth control method if you have sex.

If you miss two or more pills, consult the patient information that accompanied your prescription or call your pharmacist or doctor for advice.

How should I store this medication?

Store at room temperature.

Lomotil

Generic name: Atropine Sulfate/Diphenoxylate HCl

What is this medication?

Lomotil is a combination medicine used with other medications to treat diarrhea. Lomotil is available in tablets or liquid.

What is the most important information I should know about this medication?

- Take Lomotil exactly as prescribed by your doctor. You can develop severe breathing problems or coma if you take too much.
- Drink adequate fluids while taking Lomotil. Also, your doctor will monitor and treat your electrolyte imbalances, as needed.
- Lomotil can cause toxic megacolon (widening of the large intestine), especially in patients with ulcerative colitis (inflammatory disease of the large intestine).Tell your doctor if you have ulcerative colitis before you start taking Lomotil.
- Lomotil can increase your blood pressure severely, especially if you take it with monoamine oxidase inhibitors (MAOIs), a class of medications used to treat depression and other psychiatric conditions.
- Lomotil can cause drowsiness or dizziness. Do not drive, operate dangerous machinery, or perform activities requiring mental alertness until you know how Lomotil affects you. Also, do not drink alcohol or take medications that can cause drowsiness while taking this medication.

Who should not take this medication?

Do not take Lomotil if you are allergic to it or any of its ingredients.

Do not take Lomotil if you have certain liver diseases, or if you have diarrhea due to bacteria.

What should I tell my doctor before I take the first dose of this medication?

Tell your doctor about all prescription, over-the-counter, and herbal medications you are taking before beginning treatment with Lomotil. Also, talk to your doctor about your complete medical history, especially if you have ulcerative colitis, have liver or kidney disease, are dehydrated, are pregnant, plan to become pregnant, or are breastfeeding.

What is the usual dosage?

Please see general statement regarding dosage on page xii.

Adults and adolescents >12 years: The recommended starting dose is two tablets four times a day, or 2 teaspoonfuls of liquid four times a day.

Children 2-12 years: Your doctor will prescribe the appropriate dose of Lomotil liquid for your child, based on their weight.

How should I take this medication?
• Take Lomotil exactly as prescribed by your doctor. Tell your doctor if you do not see improvement within 48 hours of starting Lomotil.
• If your child is <13 years of age, he/she should use Lomotil liquid. Your child should not take Lomotil tablets. Use the plastic dropper provided with Lomotil liquid for measuring and giving doses to your child. Tell your child's doctor if you do not see improvement in your child's condition within 2 days of starting Lomotil.

What should I avoid while taking this medication?
Do not drive, operate dangerous machinery, or perform activities requiring mental alertness until you know how Lomotil affects you.

Do not drink alcohol or take medications that can cause drowsiness while taking Lomotil.

What are possible food and drug interactions associated with this medication?
If Lomotil is taken with certain other drugs, the effects of either could be increased, decreased, or altered. It is especially important to check with your doctor before combining Lomotil with alcohol, barbiturates (such as phenobarbital), MAOIs, or other medications that can cause drowsiness.

What are the possible side effects of this medication?
Please see general statement regarding side effects on page xiii.

Side effects may include: abdominal discomfort, allergic reactions, confusion, depression, dizziness, drowsiness, dryness of your skin and mouth, feelings of happiness or well-being, flushing, headache, increase in body temperature, intestinal blockage, itching, loss of appetite, nausea, numbness of arms or legs, rapid heartbeat, restlessness, tiredness, toxic megacolon, urinary retention (inability to urinate normally), vomiting

Can I receive this medication if I am pregnant or breastfeeding?

The effects of Lomotil during pregnancy are unknown. Lomotil can be found in your breast milk if you take it while breastfeeding. Tell your doctor immediately if you are pregnant, plan to become pregnant, or are breastfeeding.

What should I do if I miss a dose of this medication?

If you miss a dose of Lomotil, take it as soon as you remember. However, if it is almost time for your next dose, skip the one you missed and return to your regular dosing schedule. Do not take two doses at once.

How should I store this medication?

Store at room temperature.

Lopid

Generic name: Gemfibrozil

What is this medication?

Lopid is a cholesterol-lowering medicine used, in addition to an appropriate diet, to treat adults with high triglycerides. Lopid is used when diet and exercise alone have not lowered triglycerides, and when you are at risk for pancreatitis (inflammation of the pancreas). Also, Lopid can lower the risk of developing heart disease in certain people with high cholesterol.

What is the most important information I should know about this medication?

- Tell your doctor if you are taking any other medications while you are taking Lopid. Lopid may have an effect on medicines that help prevent blood clotting (such as the blood thinner warfarin). If you are taking Lopid with a blood thinner, your doctor will monitor your blood-clotting tests. Also, tell your doctor about any cholesterol-lowering medicines you may be taking as he or she will need to determine if the combination of Lopid and one of those medications is right for you.

- Lopid can cause liver problems. Your doctor will monitor your liver function.

- Lopid can increase your risk of developing gallstones. Call your doctor right away if you experience abdominal (stomach) pain, nausea, or vomiting. These may be signs of inflammation of your gallbladder or pancreas. Your doctor will also do studies to check for gallstones.

- Lopid can cause serious muscle conditions that may lead to kidney damage. Your risk can increase if you are also taking other cholesterol-lowering medicines known as statins (atorvastatin, fluvastatin, lovastatin, or pravastatin). Tell your doctor right away if you experience unexplained muscle pain, weakness, or tenderness, especially if you also have a fever or general body discomfort.

- Lopid can cause cancer, cataracts, pancreatitis, severe allergic reactions, and clotting problems.

Who should not take this medication?

Do not take Lopid if you are allergic to it or any of its ingredients.

Do not take Lopid if you have liver, gallbladder, or severe kidney problems.

Do not take Lopid if you are taking repaglinide, a medication used for diabetes.

What should I tell my doctor before I take the first dose of this medication?

Tell your doctor about all prescription, over-the-counter, and herbal medications you are taking before beginning treatment with Lopid. Also, talk to your doctor about your complete medical history, especially if you have liver, kidney, or gallbladder problems; cancer; hypothyroidism (an underactive thyroid gland); diabetes; blood disorders; muscle pain or disease; if you drink large amounts of alcohol; or are pregnant, plan to become pregnant, or are breastfeeding.

What is the usual dosage?

Please see general statement regarding dosage on page xii.

Adults: The recommended dose is 1200 milligrams a day, divided into two doses.

How should I take this medication?

- Take Lopid exactly as prescribed by your doctor.
- Take Lopid 30 minutes before the morning and evening meal.
- If you are taking Lopid with another type of cholesterol-lowering medicine called a bile acid sequestrant (such as colestipol and cholestyramine), take Lopid at least 2 hours before or after you take the other medicine.

What should I avoid while taking this medication?

Do not drink alcohol while you are taking Lopid. Alcohol can raise your triglyceride levels, and may also damage your liver while you are taking Lopid.

What are possible food and drug interactions associated with this medication?

If Lopid is taken with certain other drugs, the effects of either could be increased, decreased, or altered. It is especially important to check with your doctor before combining Lopid with the following: bile acid sequestrants, blood thinners, repaglinide, or statins.

What are the possible side effects of this medication?

Please see general statement regarding side effects on page xiii.

Side effects may include: abdominal pain, diarrhea, indigestion, inflammation of your appendix, nausea, rash, tiredness, vomiting

Can I receive this medication if I am pregnant or breastfeeding?

The effects of Lopid during pregnancy and breastfeeding are unknown. Tell your doctor immediately if you are pregnant, plan to become pregnant, or are breastfeeding.

What should I do if I miss a dose of this medication?

If you miss a dose of Lopid, take it as soon as you remember. However, if it is almost time for your next dose, skip the one you missed and return to your regular dosing schedule. Do not take two doses at once.

How should I store this medication?

Store at room temperature. Protect from light and humidity.

Lopressor

Generic name: Metoprolol Tartrate

What is this medication?

Lopressor is a medicine known as a beta-blocker, which is used to treat high blood pressure and chest pain. Lopressor is also used after a heart attack to lower the risk of death.

What is the most important information I should know about this medication?

- Take Lopressor regularly and continuously. Do not stop taking Lopressor without talking to your doctor. Abruptly stopping this medication can cause harmful effects. Your doctor should gradually reduce your dose when stopping treatment with this medication.
- Lopressor can worsen heart failure, cause breathing problems, or hide symptoms of low blood sugar levels if you have diabetes. Tell your doctor if you experience trouble breathing while you are taking Lopressor. If you have diabetes, monitor your

blood sugar frequently, especially when you first start taking Lopressor.
• Tell your doctor or dentist that you are taking Lopressor before undergoing any type of surgery.

Who should not take this medication?

Do not take Lopressor if you are allergic to it or any of its ingredients. In addition, do not take Lopressor if you have a slow heart rate, heart failure, heart block, sick sinus syndrome (abnormal heart rhythm), low blood pressure, or severe blood circulation disorders.

What should I tell my doctor before I take the first dose of this medication?

Tell your doctor about all prescription, over-the-counter, and herbal medications you are taking before beginning treatment with Lopressor. Also, talk to your doctor about your complete medical history, especially if you have allergies, heart problems or heart failure, a history of heart attack, breathing problems, pheochromocytoma (tumor of the adrenal gland), diabetes, liver or thyroid problems, or are planning to have a major surgery.

Tell your doctor if you have a history of severe allergic reactions to any allergens, because Lopressor may decrease the effectiveness of epinephrine used to treat the reaction.

What is the usual dosage?

Please see general statement regarding dosage on page xii.

High Blood Pressure

Adults: The usual starting dose is 100 milligrams (mg) once a day or in divided doses, either alone or in combination with other blood pressure-lowering medicines. Full effects should be seen in 1 week. Your doctor will increase your dose as needed until the desired effect is achieved.

Chest Pain
Adults: The usual starting dose is 50 mg twice a day. Your doctor will increase your dose as needed until the desired effect is achieved.

Heart Attack
Adults: Your doctor will prescribe the appropriate dose for you based on your condition.

If you have liver impairment, your doctor will adjust your dose appropriately.

How should I take this medication?
• Take Lopressor exactly as prescribed by your doctor. Take it with or immediately following meals.

What should I avoid while taking this medication?
Do not drive a car, operate machinery, or engage in other tasks requiring alertness until you know how Lopressor affects you.

Do not stop taking Lopressor without first talking to your doctor.

What are possible food and drug interactions associated with this medication?
If Lopressor is taken with certain other drugs, the effects of either could be increased, decreased, or altered. It is especially important to check with your doctor before combining Lopressor with the following: bupropion, cimetidine, clonidine, digoxin, diphenhydramine, fluoxetine, hydroxychloroquine, paroxetine, propafenone, quinidine, reserpine, ritonavir, terbinafine, or thioridazine.

What are the possible side effects of this medication?
Please see general statement regarding side effects on page xiii.

> **Side effects may include:** confusion, depression, diarrhea, dizziness, headache, itching, nightmares, rash, shortness of breath, short-term memory loss, slow heart rate, tiredness, trouble sleeping, vomiting

Can I receive this medication if I am pregnant or breastfeeding?

The effects of Lopressor during pregnancy are unknown. Lopressor can be found in your breast milk if you take it while breastfeeding. Tell your doctor immediately if you are pregnant, plan to become pregnant, or are breastfeeding.

What should I do if I miss a dose of this medication?

If you miss a dose of Lopressor, take it as soon as you remember. However, if it is almost time for your next dose, skip the one you missed and return to your regular dosing schedule. Do not take two doses at once.

How should I store this medication?

Store at room temperature. Protect from moisture.

Lotensin

Generic name: Benazepril HCl

What is this medication?

Lotensin is a medicine known as an angiotensin-converting enzyme (ACE) inhibitor. Lotensin is used alone or in combination with other medications to treat high blood pressure.

What is the most important information I should know about this medication?

- Lotensin can cause a rare but serious allergic reaction leading to extreme swelling of your face, eyes, lips, tongue, throat or gut (causing severe abdominal pain). You may have an increased risk of experiencing these symptoms if you have ever had an allergy to ACE inhibitor-type medicines or if you are African American. If you experience any of these symptoms, seek emergency medical attention immediately.
- Tell your doctor if you experience lightheadedness, especially during the first few weeks of Lotensin therapy. If you faint, stop taking Lotensin and tell your doctor immediately.

- Vomiting, diarrhea, fever, exercise, hot weather, alcohol, excessive perspiration, and dehydration may lead to an excessive fall in your blood pressure. Tell your doctor if you experience any of these.
- Lotensin may decrease your blood neutrophil (type of blood cells that fight infections) levels.
- Promptly report any signs of infection (such as sore throat or fever) to your doctor.
- Tell your doctor if you develop a persistent dry cough while you are taking Lotensin.

Who should not take this medication?
Do not take Lotensin if you are allergic to it or any of its ingredients.

Do not take Lotensin if you have a history of angioedema (a condition involving swelling of the face, extremities, eyes, lips, and tongue).

What should I tell my doctor before I take the first dose of this medication?
Tell your doctor about all prescription, over-the-counter, and herbal medications you are taking before beginning treatment with Lotensin. Also, talk to your doctor about your complete medical history, especially if you are pregnant or plan to become pregnant, if you have heart failure or kidney disease, or if you have ever had an allergy or sensitivity to an ACE inhibitor such as Lotensin.

What is the usual dosage?
Please see general statement regarding dosage on page xii.

Adults: The usual starting dose is 10 milligrams (mg) once a day. Your doctor may increase your daily dose to 20-40 mg a day as one dose or split into two equal doses.

Children ages ≥6 years: Your doctor will prescribe the appropriate dose for your child based on their body weight.

How should I take this medication?
- Take Lotensin exactly as prescribed by your doctor.

- Take Lotensin at the same time every day.
- Continue to take Lotensin even if you feel well. Do not take extra doses or take more often without asking your doctor.

What should I avoid while taking this medication?

Do not become pregnant or breastfeed while you are taking Lotensin.

Do not drive or operate heavy machinery until you know how Lotensin affects you.

Do not take salt substitutes or supplements containing potassium without consulting your doctor.

Do not stand or sit up quickly when you take Lotensin, especially in the morning. Sit or lie down at the first sign of dizziness, light-headedness, or fainting.

What are possible food and drug interactions associated with this medication?

If Lotensin is taken with certain other drugs, the effects of either could be increased, decreased, or altered. It is especially important to check with your doctor before combining Lotensin with any of the following: antidiabetes medications (such as insulin), diuretics (water pills) (such as amiloride, hydrochlorothiazide, spironolactone, triamterene), lithium, potassium supplements and salt substitutes containing potassium, and warfarin.

What are the possible side effects of this medication?

Please see general statement regarding side effects on page xiii.

> **Side effects may include:** cough, dizziness, drowsiness, fatigue, headache

Can I receive this medication if I am pregnant or breastfeeding?

Do not take Lotensin if you are pregnant or breastfeeding. Lotensin can harm your unborn baby. Tell your doctor immediately if you are pregnant, plan to become pregnant, or are breastfeeding.

What should I do if I miss a dose of this medication?

If you miss a dose of Lotensin, take it as soon as you remember. However, if it is almost time for your next dose, skip the one you missed and return to your regular dosing schedule. Do not take two doses at once.

How should I store this medication?

Store at room temperature. Protect from moisture.

Lotensin HCT

Generic name: Benazepril HCl/Hydrochlorothiazide

What is this medication?

Lotensin HCT is a combination medicine used to treat high blood pressure. Lotensin HCT contains two medicines: benazepril (an angiotensin-converting enzyme [ACE] inhibitor) and hydrochloro-thiazide (a diuretic [water pill]).

What is the most important information I should know about this medication?

- When taken during pregnancy, ACE inhibitors such as Lotensin HCT can cause injury and even death to the developing baby. If you are pregnant or plan to become pregnant, stop taking Lotensin HCT and contact your doctor immediately.
- Lotensin HCT can cause a rare but serious allergic reaction leading to extreme swelling of your face, lips, tongue, throat, or gut (causing severe stomach pain). If you experience any of these symptoms, seek emergency medical attention.
- Rarely, Lotensin HCT can cause a yellowing of your skin or the whites of your eyes, which can be a sign of liver injury. If this occurs, tell your doctor immediately.

- Lotensin HCT can cause lightheadedness or fainting, especially when you stand up from a lying or sitting position.
- If you experience any symptoms of infection (such as sore throat or fever) that do not go away while you are taking Lotensin HCT, tell your doctor immediately.
- Lotensin HCT can activate lupus (disease that affects the immune system) or gout (severe and painful inflammation of the joints) in certain patients.
- If you have diabetes, Lotensin HCT can increase your blood sugar levels. Check your blood sugar frequently.

Who should not take this medication?

Do not take Lotensin HCT if you are allergic to it or any of its ingredients.

Do not take Lotensin HCT if you have anuria (are unable to produce urine).

Do not take Lotensin HCT if you have a history of angioedema (a condition involving swelling of the face, extremities, eyes, lips, and tongue).

What should I tell my doctor before I take the first dose of this medication?

Tell your doctor about all prescription, over-the-counter, and herbal medications you are taking before beginning treatment with Lotensin HCT. Also, talk to your doctor if you have diabetes, heart failure, severe immune system problems, lupus, asthma, or liver or kidney disease, or if you have ever had an allergy or sensitivity to an ACE inhibitor or sulfonamide-derived medications.

What is the usual dosage?

Please see general statement regarding dosage on page xii.

Adults: The usual starting dose is 10/12.5 (10 milligrams [mg] of benazepril and 12.5 mg of hydrochlorothiazide) once a day.

Your doctor may give you a higher dose depending on your needs.

How should I take this medication?
- Take Lotensin HCT with or without food at the same time every day. Continue to use Lotensin HCT even if you feel well.
- Do not take extra doses or take more often without asking your doctor.

What should I avoid while taking this medication?
Do not become pregnant or breastfeed while you are taking Lotensin HCT.

Do not become dehydrated. Drink adequate fluids while you are taking Lotensin HCT.

Do not take salt substitutes or supplements containing potassium without consulting your doctor.

Do not stand or sit up quickly when you are taking Lotensin HCT, especially in the morning. Sit or lie down at the first sign of dizziness, lightheadedness, or fainting.

What are possible food and drug interactions associated with this medication?
If Lotensin HCT is taken with certain other drugs, the effects of either could be increased, decreased, or altered. It is especially important to check with your doctor before combining Lotensin HCT with the following: cholestyramine, colestipol, diuretics (water pills) (such as amiloride, hydrochlorothiazide, spironolactone, or triamterene), insulin, lithium, nonsteroidal anti-inflammatory drugs (NSAIDs) (such as ibuprofen or naproxen), norepinephrine, and potassium supplements or salt substitutes containing potassium.

What are the possible side effects of this medication?
Please see general statement regarding side effects on page xiii.

Side effects may include: cough, dizziness, fatigue, headache, high blood sugar, low blood pressure, nausea, rash

---

Can I receive this medication if I am pregnant or breastfeeding?
Do not take Lotensin HCT if you are pregnant or breastfeeding. Lotensin HCT can harm your unborn baby. It can be found in your breast milk if you take it while breastfeeding. Tell your doctor immediately if you are pregnant, plan to become pregnant, or are breastfeeding.

What should I do if I miss a dose of this medication?
If you miss a dose of Lotensin HCT, take it as soon as you remember. However, if it is almost time for your next dose, skip the one you missed and return to your regular dosing schedule. Do not take two doses at once.

How should I store this medication?
Store at room temperature. Protect from light.

Lorazepam: see Ativan, page 100

Losartan Potassium: see Cozaar, page 279

Lotrel
Generic name: Amlodipine Besylate/Benazepril HCl

What is this medication?
Lotrel is a combination medicine that contains two medications: amlodipine (a calcium channel blocker) and benazepril (angiotensin-converting enzyme [ACE] inhibitor). Lotrel is used alone or in combination with other medications to treat high blood pressure. Lowering of blood pressure may reduce the risk of having a stroke or heart attack.

What is the most important information I should know about this medication?
• Lotrel can cause a rare but serious allergic reaction leading to extreme swelling of your face, lips, tongue, throat, or gut

(causing severe abdominal [stomach] pain). You may have an increased risk of experiencing these symptoms if you have ever had an allergy to ACE inhibitor-type medicines or if you are African American. If you experience any of these symptoms, seek emergency medical attention right away.

- If you experience chest pain that gets worse, or that does not go away during treatment with Lotrel, get medical help right away.
- Tell your doctor if you experience lightheadedness, especially during the first few weeks of Lotrel therapy. If you faint, stop taking Lotrel and tell your doctor right away.
- If you become pregnant while you are taking Lotrel, stop taking it and call your doctor right away. Lotrel can harm your unborn baby, causing injury or even death.
- Lotrel can cause liver problems. If you experience nausea, feel more tired or weaker than usual, itching, yellowing of your skin or whites of your eyes, pain in your upper right stomach area, or "flu-like" symptoms, tell your doctor right away.
- Lotrel may decrease your white blood cell (type of blood cells that fight infections) levels, especially if you have a collagen vascular disease (such as lupus [disease that affects the immune system]) or kidney disease.
- Promptly report any signs of infection (such as sore throat or fever) to your doctor.

Who should not take this medication?
Do not take Lotrel if you are allergic to it or any of its ingredients.

Do not take Lotrel if you have a history of angioedema (a condition involving swelling of the face, extremities, eyes, lips, and tongue) related to previous treatment with similar medicines. Also, do not take Lotrel if you have a history of certain types of angioedema (such as hereditary or idiopathic).

What should I tell my doctor before I take the first dose of this medication?
Tell your doctor about all prescription, over-the-counter, and herbal medications you are taking before beginning treatment with Lotrel. Also, talk to your doctor about your complete medical history, especially if you have liver or kidney disease; a heart condition;

have diabetes; any disease that affects the immune system (such as lupus or scleroderma); ever had an allergy or sensitivity to ACE inhibitors or calcium channel blockers; are going to have surgery, allergy shots for bee stings, or kidney dialysis; or are pregnant, plan to become pregnant, or are breastfeeding.

What is the usual dosage?
Please see general statement regarding dosage on page xii.

Adults: Your doctor will prescribe the appropriate dose for you based on your previous blood pressure medication.

If you have liver impairment, your doctor will adjust your dose appropriately.

How should I take this medication?
• Take Lotrel exactly as prescribed by your doctor.
• Take Lotrel at the same time each day, with or without food. Continue to take Lotrel even if you feel well.
• Do not take extra doses or take more often without asking your doctor.

What should I avoid while taking this medication?
Do not take salt substitutes or supplements containing potassium without consulting your doctor.

What are possible food and drug interactions associated with this medication?
If Lotrel is taken with certain other drugs, the effects of either could be increased, decreased, or altered. It is especially important to check with your doctor before combining Lotrel with the following: diuretics (water pills) (such as amiloride, spironolactone, or triamterene), lithium, nonsteroidal anti-inflammatory drugs (NSAIDs) (such as ibuprofen or naproxen), potassium supplements, salt substitutes containing potassium, or simvastatin.

What are the possible side effects of this medication?
Please see general statement regarding side effects on page xiii.

Side effects may include: abdominal pain, allergic reactions, breathing problems, chest pain, cough, dizziness, feel faint, fever, "flu-like" symptoms, headache, itching, nausea, sore throat, swelling, tiredness, trouble swallowing, weakness, yellowing of your skin or whites of your eyes

Can I receive this medication if I am pregnant or breastfeeding?

Do not take Lotrel if you are pregnant or breastfeeding. Lotrel can harm your unborn baby. Tell your doctor immediately if you are pregnant, plan to become pregnant, or are breastfeeding.

What should I do if I miss a dose of this medication?

If you miss a dose of Lotrel, take it as soon as you remember. However, if it is almost time for your next dose, skip the one you missed and return to your regular dosing schedule. Do not take two doses at once.

How should I store this medication?

Store at room temperature. Protect from moisture.

Lotrisone

Generic name: Betamethasone Dipropionate/Clotrimazole

What is this medication?

Lotrisone is a topical cream (applied directly on the skin) that is used to treat fungal infections, such as tinea corporis (ringworm), tinea cruris (jock itch), and tinea pedis (athlete's foot).

What is the most important information I should know about this medication?

- Lotrisone is for external use only. Do not use it in your eyes.
- Even though Lotrisone is applied on your skin, it can still be absorbed into the bloodstream. Too much absorption can cause a serious side effect involving certain glands and hormones. To lower your risk of this happening, avoid using large amounts of Lotrisone over large areas, and do not cover it with airtight

dressings such as a plastic wrap or adhesive bandages. Your doctor may perform tests to monitor for this side effect while on Lotrisone.
- Do not use Lotrisone for any other condition other than that for which your doctor has prescribed.
- Contact your doctor if you notice irritation or any skin reactions in the area being treated.

Who should not take this medication?

Do not use Lotrisone if you are allergic to it, any of its ingredients, or other corticosteroids (such as hydrocortisone or triamcinolone) or anti-fungal medicines (such as clotrimazole or miconazole).

What should I tell my doctor before I take the first dose of this medication?

Tell your doctor about all prescription, over-the-counter, and herbal medications you are taking before beginning treatment with Lotrisone. Also, talk to your doctor about your complete medical history.

What is the usual dosage?

Please see general statement regarding dosage on page xii.

Adults and adolescents ≥17 years: Massage sufficient cream into the affected skin areas twice a day.

How should I take this medication?

- Apply Lotrisone exactly as prescribed by your doctor. Apply it in the morning and evening. Do not bandage, cover, or wrap the treated skin area.
- Do not use >45 grams of Lotrisone in one week.
- If you are applying Lotrisone in your groin area, use the medicine for 2 weeks only and apply it sparingly. Wear loose-fitting clothing to avoid tightly covering the area where Lotrisone is applied.
- If you are using Lotrisone for jock itch or ringworm, tell your doctor if there is no improvement within one week. If you are using Lotrisone for athlete's foot, tell your doctor if there is no improvement within two weeks.

What should I avoid while taking this medication?
Do not use Lotrisone in your eyes, mouth, or vagina.

Do not use Lotrisone to treat your child's diaper rash.

What are possible food and drug interactions associated with this medication?
If Lotrisone is used with certain other drugs, the effects of either could be increased, decreased, or altered. It is especially important to check with your doctor before combing Lotrisone with other products that contain corticosteroids.

What are the possible side effects of this medication?
Please see general statement regarding side effects on page xiii.

> **Side effects may include:** acne, allergic skin reaction, changes in skin color, dryness, increased hair, infection of the hair follicles, irritation, itching, skin thinning, spider veins, stretch marks

Can I receive this medication if I am pregnant or breastfeeding?
The effects of Lotrisone during pregnancy and breastfeeding are unknown. Tell your doctor immediately if you are pregnant, plan to become pregnant, or are breastfeeding.

What should I do if I miss a dose of this medication?
If you miss a dose of Lotrisone, apply it as soon as you remember. However, if it is almost time for your next dose, skip the one you missed and return to your regular dosing schedule. Do not apply two doses at once.

How should I store this medication?
Store at room temperature.

Lovastatin: *see Altoprev, page 59*

Lovastatin: *see Mevacor, page 627*

Lovaza

Generic name: Omega-3-Acid Ethyl Esters

What is this medication?

Lovaza is a medicine used in combination with a low-fat and low-cholesterol diet to lower very high triglycerides (fats) in your blood.

What is the most important information I should know about this medication?

- Taking Lovaza is not a substitute for following a healthy low-fat and low-cholesterol diet and exercising.
- Lovaza can affect blood tests for your liver or cholesterol. Your doctor will do blood tests to check your liver function, triglyceride, and cholesterol levels while you are taking Lovaza.

Who should not take this medication?

Do not take Lovaza if you are allergic to it or any of its ingredients (including soybean oil).

What should I tell my doctor before I take the first dose of this medication?

Tell your doctor about all prescription, over-the-counter, and herbal medications you are taking before beginning treatment with Lovaza. Also, talk to your doctor about your complete medical history, especially if you have diabetes; thyroid, liver, or pancreas problems; or if you are allergic to fish or shellfish. Tell your doctor if you drink more than two glasses of alcohol a day.

What is the usual dosage?

Please see general statement regarding dosage on page xii.

Adults: The usual dose is 4 capsules a day. You can take all 4 capsules at the same time or 2 capsules twice a day.

How should I take this medication?

- Your doctor will likely start you on a low-fat and low-cholesterol diet before prescribing Lovaza. Stay on this diet while you are taking Lovaza.

- Take Lovaza exactly as prescribed by your doctor. Do not take more than 4 capsules a day. Take Lovaza at the same time or times each day. Take it with or without food.
- Swallow Lovaza capsules whole. Do not break, crush, dissolve, or chew them.

What should I avoid while taking this medication?
Do not change your dose or stop taking Lovaza without first talking to your doctor.

What are possible food and drug interactions associated with this medication?
If Lovaza is taken with certain other drugs, the effects of either could be increased, decreased, or altered. It is especially important to check with your doctor before combining Lovaza with the following: aspirin, blood thinners (such as warfarin or coumarin), or nonsteroidal anti-inflammatory drugs (NSAIDs) (ibuprofen or naproxen).

What are the possible side effects of this medication?
Please see general statement regarding side effects on page xiii.

Side effects may include: burping, changes in taste, upset stomach

Can I receive this medication if I am pregnant or breastfeeding?
The effects of Lovaza during pregnancy and breastfeeding are unknown. Tell your doctor immediately if you are pregnant, plan to become pregnant, or are breastfeeding.

What should I do if I miss a dose of this medication?
If you miss a dose of Lovaza, take it as soon as you remember. However, if it is almost time for your next dose, skip the one you missed and return to your regular dosing schedule. Do not take two doses at once.

How should I store this medication?
Store at room temperature.

Lovenox

Generic name: Enoxaparin Sodium

What is this medication?
Lovenox is a medicine that reduces blood clots.

What is the most important information I should know about this medication?
- If you receive an epidural (spinal anesthesia) or undergo spinal puncture while taking Lovenox, you may be at an increased risk of developing a blood clot in or around the spine, which can result in long-term paralysis. Your risk may be further increased if you take nonsteroidal anti-inflammatory drugs (NSAIDs), platelet inhibitors, or other blood thinners (including aspirin), have an indwelling epidural catheter, a history of spinal trauma, repeated spinal anesthesia or punctures, spinal deformities, or spinal surgery.
- Contact your doctor immediately if you experience symptoms such as tingling, numbness (especially in the lower limbs), muscular weakness, pain, swelling, dizziness, vomiting, nausea, fever, unusual bleeding or bruising, and rashes or dark spots under the skin.
- Excessive bleeding (hemorrhage), leading to death, has occurred with Lovenox. The use of aspirin and other NSAIDs may enhance the risk of excessive bleeding. Be sure to tell your doctor or dentist you are on Lovenox before any surgery is scheduled and before any new medicine is taken.
- Anyone taking Lovenox should be carefully monitored by their doctor.

Who should not take this medication?
Lovenox should not be used if you are actively bleeding or have a low count of blood cells called platelets, which aid in clotting. This

condition is called "thrombocytopenia." Lovenox also should not be used if you are allergic or sensitive to heparin or pork products.

What should I tell my doctor before I take the first dose of this medication?

Tell your doctor about all prescription, over-the-counter, and herbal medications you are taking before beginning treatment with Lovenox. Also talk to your doctor about your complete medical history, especially if you have problems with clotting, uncontrolled high blood pressure, a recent ulcer, impaired vision due to diabetes, kidney problems, or excessive bleeding. Pregnant women with mechanical artificial heart valves may be at higher risk for blood clots. Treatment with Lovenox requires careful monitoring by a doctor.

What is the usual dosage?
Please see general statement regarding dosage on page xii.

Adults: The usual length of treatment varies depending on your specific medical or surgical condition. Follow your doctor's instructions on how long you should take Lovenox and at what dosing schedule.

How should I take this medication?
- Your doctor will show you the correct method for injecting Lovenox. Lovenox should be injected into fatty tissue only, which is why the abdomen is the recommended injection site. Do not inject Lovenox into the muscle, which can cause bruising and discomfort.
- Make sure you inject the whole length of the needle into the skin fold held between the thumb and forefinger; hold the skin fold throughout the injection. To minimize bruising, do not rub the injection site after completing the injection.
- Every syringe comes with a small air bubble. Do not expel the air bubble unless your doctor instructs you to adjust your dose. It is safe to give yourself the injection, even with the air bubbles.

What should I avoid while taking this medication?

Do not stop taking Lovenox without first talking to the doctor who prescribed it for you.

During your treatment with Lovenox, avoid taking aspirin, NSAIDs, or any other type of blood thinners unless your doctor tells you to. Using these medications together with Lovenox can increase your risk of bleeding.

What are possible food and drug interactions associated with this medication?

If Lovenox is used with certain other drugs, the effects of either could be increased, decreased, or altered. It is especially important to check with your doctor before combining Lovenox with the following: blood thinning medications such as warfarin and aspirin, dipyridamole, NSAIDs including ketorolac, platelet inhibitors including acetylsalicylic acid, and sulfinpyrazone.

What are the possible side effects of this medication?

Please see general statement regarding side effects on page xiii.

> **Side effects may include:** mild pain, irritation, bruising, or redness of the skin at the injection site, bleeding, anemia, diarrhea, nausea

Can I receive this medication if I am pregnant or breastfeeding?

Lovenox should be used during pregnancy only when clearly needed. If you are pregnant or plan to become pregnant, inform your doctor immediately. It is not known whether Lovenox appears in breast milk. Consult your doctor before breastfeeding.

What should I do if I miss a dose of this medication?

Lovenox should be given under special circumstances determined by your doctor. If you miss your scheduled dose, speak to your doctor for advice.

Call your doctor immediately if you think you have given yourself too much Lovenox, even if you don't see or feel any unusual symptoms right away.

How should I store this medication?
You should store your prefilled syringes at room temperature, away from light and moisture.

Lumigan
Generic name: Bimatoprost

What is this medication?
Lumigan is an eye drop used to lower pressure in the eye in people with open-angle glaucoma or high pressure in the eye.

What is the most important information I should know about this medication?
- Lumigan can darken the color of your iris (colored part of the eye), eyelid, or eyelashes. The discoloration of your eyelids or eyelashes is usually reversible; however, the discoloration of the iris is most likely permanent.
- Lumigan can also increase the length, thickness, number of eyelashes, and/or direction of eyelash growth. Tell your doctor if you notice any discoloration or changes in these areas of your eye.
- Do not allow the tip of the bottle to touch your eye or any other surface, as serious eye infections may occur if your bottle becomes contaminated. Tell your doctor immediately if you experience any eye injury, infection, conjunctivitis ("pink eye"), or eyelid reactions with Lumigan.

Who should not take this medication?
Do not use Lumigan if you are allergic to it or any of its ingredients.

What should I tell my doctor before I take the first dose of this medication?

Tell your doctor about all prescription, over-the-counter, and herbal medications you are taking before beginning treatment with Lumigan. Also, talk to your doctor about your complete medical history, especially if you have had eye surgery or other eye disorders.

What is the usual dosage?

Please see general statement regarding dosage on page xii.

Adults: Apply 1 drop into the affected eye(s) once a day in the evening.

How should I take this medication?

- Apply Lumigan exactly as prescribed by your doctor.
- Lumigan contains a preservative that may be absorbed by your contact lenses. Remove your contact lenses prior to the administration of Lumigan and reinsert them after 15 minutes.
- If you are using Lumigan with another eye drop, the drops should be applied at least 5 minutes apart.

What should I avoid while taking this medication?

Do not allow the tip of the bottle to touch your eye or any other surface, as this can contaminate Lumigan.

What are possible food and drug interactions associated with this medication?

If Lumigan is used with certain other drugs, the effects of either could be increased, decreased, or altered. It is especially important to check with your doctor before combining Lumigan with other eye drops.

What are the possible side effects of this medication?

Please see general statement regarding side effects on page xiii.

Side effects may include: burning and pain of your eye, cataracts, color changes of your iris, darkening of your eyelashes or skin around your eyes, dry eyes, eye discharge and tearing, eye or eyelid redness, growth of eyelashes, itching of your eyes, light sensitivity, swelling of your eye or eyelid, visual disturbances

Can I receive this medication if I am pregnant or breastfeeding?

The effects of Lumigan during pregnancy and breastfeeding are unknown. Tell your doctor immediately if you are pregnant, plan to become pregnant, or are breastfeeding.

What should I do if I miss a dose of this medication?

If you miss a dose of Lumigan, apply it as soon as you remember. However, if it is almost time for your next dose, skip the one you missed and return to your regular dosing schedule. Do not apply two doses at once.

How should I store this medication?

Store in the refrigerator or at room temperature.

Lunesta

Generic name: Eszopiclone

What is this medication?

Lunesta is a medicine used to treat a sleep problem called insomnia.

What is the most important information I should know about this medication?

- Lunesta is a federally controlled substance because it can be abused or lead to dependence. Keep Lunesta in a safe place to prevent misuse and abuse. Selling or giving away Lunesta may harm others, and is against the law. Tell your doctor if you have ever abused or been dependent on alcohol, prescription medicines, or street drugs.
- After taking Lunesta, you may get up out of bed while not being fully awake and do an activity (such as "sleep driving," preparing

and eating food, making phone calls, or having sex) that you
do not know you are doing. The next morning, you may not
remember that you did anything during the night. You have a
higher chance for doing these activities if you drink alcohol or
take other medicines that make you sleepy with Lunesta.

- Tell your doctor if your insomnia worsens or is not better within
7-10 days. This may mean that there is another condition causing your sleep problem.

- Do not take Lunesta unless you are able to get a full night's sleep
before you must be active again.

- Tell your doctor right away if you notice any unusual changes
in your thinking or behavior such as hallucinations, amnesia,
agitation, a lack of inhibition, depression, or suicidal thinking.

- Lunesta is used only for the temporary relief of insomnia; sleep
medicines tend to lose their effect when taken for more than
a few weeks. Taking sleeping pills for extended periods, or in
high doses, can lead to physical dependence and the danger of
a withdrawal reaction when the medication is abruptly stopped.

- Lunesta works quickly, and can impair your ability to perform
activities that require complete mental alertness or coordination
of movements. Do not drive or do other dangerous activities
after taking Lunesta until you feel fully awake.

- Some people have experienced a severe allergic reaction from
taking Lunesta, including swelling of the tongue or throat, trouble breathing, and nausea and vomiting. Tell your doctor or seek
emergency medical help right away if you develop these symptoms after taking Lunesta.

Who should not take this medication?

Do not take Lunesta if you are allergic to it or any of its ingredients.

Do not take Lunesta if you cannot get a full night's sleep.

Do not take Lunesta if you drink alcohol or take other medicines
that can make you sleepy.

What should I tell my doctor before I take the first dose of this medication?

Tell your doctor about all prescription, over-the-counter, and herbal medications you are taking before beginning treatment with Lunesta. Also, talk to your doctor about your complete medical history, especially if you have a history of depression, mental illness, suicidal thoughts, or drug or alcohol abuse or addiction; have liver disease; or are pregnant, plan to become pregnant, or are breastfeeding.

What is the usual dosage?
Please see general statement regarding dosage on page xii.

Adults: The recommended starting dose is 2 milligrams (mg) once a day at bedtime. Your doctor may increase your dose to 3 mg once a day, depending on how Lunesta affects you.

If you have liver impairment or are taking certain medications that interact with Lunesta, your doctor will adjust your dose appropriately.

Elderly: The recommended dose is 1 mg once a day at bedtime if you have difficulty falling asleep, and 2 mg once a day at bedtime if you have difficulty staying asleep.

How should I take this medication?
- Take Lunesta exactly as prescribed by your doctor. Do not take extra doses or take it more often than prescribed for you.
- Take Lunesta right before you go to bed.

What should I avoid while taking this medication?

Do not drive or do other dangerous activities after taking Lunesta until you feel fully awake.

Do not drink alcohol or take other medications that can make you sleepy while you are taking Lunesta.

Do not take Lunesta with or right after a meal.

What are possible food and drug interactions associated with this medication?

If Lunesta is taken with certain other drugs, the effects of either could be increased, decreased, or altered. It is especially important to check with your doctor before combining Lunesta with the following: alcohol, clarithromycin, itraconazole, ketoconazole, nefazodone, nelfinavir, olanzapine, other medications that can make you sleepy, ritonavir, rifampicin, or troleandomycin.

What are the possible side effects of this medication?

Please see general statement regarding side effects on page xiii.

Side effects may include: abnormal thoughts and behavior, allergic reactions, anxiety, dizziness, drowsiness, dry mouth, headache, memory loss, symptoms of the common cold, unpleasant taste in your mouth

Can I receive this medication if I am pregnant or breastfeeding?

The effects of Lunesta during pregnancy and breastfeeding are unknown. Tell your doctor immediately if you are pregnant, plan to become pregnant, or are breastfeeding.

What should I do if I miss a dose of this medication?

Lunesta should be taken under special circumstances determined by your doctor.

How should I store this medication?

Store at room temperature.

Lyrica
Generic name: Pregabalin

What is this medication?

Lyrica is a medicine used to treat seizures, pain from damaged nerves (neuropathic pain) that occurs from diabetes, shingles (painful rash caused by chickenpox virus), or spinal cord injury. Lyrica is also used to treat fibromyalgia (widespread muscle pain and weakness).

What is the most important information I should know about this medication?

- Do not stop taking Lyrica suddenly or without talking to your doctor.
- Lyrica can cause serious allergic reactions. Stop taking Lyrica and call your doctor if you experience swelling of your face, mouth, lips, tongue, gums, or neck; trouble breathing; or rash, hives, or blisters.
- Lyrica can rarely cause suicidal thoughts or actions in a very small number of people. If you have suicidal thoughts or actions, do not stop Lyrica without first talking to your doctor. Pay attention to any sudden changes in mood, behaviors, thoughts, or feelings; call your doctor right away if you have any such changes, especially if they are new, worse, or worry you.
- Lyrica may cause swelling of your hands, legs, and feet. This swelling may be a serious problem for people with heart problems.
- Tell your doctor immediately if you experience muscle problems, muscle pain, soreness, or weakness, especially if you feel sick and have a fever. Call your doctor if you have any changes in your eyesight, including blurred vision.

Who should not take this medication?

Do not take Lyrica if you are allergic to it or any of its ingredients.

What should I tell my doctor before I take the first dose of this medication?

Tell your doctor about all prescription, over-the-counter, and herbal medications you are taking before beginning treatment with Lyrica. Also, talk to your doctor about your complete medical history, especially if you have a history of depression, drug or alcohol abuse, angioedema (a condition involving swelling of the face, extremities, eyes, lips, and tongue), have kidney or heart problems, a bleeding problem or a low blood platelet count, diabetes, or are pregnant, plan to become pregnant, or are breastfeeding. Additionally, if you are a male planning to father a child, inform your doctor.

What is the usual dosage?
Please see general statement regarding dosage on page xii.

Adults: Your doctor will prescribe the appropriate dose for you based on your condition.

If you have kidney impairment, your doctor will adjust your dose appropriately.

How should I take this medication?
• Take Lyrica at the same time every day. Take it with or without food.

What should I avoid while taking this medication?
Lyrica can cause dizziness, sleepiness, fatigue, and blurred vision. Do not drive or operate machinery until you know how Lyrica affects you.

Do not drink alcohol or take medications that may cause you to feel sleepy or tired. Lyrica and alcohol, when taken together, can increase side effects, such as sleepiness and dizziness.

Do not stop taking Lyrica suddenly, because you may get headaches, nausea, diarrhea, or have trouble sleeping. Also, you may experience more frequent seizures if you already have a seizure disorder. If you need to stop taking Lyrica, your doctor will tell you how to slowly stop taking it.

What are possible food and drug interactions associated with this medication?
If Lyrica is taken with certain other drugs, the effects of either could be increased, decreased, or altered. It is especially important to check with your doctor before combining Lyrica with the following: angiotensin-converting enzyme (ACE) inhibitors (such as lisinopril), diabetes medicines known as thiazolidinediones (such as pioglitazone), or other medications that slow down your brain function (such as alprazolam, clonazepam, or phenobarbital).

What are the possible side effects of this medication?
Please see general statement regarding side effects on page xiii.

> **Side effects may include:** abnormal thinking, blurred vision, difficulty concentrating, dizziness, dry mouth, edema (swelling), sleepiness, tiredness, weight gain

Can I receive this medication if I am pregnant or breastfeeding?
The effects of Lyrica during pregnancy and breastfeeding are unknown. Tell your doctor immediately if you are pregnant, plan to become pregnant, or are breastfeeding.

What should I do if I miss a dose of this medication?
If you miss a dose of Lyrica, take it as soon as you remember. However, if it is almost time for your next dose, skip the one you missed and return to your regular dosing schedule. Do not take two doses at once.

How should I store this medication?
Store at room temperature.

Macrodantin
Generic name: Nitrofurantoin Macrocrystals

What is this medication?
Macrodantin is an antibiotic used to treat certain bacterial infections of the urinary tract.

What is the most important information I should know about this medication?
- Macrodantin can cause serious side effects, including lung problems, liver or blood disorders, and damage to your nerves. Your doctor will monitor you for these conditions.
- Macrodantin can cause diarrhea or colitis (inflammation of the colon). This can occur a couple of months after receiving the

last dose of Macrodantin. Tell your doctor right away if you have diarrhea or colitis.
- Take Macrodantin as prescribed by your doctor for the full course of treatment, even if symptoms improve earlier. Do not skip doses. Skipping doses or not completing the full course of Macrodantin can decrease its effectiveness and can lead to growth of bacteria that are resistant to the effects of Macrodantin.
- Macrodantin can cause false-positive reactions when testing for the presence of sugar in the urine using certain testing devices.

Who should not take this medication?

Do not take Macrodantin if you are unable to produce urine, produce a small amount of urine, have significant kidney impairment, or have a history of jaundice (yellowing of the skin or whites of the eyes) or liver problems associated with nitrofurantoin.

Do not take Macrodantin if you are allergic to it or any of its ingredients.

Do not take Macrodantin during the late stages of your pregnancy or labor and delivery.

What should I tell my doctor before I take the first dose of this medication?

Tell your doctor about all prescription, over-the-counter, and herbal medications you are taking before beginning treatment with Macrodantin. Also, talk to your doctor about your complete medical history, especially if you have kidney or liver disease, anemia, diabetes, electrolyte (chemicals that are important for the cells in your body to function, such as sodium and potassium) imbalances, vitamin B deficiency, debilitating diseases, are pregnant, plan to become pregnant, or are breastfeeding.

What is the usual dosage?

Please see general statement regarding dosage on page xii.

Adults: The recommended dose is 50-100 milligrams (mg) four times a day.

Children ≥1 month: Your doctor will prescribe the appropriate dose for your child, based on their weight.

How should I take this medication?
- Take Macrodantin exactly as prescribed by your doctor. You can take Macrodantin with food to improve its absorption.

What should I avoid while taking this medication?
Do not take antacid preparations containing magnesium trisilicate while taking Macrodantin.

What are possible food and drug interactions associated with this medication?
If Macrodantin is taken with certain other drugs, the effects of either could be increased, decreased, or altered. It is especially important to check with your doctor before combining Macrodantin with antacids containing magnesium trisilicate, probenecid, or sulfinpyrazone.

What are the possible side effects of this medication?
Please see general statement regarding side effects on page xiii.

Side effects may include: allergic reactions, changes in sensation, changes in vision, chest pain, chills, colitis, cough, diarrhea, difficulty breathing, dizziness, drowsiness, fever, headache, jaundice, loss of appetite, motion sickness, nausea, rash, vomiting, weakness

---

Can I receive this medication if I am pregnant or breastfeeding?
The effects of Macrodantin during pregnancy are unknown. Macrodantin can be found in your breast milk if you take it while breastfeeding. Tell your doctor if you are pregnant, plan to become pregnant, or are breastfeeding.

What should I do if I miss a dose of this medication?
If you miss a dose of Macrodantin, take it as soon as you remember. However, if it is almost time for your next dose, skip the one

you missed and return to your regular dosing schedule. Do not take two doses at once.

How should I store this medication?
Store at room temperature.

Maxzide
Generic name: Hydrochlorothiazide/Triamterene

What is this medication?
Maxzide is a combination of two diuretics (water pills) used to treat high blood pressure and other conditions that require the elimination of the excess of fluid from the body. It can be used alone or together with other blood pressure lowering medications. Maxzide is also available as Maxzide-25 MG.

What is the most important information I should know about this medication?
• Maxzide can cause high blood potassium levels. This is more likely to occur if you are elderly, severely ill, or have kidney problems or diabetes. Your doctor will monitor your blood potassium levels.
• Maxzide can cause nearsightedness and angle-closure glaucoma (high pressure in the eye). Stop taking Maxzide and tell your doctor immediately if you experience abnormal visual changes or eye pain.
• Your doctor will perform regular blood tests to check your fluids and electrolytes (chemicals that are important for the cells in your body to function, such as sodium and potassium). Tell your doctor if you experience dry mouth, thirst, weakness, fatigue, drowsiness, restlessness, muscle pain or cramps, low blood pressure, decreased urination, fast heart rate, nausea, or vomiting.
• Maxzide can cause gout (severe and painful inflammation of the joints).

Who should not take this medication?

Do not take Maxzide if you are allergic to it, any of its ingredients, or to other sulfonamide medications (such as sulfamethoxazole).

Do not take Maxzide if you have high blood potassium levels, kidney disease, or if you are unable to produce urine.

Do not take Maxzide if you are taking potassium-containing salt substitutes, potassium supplements, or other medications that prevent potassium loss (such as spironolactone or amiloride).

What should I tell my doctor before I take the first dose of this medication?

Tell your doctor about all prescription, over-the-counter, and herbal medications you are taking before beginning treatment with Maxzide. Also, talk to your doctor about your complete medical history, especially if you have allergies; asthma; diabetes; gout; kidney, liver, or thyroid problems; or if you have systemic lupus erythematosus (disease that affects the immune system).

What is the usual dosage?

Please see general statement regarding dosage on page xii.

Maxzide Tablets

Adults: The usual dose is one tablet once a day.

Maxzide-25 MG Tablets

Adults: The usual dose is one or two tablets once a day.

How should I take this medication?

• Take Maxzide exactly as prescribed by your doctor.

What should I avoid while taking this medication?

Do not take salt substitutes that contain potassium, potassium supplements, or any medicines that prevent potassium loss while you are taking Maxzide.

What are possible food and drug interactions associated with this medication?

If Maxzide is taken with certain other drugs, the effects of either could be increased, decreased, or altered. It is especially important to check with your doctor before combining Maxzide with the following: alcohol, amiloride, amphotericin B, barbiturates (such as phenobarbital), blood pressure/heart medications known as angiotensin-converting enzyme (ACE) inhibitors (such as enalapril), corticosteroids (such as prednisone), lithium, narcotic painkillers (such as hydrocodone or oxycodone), nonsteroidal anti-inflammatory drugs (NSAIDs) (such as indomethacin), norepinephrine, other blood pressure medications, potassium-containing salt substitutes, potassium supplements, spironolactone, or tubocurarine.

What are the possible side effects of this medication?

Please see general statement regarding side effects on page xiii.

> **Side effects may include:** anaphylaxis (a serious and rapid allergic reaction that may result in death if not immediately treated), anemia, change in blood potassium levels, constipation, decreased sexual performance, diarrhea, dry mouth, fast heart rate, fatigue, headache, hives, increased blood sugar levels, kidney stones, muscle cramps, nausea, rash, sensitivity to sunlight, sudden fall in blood pressure, vomiting, weakness, yellowing of your skin or whites of your eyes

Can I receive this medication if I am pregnant or breastfeeding?

The effects of Maxzide during pregnancy are unknown. Maxzide can be found in your breast milk if you take it while breastfeeding. Do not breastfeed while you are taking Maxzide. Tell your doctor immediately if you are pregnant, plan to become pregnant, or are breastfeeding.

What should I do if I miss a dose of this medication?

If you miss a dose of Maxzide, take it as soon as you remember. However, if it is almost time for your next dose, skip the one you

missed and return to your regular dosing schedule. Do not take two doses at once.

How should I store this medication?
Store at room temperature. Protect from light.

Meclizine HCl: see Antivert, page 82

Medrol
Generic name: Methylprednisolone

What is this medication?
Medrol is a steroid medicine used when your adrenal glands do not make enough hormones that help your body respond to stress or regulate your blood pressure, and water and salt intake. Medrol can also be used for conditions affecting many different parts of your body, including your skin, stomach or intestines, blood, nervous system, eyes, kidneys, lungs, or glands. In addition, this medication can be used to treat severe allergies, sudden worsening of multiple sclerosis, arthritis, or certain cancers.

What is the most important information I should know about this medication?
- Medrol can cause increased blood pressure, salt and water retention in your body, or decreased blood potassium level. Your doctor will check your blood pressure and electrolyte levels (chemicals that are important for the cells in your body to function, such as sodium and potassium) while you are taking Medrol.
- Medrol can mask some signs of infection, making it difficult for your doctor to diagnose it. Also, Medrol can lower your resistance to infections and make them harder to treat. Tell your doctor if you develop fever or other signs of infection.
- Do not expose yourself to chickenpox or measles while you are taking Medrol. This can be very serious and even fatal in children and adults who have not had chickenpox or measles. Also,

Medrol can reactivate an inactive case of tuberculosis (a bacterial infection that affects the lungs).

- Cataracts (clouding of the eye's lens), glaucoma (high pressure in the eye), other eye problems, or eye infections can occur while you are taking Medrol.

Who should not take this medication?

Do not take Medrol if you are allergic to it or any of its ingredients, or if you have a fungal infection.

What should I tell my doctor before I take the first dose of this medication?

Tell your doctor about all prescription, over-the-counter, and herbal medications you are taking before beginning treatment with Medrol. Also, talk to your doctor about your complete medical history, especially if you have any infections, cataracts, glaucoma, certain eye infections, tuberculosis, heart problems, high blood pressure, kidney or liver problems, thyroid problems, psychiatric conditions, ulcerative colitis (inflammatory disease of the large intestine), other intestinal problems, stomach ulcers, osteoporosis (thin, weak bones), myasthenia gravis (a disease characterized by long-lasting fatigue and muscle weakness), or diabetes.

What is the usual dosage?

Please see general statement regarding dosage on page xii.

Adults and children: Your doctor will prescribe the appropriate dose for you or your child based on your condition.

How should I take this medication?

- Take Medrol exactly as prescribed by your doctor.

What should I avoid while taking this medication?

Do not become exposed to chickenpox or measles.

Do not receive any live vaccines while you are taking Medrol.

Do not change your dose or stop taking Medrol without first talking to your doctor.

What are possible food and drug interactions associated with this medication?

If Medrol is taken with certain other drugs, the effects of either could be increased, decreased, or altered. It is especially important to tell your doctor if you are taking any of the following prior to treatment with Medrol: aspirin, blood thinners (such as warfarin), cyclosporine, ketoconazole, phenobarbital, phenytoin, rifampin, or troleandomycin.

What are the possible side effects of this medication?

Please see general statement regarding side effects on page xiii.

> **Side effects may include:** allergic reactions, decrease in blood potassium levels, eye problems, facial redness, headache, heart problems, high blood sugar levels, impaired wound healing, increase in blood pressure, intestinal or stomach problems, irregular menstrual periods, muscle weakness, osteoporosis

Can I receive this medication if I am pregnant or breastfeeding?

The effects of Medrol during pregnancy and breastfeeding are unknown. Tell your doctor immediately if you are pregnant, plan to become pregnant, or are breastfeeding.

What should I do if I miss a dose of this medication?

If you miss a dose of Medrol, take it as soon as you remember. However, if it is almost time for your next dose, skip the one you missed and return to your regular dosing schedule. Do not take two doses at once.

How should I store this medication?

Store at room temperature.

Medroxyprogesterone Acetate: *see Provera, page 868*

Megace

Generic name: Megestrol Acetate

What is this medication?

Megace is a medicine used to treat loss of appetite, malnutrition, or unexplained or significant weight loss in patients diagnosed with AIDS. It is available as Megace and Megace ES.

What is the most important information I should know about this medication?

- Megace can harm your unborn baby if you use it during pregnancy. If you are a woman who can become pregnant, use a reliable method of birth control during treatment with Megace. If you accidentally become pregnant, tell your doctor right away.
- Prolonged use of Megace can cause diabetes, Cushing's syndrome (a hormone disorder), and reduced adrenal function. Signs and symptoms of reduced adrenal function include low blood pressure, nausea, vomiting, dizziness, or weakness.
- Megace can cause breakthrough vaginal bleeding in women.
- Megace ES does not contain the same amount of medicine as Megace.

Who should not take this medication?

Do not take Megace if you are allergic to it or any of its ingredients, or if you are pregnant, plan to become pregnant, or are breastfeeding.

What should I tell my doctor before I take the first dose of this medication?

Tell your doctor about all prescription, over-the-counter, and herbal medications you are taking before beginning treatment with Megace. Also, talk to your doctor about your complete medical history, especially if you have a blood clotting disorder, Cushing's syndrome, reduced adrenal function, or diabetes.

What is the usual dosage?

Please see general statement regarding dosage on page xii.

Megace
Adults: The recommended initial dose is 800 milligrams (mg) (20 milliliters [mL]) a day.

Megace ES
Adults: The recommended initial dose is 625 mg (5 mL or one teaspoon) a day.

How should I take this medication?
- Take Megace exactly as prescribed by your doctor.
- Shake the container well before you take the medicine.
- If you are taking Megace, a measuring cup with 10 mL and 20 mL markings is provided to you.

What should I avoid while taking this medication?
Do not become pregnant while you are taking Megace.

What are possible food and drug interactions associated with this medication?
If Megace is taken with certain other drugs, the effects of either could be increased, decreased, or altered. It is especially important to check with your doctor before combining Megace with indinavir.

What are the possible side effects of this medication?
Please see general statement regarding side effects on page xiii.

Side effects may include: anemia, decreased sex drive, diarrhea, fever, gas, headache, high blood sugar levels, impotence, increased blood pressure, lack of strength, nausea, rash, sleeplessness, upset stomach, vomiting

---

Can I receive this medication if I am pregnant or breastfeeding?
Do not take Megace if you are pregnant or breastfeeding. Tell your doctor immediately if you are pregnant, plan to become pregnant, or are breastfeeding.

What should I do if I miss a dose of this medication?

If you miss a dose of Megace, take it as soon as you remember. However, if it is almost time for your next dose, skip the one you missed and return to your regular dosing schedule. Do not take two doses at once.

How should I store this medication?

Store at room temperature. Protect from heat.

Megestrol Acetate: *see Megace, page 612*

Meloxicam: *see Mobic, page 646*

Memantine HCl: *see Namenda, page 668*

Memantine HCl: *see Namenda XR, page 671*

Metaxalone: *see Skelaxin, page 938*

Metformin HCl: *see Glucophage, page 421*

Metformin HCl/Pioglitazone HCl: *see Actoplus Met, page 18*

Metformin HCl/Sitagliptin: *see Janumet, page 488*

Metformin HCl/Sitagliptin: *see Janumet XR, page 491*

Methadone HCl: *see Methadose, page 614*

Methadose

Generic name: Methadone HCl

What is this medication?

Methadose is a medicine that contains the narcotic painkiller methadone. Methadose is used to control withdrawal symptoms during detoxification of opioid dependence. It is also used for maintenance treatment of opioid dependence. Methadose is available as tablets, a liquid, and a sugar free liquid. Methadose tablets are also used to treat moderate to severe around-the-clock pain.

Methadose is a federally controlled narcotic with potential for abuse.

What is the most important information I should know about this medication?

- Methadose has abuse potential. Mental and physical dependence can occur with the use of Methadose when it is used improperly.
- Methadose can cause life-threatening breathing and heart problems. Tell your doctor or get medical help right away if you experience trouble breathing; extreme drowsiness and your breathing slows down; slow shallow breathing (little chest movement with breathing); fast, slow, or irregular heartbeat; or if you feel faint, very dizzy, or confused.
- Methadose can cause your blood pressure to drop, making you feel dizzy if you get up too fast from sitting or lying down.

Who should not take this medication?

Do not take Methadose if you are allergic to it or any of its ingredients.

Do not take Methadose if you have a blockage or narrowing of your stomach or intestines, or if you have severe asthma or other lung problems.

What should I tell my doctor before I take the first dose of this medication?

Tell your doctor about all prescription, over-the-counter, and herbal medications you are taking before beginning treatment with Methadose. Also, talk to your doctor about your complete medical history, especially if you have ever had head injury, seizures, problems urinating, pancreas or gallbladder problems, mental health problems, lung or breathing problems, or heart, liver, kidney, or thyroid problems. Also, tell your doctor if you have a history of alcohol or drug abuse.

What is the usual dosage?

Please see general statement regarding dosage on page xii.

Adults: Your doctor will prescribe the appropriate dose for you and adjust your dose based on your condition, previous treatment with painkillers, and your tolerance for narcotics.

How should I take this medication?

- Take Methadose exactly as prescribed by your doctor. Do not change your dose or stop taking Methadose without first talking to your doctor.
- When you stop taking Methadose, flush the remaining tablets down the toilet.

What should I avoid while taking this medication?

Do not drive or operate heavy machinery until you know how Methadose affects you.

Do not drink alcohol or take prescription or over-the-counter medicines that contain alcohol while you are taking Methadose.

What are possible food and drug interactions associated with this medication?

If Methadose is taken with certain other drugs, the effects of either could be increased, decreased, or altered. Methadose may interact with numerous medications. Therefore, it is very important that you tell your doctor about any other medications you are taking.

What are the possible side effects of this medication?

Please see general statement regarding side effects on page xiii.

Side effects may include: constipation, dizziness, drowsiness, headache, lightheadedness, nausea, sleepiness, sweating, tiredness, vomiting

Can I receive this medication if I am pregnant or breastfeeding?

The effects of Methadose during pregnancy are unknown. Methadose can be found in your breast milk if you take it while breastfeeding. Tell your doctor immediately if you are pregnant, plan to become pregnant, or are breastfeeding.

What should I do if I miss a dose of this medication?

If you take Methadose for pain and miss a dose, take it as soon as you remember. However, if it is almost time for your next dose, skip the one you missed and return to your regular dosing schedule. Do not take two doses at once.

If you take Methadose for opioid addiction and miss a dose, take your next dose on the following day as scheduled.

How should I store this medication?

Store at room temperature. Protect from light.

Methimazole: *see Tapazole, page 964*

Methocarbamol: *see Robaxin, page 908*

Methotrexate

Generic name: Methotrexate

What is this medication?

Methotrexate is a medicine used to treat certain cancers of the uterus, breast, head and neck, or lung; or to treat certain types of blood cancer or lymphomas. Also, methotrexate is used to treat the symptoms of severe psoriasis (immune disorder that affects the skin). It is also used to manage severe, active rheumatoid arthritis (a type of arthritis that involves inflammation of the joints) or arthritis in children who had an insufficient response to other treatments for arthritis. Methotrexate is available in tablets or is administered intramuscularly (injected into the muscle), intravenously (through a vein in your arm), or intrathecally (within the spinal canal).

What is the most important information I should know about this medication?

- Methotrexate decreases your blood cell counts (such as white blood cells, platelets [type of blood cells that form clots to help stop bleeding], and red blood cells). Tell your doctor right away if you develop a fever, other signs of infection (such as chills, cough, or burning pain on urination), or bleeding while on methotrexate therapy. Your doctor will perform frequent blood tests while you are taking methotrexate to monitor your blood counts.

- Methotrexate can cause intestinal or stomach toxicity, especially if you take it with nonsteroidal anti-inflammatory drugs (NSAIDs). It can also cause diarrhea, ulcers, stomach bleeding, or liver problems, especially if you receive it for a long time. Your doctor will monitor you for these symptoms.

- Methotrexate can cause lung toxicity or severe skin reactions, which can occur any time during treatment with methotrexate. Tell your doctor right away if you develop breathing problems, especially a dry cough, or rash.

- Methotrexate can cause harm to your unborn baby. Do not become pregnant while receiving treatment with methotrexate and for 1 month afterwards, and use effective forms of birth control during this time. Men should also not father a child while receiving treatment with methotrexate and for 3 months afterwards. During this time, men with female partners of childbearing potential should use effective forms of birth control.

Who should not take this medication?

Do not take methotrexate if you are allergic to it or any of its ingredients.

Do not take methotrexate if you are pregnant, plan to become pregnant, or are breastfeeding.

If you have psoriasis or rheumatoid arthritis, do not take methotrexate if you have a history of alcoholism, long-term liver disease, conditions that weaken your immune system, blood problems or your bone marrow does not make enough blood cells.

What should I tell my doctor before I take the first dose of this medication?

Tell your doctor about all prescription, over-the-counter, and herbal medications you are taking before beginning treatment with methotrexate. Also, talk to your doctor about your complete medical history, especially if you have kidney problems or are receiving dialysis; liver problems; fluid in your stomach area; lung problems, including fluid in your lungs; or are pregnant, plan to become pregnant, or are breastfeeding.

What is the usual dosage?
Please see general statement regarding dosage on page xii.

Your doctor might prescribe different doses than those listed below based on your condition and its severity.

Cancer
Adults: Your doctor will administer the appropriate dose for you based on your height, weight, and type of cancer.

Psoriasis
Adults: The recommended starting dose is 10-25 milligrams (mg) once a week, or 2.5 mg every 12 hours for 3 doses once a week.

Rheumatoid Arthritis
Adults: The recommended starting dose is 7.5 mg once a week, or 2.5 mg every 12 hours for 3 doses once a week.

Juvenile Rheumatoid Arthritis
Children 2-16 years: Your doctor will prescribe the appropriate dose for your child, based on their weight.

How should I take this medication?
- Take methotrexate exactly as prescribed by your doctor. Do not take more methotrexate than prescribed without talking to your doctor.

- For severe psoriasis, rheumatoid arthritis, and juvenile rheumatoid arthritis, methotrexate should be taken weekly, not every day. If you take too much methotrexate, call your doctor or seek emergency medical help right away.
- Your doctor will administer methotrexate intramuscularly, intravenously, or intrathecally to you.

What should I avoid while taking this medication?

Do not become pregnant or breastfeed while being treated with methotrexate.

Do not drink alcohol or receive certain live vaccines.

Do not miss your scheduled follow-up appointments with your doctor.

What are possible food and drug interactions associated with this medication?

If methotrexate is taken with certain other drugs, the effects of either could be increased, decreased, or altered. It is especially important to check with your doctor before combining methotrexate with the following: certain antibiotics (such as chloramphenicol, penicillins, tetracycline, or trimethoprim/sulfamethoxazole), certain medications that can cause liver toxicity (such as azathioprine, retinoids, or sulfasalazine), NSAIDs, phenylbutazone, phenytoin, probenecid, salicylates, or theophylline.

What are the possible side effects of this medication?

Please see general statement regarding side effects on page xiii.

Side effects may include: abdominal distress, chills, decreased white blood cell count, dizziness, fever, infection, inflammation of the lining in your mouth, nausea, rash, tiredness

---

Can I receive this medication if I am pregnant or breastfeeding?

Methotrexate can cause harm to your baby if you take it during pregnancy or breastfeeding. Do not take methotrexate if you are pregnant or breastfeeding. Tell your doctor immediately if you are pregnant, plan to become pregnant, or are breastfeeding.

What should I do if I miss a dose of this medication?

If you miss a dose of methotrexate, take it as soon as you remember. However, if it is almost time for your next dose, skip the one you missed and return to your regular dosing schedule. Do not take two doses at once.

Methotrexate injection should be given under special circumstances determined by your doctor. If you miss your scheduled appointment, contact your doctor for advice.

How should I store this medication?

Store at room temperature.

Your doctor will store methotrexate injection for you.

Methotrexate: *see Methotrexate, page 617*

Methylphenidate HCl: *see Concerta, page 261*

Methylphenidate HCl: *see Ritalin, page 905*

Methylprednisolone: *see Medrol, page 609*

Metoclopramide

Generic name: Metoclopramide

What is this medication?

Metoclopramide is a medicine used as a short-term treatment to relieve the heartburn symptoms of gastroesophageal reflux disease (GERD) when certain other treatments do not work. Also, metoclopramide is used to relieve the symptoms of diabetic gastroparesis (slow stomach emptying in people with diabetes). Metoclopramide

tablets can also be found under the brand name Reglan. Metoclopramide is also available as a suspension.

What is the most important information I should know about this medication?

- Metoclopramide can cause tardive dyskinesia (abnormal muscle movements, including tremor, shuffling, and uncontrolled,
  involuntary movements) which happens mostly in your face
  muscles. Also, metoclopramide can cause uncontrolled spasms
  of your muscles or Parkinson's-like symptoms. Tell your doctor immediately if you have movements that you cannot stop or
  control (such as lip smacking or puckering, chewing, frowning
  or scowling, sticking out your tongue, blinking and moving your
  eyes, body stiffness, or shaking of your arms and legs).
- In rare cases, metoclopramide can cause neuroleptic malignant
  syndrome (NMS) (a life-threatening brain disorder). NMS is a
  medical emergency. Tell your doctor immediately if you experience a high fever, muscle rigidity, confusion, fast or irregular
  heartbeats, or sweating more than usual.
- Metoclopramide can cause serious side effects, such as depression or thoughts about suicide, high blood pressure, or excessive body water. Tell your doctor if you have or had a history of
  depression or mental illness, high blood pressure, liver problems, heart failure or heart rhythm problems.
- After you stop taking metoclopramide, you can experience
  withdrawal symptoms, such as dizziness, nervousness, or
  headaches.

Who should not take this medication?

Do not take metoclopramide if you are allergic to it or any of its
ingredients.

Do not take metoclopramide if you have stomach or intestine
problems, pheochromocytoma (tumor of the adrenal gland), or
seizures.

Do not take metoclopramide if you take other medicines that can
cause uncontrolled movements.

What should I tell my doctor before I take the first dose of this medication?

Tell your doctor about all prescription, over-the-counter, and herbal medications you are taking before beginning treatment with metoclopramide. Also, talk to your doctor about your complete medical history, especially if you have kidney or liver disease, depression or mental illness, high blood pressure, heart failure or heart rhythm problems, diabetes, breast cancer, or Parkinson's disease.

What is the usual dosage?

Please see general statement regarding dosage on page xii.

GERD

Adults: The recommended dose is 10-15 milligrams (mg) 30 minutes before each meal and at bedtime. Do not take metoclopramide more than four times a day. Your doctor will prescribe the appropriate dose for you based on your condition.

Diabetic Gastroparesis

Adults: The recommended dose is 10 mg 30 minutes before each meal and at bedtime for 2-8 weeks.

If you have kidney impairment, your doctor will adjust your dose appropriately.

How should I take this medication?

- Take metoclopramide exactly as prescribed by your doctor. Do not take metoclopramide for more than 12 weeks.

What should I avoid while taking this medication?

Do not drink alcohol while you are taking metoclopramide. Alcohol can worsen some side effects, such as feeling sleepy.

Do not drive, work with machines, or engage in dangerous tasks until you know how metoclopramide affects you. This medication can cause sleepiness.

What are possible food and drug interactions associated with this medication?

If metoclopramide is taken with certain other drugs, the effects of either could be increased, decreased, or altered. It is especially important to check with your doctor before combining metoclopramide with the following: acetaminophen, alcohol, anticholinergics (such as atropine or oxybutynin), cyclosporine, digoxin, insulin, levodopa, monoamine oxidase inhibitors (MAOIs), a class of drugs used to treat depression and other psychiatric conditions (such as phenelzine), narcotic painkillers (such as hydrocodone or oxycodone), other medicines that contain metoclopramide (such as Reglan ODT), sedatives (such as lorazepam or phenobarbital), tetracycline, or tranquilizers (such as chlorpromazine).

What are the possible side effects of this medication?

Please see general statement regarding side effects on page xiii.

> **Side effects may include:** confusion, dizziness, feeling exhausted, headache, restlessness, sleepiness, tiredness, trouble sleeping

Can I receive this medication if I am pregnant or breastfeeding?

The effects of metoclopramide during pregnancy are unknown. Metoclopramide can be found in your breast milk if you take it while breastfeeding. Tell your doctor immediately if you are pregnant, plan to become pregnant, or are breastfeeding.

What should I do if I miss a dose of this medication?

If you miss a dose of metoclopramide, take it as soon as you remember. However, if it is almost time for your next dose, skip the one you missed and return to your regular dosing schedule. Do not take two doses at once.

How should I store this medication?

Store at room temperature.

Metoclopramide: see Metoclopramide, page 621

Metoprolol Succinate: see Toprol-XL, page 1006

Metoprolol Tartrate: see Lopressor, page 575

Metrogel-Vaginal
Generic name: Metronidazole

What is this medication?
Metrogel-Vaginal is a vaginal cream used to treat certain bacterial vaginal infections in women.

What is the most important information I should know about this medication?
- Metrogel-Vaginal is not for use in your eyes, mouth, or skin.
- Metrogel-Vaginal can cause seizures and peripheral neuropathy (a condition characterized by a sensation of numbness or tingling of your hands and feet). If you experience abnormal nerve symptoms, stop using Metrogel-Vaginal and tell your doctor immediately.
- Metrogel-Vaginal can cause burning and irritation of your eyes. If Metrogel-Vaginal accidentally gets in contact with your eyes, rinse your eyes thoroughly with cool tap water.

Who should not take this medication?
Do not use Metrogel-Vaginal if you are allergic to it, any of its ingredients, or to similar products.

What should I tell my doctor before I take the first dose of this medication?
Tell your doctor about all prescription, over-the-counter, and herbal medications you are taking before beginning treatment with Metrogel-Vaginal. Also, talk to your doctor about your complete medical history, especially if you have a history of seizures, brain and spinal cord problems, liver problems, alcohol abuse, or are pregnant, plan to become pregnant, or are breastfeeding.

What is the usual dosage?
Please see general statement regarding dosage on page xii.

Adults: Insert 1 applicatorful into your vagina 1-2 times a day for 5 days.

How should I take this medication?
- Use Metrogel-Vaginal exactly as prescribed by your doctor. Do not apply extra doses or use more often without asking your doctor.
- Please review the instructions that came with your prescription on how to properly insert the applicator.
- If your doctor prescribed once a day dosing, use Metrogel-Vaginal at bedtime.

What should I avoid while taking this medication?
Do not use Metrogel-Vaginal if you have taken disulfiram within the last 2 weeks.

Do not drink alcohol while on Metrogel-Vaginal therapy.

Do not have vaginal intercourse during treatment with Metrogel-Vaginal.

What are possible food and drug interactions associated with this medication?
If Metrogel-Vaginal is used with certain other drugs, the effects of either could be increased, decreased, or altered. It is especially important to check with your doctor before combining Metrogel-Vaginal with the following: blood thinners (such as warfarin), disulfuram, cimetidine, or lithium.

What are the possible side effects of this medication?
Please see general statement regarding side effects on page xiii.

> **Side effects may include:** bloating, dry mouth, headache, inflammation of your vagina, irritation, itching, nausea, pelvic discomfort, rash, stomach discomfort, vaginal discharge, vaginal irritation, vomiting

Can I receive this medication if I am pregnant or breastfeeding?

The effects of Metrogel-Vaginal during pregnancy and breastfeeding are unknown. Tell your doctor immediately if you are pregnant, plan to become pregnant, or are breastfeeding.

What should I do if I miss a dose of this medication?

If you miss a dose of Metrogel-Vaginal, apply it as soon as you remember. However, if it is almost time for your next dose, skip the one you missed and return to your regular dosing schedule. Do not apply two doses at once.

How should I store this medication?

Store at room temperature, away from extreme heat or cold.

Metronidazole: *see Metrogel-Vaginal, page 625*

Mevacor

Generic name: Lovastatin

What is this medication?

Mevacor belongs to a class of medicines called "statins," which are used to lower your cholesterol when a low-fat diet is not enough. Mevacor lowers your total cholesterol and the "bad" low-density lipoprotein (LDL) cholesterol, thereby helping to slow the hardening of your arteries, lower your risk of a heart attack or unstable chest pain, or the need for procedures to restore the blood flow back to the heart or to another part of the body.

What is the most important information I should know about this medication?

- Taking Mevacor is not a substitute for following a healthy low-fat and low-cholesterol diet and exercising to lower your cholesterol.
- Do not take Mevacor if you are pregnant, think you may be pregnant, plan to become pregnant, or are breastfeeding.

- Mevacor can cause muscle pain, tenderness, weakness, fatigue, loss of appetite, right upper abdominal discomfort, dark urine, or yellowing of your skin or whites of your eyes. Call your doctor right away if you notice any of these symptoms.

Who should not take this medication?

Do not take Mevacor if you are allergic to it or any of its ingredients, or if you currently have liver disease. Also, do not take Mevacor in combination with anti-HIV medications (such as indinavir), boceprevir, clarithromycin, erythromycin, itraconazole, ketoconazole, nefazodone, posaconazole, telaprevir, or telithromycin.

Do not take Mevacor if you are pregnant, plan to become pregnant, or are breastfeeding.

What should I tell my doctor before I take the first dose of this medication?

Tell your doctor about all prescription, over-the-counter, and herbal medications you are taking before beginning treatment with Mevacor. Also, talk to your doctor about your complete medical history, especially if you drink excessive amounts of alcohol or you have liver, kidney, thyroid, or heart problems, muscle aches or weakness; or diabetes. Tell your doctor if you are pregnant, plan to become pregnant, or are breastfeeding.

What is the usual dosage?

Please see general statement regarding dosage on page xii.

Adults: The usual starting dose is 20 milligrams (mg) once a day in the evening. Your doctor will check your blood cholesterol levels during treatment with Mevacor and will change your dose based on the results.

Adolescents 10-17 years: The usual dose is 10-40 mg once a day in the evening. Your doctor will check your blood cholesterol levels during treatment with Mevacor and will change your dose based on the results.

If you have kidney impairment or you are taking other medications, your doctor will adjust your dose appropriately.

How should I take this medication?
- Your doctor will likely start you on a low-cholesterol diet before prescribing Mevacor. Stay on this diet while you are taking Mevacor.
- Take Mevacor with your evening meal.

What should I avoid while taking this medication?
Do not drink large amounts of grapefruit juice (>1 quart a day) while you are taking Mevacor.

What are possible food and drug interactions associated with this medication?
If Mevacor is taken with certain other drugs, the effects of either could be increased, decreased, or altered. It is especially important to check with your doctor before combining Mevacor with the following: alcohol, amiodarone, cholesterol-lowering medicines known as fibrates (such as fenofibrate or gemfibrozil), cimetidine, colchicine, cyclosporine, danazol, diltiazem, grapefruit juice, niacin, ranolazine, spironolactone, verapamil, or voriconazole.

What are the possible side effects of this medication?
Please see general statement regarding side effects on page xiii.

Side effects may include: constipation, gas, headache

Can I receive this medication if I am pregnant or breastfeeding?
Do not take Mevacor during pregnancy or breastfeeding. Tell your doctor immediately if you are pregnant, plan to become pregnant, or are breastfeeding.

What should I do if I miss a dose of this medication?
If you miss a dose of Mevacor, take it as soon as you remember. However, if it is almost time for your next dose, skip the one you

missed and return to your regular dosing schedule. Do not take two doses at once.

How should I store this medication?
Store at room temperature. Protect from light.

Micardis
Generic name: Telmisartan

What is this medication?
Micardis is a medicine used alone or in combination with other medications to treat high blood pressure. Micardis is also used to lower the risk of heart attack, stroke, or death from heart problems in people who are 55 years or older with high risk of developing heart problems.

What is the most important information I should know about this medication?
- Micardis can cause low blood pressure, especially if you take diuretics (water pills), are on a low-salt diet, or receive dialysis. If you feel faint or dizzy, lie down and call your doctor right away.
- Micardis can cause a serious allergic reaction. Tell your doctor right away if you experience swelling of your face, throat, or tongue; difficulty breathing; or skin rash.
- Micardis can worsen your kidney function if you already have kidney problems. Tell your doctor if you develop swelling in your feet, ankles, or hands, or unexplained weight gain.

Who should not take this medication?
Do not take Micardis if you are allergic to it or any of its ingredients. Do not take Micardis if you are pregnant, plan to become pregnant, or are breastfeeding.

What should I tell my doctor before I take the first dose of this medication?
Tell your doctor about all prescription, over-the-counter, and herbal medications you are taking before beginning treatment with

Micardis. Also, talk to your doctor about your complete medical history, especially if you have kidney, liver, or heart problems.

What is the usual dosage?
Please see general statement regarding dosage on page xii.

High Blood Pressure
Adults: The usual starting dose is 40 milligrams (mg) once a day. Your doctor will increase your dose as needed until the desired effect is achieved.

Heart Disease Risk Reduction
Adults: The usual dose is 80 mg once a day.

If you have liver impairment, your doctor will adjust your dose appropriately.

How should I take this medication?
• Take Micardis exactly as prescribed by your doctor. Take it at the same time every day, with or without food.

What should I avoid while taking this medication?
Do not become pregnant or breastfeed while you are taking Micardis.

Do not change your dose unless your doctor tells you to.

What are possible food and drug interactions associated with this medication?
If Micardis is taken with certain other drugs, the effects of either could be increased, decreased, or altered. It is especially important to check with your doctor before combining Micardis with the following: certain diuretics (such as amiloride, spironolactone, or triamterene), digoxin, lithium, nonsteroidal anti-inflammatory drugs (such as ibuprofen or naproxen), potassium supplements, ramipril, or salt substitutes that contain potassium.

What are the possible side effects of this medication?
Please see general statement regarding side effects on page xiii.

> **Side effects may include:** back pain, diarrhea, inflammation of your sinuses

Can I receive this medication if I am pregnant or breastfeeding?

Do not take Micardis if you are pregnant or breastfeeding. Micardis can harm your unborn baby. Tell your doctor immediately if you are pregnant, plan to become pregnant, or are breastfeeding.

What should I do if I miss a dose of this medication?

If you miss a dose of Micardis, take it as soon as you remember. However, if it is almost time for your next dose, skip the one you missed and return to your regular dosing schedule. Do not take two doses at once.

How should I store this medication?

Store at room temperature.

Micardis HCT

Generic name: Hydrochlorothiazide/Telmisartan

What is this medication?

Micardis HCT is a combination medicine used to treat high blood pressure. Micardis HCT contains two medicines: telmisartan (an angiotensin receptor blocker [ARB]) and hydrochlorothiazide (a diuretic [water pill]).

What is the most important information I should know about this medication?

- When taken during pregnancy, ARBs such as Micardis HCT can cause injury to the unborn baby. If you are pregnant or plan to become pregnant, stop taking Micardis HCT and contact your doctor right away.
- Micardis HCT can cause low blood pressure, especially if you take diuretics or are on a low-salt diet. If you feel faint or dizzy, lie down and call your doctor right away.

- Micardis HCT can cause an allergic reaction. Tell your doctor if you experience swelling of your face, lips, tongue, or throat.
- Micardis HCT can activate lupus (disease that affects the immune system) or gout (severe and painful inflammation of the joints) and increase cholesterol and triglyceride levels in certain patients.
- Micardis HCT can cause problems seeing objects that are farther away, as well as acute angle-closure glaucoma (high pressure in the eye). Tell your doctor immediately if you experience abnormal visual changes or eye pain.
- Micardis HCT can cause imbalances in fluids and electrolytes (chemicals that are important for the cells in your body to function, such as sodium and potassium). Signs and symptoms of this include dry mouth, thirst, weakness, fatigue, drowsiness, restlessness, confusion, seizures, muscle pain or cramps, low blood pressure, decreased urination, fast heart rate, nausea, and vomiting. Your doctor will monitor your blood electrolyte levels periodically during treatment with Micardis HCT.
- If you have diabetes, Micardis HCT can increase your blood sugar levels. Check your blood sugar frequently.

Who should not take this medication?

Do not take Micardis HCT if you are allergic to it or any of its ingredients, or to a sulfonamide-derived medication.

Do not take Micardis HCT if you are unable to produce urine.

What should I tell my doctor before I take the first dose of this medication?

Tell your doctor about all prescription, over-the-counter, and herbal medications you are taking before beginning treatment with Micardis HCT. Also, talk to your doctor if you have diabetes, heart failure, severe immune system problems, lupus, gout, asthma, or liver or kidney disease, or if you have ever had an allergy or sensitivity to an ARB or sulfonamide-derived medication.

What is the usual dosage?

Please see general statement regarding dosage on page xii.

Adults: The usual starting dose is 40/12.5 (40 milligrams [mg] of telmisartan and 12.5 mg of hydrochlorothiazide) once a day. Your doctor may give you a higher dose, depending on your needs.

How should I take this medication?
• You can take Micardis HCT tablets with or without food.

What should I avoid while taking this medication?
Do not become pregnant or breastfeed while you are taking Micardis HCT.

Do not become dehydrated. Drink adequate amounts of fluids while you are taking Micardis HCT to avoid becoming dehydrated.

What are possible food and drug interactions associated with this medication?
If Micardis HCT is taken with certain other drugs, the effects of either could be increased, decreased, or altered. It is especially important to check with your doctor before combining Micardis HCT with the following: alcohol, barbiturates (such as phenobarbital), cholestyramine, colestipol, diabetes medicines (such as insulin), digoxin, lithium, narcotic painkillers (such as hydrocodone or oxycodone), nonsteroidal anti-inflammatory drugs (NSAIDs) (such as ibuprofen or naproxen), norepinephrine, other blood pressure medications, potassium supplements, ramipril, salt substitutes that contain potassium, steroids, tubocurarine, or blood thinners (such as warfarin).

What are the possible side effects of this medication?
Please see general statement regarding side effects on page xiii.

> **Side effects may include:** diarrhea, dizziness, fatigue, "flu-like" symptoms, inflammation of your sinuses, nausea, upper respiratory tract infection

Can I receive this medication if I am pregnant or breastfeeding?
Do not take Micardis HCT if you are pregnant or breastfeeding. Micardis HCT can harm your unborn baby. It can be found in your

Visual Identification Guide

Visual Identification Guide

To help you ensure that you're taking the right medication as prescribed by your physician, this section provides full-color, actual-sized photographs of tablets and capsules.

Products in this section are arranged alphabetically by brand name; you will also find each medication's generic name, as well as its strength and the name of its manufacturer.

For more information about any of the products in this section, please turn to the Product Information section.

While every effort has been made to guarantee faithful reproduction of the photos in this section, changes in size, color, and design are always a possibility. Also, please note that there may be other dosage forms and strengths not pictured here. When in doubt, be sure to confirm a product's identity with your doctor or your pharmacist or by consulting the manufacturer's website.

ABILIFY

(aripiprazole) injection
BRISTOL-MYERS SQUIBB

9.75 mg/1.3 mL

ABILIFY

(aripiprazole)
BRISTOL-MYERS SQUIBB

1 mg/mL

Oral Solution

ABILIFY

(aripiprazole) tablets
BRISTOL-MYERS SQUIBB

2 mg

5 mg

10 mg

15 mg

20 mg

30 mg

ABILIFY DISCMELT

(aripiprazole)
BRISTOL-MYERS SQUIBB

10 mg

15 mg

Orally Disintegrating Tablets

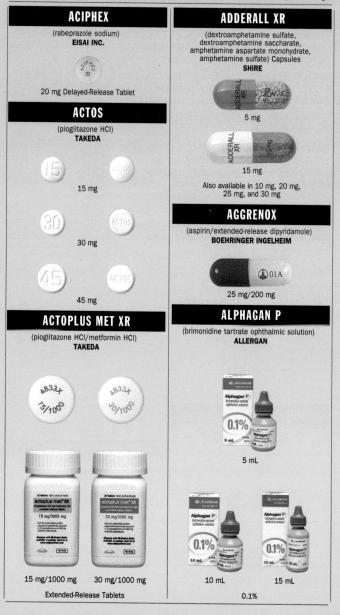

ACIPHEX

(rabeprazole sodium)
EISAI INC.

20 mg Delayed-Release Tablet

ACTOS

(pioglitazone HCl)
TAKEDA

15 mg

30 mg

45 mg

ACTOPLUS MET XR

(pioglitazone HCl/metformin HCl)
TAKEDA

15 mg/1000 mg   30 mg/1000 mg

Extended-Release Tablets

ADDERALL XR

(dextroamphetamine sulfate,
dextroamphetamine saccharate,
amphetamine aspartate monohydrate,
amphetamine sulfate) Capsules
SHIRE

5 mg

15 mg

Also available in 10 mg, 20 mg,
25 mg, and 30 mg

AGGRENOX

(aspirin/extended-release dipyridamole)
BOEHRINGER INGELHEIM

25 mg/200 mg

ALPHAGAN P

(brimonidine tartrate ophthalmic solution)
ALLERGAN

5 mL

10 mL   15 mL

0.1%

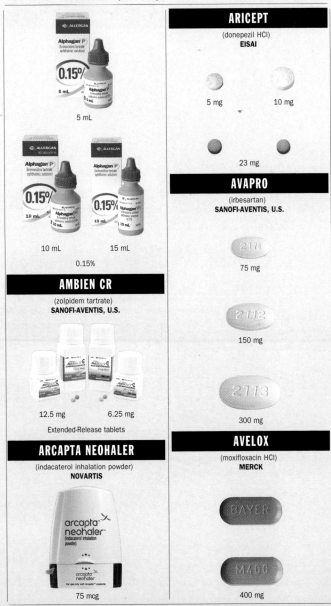

5 mL

10 mL   15 mL

0.15%

AMBIEN CR

(zolpidem tartrate)
SANOFI-AVENTIS, U.S.

12.5 mg   6.25 mg

Extended-Release tablets

ARCAPTA NEOHALER

(indacaterol inhalation powder)
NOVARTIS

75 mcg

ARICEPT

(donepezil HCl)
EISAI

5 mg   10 mg

23 mg

AVAPRO

(irbesartan)
SANOFI-AVENTIS, U.S.

75 mg

150 mg

300 mg

AVELOX

(moxifloxacin HCl)
MERCK

400 mg

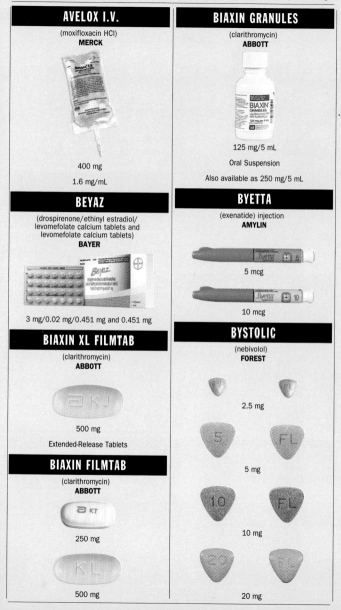

AVELOX I.V.
(moxifloxacin HCl)
MERCK

400 mg

1.6 mg/mL

BEYAZ
(drospirenone/ethinyl estradiol/
levomefolate calcium tablets and
levomefolate calcium tablets)
BAYER

3 mg/0.02 mg/0.451 mg and 0.451 mg

BIAXIN XL FILMTAB
(clarithromycin)
ABBOTT

500 mg

Extended-Release Tablets

BIAXIN FILMTAB
(clarithromycin)
ABBOTT

250 mg

500 mg

BIAXIN GRANULES
(clarithromycin)
ABBOTT

125 mg/5 mL

Oral Suspension

Also available as 250 mg/5 mL

BYETTA
(exenatide) injection
AMYLIN

5 mcg

10 mcg

BYSTOLIC
(nebivolol)
FOREST

2.5 mg

5 mg

10 mg

20 mg

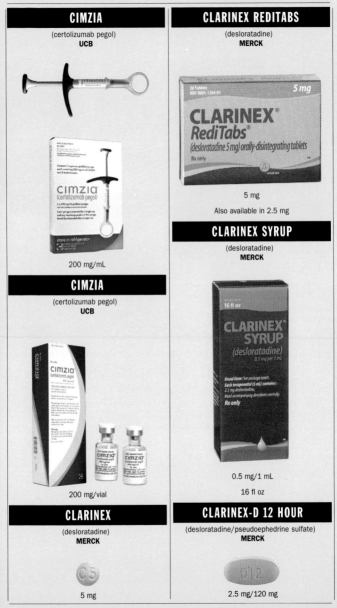

CIMZIA

(certolizumab pegol)
UCB

200 mg/mL

CIMZIA

(certolizumab pegol)
UCB

200 mg/vial

CLARINEX

(desloratadine)
MERCK

5 mg

CLARINEX REDITABS

(desloratadine)
MERCK

5 mg

Also available in 2.5 mg

CLARINEX SYRUP

(desloratadine)
MERCK

0.5 mg/1 mL

16 fl oz

CLARINEX-D 12 HOUR

(desloratadine/pseudoephedrine sulfate)
MERCK

2.5 mg/120 mg

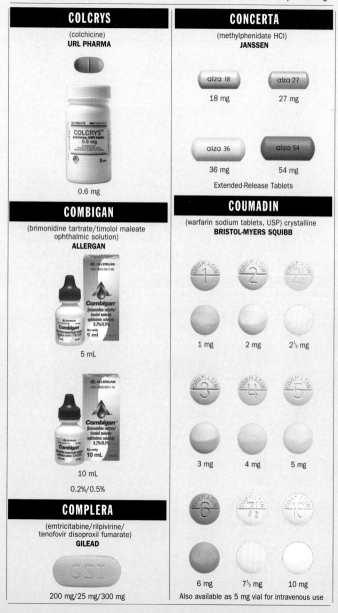

COLCRYS

(colchicine)
URL PHARMA

0.6 mg

COMBIGAN

(brimonidine tartrate/timolol maleate
ophthalmic solution)
ALLERGAN

5 mL

10 mL

0.2%/0.5%

COMPLERA

(emtricitabine/rilpivirine/
tenofovir disoproxil fumarate)
GILEAD

200 mg/25 mg/300 mg

CONCERTA

(methylphenidate HCl)
JANSSEN

alza 18   alza 27
18 mg   27 mg

alza 36   alza 54
36 mg   54 mg

Extended-Release Tablets

COUMADIN

(warfarin sodium tablets, USP) crystalline
BRISTOL-MYERS SQUIBB

1 mg   2 mg   2½ mg

3 mg   4 mg   5 mg

6 mg   7½ mg   10 mg

Also available as 5 mg vial for intravenous use

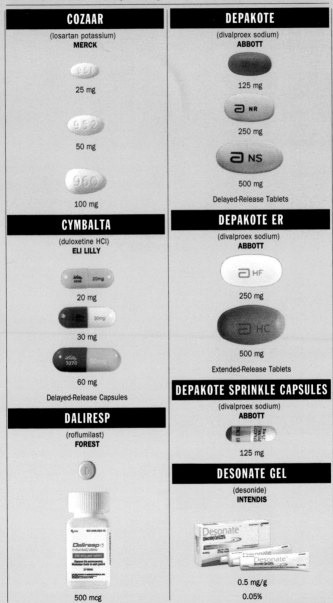

COZAAR

(losartan potassium)
MERCK

25 mg

50 mg

100 mg

CYMBALTA

(duloxetine HCl)
ELI LILLY

20 mg

30 mg

60 mg

Delayed-Release Capsules

DALIRESP

(roflumilast)
FOREST

500 mcg

DEPAKOTE

(divalproex sodium)
ABBOTT

125 mg

250 mg

500 mg

Delayed-Release Tablets

DEPAKOTE ER

(divalproex sodium)
ABBOTT

250 mg

500 mg

Extended-Release Tablets

DEPAKOTE SPRINKLE CAPSULES

(divalproex sodium)
ABBOTT

125 mg

DESONATE GEL

(desonide)
INTENDIS

0.5 mg/g

0.05%

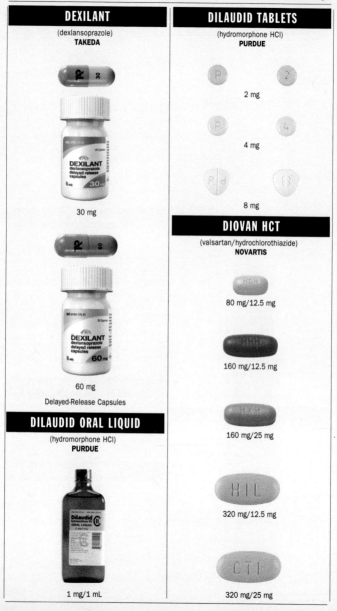

DEXILANT

(dexlansoprazole)
TAKEDA

30 mg

60 mg

Delayed-Release Capsules

DILAUDID ORAL LIQUID

(hydromorphone HCl)
PURDUE

1 mg/1 mL

DILAUDID TABLETS

(hydromorphone HCl)
PURDUE

2 mg

4 mg

8 mg

DIOVAN HCT

(valsartan/hydrochlorothiazide)
NOVARTIS

80 mg/12.5 mg

160 mg/12.5 mg

160 mg/25 mg

320 mg/12.5 mg

320 mg/25 mg

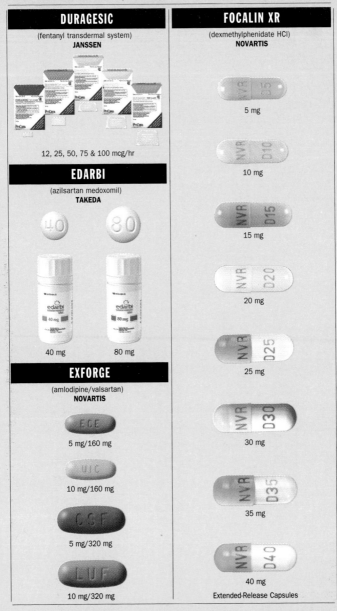

DURAGESIC

(fentanyl transdermal system)
JANSSEN

12, 25, 50, 75 & 100 mcg/hr

EDARBI

(azilsartan medoxomil)
TAKEDA

40 mg 80 mg

EXFORGE

(amlodipine/valsartan)
NOVARTIS

5 mg/160 mg

10 mg/160 mg

5 mg/320 mg

10 mg/320 mg

FOCALIN XR

(dexmethylphenidate HCl)
NOVARTIS

5 mg

10 mg

15 mg

20 mg

25 mg

30 mg

35 mg

40 mg

Extended-Release Capsules

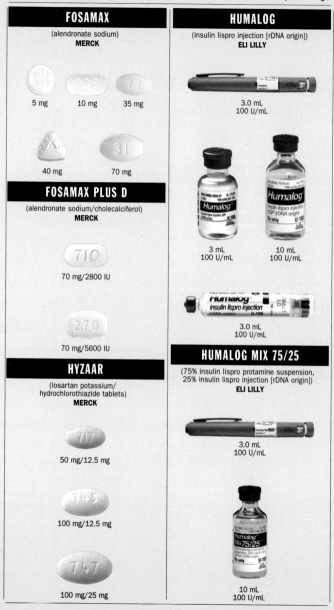

FOSAMAX

(alendronate sodium)
MERCK

5 mg   10 mg   35 mg

40 mg   70 mg

FOSAMAX PLUS D

(alendronate sodium/cholecalciferol)
MERCK

70 mg/2800 IU

70 mg/5600 IU

HYZAAR

(losartan potassium/
hydrochlorothiazide tablets)
MERCK

50 mg/12.5 mg

100 mg/12.5 mg

100 mg/25 mg

HUMALOG

(insulin lispro injection [rDNA origin])
ELI LILLY

3.0 mL
100 U/mL

3 mL
100 U/mL

10 mL
100 U/mL

3.0 mL
100 U/mL

HUMALOG MIX 75/25

(75% insulin lispro protamine suspension,
25% insulin lispro injection [rDNA origin])
ELI LILLY

3.0 mL
100 U/mL

10 mL
100 U/mL

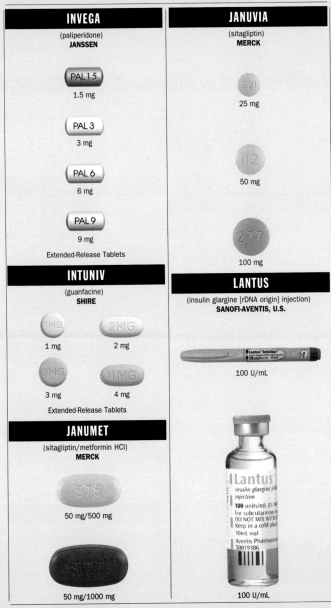

INVEGA

(paliperidone)
JANSSEN

PAL 1.5
1.5 mg

PAL 3
3 mg

PAL 6
6 mg

PAL 9
9 mg

Extended-Release Tablets

INTUNIV

(guanfacine)
SHIRE

1MG
1 mg

2MG
2 mg

3MG
3 mg

4MG
4 mg

Extended-Release Tablets

JANUMET

(sitagliptin/metformin HCl)
MERCK

575
50 mg/500 mg

577
50 mg/1000 mg

JANUVIA

(sitagliptin)
MERCK

221
25 mg

112
50 mg

277
100 mg

LANTUS

(insulin glargine [rDNA origin] injection)
SANOFI-AVENTIS, U.S.

Lantus® SoloStar
100 U/mL

Lantus
insulin glargine (rDNA)
injection
100 units/mL (U-100)
For subcutaneous in
DO NOT MIX WITH
Keep in a cold place
10mL vial
Aventis Pharmaceu
50019386

100 U/mL

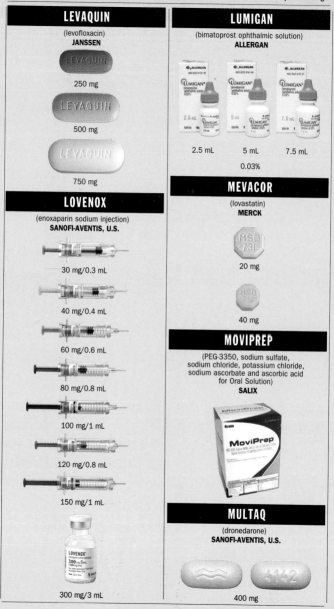

LEVAQUIN
(levofloxacin)
JANSSEN

250 mg

500 mg

750 mg

LOVENOX
(enoxaparin sodium injection)
SANOFI-AVENTIS, U.S.

30 mg/0.3 mL

40 mg/0.4 mL

60 mg/0.6 mL

80 mg/0.8 mL

100 mg/1 mL

120 mg/0.8 mL

150 mg/1 mL

300 mg/3 mL

LUMIGAN
(bimatoprost ophthalmic solution)
ALLERGAN

2.5 mL   5 mL   7.5 mL

0.03%

MEVACOR
(lovastatin)
MERCK

20 mg

40 mg

MOVIPREP
(PEG-3350, sodium sulfate,
sodium chloride, potassium chloride,
sodium ascorbate and ascorbic acid
for Oral Solution)
SALIX

MULTAQ
(dronedarone)
SANOFI-AVENTIS, U.S.

400 mg

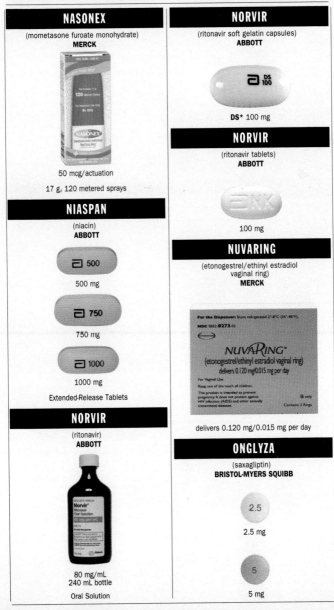

NASONEX

(mometasone furoate monohydrate)
MERCK

50 mcg/actuation

17 g, 120 metered sprays

NIASPAN

(niacin)
ABBOTT

500 mg

750 mg

1000 mg

Extended-Release Tablets

NORVIR

(ritonavir)
ABBOTT

80 mg/mL
240 mL bottle

Oral Solution

NORVIR

(ritonavir soft gelatin capsules)
ABBOTT

DS* 100 mg

NORVIR

(ritonavir tablets)
ABBOTT

100 mg

NUVARING

(etonogestrel/ethinyl estradiol
vaginal ring)
MERCK

delivers 0.120 mg/0.015 mg per day

ONGLYZA

(saxagliptin)
BRISTOL-MYERS SQUIBB

2.5 mg

5 mg

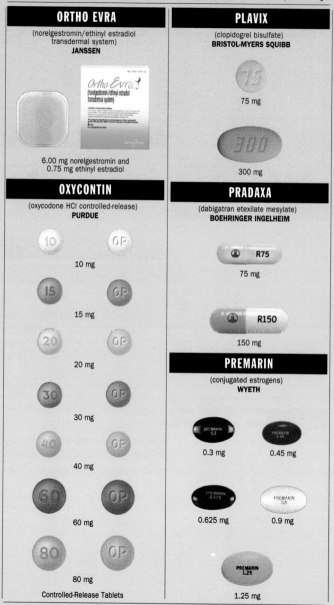

ORTHO EVRA

(norelgestromin/ethinyl estradiol transdermal system)
JANSSEN

6.00 mg norelgestromin and
0.75 mg ethinyl estradiol

OXYCONTIN

(oxycodone HCl controlled-release)
PURDUE

10 mg

15 mg

20 mg

30 mg

40 mg

60 mg

80 mg

Controlled-Release Tablets

PLAVIX

(clopidogrel bisulfate)
BRISTOL-MYERS SQUIBB

75 mg

300 mg

PRADAXA

(dabigatran etexilate mesylate)
BOEHRINGER INGELHEIM

R75
75 mg

R150
150 mg

PREMARIN

(conjugated estrogens)
WYETH

PREMARIN 0.3
0.3 mg

PREMARIN 0.45
0.45 mg

PREMARIN 0.625
0.625 mg

PREMARIN 0.9
0.9 mg

PREMARIN 1.25
1.25 mg

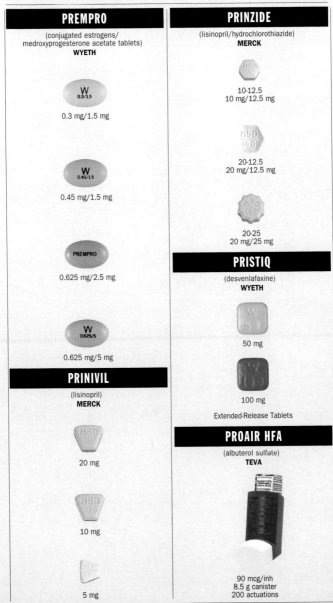

PREMPRO

(conjugated estrogens/
medroxyprogesterone acetate tablets)
WYETH

W
0.3/1.5

0.3 mg/1.5 mg

W
0.45/1.5

0.45 mg/1.5 mg

PREMPRO

0.625 mg/2.5 mg

W
0.625/5

0.625 mg/5 mg

PRINIVIL

(lisinopril)
MERCK

MSD 207

20 mg

MSD 106

10 mg

MSD 19

5 mg

PRINZIDE

(lisinopril/hydrochlorothiazide)
MERCK

MSD 145

10-12.5
10 mg/12.5 mg

MSD 140

20-12.5
20 mg/12.5 mg

MSD 142

20-25
20 mg/25 mg

PRISTIQ

(desvenlafaxine)
WYETH

W
50

50 mg

W
100

100 mg

Extended-Release Tablets

PROAIR HFA

(albuterol sulfate)
TEVA

90 mcg/inh
8.5 g canister
200 actuations

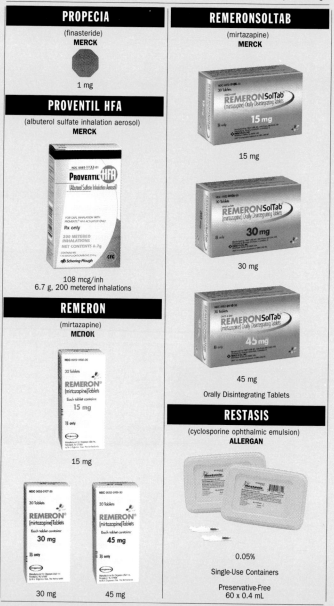

PROPECIA

(finasteride)
MERCK

1 mg

PROVENTIL HFA

(albuterol sulfate inhalation aerosol)
MERCK

108 mcg/inh
6.7 g, 200 metered inhalations

REMERON

(mirtazapine)
MERCK

15 mg

30 mg   45 mg

REMERONSOLTAB

(mirtazapine)
MERCK

15 mg

30 mg

45 mg

Orally Disintegrating Tablets

RESTASIS

(cyclosporine ophthalmic emulsion)
ALLERGAN

0.05%

Single-Use Containers

Preservative-Free
60 x 0.4 mL

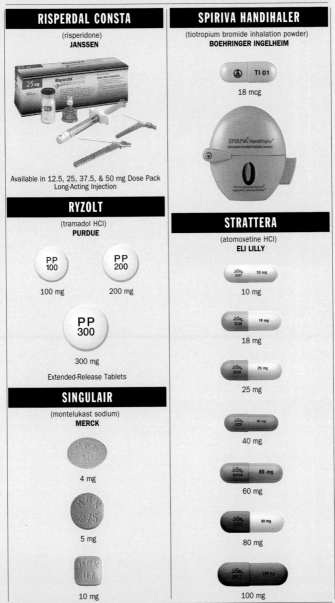

RISPERDAL CONSTA
(risperidone)
JANSSEN

Available in 12.5, 25, 37.5, & 50 mg Dose Pack
Long-Acting Injection

RYZOLT
(tramadol HCl)
PURDUE

PP 100 — 100 mg

PP 200 — 200 mg

PP 300 — 300 mg

Extended-Release Tablets

SINGULAIR
(montelukast sodium)
MERCK

MRK 711 — 4 mg

MRK 275 — 5 mg

MRK 117 — 10 mg

SPIRIVA HANDIHALER
(tiotropium bromide inhalation powder)
BOEHRINGER INGELHEIM

TI 01 — 18 mcg

STRATTERA
(atomoxetine HCl)
ELI LILLY

Lilly 3227 — 10 mg

Lilly 3238 — 18 mg

Lilly 3228 — 25 mg

Lilly 3229 — 40 mg

Lilly 3239 — 60 mg

80 mg

100 mg

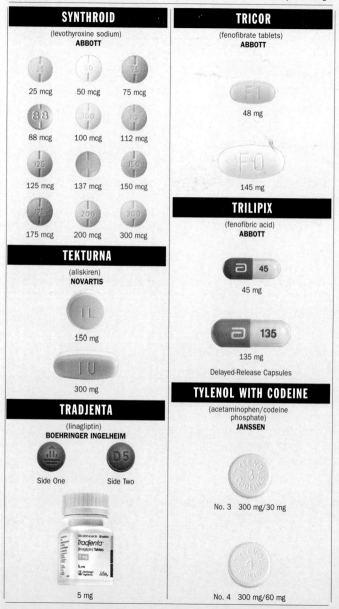

SYNTHROID

(levothyroxine sodium)
ABBOTT

25 mcg   50 mcg   75 mcg

88 mcg   100 mcg   112 mcg

125 mcg   137 mcg   150 mcg

175 mcg   200 mcg   300 mcg

TEKTURNA

(aliskiren)
NOVARTIS

150 mg

300 mg

TRADJENTA

(linagliptin)
BOEHRINGER INGELHEIM

Side One   Side Two

5 mg

TRICOR

(fenofibrate tablets)
ABBOTT

48 mg

145 mg

TRILIPIX

(fenofibric acid)
ABBOTT

45 mg

135 mg

Delayed-Release Capsules

TYLENOL WITH CODEINE

(acetaminophen/codeine phosphate)
JANSSEN

No. 3   300 mg/30 mg

No. 4   300 mg/60 mg

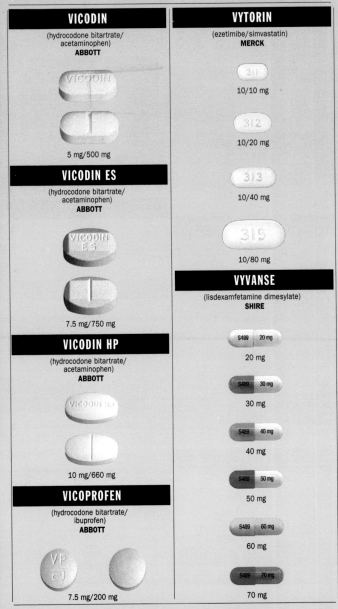

VICODIN

(hydrocodone bitartrate/
acetaminophen)
ABBOTT

5 mg/500 mg

VICODIN ES

(hydrocodone bitartrate/
acetaminophen)
ABBOTT

7.5 mg/750 mg

VICODIN HP

(hydrocodone bitartrate/
acetaminophen)
ABBOTT

10 mg/660 mg

VICOPROFEN

(hydrocodone bitartrate/
ibuprofen)
ABBOTT

7.5 mg/200 mg

VYTORIN

(ezetimibe/simvastatin)
MERCK

10/10 mg

10/20 mg

10/40 mg

10/80 mg

VYVANSE

(lisdexamfetamine dimesylate)
SHIRE

20 mg

30 mg

40 mg

50 mg

60 mg

70 mg

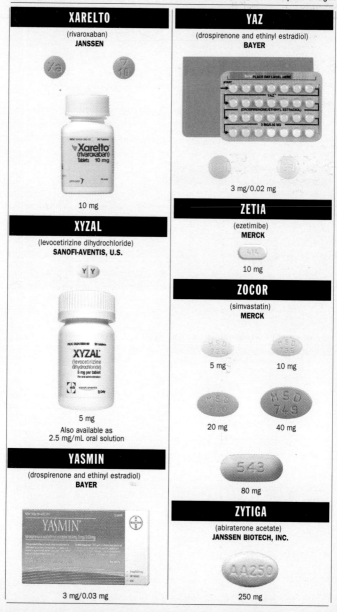

XARELTO
(rivaroxaban)
JANSSEN

10 mg

XYZAL
(levocetirizine dihydrochloride)
SANOFI-AVENTIS, U.S.

5 mg
Also available as
2.5 mg/mL oral solution

YASMIN
(drospirenone and ethinyl estradiol)
BAYER

3 mg/0.03 mg

YAZ
(drospirenone and ethinyl estradiol)
BAYER

3 mg/0.02 mg

ZETIA
(ezetimibe)
MERCK

10 mg

ZOCOR
(simvastatin)
MERCK

5 mg

10 mg

20 mg

40 mg

80 mg

ZYTIGA
(abiraterone acetate)
JANSSEN BIOTECH, INC.

250 mg

breast milk if you take it while breastfeeding. Tell your doctor immediately if you are pregnant, plan to become pregnant, or are breastfeeding.

What should I do if I miss a dose of this medication?
If you miss a dose of Micardis HCT, take it as soon as you remember. However, if it is almost time for your next dose, skip the one you missed and return to your regular dosing schedule. Do not take two doses at once.

How should I store this medication?
Store at room temperature.

Micro-K
Generic name: Potassium Chloride

What is this medication?
Micro-K is a potassium supplement that helps prevent and treat low blood potassium levels in your body.

What is the most important information I should know about this medication?
• Micro-K can increase your blood potassium to levels higher than normal, which can result in a heart attack. Your risk is higher if you have kidney disease or any other condition that does not allow potassium to be eliminated from your body. Your doctor will perform blood tests regularly to monitor your blood potassium levels.
• Micro-K can cause serious stomach and intestinal problems. Tell your doctor right away if you experience vomiting, abdominal pain, stomach bloating, or tarry stools.

Who should not take this medication?
Do not take Micro-K if you are allergic to it or any of its ingredients.

Do not take Micro-K if you have high blood potassium levels or any condition that stops or slows the passage of capsules through your stomach or intestinal tract.

What should I tell my doctor before I take the first dose of this medication?

Tell your doctor about all prescription, over-the-counter, and herbal medications you are taking before beginning treatment with Micro-K. Also, talk to your doctor about your complete medical history, especially if you have stomach problems, heart disease, kidney problems, or metabolic acidosis (a condition in which there is too much acid in the body).

What is the usual dosage?

Please see general statement regarding dosage on page xii.

Prevention of Low Potassium Levels
Adults: The usual dose is 20 milliequivalents (mEq) once a day.

Treatment of Low Potassium Levels
Adults: The usual dose is 40-100 mEq a day in divided doses.

Your doctor will increase your dose as appropriate.

How should I take this medication?

- Take Micro-K exactly as prescribed by your doctor. Take each dose of Micro-K with meals and with a full glass of water or other liquid. Do not take more than 20 mEq in a single dose.
- Swallow Micro-K capsules whole. Do not crush, chew, or suck on them.
- If you have difficulty swallowing whole capsules, open the capsule and sprinkle the medicine onto a spoonful of soft food (such as applesauce or pudding). Swallow the food and medicine mixture right away. Drink a glass of water or juice after you swallow the mixture to be sure you have taken all the medicine. Do not store any of the mixture for later use.

What should I avoid while taking this medication?

Do not change your dose of Micro-K without first talking to your doctor.

What are possible food and drug interactions associated with this medication?

If Micro-K is taken with certain other drugs, the effects of either could be increased, decreased, or altered. It is especially important to check with your doctor before combining Micro-K with the following: blood pressure medicines known as angiotensin converting enzyme (ACE) inhibitors (such as captopril or lisinopril) or certain diuretics (water pills) (such as amiloride or triamterene).

What are the possible side effects of this medication?

Please see general statement regarding side effects on page xiii.

Side effects may include: abdominal discomfort, diarrhea, gas, nausea, vomiting

Can I receive this medication if I am pregnant or breastfeeding?

The effects of Micro-K during pregnancy are unknown. You can continue to take Micro-K while you are breastfeeding. Tell your doctor immediately if you are pregnant, plan to become pregnant, or are breastfeeding.

What should I do if I miss a dose of this medication?

If you miss a dose of Micro-K, take it as soon as you remember. However, if it is almost time for your next dose, skip the one you missed and return to your regular dosing schedule. Do not take two doses at once.

How should I store this medication?

Store at room temperature.

Minocin

Generic name: Minocycline HCl

What is this medication?

Minocin is an antibiotic used to treat certain bacterial infections of the respiratory (lung) tract, urethra, rectum, or skin; Rocky Mountain spotted fever or other types of fever; severe acne; or certain sexually transmitted diseases (such as chlamydia, gonorrhea, or syphilis). Minocin can be used to treat certain bacterial infection for people who are allergic to penicillin or cannot take penicillin antibiotics. It may also be used to treat other bacterial infections as determined by your doctor.

What is the most important information I should know about this medication?

- Minocin can cause permanent discoloration (yellow-gray brown) of the teeth if it is taken during tooth development (during the last half of pregnancy, infancy, and childhood to the age of 8 years). Minocin can also impair the bone growth of a baby

- Minocin can also cause other serious side effects. Stop taking Minocin and call your doctor if you develop unusual headaches blurred vision, rash, joint pain, or feel very tired.

- Minocin can make your skin more sensitive to light. If you notice skin eruptions developing, stop the medication and call your doctor immediately. You may consider using sunscreen or sun block when taking Minocin.

- Minocin can cause central nervous system (CNS) effects, including lightheadedness, dizziness, and a spinning feeling (vertigo). Do not drive or operate machinery if you experience these symptoms.

- Diarrhea is a common problem when taking antibiotics; it usually ends when the antibiotic is stopped. Sometimes after starting treatment with antibiotics, people may develop watery and bloody stools (with or without stomach cramps and fever) even as late as two or more months after having taken the last dose of the antibiotic. Contact your doctor right away if this occurs.

- Take Minocin as prescribed by your doctor for the full course of treatment, even if your symptoms improve earlier. Do not skip doses. Skipping doses or not completing the full course of Minocin can decrease its effectiveness and can lead to the growth of bacteria that are resistant to the effects of Minocin.

Who should not take this medication?

Do not take Minocin if you are allergic to it, any of its ingredients, or similar antibiotics (such as tetracycline).

Do not take Minocin to treat viral infections, such as the common cold.

What should I tell my doctor before I take the first dose of this medication?

Tell your doctor about all prescription, over-the-counter, and herbal medications you are taking before beginning treatment with Minocin. Also, talk to your doctor about your complete medical history, especially if you have allergies, have liver or kidney disease, are pregnant, plan to become pregnant, or are breastfeeding.

What is the usual dosage?

Please see general statement regarding dosage on page xii.

Adults: The usual starting dose is 200 milligrams (mg), followed by 100 mg every 12 hours. Your doctor may prescribe a different dose based on the type and severity of your infection.

Children >8 years: Your doctor will prescribe the appropriate dose for your child, based on their weight and the severity of their infection.

How should I take this medication?

- Take Minocin exactly as prescribed by your doctor. Take Minocin with a full glass of fluid to wash down the medication and to reduce the risk of irritation and ulceration of your esophagus. Take it with or without food.
- Swallow Minocin capsules whole. Do not cut, crush, or chew them.

What should I avoid while taking this medication?

Do not expose yourself to excessive sunlight or artificial ultraviolet light while you are taking Minocin.

Do not drive or operate machinery if you experience CNS effect while you are taking Minocin.

What are possible food and drug interactions associated with this medication?

If Minocin is used with certain other drugs, the effects of either could be increased, decreased, or altered. It is especially important to check with your doctor before combining Minocin with the following: antacids containing aluminum, calcium, or magnesium; birth control pills; blood thinners (such as warfarin); certain migraine medicines; iron-containing preparations; isotretinoin; methoxyflurane; or penicillin.

What are the possible side effects of this medication?

Please see general statement regarding side effects on page xiii.

> **Side effects may include:** allergic reactions, anemia, cough, decreased hearing, diarrhea, dizziness, fever, headache, joint or muscle pain, liver or kidney problems, loss of appetite, nausea, rash, ringing in your ears, shortness of breath, upset stomach, vaginal infection, vomiting

Can I receive this medication if I am pregnant or breastfeeding?

Minocin can harm your unborn baby if you take it during pregnancy. Minocin can be found in your breast milk if you take it while breastfeeding. Do not breastfeed while you are taking Minocin. Tell your doctor immediately if you are pregnant, plan to become pregnant, or are breastfeeding.

What should I do if I miss a dose of this medication?

If you miss a dose of Minocin, take it as soon as you remember. However, if it is almost time for your next dose, skip the one you missed and return to your regular dosing schedule. Do not take two doses at once.

How should I store this medication?
Store at room temperature. Protect from light, moisture, and excessive heat.

Minocycline HCI: see Minocin, page 638

Miralax
Generic name: Polyethylene Glycol 3350

What is this medication?
Miralax is a medicine used to treat constipation. Miralax produces a bowel movement in 1 to 3 days.

What is the most important information I should know about this medication?
- Miralax is not for prolonged use. Tell your doctor if you need to use a laxative for longer than 1 week.
- Stop use and ask a doctor if you have rectal bleeding; if your nausea, bloating, cramping, or abdominal pain becomes worse; or if you get diarrhea.

Who should not take this medication?
Do not use Miralax if you are allergic to polyethylene glycol.

Do not use Miralax if you have kidney disease, except under the advice and supervision of your doctor.

What should I tell my doctor before I take the first dose of this medication?
Tell your doctor about all prescription, over-the-counter, and herbal medications you are taking before beginning treatment with Miralax. Also talk to your doctor about your complete medical history, especially if you have kidney problems, irritable bowel syndrome (abdominal pain accompanied by diarrhea and constipation associated with stress), nausea, vomiting, abdominal pain, or a sudden change in bowel habits that lasts more than 2 weeks.

What is the usual dosage?
Please see general statement regarding dosage on page xii.

> ***Adults and adolescents ≥17 years:*** The recommended dose is 17 grams once a day.

How should I take this medication?
• Take Miralax once a day. Fill the bottle top to the indicated line, the white section in the cap, to get the correct dose (17 grams). Stir and dissolve Miralax powder in 4 to 8 ounces of a beverage (cold, hot, or room temperature). Drink the mixture completely.

What should I avoid while taking this medication?
Do not take a larger dose or more often than your doctor tells you. Unless your doctor directs otherwise, do not use Miralax for more than 7 days.

Do not use Miralax if foil seal under cap, printed with "SEALED for YOUR PROTECTION," is missing, open, or broken.

What are possible food and drug interactions associated with this medication?
No significant interactions have been reported with Miralax at this time. However, always tell your doctor about any medicines you take, including over-the-counter medications, vitamins, and herbal supplements.

What are the possible side effects of this medication?
Please see general statement regarding side effects on page xiii.

> **Side effects may include:** abdominal pain, bloating, cramping, diarrhea, more frequent stools, nausea, rectal bleeding

Can I receive this medication if I am pregnant or breastfeeding?
The effects of Miralax during pregnancy and breastfeeding are unknown. Tell your doctor immediately if you are pregnant, plan to become pregnant, or are breastfeeding.

What should I do if I miss a dose of this medication?
If you miss a dose of Miralax, take it as soon as you remember. However, if it is almost time for your next dose, skip the one you missed and return to your regular dosing schedule. Do not take two doses at once.

How should I store this medication?
Store at room temperature.

Mirapex
Generic name: Pramipexole Dihydrochloride

What is this medication?
Mirapex is a medicine used to treat restless legs syndrome (RLS) and the signs and symptoms of Parkinson's disease.

What is the most important information I should know about this medication?
- Mirapex can cause you to fall asleep (even if you don't feel sleepy) while you are doing daily activities (such as driving, talking to other people, watching TV, or eating). Some people taking Mirapex have had car accidents because they fell asleep while driving. You could fall asleep without any warning. Do not drive a car, operate a machine, or do anything that requires you to be alert until you know how Mirapex affects you. Tell your doctor right away if you experience anything described here or if you feel sleepier than is normal for you. .
- Mirapex can cause you to develop unusual urges or behavior such as gambling, compulsive eating, compulsive buying, and increased sex drive. If you or your family members notice that you are developing unusual urges or behavior, tell your doctor immediately.

Who should not take this medication?
Do not take Mirapex if you are allergic to it or any of its ingredients.

What should I tell my doctor before I take the first dose of this medication?

Tell your doctor about all prescription, over-the-counter, and herbal medications you are taking before beginning treatment with Mirapex. Also, talk to your doctor about your complete medical history, expecially if you feel sleepy during the day from a sleep problem other than RLS, have low blood pressure, feel dizzy or faint (especially when getting up from a lying or sitting position), have trouble controlling your muscles, or have kidney problems. Tell your doctor if you are pregnant, plan to become pregnant, or are breastfeeding.

What is the usual dosage?

Please see general statement regarding dosage on page xii.

Parkinson's Disease
Adults: Your doctor will prescribe the appropriate dose for you.

Restless Legs Syndrome
Adults: The usual starting dose is 0.125 milligrams (mg) taken once a day 2-3 hours before bedtime. Your doctor may increase your dose every 4-7 days, up to a maximum of 0.5 mg a day.

How should I take this medication?

- Take Mirapex exactly as your doctor tells you to. Do not take more or less Mirapex than your doctor tells you to.
- Be sure to tell your doctor right away if you stop taking Mirapex for any reason. Do not start taking Mirapex again before talking to your doctor.
- You can take Mirapex with or without food. Taking Mirapex with food can lower your chances of having nausea.

What should I avoid while taking this medication?

Do not drive a car, operate machinery, or do anything that requires you to be alert until you know how Mirapex affects you.

Do not drink alcohol while you are taking Mirapex. It can increase your chances of feeling sleepy or falling asleep when you should be awake.

What are possible food and drug interactions associated with this medication?

If Mirapex is taken with certain other drugs, the effects of either could be increased, decreased, or altered. It is especially important to check with your doctor before combining Mirapex with the following: amantadine; carbidopa/levodopa; cimetidine; diltiazem; metoclopramide; quinidine; quinine; ranitidine; tranquilizers or sedatives that belong to classes of medications known as phenothiazines, butyrophenones, or thioxanthenes; triamterene; or verapamil.

What are the possible side effects of this medication?

Please see general statement regarding side effects on page xiii.

> **Side effects may include:** abnormal movements, confusion, constipation, dizziness, fainting, hallucinations (your chances of experiencing hallucinations are greater if you are >65 years old), insomnia, low blood pressure when you sit or stand up quickly, muscle weakness, nausea, sleepiness, sweating

Can I receive this medication if I am pregnant or breastfeeding?

The effects of Mirapex during pregnancy and breastfeeding are unknown. Tell your doctor immediately if you are pregnant, plan to become pregnant, or are breastfeeding.

What should I do if I miss a dose of this medication?

If you miss a dose of Mirapex, skip the one you missed and return to your regular dosing schedule. Do not take two doses at once.

How should I store this medication?

Store tablets at room temperature.

Mirtazapine: *see Remeron, page 879*

Mobic

Generic name: Meloxicam

What is this medication?

Mobic is a nonsteroidal anti-inflammatory drug (NSAID) used to treat osteoarthritis, rheumatoid arthritis in adults, and juvenile rheumatoid arthritis. Mobic is available in tablets and an oral suspension.

What is the most important information I should know about this medication?

- Mobic can cause serious problems (such as heart attack or stroke). Your risk can increase when this medication is used for long periods of time and if you have heart disease. Tell your doctor if you experience chest pain, shortness of breath, weakness, or slurred speech.
- Mobic can cause high blood pressure and heart failure or worsen existing high blood pressure. Tell your doctor if you experience weight gain or swelling.
- Mobic can cause discomfort, ulcers, or bleeding in your stomach or intestines. Your risk can increase with long-term use, smoking, drinking alcohol, older age, or with certain medications. Tell your doctor immediately if you experience stomach pain or if you have bloody vomit or stools.
- Long-term use of Mobic can cause kidney injury. Your risk can increase if you have kidney impairment; heart failure; liver problems; are taking certain medications, including diuretics (water pills) (such as furosemide or hydrochlorothiazide) or blood/heart medications known as angiotensin-converting enzyme (ACE) inhibitors (such as lisinopril); or are elderly.
- Mobic can also cause liver injury. Stop taking Mobic and call your doctor if you experience nausea, tiredness, weakness, itchiness, yellowing of your skin or whites of your eyes, right upper abdominal tenderness, or "flu-like" symptoms.
- Mobic can cause a serious allergic reaction. Stop taking Mobic and tell your doctor right away if you experience difficulty breathing or swelling of your face or throat.
- Stop taking Mobic and tell your doctor right away if you experience serious skin reactions, such as rash, blisters, fever, or itchiness.

Who should not take this medication?

Do not take Mobic if you are allergic to it or any of its ingredients.

Do not take Mobic if you have experienced asthma, hives, or allergic-type reactions after taking aspirin or other NSAIDs (such as ibuprofen or naproxen).

Do not take Mobic right before or after a heart surgery called a coronary artery bypass graft (CABG).

What should I tell my doctor before I take the first dose of this medication?

Tell your doctor about all prescription, over-the-counter, and herbal medications you are taking before beginning treatment with Mobic. Also, talk to your doctor about your complete medical history, especially if you have any of the following: allergies to medications, heart problems, history of asthma, high blood pressure, kidney or liver disease, or stomach problems, or are pregnant, plan to become pregnant, or are breastfeeding.

What is the usual dosage?

Please see general statement regarding dosage on page xii.

Osteoarthritis and Rheumatoid Arthritis

Adults: The recommended dose is 7.5 milligrams once a day. Your doctor will increase your dose as needed until the desired effect is achieved.

Juvenile Rheumatoid Arthritis

Children 2-17 years: Your doctor will prescribe the appropriate dose for your child, based on their weight.

How should I take this medication?

- Take Mobic exactly as prescribed by your doctor. Take it with or without food.
- Shake the oral suspension gently before you or your child take the medicine.

What should I avoid while taking this medication?

Do not take aspirin or other NSAIDs in combination with Mobic.

What are possible food and drug interactions associated with this medication?

If Mobic is taken with certain other drugs, the effects of either could be increased, decreased, or altered. It is especially important to check with your doctor before combining Mobic with the following: ACE inhibitors, aspirin, blood thinners (such as warfarin), cholestyramine, cyclosporine, diuretics, Kayexalate, lithium, methotrexate, or steroids.

What are the possible side effects of this medication?

Please see general statement regarding side effects on page xiii.

> **Side effects may include:** constipation, diarrhea, dizziness, gas, heartburn, nausea, stomach pain, vomiting

Can I receive this medication if I am pregnant or breastfeeding?

Do not take Mobic if you are in the late stage of your pregnancy (≥30 weeks) or if you are breastfeeding. The effects of Mobic during early pregnancy are unknown. Tell your doctor immediately if you are pregnant, plan to become pregnant, or are breastfeeding.

What should I do if I miss a dose of this medication?

If you miss a dose of Mobic, take it as soon as you remember. However, if it is almost time for your next dose, skip the one you missed and return to your regular dosing schedule. Do not take two doses at once.

How should I store this medication?

Store at room temperature.

Mometasone Furoate Monohydrate: *see Nasonex, page 677*

Monodox
Generic name: Doxycycline Monohydrate

What is this medication?
Monodox is an antibiotic used to treat certain bacterial infections of the respiratory (lung) tract, urethra, rectum, or skin; Rocky Mountain spotted fever or other types of fever; or certain sexually transmitted diseases (such as chlamydia, gonorrhea, or syphilis). Monodox can be used to treat certain bacterial infections for people who are allergic to penicillin or cannot take penicillin antibiotics. It may also be used to treat other bacterial infections, as determined by your doctor.

What is the most important information I should know about this medication?
- Monodox can cause permanent discoloration (yellow-gray-brown) of the teeth if it is taken during tooth development (during the last half of the pregnancy, infancy, and childhood to the age of 8 years). Monodox can also impair the bone growth of a baby.
- Monodox can cause diarrhea or colitis (inflammation of the colon). This can occur a couple of months after receiving the last dose of Monodox. Tell your doctor immediately if you have diarrhea or colitis.
- Monodox may make your skin more sensitive to light. If you notice skin eruptions developing, stop the medication and call your doctor immediately. You may consider using sunscreen or sunblock when taking Monodox.
- Drink plenty of fluids while you are taking Monodox to reduce the risk of irritation and ulceration of your esophagus.
- Monodox can increase your chance of getting a certain fungal infection of your vagina called vaginal candidiasis.
- Use Monodox as prescribed by your doctor for the full course of treatment, even if symptoms improve earlier. Do not skip doses. Skipping doses or not completing the full course of Monodox can decrease its effectiveness and can lead to growth of bacteria that are resistant to the effects of Monodox.

Who should not take this medication?

Do not take Monodox if you are allergic to it, any of its ingredients, or similar antibiotics (such as tetracycline).

Do not take Monodox to treat viral infections, such as the common cold.

What should I tell my doctor before I take the first dose of this medication?

Tell your doctor about all prescription, over-the-counter, and herbal medications you are taking before beginning treatment with Monodox. Also, talk to your doctor about your complete medical history, especially if you have allergies, have liver or kidney disease, are pregnant, plan to become pregnant, or are breastfeeding.

What is the usual dosage?

Please see general statement regarding dosage on page xii.

Your doctor might prescribe different doses than those listed below based on the type and severity of your infection.

Adults: The recommended starting dose is 200 milligrams (mg), divided into smaller doses taken 2 or 4 times on the first day. This is followed by a maintenance dose of 100 mg a day.

Children >8 years: Your doctor will prescribe the appropriate dose for your child, based on their weight and the severity of their infection.

How should I take this medication?

• Take Monodox exactly as prescribed by your doctor. Take this medication with plenty of fluids to wash down the medication and to reduce the risk of irritation and ulceration of your esophagus. You can take Monodox with food if stomach irritation occurs.

What should I avoid while taking this medication?

Do not expose yourself to excessive sunlight or artificial ultraviolet light while you are taking Monodox.

What are possible food and drug interactions associated with this medication?

If Monodox is used with certain other drugs, the effects of either could be increased, decreased, or altered. It is especially important to check with your doctor before combining Monodox with the following: antacids containing aluminum, calcium, or magnesium; birth control pills; bismuth subsalicylate; blood thinners (such as warfarin); iron-containing preparations; methoxyflurane; penicillin; or seizure medications (such as carbamazepine, phenobarbital, or phenytoin).

What are the possible side effects of this medication?

Please see general statement regarding side effects on page xiii.

> **Side effects may include:** allergic reactions, colitis, diarrhea, difficulty swallowing, flu symptoms, headache, joint pain, loss of appetite, nausea, rash, swelling of your tongue, vomiting

Can I receive this medication if I am pregnant or breastfeeding?

The effects of Monodox during pregnancy are unknown. Monodox can be found in your breast milk if you take it during breastfeeding. Do not take Monodox while breastfeeding. Tell your doctor immediately if you are pregnant, plan to become pregnant, or are breastfeeding.

What should I do if I miss a dose of this medication?

If you miss a dose of Monodox, take it as soon as you remember. However, if it is almost time for your next dose, skip the one you missed and return to your regular dosing schedule. Do not take two doses at once.

How should I store this medication?

Store at room temperature. Protect from light.

Montelukast Sodium: *see Singulair, page 934*

Morphine sulfate

Generic name: Morphine Sulfate

What is this medication?

Morphine sulfate is a narcotic pain medicine used to relieve moderate to severe pain that is expected to last a short period of time, and pain that continues around-the-clock and is expected to last for a long period of time. This medication is available as an oral solution to be taken by mouth.

Morphine sulfate is a federally controlled substance because it has abuse potential.

What is the most important information I should know about this medication?

- Morphine sulfate has abuse potential. Mental and physical dependence can occur with the use of morphine sulfate when it is used improperly for long periods of time.
- Keep morphine sulfate in a safe place away from children. Accidental use by a child is a medical emergency and can cause death. If a child accidentally takes morphine sulfate, get emergency help immediately.
- Morphine sulfate can cause serious breathing problems that can become life-threatening, especially when it is used in the wrong way for long periods of time. Tell your doctor if you have any lung or breathing problems (such as asthma); your doctor will continuously monitor you.
- Morphine sulfate can reduce your blood pressure. This is more likely to happen if you have certain heart problems, or are taking other medications that can reduce your blood pressure.
- Morphine sulfate can impair your mental and physical abilities. Do not drive, operate heavy machinery, or do other dangerous activities until you know how morphine sulfate affects you. Also, do not drink alcohol or take other medications that can affect your brain (such as medications that make you drowsy or narcotic painkillers) while using morphine sulfate.

Who should not take this medication?

Do not take morphine sulfate if you are allergic to it, any of its ingredients, or if you are having an asthma attack, have severe asthma, trouble breathing, or lung problems.

Do not take morphine sulfate if you have paralytic ileus (impairment of the small intestines).

What should I tell my doctor before I take the first dose of this medication?

Tell your doctor about all prescription, over-the-counter, and herbal medications you are taking before beginning treatment with morphine sulfate. Also, talk to your doctor about your allergies and complete medical history, especially if you have breathing problems; brain problems, head injury, or seizures; severe liver or kidney problems; adrenal gland problems; hypothyroidism (an underactive thyroid gland); urinary blockage; alcoholism; mental problems or hallucinations; constipation or bowel problems; pancreatitis (inflammation of the pancreas); history of or a present drug abuse or addiction problem; or a family history of drug abuse or addiction problem.

What is the usual dosage?

Please see general statement regarding dosage on page xii.

Adults ≥18 years: The recommended starting dose is 10-20 milligrams (mg) every 4 hours as needed for pain. Your doctor will adjust the dose for you based on the severity of your pain and your response to this medication.

How should I take this medication?

- Take morphine sulfate exactly as prescribed by your doctor. Know the exact dose and strength of morphine sulfate your doctor prescribed for you.
- Use the oral syringe provided with your morphine sulfate oral solution to help make sure you measure the right amount. Your doctor should show you the correct way to measure the right amount of morphine sulfate. Do not stop taking morphine sulfate abruptly without talking to your doctor.

- Please review the instructions that came with your prescription on how to properly use the syringe to take morphine sulfate oral solution.

What should I avoid while taking this medication?

Do not drive, operate heavy machinery, or do other dangerous activities until you know how morphine sulfate affects you.

Do not drink alcohol while you are taking morphine sulfate.

What are possible food and drug interactions associated with this medication?

If morphine sulfate is taken with certain other drugs, the effects of either could be increased, decreased, or altered. It is especially important to check with your doctor before combining morphine sulfate with the following: alcohol, antihistamines (such as diphenhydramine), certain antipsychotic medications (such as clozapine or fluphenazine), cimetidine; monoamine oxidase inhibitors (MAOIs), a class of drugs used to treat depression and other psychiatric conditions (such as phenelzine), other narcotic painkillers (such as oxycodone), quinidine, or other medications that slow down your brain function (such as alprazolam, diazepam, or phenobarbital).

What are the possible side effects of this medication?

Please see general statement regarding side effects on page xiii.

> **Side effects may include:** breathing problems, constipation, decrease in blood pressure, dizziness, drowsiness, heart problems, lightheadedness, nausea, sweating, vomiting

Can I receive this medication if I am pregnant or breastfeeding?

The effects of morphine sulfate during pregnancy are unknown. Morphine sulfate can be found in your breast milk if you use it during breastfeeding. Do not take morphine sulfate while you are breastfeeding. Tell your doctor immediately if you are pregnant, plan to become pregnant, or are breastfeeding.

What should I do if I miss a dose of this medication?

If you miss a dose of morphine sulfate, take it as soon as you remember. However, if it is almost time for your next dose, skip the one you missed and return to your regular dosing schedule. Do not take two doses at once.

How should I store this medication?

Store at room temperature. Protect from light and moisture.

Morphine Sulfate: see Morphine sulfate, page 652

Morphine Sulfate: see MS Contin, page 659

Moviprep

Generic name: Ascorbic Acid/Polyethylene Glycol 3350/Potassium Chloride/Sodium Ascorbate/Sodium Chloride/Sodium Sulfate

What is this medication?

Moviprep is a medicine used for colon cleansing in preparation for a colonoscopy.

What is the most important information I should know about this medication?

- Moviprep can cause seizures and abnormal heart rhythms. Be sure to drink plenty of fluids before, during, and after you take Moviprep.

Who should not take this medication?

Do not take Moviprep if you are allergic to it or any of its ingredients, if you have a blockage in your bowel, an opening in the wall of your stomach or intestine, or a very dilated intestine.

What should I tell my doctor before I take the first dose of this medication?

Tell your doctor about all prescription, over-the-counter, and herbal medications you are taking before beginning treatment with

Moviprep. Also, talk to your doctor about your complete medical history, especially if you have kidney impairment, difficulty swallowing, glucose-6-phosphate dehydrogenase (G6PD) deficiency (lack of an enzyme responsible for the breakdown of red blood cells), or have any stomach disorders. In addition, tell your doctor if you have phenylketonuria (an inability to process phenylalanine, a protein in your body).

What is the usual dosage?
Please see general statement regarding dosage on page xii.

Split-Dose Regimen
Adults: The evening before your colonoscopy, drink the first liter of Moviprep over one hour (one 8-ounce glass every 15 minutes), and then drink 16 ounces of clear liquid. Then, on the morning of the colonoscopy, drink the second liter of Moviprep over one hour, and then drink 16 ounces of clear liquid at least one hour prior to the start of the colonoscopy.

Evening-Only (Full-Dose) Regimen
Adults: Around 6 o'clock the evening before your colonoscopy, drink the first liter of Moviprep over one hour (one 8-ounce glass every 15 minutes), and then about an hour and a half later, drink the second liter of Moviprep over one hour. In addition, drink approximately 32 ounces of clear liquid during the evening before the colonoscopy.

How should I take this medication?
- Take Moviprep exactly as prescribed by your doctor. Please review the instructions that came with your prescription on how to properly take Moviprep.

What should I avoid while taking this medication?
Do not eat solid foods after you have taken Moviprep until after your colonoscopy.

Do not take any medication within one hour of starting each dose of Moviprep.

What are possible food and drug interactions associated with this medication?

If Moviprep is taken with certain other drugs, the effects of either could be increased, decreased, or altered. It is important to check with your doctor before combining Moviprep with any other medication.

What are the possible side effects of this medication?

Please see general statement regarding side effects on page xiii.

> **Side effects may include:** anal discomfort, difficulty sleeping, general feeling of discomfort, hunger, nausea, stomach discomfort or pain, thirst, vomiting

Can I receive this medication if I am pregnant or breastfeeding?

The effects of Moviprep during pregnancy and breastfeeding are unknown. Tell your doctor immediately if you are pregnant, plan to become pregnant, or are breastfeeding.

What should I do if I miss a dose of this medication?

Moviprep should be given under special circumstances determined by your doctor. If you miss your scheduled dose, contact your doctor or pharmacist for advice.

How should I store this medication?

Store pouches at room temperature. If mixed, refrigerate and use the solution within 24 hours.

Moxeza

Generic name: Moxifloxacin HCl

What is this medication?

Moxeza is an antibiotic eyedrop that is used to treat bacterial conjunctivitis (pink eye).

What is the most important information I should know about this medication?

- Prolonged use of Moxeza may lead to an overgrowth of bacteria and possibly fungi.
- Do not wear contact lenses if you have signs of an eye infection.
- Do not touch the dropper tip to any surface to avoid contaminating the contents.
- Contact your doctor if your condition gets worse, because this may be a sign of a different or more serious infection.

Who should not take this medication?

Do not use Moxeza if you are allergic to it or any of its ingredients.

What should I tell my doctor before I take the first dose of this medication?

Tell your doctor about all prescription, over-the-counter, and herbal medications you are taking before beginning treatment with Moxeza. Also, talk to your doctor about your complete medical history, especially if you wear contact lenses, are pregnant, plan to become pregnant, or are breastfeeding.

What is the usual dosage?

Please see general statement regarding dosage on page xii.

Adults and children ≥4 months: Apply one drop in the affected eye(s) twice a day for 7 days.

How should I take this medication?

- Take Moxeza as directed by your doctor.

What should I avoid while taking this medication?

Do not wear contact lenses if you have signs of an eye infection.

What are possible food and drug interactions associated with this medication?

No significant interactions have been reported with Moxeza at this time. However, always tell your doctor about any medicines you take, including over-the-counter drugs, vitamins, and herbal supplements.

What are the possible side effects of this medication?
Please see general statement regarding side effects on page xiii.

> **Side effects may include:** eye irritation, fever, pink eye

Can I receive this medication if I am pregnant or breastfeeding?
The effects of Moxeza during pregnancy and breastfeeding are unknown. Tell your doctor immediately if you are pregnant, plan to become pregnant, or are breastfeeding.

What should I do if I miss a dose of this medication?
If you miss a dose of Moxeza, apply it as soon as you remember. However, if it is almost time for your next dose, skip the one you missed and return to your regular dosing schedule. Do not apply two doses at once.

How should I store this medication?
Store at room temperature. Protect from freezing.

Moxifloxacin HCl: *see Avelox, page 113*

Moxifloxacin HCl: *see Moxeza, page 657*

Moxifloxacin HCl: *see Vigamox, page 1074*

MS Contin
Generic name: Morphine Sulfate

What is this medication?
MS Contin is a pain medicine that contains the narcotic painkiller morphine. MS Contin is used to treat moderate to severe around-the-clock pain.

MS Contin is a federally controlled substance because it has abuse potential.

What is the most important information I should know about this medication?

- MS Contin has abuse potential. Mental and physical dependence can occur with the use of MS Contin when it is used improperly.
- MS Contin can cause serious breathing problems that can become life-threatening, especially when it is used in the wrong way.
- MS Contin can cause low blood pressure. You can experience dizziness, lightheadedness, or fainting. To prevent this, carefully get up from a sitting or lying position. Sit or lie down at the first sign of any of these symptoms.
- MS Contin can cause allergic reactions or anaphylaxis (a serious and rapid allergic reaction that may result in death if not immediately treated). Stop taking MS Contin and tell your doctor immediately if you develop a rash, difficulty breathing, or swelling of your face, mouth, or throat.

Who should not take this medication?

Do not take MS Contin if you are allergic to it or any of its ingredients.

Do not take MS Contin if you have severe asthma, trouble breathing, or other lung problems.

Do not take MS Contin if you have paralytic ileus (bowel blockage) or narrowing of the stomach or small intestine.

What should I tell my doctor before I take the first dose of this medication?

Tell your doctor about all prescription, over-the-counter, and herbal medications you are taking before beginning treatment with MS Contin. Also, talk to your doctor about your complete medical history, especially if you have trouble breathing or lung problems; head injury; liver or kidney disease; thyroid problems; seizures; problems urinating; pancreas, gallbladder, or mental health problems; or a history of alcohol or drug abuse.

What is the usual dosage?
Please see general statement regarding dosage on page xii.

Adults: Your doctor will prescribe the appropriate dose for you based on your condition, previous treatment with painkillers, and your tolerance for narcotics.

If you are elderly or have hepatic impairment, your doctor will adjust your dose appropriately.

How should I take this medication?
- Take Ms Contin exactly as prescribed by your doctor. Do not change your dose or stop taking MS Contin without first talking to your doctor.
- Take each dose at the same time every day.
- Swallow MS Contin tablets whole. Do not cut, break, chew, crush, dissolve, or inject them.

What should I avoid while taking this medication?
Do not drink alcohol or take other medications that contain alcohol while you are taking MS Contin.

Do not drive or operate heavy machinery until you know how MS Contin affects you.

Do not share MS Contin with others.

What are possible food and drug interactions associated with this medication?
If MS Contin is taken with certain other drugs, the effects of either could be increased, decreased, or altered. It is especially important to check with your doctor before combining MS Contin with the following: alcohol, anticholinergics (such as ipratropium or oxybutynin), antidepressant medications known as monoamine oxidase inhibitors (such as selegiline or phenelzine), butorphanol, cimetidine, diuretics (water pills), general anesthetics, muscle relaxants (such as tubocurarine), nalbuphine, pentazocine, phenothiazines (such as chlorpromazine or mesoridazine), quinidine,

sedative-hypnotics (such as alprazolam or diazepam), tranquilizers (such as chlordiazepoxide).

What are the possible side effects of this medication?

Please see general statement regarding side effects on page xiii.

> **Side effects may include:** abdominal pain, constipation, dizziness, headache, nausea, sleepiness, tiredness, vomiting

Can I receive this medication if I am pregnant or breastfeeding?

The effects of MS Contin during pregnancy are unknown. MS Contin can be found in your breast milk if you take it while breastfeeding. Do not breastfeed while you are taking MS Contin. Tell your doctor immediately if you are pregnant, plan to become pregnant, or are breastfeeding.

What should I do if I miss a dose of this medication?

If you miss a dose of MS Contin, take it as soon as you remember and then take your next dose 8 or 12 hours later as directed by your doctor. However, if it is almost time for your next dose, skip the one you missed and return to your regular dosing schedule. Do not take more than one dose in 8 hours.

How should I store this medication?

Store at room temperature.

Multaq

Generic name: Dronedarone

What is this medication?

Multaq is a medicine used to lower the chance that you would need to go into the hospital for atrial fibrillation (an irregular, fast heartbeat). This medication is used if you have had atrial fibrillation in the past but are now in normal rhythm.

What is the most important information I should know about this medication?

- Do not take Multaq if you have symptoms of heart failure that recently worsened or if you have severe heart failure; doing so can be life-threatening. Tell your doctor immediately if you experience shortness of breath, wheezing, chest tightness; coughing up frothy mucus at rest, nighttime, or after minor exercise; trouble sleeping or waking up at night because of breathing problems; rapid weight gain; or swelling of your feet or legs.

- Do not take Multaq if you have a type of atrial fibrillation called permanent atrial fibrillation, which is when your heartbeat will not or cannot be changed back to a normal rhythm. Your doctor will monitor your heart rhythm regularly. Tell your doctor immediately if you notice that your pulse is irregular.

- Multaq can cause severe liver problems. Your doctor will monitor your liver function before you start taking Multaq and during treatment. Tell your doctor immediately if you develop loss of appetite, nausea, vomiting, fever, feeling unwell, unusual tiredness, itching, yellowing of your skin or the whites of your eyes, unusual darkening of your urine, or pain or discomfort in your right upper stomach area.

Who should not take this medication?

Do not take Multaq if you have severe heart failure or heart failure with symptoms that recently worsened, permanent atrial fibrillation, severe liver impairment or liver problems after previous use of amiodarone (a medicine for abnormal heartbeat), sick sinus syndrome (abnormal heart rhythm) or heart block (unless you have a pacemaker), or abnormally slow heartbeat. Also, do not take Multaq if you are pregnant, plan to become pregnant, or are breastfeeding.

Do not take Multaq if you take certain medicines that can change the amount of Multaq that gets in your body (such as clarithromycin, cyclosporine, itraconazole, ketoconazole, nefazodone, ritonavir, telithromycin, or voriconazole), or if you take certain medicines that can cause other dangerous abnormal heartbeats (such as amiodarone, chlorpromazine, disopyramide, dofetilide, erythromycin, flecainide, fluphenazine, procainamide, propafenone, quinidine, sotalol, or thioridazine).

What should I tell my doctor before I take the first dose of this medication?

Tell your doctor about all prescription, over-the-counter, and herbal medications you are taking before beginning treatment with Multaq. Also, talk to your doctor about your complete medical history, especially if you have other heart problems, have liver or kidney impairment, have low blood potassium or magnesium levels, are pregnant, plan to become pregnant, or are breastfeeding.

What is the usual dosage?

Please see general statement regarding dosage on page xii.

Adults: The recommended dose is 400 milligrams twice a day.

How should I take this medication?

- Take Multaq exactly as prescribed by your doctor.
- You can take Multaq two times a day with food, once with your morning meal and once with your evening meal.
- Do not stop taking this medication even if you are feeling well for a long time.

What should I avoid while taking this medication?

Do not drink grapefruit juice while you are taking Multaq. Grapefruit juice can increase the amount of Multaq in your blood and increase your risk of experiencing side effects.

What are possible food and drug interactions associated with this medication?

If Multaq is taken with certain other drugs, the effects of either could be increased, decreased, or altered. It is especially important to check with your doctor before combining Multaq with the following: blood pressure/heart medications known as beta-blockers (such as propranolol) or calcium channel blockers (such as diltiazem, nifedipine, or verapamil), blood thinners (such as dabigatran or warfarin), certain antibiotics (such as rifampin), certain medicines that can cause other dangerous abnormal heartbeats, certain medicines that can change the amount of Multaq that gets in your body, cholesterol medications (such as simvastatin), digoxin, grapefruit juice, pantoprazole, seizure medications (such as carbamazepine, phenobarbital, or phenytoin), sirolimus, St. John's wort, or tacrolimus.

What are the possible side effects of this medication?
Please see general statement regarding side effects on page xiii.

> **Side effects may include:** abdominal pain, diarrhea, indigestion, itching, nausea, rash, redness of your skin, slowed heartbeat, tiredness, vomiting, weakness

Can I receive this medication if I am pregnant or breastfeeding?
Do not take Multaq if you are pregnant or breastfeeding. Multaq can cause harm to your unborn baby if you use it during pregnancy. Tell your doctor immediately if you are pregnant, plan to become pregnant, or are breastfeeding.

What should I do if I miss a dose of this medication?
If you miss a dose of Multaq, skip the one you missed and return to your regular dosing schedule. Do not try to make up for a missed dose. Do not take two doses at once.

How should I store this medication?
Store at room temperature.

Mupirocin Calcium: see Bactroban, page 131

Nabumetone
Generic name: Nabumetone

What is this medication?
Nabumetone is a nonsteroidal anti-inflammatory drug (NSAID) used to treat osteoarthritis and rheumatoid arthritis.

What is the most important information I should know about this medication?

- Nabumetone can cause serious problems (such as heart attack or stroke). Your risk can increase when this medication is used for long periods of time and if you have heart disease. Tell your doctor if you experience chest pain, shortness of breath, weakness, or slurred speech.
- Nabumetone can cause high blood pressure and heart failure or worsen existing high blood pressure. Tell your doctor if you experience weight gain or swelling.
- Nabumetone can cause discomfort, ulcers, or bleeding in your stomach or intestines. Your risk can increase with long-term use, smoking, drinking alcohol, older age, or with certain medications. Tell your doctor immediately if you experience stomach pain or if you have bloody vomit or stools.
- Long-term use of nabumetone can cause kidney injury. Your risk can increase if you have kidney impairment; heart failure; liver problems; are taking certain medications, including diuretics (water pills) (such as furosemide or hydrochlorothiazide); or are elderly.
- Nabumetone can also cause liver injury. Stop taking nabumetone and call your doctor if you experience nausea, tiredness, weakness, itchiness, yellowing of your skin or whites of your eyes, right upper abdominal tenderness, or "flu-like" symptoms.
- Nabumetone can cause a serious allergic reaction. Stop taking nabumetone and tell your doctor right away if you experience difficulty breathing or swelling of your face or throat.
- Stop taking nabumetone and tell your doctor right away if you experience serious skin reactions, such as rash, blisters, fever, or itchiness.

Who should not take this medication?

Do not take nabumetone if you are allergic to it or any of its ingredients.

Do not take nabumetone if you have experienced asthma, hives, or allergic-type reactions after taking aspirin or other NSAIDs (such as ibuprofen or naproxen).

Do not take nabumetone right before or after a heart surgery called a coronary artery bypass graft (CABG).

What should I tell my doctor before I take the first dose of this medication?

Tell your doctor about all prescription, over-the-counter, and herbal medications you are taking before beginning treatment with nabumetone. Also, talk to your doctor about your complete medical history, especially if you have any of the following: allergies to medications, heart problems, history of asthma, high blood pressure, kidney or liver disease, or stomach problems, or are pregnant, plan to become pregnant, or are breastfeeding.

What is the usual dosage?

Please see general statement regarding dosage on page xii.

Adults: The recommended starting dose is 1000 milligrams once a day. Your doctor will increase your dose as needed until the desired effect is achieved.

How should I take this medication?

▪ Take nabumetone exactly as prescribed by your doctor. Take it with or without food.

What should I avoid while taking this medication?

Do not take aspirin or other NSAIDs in combination with nabumetone.

Do not expose your skin to sunlamps, tanning beds, and the sun while you are taking nabumetone. Nabumetone can make your skin more sensitive to light and cause sunburns. Wear sunscreen or protective clothing if you are going to be outside for long periods.

What are possible food and drug interactions associated with this medication?

If nabumetone is taken with certain other drugs, the effects of either could be increased, decreased, or altered. It is especially important to check with your doctor before combining nabumetone with the following: aspirin, blood/heart medications known as angiotensin-converting enzyme (ACE) inhibitors (such as lisino-pril), blood thinners (such as warfarin), diuretics, lithium, metho-trexate, or steroids.

What are the possible side effects of this medication?

Please see general statement regarding side effects on page xiii.

> **Side effects may include:** constipation, diarrhea, dizziness, gas, heartburn, nausea, stomach pain, vomiting

Can I receive this medication if I am pregnant or breastfeeding?

Do not take nabumetone if you are in the late stage of your preg-nancy or if you are breastfeeding. The effects of nabumetone dur-ing early pregnancy are unknown. Tell your doctor immediately if you are pregnant, plan to become pregnant, or are breastfeeding.

What should I do if I miss a dose of this medication?

If you miss a dose of nabumetone, take it as soon as you remem-ber. However, if it is almost time for your next dose, skip the one you missed and return to your regular dosing schedule. Do not take two doses at once.

How should I store this medication?

Store at room temperature.

Nabumetone: *see Nabumetone, page 665*

Namenda

Generic name: Memantine HCl

What is this medication?

Namenda is a medicine that is used to treat patients with Alzheim-er's disease. Namenda is available in tablets and an oral solution.

What is the most important information I should know about this medication?

- If you accidentally take more Namenda than you should, inform your doctor immediately. You may require medical attention. Some people who have accidentally taken too much memantine (the active ingredient in Namenda) have experienced dizziness, unsteadiness, weakness, tiredness, confusion, or other symptoms.
- If you have, or ever had seizures or difficulty passing urine, your doctor will need to monitor you more closely while you are taking Namenda.

Who should not take this medication?

Do not take Namenda if you are allergic to it or any of its ingredients.

What should I tell my doctor before I take the first dose of this medication?

Tell your doctor about all prescription, over-the-counter, and herbal medications you are taking before beginning treatment with Namenda. Also, talk to your doctor about your complete medical history, especially if you have kidney or liver disease, history of seizures or difficulty urinating, or if you have a urinary tract infection.

What is the usual dosage?

Please see general statement regarding dosage on page xii.

Adults: The recommended starting dose is 5 milligrams (mg) once a day.

How should I take this medication?

- Take Namenda exactly as prescribed by your doctor. Do not take extra doses or take more often without asking your doctor.
- Take Namenda with or without food.
- If you are taking Namenda oral solution, your doctor or pharmacist will provide you with instructions on how to use the dosing device. Do not mix Namenda oral solution with any other liquid.

What should I avoid while taking this medication?

Do not consume food or medicines (such as sodium bicarbonate) that make your urine alkaline. Urine that is alkaline will affect how your body eliminates Namenda and may increase your risk for side effects. Talk to your doctor about what foods and medicines should be avoided.

What are possible food and drug interactions associated with this medication?

If Namenda is taken with certain other drugs, the effects of either could be increased, decreased, or altered. It is especially important to check with your doctor before combining Namenda with the following: amantadine, carbonic anhydrase inhibitors (such as acetazolamide or methazolamide), cimetidine, dextromethorphan, diuretics (water pills) (such as hydrochlorothiazide or triamterene), ketamine, metformin, nicotine, quinidine, ranitidine, or sodium bicarbonate.

What are the possible side effects of this medication?

Please see general statement regarding side effects on page xiii.

Side effects may include: back pain, confusion, constipation, cough, dizziness, hallucinations, headache, high blood pressure, pain, shortness of breath, tiredness, vomiting

Can I receive this medication if I am pregnant or breastfeeding?

The effects of Namenda during pregnancy and breastfeeding are unknown. Tell your doctor immediately if you are pregnant, plan to become pregnant, or are breastfeeding.

What should I do if I miss a dose of this medication?

If you miss a dose of Namenda, take it as soon as you remember. However, if it is almost time for your next dose, skip the one you missed and return to your regular dosing schedule. Do not take two doses at once.

How should I store this medication?

Store at room temperature.

Namenda XR

Generic name: Memantine HCl

What is this medication?

Namenda XR is a medicine that is used to treat patients with Alzheimer's disease.

What is the most important information I should know about this medication?

- If you accidentally take more Namenda XR than you should, inform your doctor immediately. You may require medical attention. Some people who have accidentally taken too much memantine (the active ingredient in Namenda XR) have experienced dizziness, unsteadiness, weakness, tiredness, confusion, or other symptoms.
- If you have, or ever had seizures or difficulty passing urine, your doctor will need to monitor you more closely while you are taking Namenda XR.

Who should not take this medication?

Do not take Namenda XR if you are allergic to it or any of its ingedients.

What should I tell my doctor before I take the first dose of this medication?

Tell your doctor about all prescription, over-the-counter, and herbal medications you are taking before beginning treatment with Namenda XR. Also, talk to your doctor about your complete medical history, especially if you have kidney or liver disease, history of seizures or difficulty urinating, or if you have a urinary tract infection.

What is the usual dosage?

Please see general statement regarding dosage on page xii.

Adults: The starting dose is 7 milligrams (mg) once a day.

If you have severe kidney impairment, your doctor will adjust your dose appropriately.

How should I take this medication?

- Take Namenda XR exactly as prescribed by your doctor. Do not take extra doses or take more often without asking your doctor.
- Take Namenda XR with or without food.
- Swallow Namenda XR capsules whole. Do not crush, divide, or chew the capsules. Alternatively, open the capsule and sprinkle the contents on applesauce before swallowing. Take the contents of the entire capsule. Do not divide the dose.

What should I avoid while taking this medication?

Do not consume food or medicines (such as sodium bicarbonate) that make your urine alkaline. Urine that is alkaline will affect how your body eliminates Namenda XR and may increase your risk for side effects. Talk to your doctor about what foods and medicines should be avoided.

What are possible food and drug interactions associated with this medication?

If Namenda XR is taken with certain other drugs, the effects of either could be increased, decreased, or altered. It is especially important to check with your doctor before combining Namenda XR with the following: amantadine, carbonic anhydrase inhibitors (such as acetazolamide or methazolamide), cimetidine, dextromethorphan, diuretics (water pills) (such as hydrochlorothiazide or triamterene), ketamine, metformin, nicotine, quinidine, ranitidine, sodium bicarbonate.

What are the possible side effects of this medication?

Please see general statement regarding side effects on page xiii.

> **Side effects may include:** anxiety, back pain, constipation, diarrhea, dizziness, drowsiness, headache, high blood pressure, influenza, weight gain

Can I receive this medication if I am pregnant or breastfeeding?

The effects of Namenda XR during pregnancy and breastfeeding are unknown. Tell your doctor immediately if you are pregnant, plan to become pregnant, or are breastfeeding.

What should I do if I miss a dose of this medication?

If you miss a dose of Namenda XR, take it as soon as you remember. However, if it is almost time for your next dose, skip the one you missed and return to your regular dosing schedule. Do not take two doses at once.

If you forget to take Namenda XR for several days, do not take the next dose until you have talked to your doctor.

How should I store this medication?

Store at room temperature.

Naprosyn

Generic name: Naproxen Sodium

What is this medication?

Naprosyn is a nonsteroidal anti-inflammatory drug (NSAID) used to treat rheumatoid arthritis, osteoarthritis, ankylosing spondylitis (arthritis of the spine), juvenile arthritis, tendinitis, bursitis (inflammation and pain around joints), acute gout (severe and painful inflammation of the joints), and pain. In addition, Naprosyn is used to treat pain associated with menstrual periods. Naprosyn is available as tablets, an oral suspension, and EC-Naprosyn delayed-release tablets (releases medicine into your body at a later time from when you take it).

What is the most important information I should know about this medication?

- Naprosyn can cause serious problems (such as heart attack or stroke). Your risk can increase when this medication is used for long periods of time and if you have heart disease. Tell your doctor if you experience chest pain, shortness of breath, weakness, or slurred speech.

- Naprosyn can cause high blood pressure and heart failure or worsen existing high blood pressure. Tell your doctor if you experience weight gain or swelling.
- Naprosyn can cause discomfort, ulcers, or bleeding in your stomach or intestines. Your risk can increase with long-term use, smoking, drinking alcohol, older age, poor health, or with certain medications. Tell your doctor immediately if you experience stomach pain or if you have bloody vomit or stools.
- Long-term use of Naprosyn can cause kidney injury. Your risk can increase if you have kidney impairment; heart failure; liver problems; are taking certain medications, including diuretics (water pills) (such as furosemide or hydrochlorothiazide) or blood/heart medications known as angiotensin-converting enzyme (ACE) inhibitors (such as lisinopril); or are elderly.
- Naprosyn can also cause liver injury. Stop taking Naprosyn and call your doctor if you experience nausea, tiredness, weakness, itchiness, yellowing of your skin or whites of your eyes, right upper abdominal tenderness, or "flu-like" symptoms.
- Naprosyn can cause a serious allergic reaction. Stop taking Naprosyn and tell your doctor right away if you experience difficulty breathing or swelling of your face, mouth, or throat.
- Stop taking Naprosyn and tell your doctor right away if you experience serious skin reactions, such as rash, blisters, fever, or itchiness.

Who should not take this medication?

Do not take Naprosyn if you are allergic to it or any of its ingredients, or if you have experienced asthma, rash, or allergic-type reactions after taking aspirin or other NSAIDs (such as ibuprofen).

Do not take Naprosyn right before or after a heart surgery called a coronary artery bypass graft (CABG).

What should I tell my doctor before I take the first dose of this medication?

Tell your doctor about all prescription, over-the-counter, and herbal medications you are taking before beginning treatment with

Naprosyn. Also, talk to your doctor about your complete medical history, especially if you have any of the following: allergies to medications, heart problems, history of asthma, high blood pressure, kidney or liver disease, or stomach problems, or are pregnant, plan to become pregnant, or are breastfeeding.

What is the usual dosage?

Please see general statement regarding dosage on page xii.

Rheumatoid Arthritis, Osteoarthritis, and Ankylosing Spondylitis

Naprosyn
Adults: The recommended starting dose is 250 milligrams (mg) twice a day, 375 mg twice a day, or 500 mg twice a day.

EC-Naprosyn
Adults: The recommended starting dose is 375 mg twice a day or 500 mg twice a day.

Acute Gout

Naprosyn
Adults: The recommended starting dose is 750 mg, followed by 250 mg every 8 hours.

Pain, Menstrual Pain, Tendonitis, and Bursitis

Naprosyn
Adults: Your doctor will prescribe the appropriate dose for you.

Juvenile Arthritis

Naprosyn oral suspension
Children ≥2 years: Your doctor will prescribe the appropriate dose for your child, based on their weight.

Your doctor will adjust your dose appropriately.

If you are elderly, or have liver or kidney impairment, your doctor will adjust your dose approrpriately.

How should I take this medication?
- Take Naprosyn exactly as prescribed by your doctor.
- Swallow EC-Naprosyn tablets whole. Do not break, crush, or chew them.
- Shake the Naprosyn oral suspension gently before you give the medicine to your child.

What should I avoid while taking this medication?
Do not take Naprosyn with other medications called Anaprox, Anaprox DS, Aleve, or other medications that contain naproxen, since all these medicines contain the same active ingredient.

What are possible food and drug interactions associated with this medication?
If Naprosyn is taken with certain other drugs, the effects of either could be increased, decreased, or altered. It is especially important to check with your doctor before combining Naprosyn with the following: ACE inhibitors, antacids, aspirin, blood pressure/heart medications known as beta blockers (such a propranolol), blood thinners (such as warfarin), certain antibiotics (such as trimethoprim/sulfamethoxazole or sulfisoxazole), certain antidepressants (such as fluoxetine or paroxetine), cholestyramine, diabetes medicines (such as glipizide or glyburide), diuretics, lithium, methotrexate, phenytoin, probenecid, or sucralfate.

What are the possible side effects of this medication?
Please see general statement regarding side effects on page xiii.

> **Side effects may include:** constipation, diarrhea, dizziness, gas, heartburn, nausea, stomach pain, vomiting

Can I receive this medication if I am pregnant or breastfeeding?
Do not take Naprosyn if you are in the late stage of your pregnancy or if you are breastfeeding. The effects of Naprosyn during early

pregnancy are unknown. Tell your doctor immediately if you are pregnant, plan to become pregnant, or are breastfeeding.

What should I do if I miss a dose of this medication?
If you miss a dose of Naprosyn, take it as soon as you remember. However, if it is almost time for your next dose, skip the one you missed and return to your regular dosing schedule. Do not take two doses at once.

How should I store this medication?
Store at room temperature.

Naproxen Sodium: *see Anaprox, page 76*

Naproxen Sodium: *see Naprosyn, page 673*

Nasonex
Generic name: Mometasone Furoate Monohydrate

What is this medication?
Nasonex is a medicine used to prevent and treat nasal symptoms (such as stuffy and runny nose, itching, or sneezing) of seasonal or year-round allergies. Nasonex is also used to treat nasal polyps (non-cancerous growth·in the nose). Nasonex is available as a nasal spray.

What is the most important information I should know about this medication?
• Nasonex is for use in your nose only.
• Nasonex can cause nosebleeds, infections in your nose and throat, form a hole in the wall between your nostrils, or impair wound healing. Do not use Nasonex if you have a sore in your nose, have had nasal surgery, or a recent nasal injury until healing has occurred. Tell your doctor if you have any redness or white colored patches in your nose and throat.

- Cataracts (clouding of the eye's lens) or glaucoma (high pressure in the eye) can occur while you are using Nasonex. Tell your doctor if you experience a change in your vision.
- If you use Nasonex, you can have a higher risk of getting an infection. Do not expose yourself to chickenpox or measles while you are using Nasonex. Tell your doctor if you experience any signs or symptoms of infection (such as a fever, pain, aches, chills, feeling tired, nausea, or vomiting).
- Nasonex can cause slowed or delayed growth in children. Check your child's growth regularly during treatment with Nasonex.
- A decrease in nasal symptoms may occur 1-2 days after starting treatment with Nasonex. The full benefit of Nasonex is usually achieved within 1-2 weeks. Tell your doctor if your symptoms do not improve within that time, or if your condition worsens.

Who should not take this medication?
Do not use Nasonex if you are allergic to it or any of its ingredients.

What should I tell my doctor before I take the first dose of this medication?
Tell your doctor about all prescription, over-the-counter, and herbal medications you are taking before beginning treatment with Nasonex. Also, talk to your doctor about your complete medical history, especially if you recently have had nasal sores, surgery, or injury; have eye or vision problems; have tuberculosis (a bacterial infection that affects the lungs), or any type of infection, or had exposure to chickenpox or measles; or if you have other medical conditions that require long-term steroid treatment.

What is the usual dosage?
Please see general statement regarding dosage on page xii.

Treatment of Allergy Symptoms
Adults and adolescents ≥12 years: The recommended dose is 2 sprays in each nostril once a day.

Children 2-11 years: The recommended dose is 1 spray in each nostril once a day.

Prevention of Allergy Symptoms
Adults and adolescents ≥12 years: The recommended dose is 2 sprays in each nostril once a day.

Nasal Polyps
Adults: The recommended dose is 2 sprays in each nostril twice a day.

How should I take this medication?
- Use Nasonex exactly as prescribed by your doctor. Shake the bottle gently before each use.
- If you are using the nasal spray unit for the first time, you must prime it (to release into the air the dose that is already in the unit). To do this, press the pump 10 times or until a fine spray appears. If it has not been used for 1 week or longer, you must prime the pump by pressing 2 times or until you see a fine mist.
- Gently blow your nose to clear your nostrils. Close one nostril and tilt your head forward slightly when you spray Nasonex into each of your nostrils. Gently breathe in through your nostril and while breathing in press down on the applicator to release a spray.
- Please review the instructions that came with your prescription on how to properly use Nasonex.

What should I avoid while taking this medication?
Do not spray Nasonex into your eyes.

Do not apply extra doses or stop using Nasonex without talking to your doctor.

What are possible food and drug interactions associated with this medication?
No significant interactions have been reported with Nasonex at this time. However, always tell your doctor about any medicines you take, including over-the-counter medications, vitamins, and herbal supplements.

What are the possible side effects of this medication?
Please see general statement regarding side effects on page xiii.

> **Side effects may include:** cough, headache, nosebleeds, sore throat, viral infections

Can I receive this medication if I am pregnant or breastfeeding?

The effects of Nasonex during pregnancy and breastfeeding are unknown. Tell your doctor immediately if you are pregnant, plan to become pregnant, or are breastfeeding.

What should I do if I miss a dose of this medication?

If you miss a dose of Nasonex, apply it as soon as you remember. However, if it is almost time for your next dose, skip the one you missed and return to your regular dosing schedule. Do not apply two doses at once.

How should I store this medication?

Store at room temperature. Protect from light.

Nebivolol: see Bystolic, page 167

Neurontin

Generic name: Gabapentin

What is this medication?

Neurontin is a medicine used to treat seizures and pain from damaged nerves (neuropathic pain) that follows healing from shingles (painful rash caused by chickenpox virus). Neurontin is available as capsules, tablets, and an oral solution.

What is the most important information I should know about this medication?

• Do not stop taking Neurontin without first talking to your doctor. Stopping Neurontin suddenly can cause serious health problems.
• Neurontin can cause suicidal thoughts or actions in a very small number of people. Tell your doctor immediately if you

experience any of the following symptoms, especially if they are new, worse, or worry you: thoughts about suicide or dying, attempts to commit suicide, new or worse depression, new or worse anxiety, feeling agitated or restless, panic attacks, trouble sleeping, new or worse irritability, acting aggressive, being angry, or violent.

- Using Neurontin in children 3-12 years can cause emotional changes, aggressive behavior, problems with concentration, restlessness, changes in their school performance, or hyperactivity.
- Neurontin can cause a serious or life-threatening allergic reaction that may affect your skin or other parts of your body, such as your liver or blood cells. You may or may not develop a rash when you get this type of reaction.
- Tell your doctor right away if you experience skin rash, hives, fever, swollen glands that do not go away, swelling of your lips and tongue, yellowing of your skin or of the whites of the eyes, unusual bruising or bleeding, severe fatigue or weakness, unexpected muscle pain, or frequent infections.

Who should not take this medication?

Do not take Neurontin if you are allergic to it or any of its ingredients.

What should I tell my doctor before I take the first dose of this medication?

Tell your doctor about all prescription, over-the-counter, and herbal medications you are taking before beginning treatment with Neurontin. Also, talk to your doctor about your complete medical history, especially if you have a history of mental or mood problems, suicidal thoughts, or you have kidney, liver, or heart disease.

What is the usual dosage?

Please see general statement regarding dosage on page xii.

If your Neurontin dose is reduced, discontinued, or substituted with another medication, your doctor will gradually do this over a minimum of 1 week.

Seizures

Adults and adolescents ≥12 years: The usual daily dose is between 900 and 1800 milligrams (mg). This dose is taken in divided doses three times a day. The time between doses should not exceed 12 hours.

Children 3-12 years: Your doctor will prescribe the appropriate dose for your child, based on their weight.

Nerve Pain Associated with Shingles

Adults: The usual starting dose is a single 300-mg dose on the first day, followed by 300 mg twice a day on the second day, and 300 mg three times a day on the third day. Your doctor may increase your total daily dose as needed.

If you have kidney impairment, your doctor will adjust your dose appropriately.

How should I take this medication?

- Take Neurontin exactly as prescribed by your doctor. Do not take extra doses or take more often without asking your doctor.
- Do not change your dose of Neurontin without talking to your doctor. If you break a tablet in half, the unused half of the tablet should be taken at your next scheduled dose. Half tablets not used within several days of breaking should be thrown away. If taking capsules, always swallow them whole with plenty of water.
- Take Neurontin with or without food. If you take an antacid containing aluminum and magnesium, you should wait at least 2 hours before taking your next dose of Neurontin.

What should I avoid while taking this medication?

Do not drink alcohol or take other medicines that make you sleepy or dizzy while taking Neurontin without first talking to your doctor. Taking Neurontin with alcohol or drugs that cause sleepiness or dizziness may make your sleepiness or dizziness worse.

Do not drive, operate heavy machinery, or engage in other danger-ous activities until you know how Neurontin affects you. Neurontin can slow your thinking and motor skills.

What are possible food and drug interactions associated with this medication?

If Neurontin is taken with certain other drugs, the effects of either could be increased, decreased, or altered. It is especially important to check with your doctor before combining Neurontin with the fol-lowing: antacids, cimetidine, hydrocodone, morphine, or naproxen.

What are the possible side effects of this medication?

Please see general statement regarding side effects on page xiii.

> **Side effects may include:** difficulty speaking, dizziness, double vision, drowsiness, fever, jerky movements, lack of coordination, temporary loss of memory, tiredness, tremor, unusual eye move-ment, viral infection

Can I receive this medication if I am pregnant or breastfeeding?

The effects of Neurontin during pregnancy and breastfeeding are unknown. Tell your doctor immediately if you are pregnant, plan to become pregnant, or are breastfeeding.

What should I do if I miss a dose of this medication?

If you miss a dose of Neurontin, take it as soon as you remember. However, if it is almost time for your next dose, skip the one you missed and return to your regular dosing schedule. Do not take two doses at once.

How should I store this medication?

Store the capsules or tablets at room temperature. Store the oral solution in the refrigerator.

Nexium

Generic name: Esomeprazole Magnesium

What is this medication?

Nexium is a medicine called a proton pump inhibitor (PPI). It reduces the amount of acid in your stomach. Nexium is used in adults to treat heartburn and other symptoms associated with gastroesophageal reflux disease (GERD), erosive esophagitis (inflammation and ulceration of the esophagus [the tube that connects your mouth and stomach]), and maintain healing of erosive esophagitis.

Nexium is also used to reduce the risk of stomach ulcers in people on continuous therapy with nonsteroidal anti-inflammatory drugs (NSAIDs) (such as ibuprofen or naproxen); for long-term treatment of conditions where the stomach makes too much acid, such as Zollinger-Ellison syndrome; and with other medicines to eliminate the bacteria that often causes ulcers (known as *Helicobacter pylori*).

In addition, Nexium is used to treat GERD in children and adolescents, and erosive esophagitis in infants and children.

Nexium is available as capsules and an oral suspension.

What is the most important information I should know about this medication?

- Nexium can cause low magnesium levels in your body. Tell your doctor immediately if you have seizures, dizziness, abnormal or fast heartbeat, jitteriness, jerking movements or shaking, muscle weakness, spasms of your hands and feet, cramps or muscle aches, or spasm of your voice box.
- Tell your doctor if you experience any symptoms of a serious allergic reaction with Nexium (such as rash, face swelling, throat tightness, or difficulty breathing).
- People who are taking multiple daily doses of Nexium for a long period of time may have an increased risk of fractures of the hip, wrist, or spine.

Who should not take this medication?

Do not take Nexium if you are allergic to it, any of its ingredients, or to any other PPI.

What should I tell my doctor before I take the first dose of this medication?

Tell your doctor about all prescription, over-the-counter, and herbal medications you are taking before beginning treatment with Nexium. Also, talk to your doctor about your complete medical history, especially if you have low magnesium levels, any allergies, or liver problems. Tell your doctor if you are pregnant, plan to become pregnant, or are breastfeeding.

What is the usual dosage?

Please see general statement regarding dosage on page xii.

Healing of Erosive Esophagitis

Adults: The recommended dose is 20 milligrams (mg) or 40 mg once a day for 4-8 weeks. Depending on your response, your doctor may suggest another 4-8 weeks of treatment.

Children 1-11 years: Depending on your child's weight, the recommended dose is 10 mg or 20 mg once a day for 8 weeks.

Infants 1 month-<1 year: Depending on your child's weight, the recommended dose is 2.5 mg, 5 mg, or 10 mg once a day for up to 6 weeks.

Maintenance of Healing of Erosive Esophagitis

Adults: The recommended dose is 20 mg once a day.

Symptomatic GERD

Adults: The recommended dose is 20 mg once a day for 4 weeks.

Adolescents 12-17 years: The recommended dose is 20 mg or 40 mg once a day for up to 8 weeks.

Children 1-11 years: The recommended dose is 10 mg once a day for up to 8 weeks.

Prevention of Stomach Ulcer Due to NSAIDs
Adults: The recommended dose is 20 mg or 40 mg once a day for up to 6 months.

Prevention of Duodenal Ulcer Due to *H. pylori* Infection
Adults: This treatment involves taking three different medications. The usual dose for the triple therapy is: Nexium 40 mg once a day for 10 days, amoxicillin 1000 mg twice a day for 10 days, and clarithromycin 500 mg twice a day for 10 days.

Treatment of Excess Stomach Acid (Such as Zollinger-Ellison Syndrome)
Adults: The recommended dose is 40 mg twice a day. Your doctor might prescribe a different dose or duration based on your condition.

How should I take this medication?
- Take Nexium exactly as prescribed by your doctor. Do not change your dose or stop taking it without first talking to your doctor. Take Nexium at least 1 hour before a meal.
- Swallow Nexium capsules whole. If you have trouble with this, open the capsule and empty the contents into a tablespoon of applesauce. Swallow the applesauce mixture immediately. Do not chew the mixture or store it for later use.
- Your doctor will give you instructions on how to prepare the Nexium oral suspension.
- Please review to instructions that came with your prescription on how to properly take Nexium.

What should I avoid while taking this medication?
Do not chew or crush the capsules. This will damage them and the medicine will not work.

What are possible food and drug interactions associated with this medication?
If Nexium is taken with certain other drugs, the effects of either could be increased, decreased, or altered. It is especially important to check with your doctor before combining Nexium with the following: atazanavir, cilostazol, diazepam, digoxin, erlotinib,

ketoconazole, methotrexate, nelfinavir, products that contain iron, rifampin, saquinavir, St. John's wort, tacrolimus, voriconazole, or warfarin.

What are the possible side effects of this medication?
Please see general statement regarding side effects on page xiii.

> **Side effects may include:** abdominal pain, constipation, diarrhea, drowsiness, dry mouth, gas, headache, nausea

Can I receive this medication if I am pregnant or breastfeeding?
The effects of Nexium during pregnancy and breastfeeding are unknown. Tell your doctor immediately if you are pregnant, plan to become pregnant, or are breastfeeding.

What should I do if I miss a dose of this medication?
If you miss a dose of Nexium, take it as soon as you remember. However, if it is almost time for your next dose, skip the one you missed and return to your regular dosing schedule. Do not take two doses at once.

How should I store this medication?
Store at room temperature.

Niacin: *see Niaspan, page 687*

Niaspan
Generic name: Niacin

What is this medication?
Niaspan is a medicine used alone or in combination with other cholesterol-lowering medicines to lower your cholesterol when a low-fat diet is not enough. Niaspan increases "good" high-density lipoprotein (HDL) cholesterol in your body and lowers the "bad"

low-density lipoprotein (LDL) cholesterol and fats (triglycerides). Niaspan is also used to lower the risk of heart attack in people who have had a heart attack and have high cholesterol. In addition, Niaspan is used with another cholesterol-lowering medicine called bile acid resins (such as colestipol and cholestyramine) to slow the buildup of fat deposits in the arteries of people with coronary artery disease (narrowing of the small blood vessels that supply blood and oxygen to the heart) and high cholesterol.

What is the most important information I should know about this medication?

- Taking Niaspan is not a substitute for following a healthy low-fat and low-cholesterol diet and exercising to lower your cholesterol.
- Flushing is the most common side effect of Niaspan. Symptoms of flushing include warmth, redness, itching, or tingling of your skin. This is more likely to happen when you first start taking Niaspan or when your dose of Niaspan is increased. If you wake up at night because of flushing, get up slowly, especially if you feel dizzy or faint, or if you take blood pressure medicines.
- To lower your chance of flushing, take Niaspan with a low-fat snack, do not drink hot beverages (such as coffee), alcohol, or eat spicy food around the time you take Niaspan, and ask your doctor if you can take aspirin before you take Niaspan.
- Niaspan can cause muscle pain, tenderness, weakness, fatigue, loss of appetite, right upper abdominal discomfort, dark urine, light colored stools, itchy skin, nausea, or yellowing of your skin or whites of your eyes. Call your doctor right away if you notice any of these symptoms. Your risk for these effects may be higher if you take Niaspan with other cholesterol-lowering medicines known as "statins" (such as lovastatin or simvastatin).
- Niaspan can increase your blood sugar levels. If you have diabetes or are at risk for diabetes, monitor your blood sugar regularly, as determined by your doctor.

Who should not take this medication?

Do not take Niaspan if you are allergic to it or any of its ingredients.

Do not take Niaspan if you have liver disease, stomach ulcers, or bleeding problems.

What should I tell my doctor before I take the first dose of this medication?

Tell your doctor about all prescription, over-the-counter, and herbal medications you are taking before beginning treatment with Niaspan. Also, talk to your doctor about your complete medical history, especially if you have chest pain (angina), diabetes, gout (severe and painful inflammation of the joints), heart, kidney, liver, or thyroid problems, stomach ulcers, or if you recently had a heart attack. Tell your doctor if you drink large amounts of alcohol or if you are taking vitamins or other supplements that contain niacin or nicotinamide.

What is the usual dosage?

Please see general statement regarding dosage on page xii.

Adults: The usual starting dose is 500 milligrams (mg) once a day at bedtime. Your doctor will increase your dose appropriately.

How should I take this medication?

- Your doctor will likely start you on a low-cholesterol diet before prescribing Niaspan. Stay on this diet while you are taking Niaspan.
- Take Niaspan exactly as prescribed by your doctor. Take it once a day at bedtime after a low-fat snack.
- Swallow Niaspan tablets whole. Do not crush, chew, or break them.
- If you are taking Niaspan with a bile acid resin, take the medicines at least 4-6 hours apart.

What should I avoid while taking this medication?

Do not take Niaspan on an empty stomach.

Do not change your dose or stop taking Niaspan without first talking to your doctor.

What are possible food and drug interactions associated with this medication?

If Niaspan is taken with certain other drugs, the effects of either could be increased, decreased, or altered. It is especially important to check with your doctor before combining Niaspan with the following: alcohol, blood pressure medications, statins, or vitamins or supplements that contain large doses of niacin or nicotinamide.

What are the possible side effects of this medication?

Please see general statement regarding side effects on page xiii.

> **Side effects may include:** diarrhea, flushing, increased cough, nausea, rash, vomiting

Can I receive this medication if I am pregnant or breastfeeding?

The effects of Niaspan during pregnancy are unknown. Niaspan can be found in your breast milk if you take it while breastfeeding. Do not breastfeed while you are taking Niaspan. Tell your doctor immediately if you are pregnant, plan to become pregnant, or are breastfeeding.

What should I do if I miss a dose of this medication?

If you miss a dose of Niaspan, take it as soon as you remember. However, if it is almost time for your next dose, skip the one you missed and return to your regular dosing schedule. Do not take your dose in the morning or take two doses at once.

How should I store this medication?

Store at room temperature.

Nifedical XL
Generic name: Nifedipine

What is this medication?
Nifedical XL is a medicine known as a calcium channel blocker, which is used alone or in combination with other medications to treat high blood pressure. Nifedical XL is also used to treat chest pain.

What is the most important information I should know about this medication?
- Your blood pressure can become lower than normal during treatment with Nifedical XL. Tell your doctor if you experience dizziness, lightheadedness, or fainting while on Nifedical XL.
- Although this happens rarely, patients with severe heart disease can experience an increase in the frequency and duration of chest pain, or even have a heart attack, when starting treatment with Nifedical XL or if the dose is increased.
- Nifedical XL can cause heart failure. Tell your doctor if you have any heart conditions.
- Nifedical XL can cause serious stomach problems. Your risk can increase if you already have stomach problems or are taking certain medications.
- Nifedical XL can cause edema (swelling) of your lower legs and arms. Tell your doctor right away if you experience any swelling.

Who should not take this medication?
Do not take Nifedical XL if you are allergic to it or any of its ingredients.

What should I tell my doctor before I take the first dose of this medication?
Tell your doctor about all prescription, over-the-counter, and herbal medications you are taking before beginning treatment with Nifedical XL. Also, talk to your doctor about your complete medical history, especially if you have heart disease, liver or stomach problems, acid reflux, an underactive thyroid, or diabetes. Tell your doctor if you have a history of colon cancer or have ever had gastric bypass surgery.

What is the usual dosage?

Please see general statement regarding dosage on page xii.

High Blood Pressure and Chest Pain

Adults: The usual starting dose is 30 milligrams (mg) or 60 mg once a day. Your doctor may give you a higher dose depending on your needs.

How should I take this medication?

• Swallow Nifedical XL tablets whole. Do not chew, crush, or divide them.

What should I avoid while taking this medication?

Do not stop taking Nifedical XL without first talking to your doctor.

What are possible food and drug interactions associated with this medication?

If Nifedical XL is used with certain other drugs, the effects of either could be increased, decreased, or altered. It is especially important to check with your doctor before combining Nifedical XL with the following: blood pressure/heart medications known as beta-blockers (such as atenolol or metoprolol), blood thinners (such as warfarin), cimetidine, or digoxin.

What are the possible side effects of this medication?

Please see general statement regarding side effects on page xiii.

> **Side effects may include:** constipation, fatigue, headache, nausea, swelling

Can I receive this medication if I am pregnant or breastfeeding?

The effects of Nifedical XL during pregnancy and breastfeeding are unknown. Tell your doctor immediately if you are pregnant, plan to become pregnant, or are breastfeeding.

What should I do if I miss a dose of this medication?
If you miss a dose of Nifedical XL, take it as soon as you remember. However, if it is almost time for your next dose, skip the one you missed and return to your regular dosing schedule. Do not take two doses at once.

How should I store this medication?
Store at room temperature. Protect from moisture and humidity.

Nifedipine: *see Nifedical XL, page 691*

Nifedipine: *see Procardia XL, page 844*

Nitrofurantoin Macrocrystals: *see Macrodantin, page 603*

Nitroglycerin: *see Nitrostat, page 693*

Nitrostat
Generic name: Nitroglycerin

What is this medication?
Nitrostat is a medicine used to prevent or relieve an attack of angina (chest pain) caused by coronary artery disease.

What is the most important information I should know about this medication?
- Nitrostat can cause a severe decrease in blood pressure. This is most likely to occur while rising from a seated position. This effect can occur more frequently if you consume alcohol. Tell your doctor immediately if you experience dizziness or lightheadedness.
- Headache is a common side effect of Nitrostat. If you get headaches while you are using Nitrostat, this is a sign that the medicine is working properly. You should not try to avoid headaches by changing the time you take Nitrostat.

• Stop taking Nitrostat and tell your doctor immediately if you experience blurred vision or dry mouth.

Who should not take this medication?

Do not take Nitrostat if you are allergic to it, any of its ingredients,
or other nitrates or nitrites. Also, do not use Nitrostat if you had a
very recent heart attack, have severe anemia, have increased pressure in your head, or are taking a medicine for impotence (such as
sildenafil, tadalafil, or vardenafil).

What should I tell my doctor before I take the first dose of this medication?

Tell your doctor about all prescription, over-the-counter, and herbal
medications you are taking before beginning treatment with Nitrostat. Also, talk to your doctor about your complete medical history,
especially if you are allergic to nitrates, have heart failure or any
other heart condition, are pregnant, plan to become pregnant, or
are breastfeeding.

What is the usual dosage?
Please see general statement regarding dosage on page xii.

Adults: The recommended dose is 1 tablet at the first sign of
chest pain. If your doctor prescribes this to prevent angina, take
this medication 5-10 minutes before activities that might cause
chest pain.

How should I take this medication?

• Take Nitrostat exactly as prescribed by your doctor. Nitrostat is
a sublingual tablet that dissolves under your tongue or in your
oral cavity. You may feel a burning or tingling sensation in your
mouth when you take Nitrostat.
• Sit down when you take Nitrostat and use caution when you
stand up. You can repeat your dose every 5 minutes, until your
chest pain is relieved. If your chest pain persists after a total of
3 tablets in a 15-minute period, or is different than the pain you
typically experience, get emergency medical help immediately.

What should I avoid while taking this medication?
Do not consume alcohol while you are taking Nitrostat.

Do not chew, crush, or swallow Nitrostat tablets.

What are possible food and drug interactions associated with this medication?
If Nitrostat is used with certain other drugs, the effects of either could be increased, decreased, or altered. It is especially important to check with your doctor before combining Nitrostat with the following: alcohol, alteplase, aspirin, blood pressure/heart medications known as beta-blockers (such as propranolol) or calcium channel blockers (such as amlodipine), certain antidepressants (such as amitriptyline, desipramine, or doxepin), ergotamine, or medicine for impotence.

What are the possible side effects of this medication?
Please see general statement regarding side effects on page xiii.

> **Side effects may include:** allergic reactions (such as rash), balance problems, decrease in blood pressure, dizziness, fainting, flushing, headache, increased chest pain, irregular heartbeat, lightheadedness, nausea, paleness, skin rash, sweating, vomiting, weakness

Can I receive this medication if I am pregnant or breastfeeding?
The effects of Nitrostat during pregnancy and breastfeeding are unknown. Tell your doctor immediately if you are pregnant, plan to become pregnant, or are breastfeeding.

What should I do if I miss a dose of this medication?
Nitrostat should be given only as needed.

How should I store this medication?
Store at room temperature. Keep in the original container and tightly capped.

Nizoral

Generic name: Ketoconazole

What is this medication?

Nizoral is a medicine used to treat certain serious fungal infections in your blood and body. These infections are called candidiasis, candiduria, blastomycosis, coccidioidomycosis, histoplasmosis, chromomycosis, and paracoccidioidomycosis.

What is the most important information I should know about this medication?

- Nizoral can cause serious or even fatal liver damage. Your doctor will monitor your liver function before and after you start taking Nizoral. Tell your doctor right away if you experience unusual tiredness, loss of appetite, nausea or vomiting, yellowing of your skin or whites of your eyes, dark urine, or pale stools.
- Nizoral can cause serious irregular heartbeat when it is taken with astemizole, cisapride, or terfenadine.
- Nizoral can cause serious allergic reactions. Tell your doctor or seek emergency help right away if you develop difficulty breathing, tightness in your chest, swelling of your eyelids, face, or lips, or rash.
- Nizoral requires acidity to be dissolved. Tell your doctor if you have a condition of absent or no gastric acid production in the stomach (achlorhydria). Take antacids or other medications that lower the acid in your stomach at least 2 hours after taking Nizoral. You can dissolve Nizoral in an acidic solution (hydrochloric acid) as directed by your doctor.
- Nizoral can lower your testosterone or corticosteroid (natural substances found in the body that help fight inflammation) levels. Your doctor will monitor you for this.
- Do not take more Nizoral than prescribed by your doctor.
- Take Nizoral as prescribed by your doctor for the full course of treatment, even if symptoms improve earlier. Do not skip doses. Complete the full course of Nizoral. Skipping doses or not completing the full course of Nizoral can decrease its effectiveness and can make the infection harder to treat in the future.

Who should not take this medication?

Do not take Nizoral if you are allergic to it or any of its ingredients.

Do not take Nizoral together with astemizole, cisapride, terfenadine, or triazolam.

What should I tell my doctor before I take the first dose of this medication?

Tell your doctor about all prescription, over-the-counter, and herbal medications you are taking before beginning treatment with Nizoral. Also, talk to your doctor about your complete medical history, especially if you have achlorhydria, have liver or blood problems, are pregnant, plan to become pregnant, or are breastfeeding.

What is the usual dosage?

Please see general statement regarding dosage on page xii.

Adults: The recommended starting dose is 200 milligrams (mg) once a day.

Children >2 years: Your doctor will prescribe the appropriate dose for your child, based on their weight.

How should I take this medication?

• Take Nizoral exactly as prescribed by your doctor. You can take Nizoral with or without food. You can take Nizoral tablets with meals to avoid stomach upset.

What should I avoid while taking this medication?

Do not drink alcohol while taking Nizoral.

Do not take antacids or other medications that lower the acid in your stomach within 2 hours after you take Nizoral.

Do not take astemizole, cisapride, terfenadine, or triazolam while taking Nizoral.

What are possible food and drug interactions associated with this medication?

If Nizoral is taken with certain other drugs, the effects of either could be increased, decreased, or altered. Nizoral may interact with numerous medications. Therefore, it is very important that you tell your doctor about any other medications you are taking.

What are the possible side effects of this medication?

Please see general statement regarding side effects on page xiii.

> **Side effects may include:** abdominal pain, allergic reactions, chills, diarrhea, dizziness, enlargement of breasts, fever, head-ache, impotence, light sensitivity, nausea, sleepiness, vomiting, itching

Can I receive this medication if I am pregnant or breastfeeding?

The effects of Nizoral during pregnancy are unknown. Nizoral can be found in your breast milk if you take it during breastfeeding. Do not breastfeed while taking Nizoral. Tell your doctor immediately if you are pregnant, plan to become pregnant, or are breastfeeding.

What should I do if I miss a dose of this medication?

If you miss a dose of Nizoral, take it as soon as you remember. However, if it is almost time for your next dose, skip the one you missed and return to your regular dosing schedule. Do not take two doses at once.

How should I store this medication?

Store at room temperature. Protect from moisture.

Nortriptyline HCl: *see Pamelor, page 761*

Norvasc
Generic name: Amlodipine Besylate

What is this medication?

Norvasc is a medicine known as a calcium channel blocker, which is used to treat high blood pressure and chest pain, either alone or in combination with other medicines. Norvasc is also used in people with coronary artery disease (narrowing of the small blood vessels that supply blood and oxygen to the heart) to lower the risk of hospitalization due to chest pain or the need for procedures to restore the blood flow back to the heart or to another part of the body.

What is the most important information I should know about this medication?

- Your blood pressure can become lower than normal during treatment with Norvasc. Tell your doctor if you experience dizziness, lightheadedness, or fainting while on Norvasc.
- Although this happens rarely, patients with severe heart disease can experience worsening of chest pain, or even have a heart attack, when starting treatment with Norvasc or if the dose is increased. If this happens, call your doctor right away or go directly to an emergency room.

Who should not take this medication?

Do not take Norvasc if you are allergic to it or any of its ingredients.

What should I tell my doctor before I take the first dose of this medication?

Tell your doctor about all prescription, over-the-counter, and herbal medications you are taking before beginning treatment with Norvasc. Also, talk to your doctor about your complete medical history, especially if you have liver problems, heart disease, or are pregnant, plan to become pregnant, or are breastfeeding.

What is the usual dosage?

Please see general statement regarding dosage on page xii.

High Blood Pressure
Adults: The usual starting dose is 5 milligrams (mg) once a day.

Children 6-17 years: The usual dose is 2.5 mg-5 mg once a day.

Chest Pain and Coronary Artery Disease
Adults: The usual dose is 5 mg-10 mg once a day.

If you are elderly or have liver impairment, your doctor will adjust your dose appropriately.

How should I take this medication?
• Take Norvasc once a day, at the same time every day. Take it with or without food.

What should I avoid while taking this medication?
Do not stop taking your other prescription medicines, including any other blood pressure medicines while you are taking Norvasc, without first talking to your doctor.

What are possible food and drug interactions associated with this medication?
If Norvasc is taken with certain other drugs, the effects of either could be increased, decreased, or altered. It is especially important to check with your doctor before combining Norvasc with the following: diltiazem, itraconazole, ketoconazole, ritonavir, or simvastatin.

What are the possible side effects of this medication?
Please see general statement regarding side effects on page xiii.

Side effects may include: dizziness; extreme sleepiness; flushing of your face; fluttery, throbbing, or irregular heartbeat; headache; nausea; stomach pain; swelling of your legs or ankles; tiredness

---

Can I receive this medication if I am pregnant or breastfeeding?

The effects of Norvasc during pregnancy and breastfeeding are unknown. Do not take Norvasc if you are breastfeeding. Tell your doctor immediately if you are pregnant, plan to become pregnant, or are breastfeeding.

What should I do if I miss a dose of this medication?

If you miss a dose of Norvasc, take it as soon as you remember. However, if it is almost time for your next dose, skip the one you missed and return to your regular dosing schedule. Do not take two doses at once.

How should I store this medication?

Store at room temperature.

Norvir

Generic name: Ritonavir

What is this medication?

Norvir is in a class of medicines called protease inhibitors. Norvir is used in combination with other medicines to treat people with human immunodeficiency virus (HIV) infection (or AIDS). Norvir is available in capsules, tablets, and oral solution.

What is the most important information I should know about this medication?

- Norvir is not a cure for AIDS or HIV infection. You may continue to experience symptoms and develop complications, including infections such as pneumonia and herpes virus infections.
- Norvir does not reduce the risk of passing HIV to others through sexual contact or blood contamination.
- When your Norvir supply starts to run low, get more from your doctor or pharmacy. This is very important because the amount of virus in your blood may increase if the medicine is stopped for even a short time. The virus may develop resistance to Norvir and become harder to treat.

Who should not take this medication?

Do not take Norvir if you have had a serious allergic reaction to Norvir or any of its ingredients.

Do not take Norvir with: alfuzosin hydrochloride, amiodarone, cisapride, dihydroergotamine, ergonovine, ergotamine, flecainide, lovastatin, methylergonovine, oral midazolam, pimozide, propafenone, quinidine, sildenafil, simvastatin, St. John's wort, triazolam, or voriconazole.

What should I tell my doctor before I take the first dose of this medication?

Tell your doctor about all prescription, over-the-counter, and herbal medications you are taking before beginning treatment with Norvir. Also, talk to your doctor about your complete medical history, especially if you have liver or heart problems, diabetes, bleeding problems or hemophilia (a bleeding disorder), or if you are pregnant, plan to become pregnant, or are breastfeeding.

What is the usual dosage?

Please see general statement regarding dosage on page xii.

Adults: The recommended dose is 600 milligrams (mg) twice a day.

Your doctor may start you at 300 mg twice a day to avoid side effects. Your doctor will increase your dose every 2-3 days by 100 mg up to the recommended dose.

Children ≥1 month: Your doctor will prescribe the appropriate dose for your child based on their body weight.

How should I take this medication?

• You should stay under a doctor's care when taking Norvir.
• Take Norvir exactly as prescribed by your doctor. Do not change your dose or stop your treatment without talking to your doctor first.
• Take Norvir with food or meals.

- Swallow Norvir tablets whole. Do not chew, break, or crush the tablets before swallowing.
- If you are taking Norvir oral solution, shake it well before each use. Use a special spoon or dosing syringe to measure each dose of the oral solution accurately. A household teaspoon may not hold the correct amount of oral solution. If you want to improve the taste, you can mix the liquid with 8 ounces of chocolate milk, Ensure, or Advera. Take Norvir oral solution within one hour of mixing with these fluids.

What should I avoid while taking this medication?
Do not have sex without protection (such as a condom).

Do not share needles or other injection equipment with another person.

Do not share personal items that can have blood or body fluids on them (such as toothbrushes and razor blades).

Do not breastfeed.

What are possible food and drug interactions associated with this medication?
If Norvir is taken with certain other drugs, the effects of either could be increased, decreased, or altered. Norvir may interact with numerous other medications. Therefore, it is very important that you tell your doctor about any other medications you are taking.

What are the possible side effects of this medication?
Please see general statement regarding side effects on page xiii.

Side effects may include: abdominal pain; changes in your taste; diarrhea; dizziness; feeling weak or tired; headache; loss of appetite; nausea; tingling feeling or numbness in the hands, feet, or around the lips; vomiting

Can I receive this medication if I am pregnant or breastfeeding?

The effects of Norvir during pregnancy and breastfeeding are unknown. It is recommended that you do not breastfeed your baby if you are infected with HIV. Tell your doctor immediately if you are pregnant, plan to become pregnant, or are breastfeeding.

What should I do if I miss a dose of this medication?

If you miss a dose of Norvir, take it as soon as you remember. However, if it is almost time for your next dose, skip the one you missed and return to your regular dosing schedule. Do not take two doses at once.

How should I store this medication?

Store capsules in the refrigerator. Capsules can be stored at room temperature if used within 30 days. Protect from light and keep away from heat.

Store tablets at room temperature.

Store oral solution at room temperature. Do not refrigerate. Keep away from heat. Shake well before each use.

Keep capsules, tablets, and oral solution in its original container.

Novolog

Generic name: Insulin Aspart, rDNA origin

What is this medication?

Novolog is a medicine that is a fast-acting insulin. Novolog is used to control high blood sugar in people with diabetes. Novolog comes as a prefilled pen, vial, and a cartridge.

What is the most important information I should know about this medication?

• Do not change the type of insulin you use unless told to do so by your doctor. Your insulin dose and the time you take your dose can change with different types of insulin. Make sure you have the right type and strength of insulin prescribed for you.

- Do not make any changes to your insulin dose unless you have talked to your doctor. Your insulin needs may change because of illness, stress, other medicines, or changes in your diet or activity level.

- Novolog can cause you to experience low blood sugar. Therefore, it is important to use it as prescribed by your doctor. Symptoms of low blood sugar include: hunger, dizziness, feeling shaky or shakiness, lightheadedness, sweating, irritability, headache, fast heartbeat, or confusion. Always carry a quick source of sugar to treat low blood sugar (such as glucose tablets, hard candy, or juice).

- Novolog starts working faster than other insulins. You should inject it 5-10 minutes or less before a meal. If you do not plan to eat within 5-10 minutes, delay the injection until the correct time (5-10 minutes before eating).

- If you forget to inject your dose of Novolog, your blood sugar may get too high. If your high blood sugar is not treated, it can lead to serious problems (such as passing out or loss of consciousness, coma, or even death). Follow your doctor's instructions for treating high blood sugar. Symptoms of high blood sugar include: increased thirst, frequent urination, drowsiness, loss of appetite, difficulty breathing, fruity smelling breath, nausea, vomiting, or stomach ache.

Who should not take this medication?

Do not take Novolog if you are allergic to it or any of its ingredients. Also, do not use Novolog if your blood sugar is too low.

What should I tell my doctor before I take the first dose of this medication?

Tell your doctor about all prescription, over-the-counter, and herbal medications you are taking before beginning treatment with Novolog. Also, talk to your doctor about your complete medical history, especially if you have kidney or liver problems, or are pregnant, plan to become pregnant, or are breastfeeding.

What is the usual dosage?

Please see general statement regarding dosage on page xii.

Adults and children ≥2 years: Your doctor will determine your dose based on your blood sugar levels.

How should I take this medication?

- Inject Novolog exactly as prescribed by your doctor. Use the proper injection technique taught to you by your doctor. Read the User Manual that comes with your Novolog Prefilled Pen for detailed instructions.
- Inject Novolog 5-10 minutes before you eat. Inject it under the skin of your stomach area, upper arm, upper leg, or buttocks. Never inject Novolog into a muscle or vein. Change your injection site with each dose.
- Only use Novolog that is clear and colorless.
- Your doctor may tell you to mix your Novolog with a longer-acting human insulin. When mixing these two types of insulin, draw Novolog into the syringe first. Do not dilute or mix Novolog with any other insulin in the same external insulin pump.

What should I avoid while taking this medication?

Do not drink alcohol while using Novolog. Alcohol may affect your blood sugar.

Do not drive or operate machinery if you have trouble paying attention or have slower reaction times if you have low blood sugar.

Do not inject Novolog in the same place twice; rotate the injection sites.

Do not use Novolog in the same external pump with other insulin products.

Do not share Novolog with anyone else, even if they have diabetes. It may harm them.

What are possible food and drug interactions associated with this medication?

If Novolog is used with certain other drugs, the effects of either could be increased, decreased, or altered. Novolog may interact with numerous medications. Therefore, it is very important that you tell your doctor about any other medications you are taking.

What are the possible side effects of this medication?

Please see general statement regarding side effects on page xiii.

> **Side effects may include:** allergic reactions, injection-site reactions, itching, low blood sugar, rash, skin thickening or pitting at the injection site, swelling of your hands and feet, vision changes, weight gain

Can I receive this medication if I am pregnant or breastfeeding?

The effects of Novolog during pregnancy and breastfeeding are unknown. Tell your doctor immediately if you are pregnant, plan to become pregnant, or are breastfeeding.

What should I do if I miss a dose of this medication?

It is very important to follow your insulin regimen exactly as prescribed by your doctor. Do not miss any doses. Ask your doctor for specific instructions to follow in case you ever miss a dose of insulin.

How should I store this medication?

Store unopened Novolog in the refrigerator (not the freezer). Protect from extreme heat, cold, or light.

After you open Novolog vials, store them in the refrigerator or at room temperature for 28 days.

After you start using Novolog cartridges or prefilled pens, do not refrigerate them. Keep them at room temperature, away from direct heat and light for up to 28 days.

Novolog Mix 70/30
Generic name: Insulin Aspart Protamine/Insulin Aspart, rDNA origin

What is this medication?
Novolog Mix 70/30 is a medicine that contains a mixture of fast-acting and longer-acting insulins. It is used to control high blood sugar in people with diabetes. Novolog Mix 70/30 comes as a pre-filled pen and a vial.

What is the most important information I should know about this medication?
- Do not change the type of insulin you use unless told to do so by your doctor. Your insulin dose and the time you take your dose can change with different types of insulin. Make sure you have the right type and strength of insulin prescribed for you.
- Do not make any changes with your insulin dose unless you have talked to your doctor. Your insulin needs may change because of illness, stress, other medicines, or changes in your diet or activity level.
- Novolog Mix 70/30 can cause you to experience low blood sugar. Therefore, it is important to take it as prescribed by your doctor. Symptoms of low blood sugar include: hunger, dizziness, feeling shaky or shakiness, lightheadedness, sweating, irritability, headache, fast heartbeat, or confusion. Always carry a quick source of sugar to treat low blood sugar (such as glucose tablets, hard candy, or juice).
- If you forget to inject your dose of Novolog Mix 70/30, your blood sugar may get too high. If your high blood sugar is not treated, it can lead to serious problems (such as passing out or loss of consciousness, coma, or even death). Follow your doctor's instructions for treating high blood sugar. Symptoms of high blood sugar include: increased thirst, frequent urination, drowsiness, loss of appetite, difficulty breathing, fruity smell in your breath, nausea, vomiting, or stomach ache.
- If you have type 1 diabetes, you should inject Novolog Mix 70/30 up to 15 minutes before a meal. If you have type 2 diabetes, inject Novolog Mix 70/30 up to 15 minutes before or after starting your meal. If you do not plan to eat within 15 minutes, delay the injection until the correct time (15 minutes before eating).

Who should not take this medication?

Do not inject Novolog Mix 70/30 if you are allergic to it or any of its ingredients. Also, do not inject Novolog Mix 70/30 if your blood sugar is too low.

What should I tell my doctor before I take the first dose of this medication?

Tell your doctor about all prescription, over-the-counter, and herbal medications you are taking before beginning treatment with Novolog Mix 70/30. Also, talk to your doctor about your complete medical history, especially if you have kidney or liver problems, are pregnant, plan to become pregnant, or are breastfeeding.

What is the usual dosage?

Please see general statement regarding dosage on page xii.

Adults: Your doctor will determine your dose based on your blood sugar levels.

How should I take this medication?

- Administer Novolog Mix 70/30 exactly as prescribed by your doctor. Use the proper injection technique taught to you by your doctor. Read the User Manual that comes with your Novolog Mix 70/30 FlexPen for detailed instructions.
- Mix Novolog Mix 70/30 well before each use. For Novolog Mix 70/30 in a vial, carefully shake or rotate the vial until completely mixed. For prefilled pens, carefully follow the User Manual for instructions on how to mix the pen. Novolog Mix 70/30 should be white or cloudy after you mix it well. If it is not evenly mixed or has solid particles or clumps in it, return it to the pharmacy for a replacement.
- If you have type 1 diabetes, you should inject Novolog Mix 70/30 up to 15 minutes before a meal. If you have type 2 diabetes, you should inject Novolog Mix 70/30 up to 15 minutes before or after starting your meal. Inject Novolog Mix 70/30 under the skin of your stomach area, upper arms, buttocks, or upper legs. Novolog Mix 70/30 may affect your blood sugar levels faster if you inject it under the skin of your stomach area. Never inject

Novolog Mix 70/30 into a muscle or vein. Change your injection site with each dose.

What should I avoid while taking this medication?

Do not drink alcohol while using Novolog Mix 70/30. Alcohol may affect your blood sugar.

Do not drive or operate machinery if you have trouble paying attention or reacting when you have low blood sugar.

Do not inject Novolog Mix 70/30 in the same place twice; rotate the injection sites.

Do not use Novolog Mix 70/30 in the same syringe with other insulin products, and do not use it in an insulin pump.

Do not share Novolog Mix 70/30 with anyone else, even if they have diabetes. It may harm them.

What are possible food and drug interactions associated with this medication?

If Novolog Mix 70/30 is used with certain other drugs, the effects of either could be increased, decreased, or altered. Novolog Mix 70/30 may interact with numerous medications. Therefore, it is very important that you tell your doctor about any other medications you are taking.

What are the possible side effects of this medication?

Please see general statement regarding side effects on page xiii.

Side effects may include: allergic reactions, injection-site reactions, itching, low blood sugar, rash, skin thickening or pitting at the injection site, swelling of your hands and feet, vision changes, weight gain

---

Can I receive this medication if I am pregnant or breastfeeding?

The effects of Novolog Mix 70/30 during pregnancy and breast-feeding are unknown. Tell your doctor immediately if you are pregnant, plan to become pregnant, or are breastfeeding.

What should I do if I miss a dose of this medication?

It is very important to follow your insulin regimen exactly as pre-scribed by your doctor. Do not miss any doses. Ask your doctor for specific instructions to follow in case you ever miss a dose of insulin.

How should I store this medication?

Store unopened Novolog Mix 70/30 vials in the refrigerator (not the freezer). Protect from extreme heat, cold, or light.

After you open Novolog Mix 70/30, store the vials in the refrigera-tor or at room temperature for 28 days. After you open Novolog Mix 70/30 prefilled pens, do not refrigerate them. Keep them at room temperature, away from direct heat and light for up to 14 days.

Nuvaring

Generic name: Ethinyl Estradiol/Etonogestrel

What is this medication?

Nuvaring is a flexible birth control vaginal ring that is used to pre-vent pregnancy.

What is the most important information I should know about this medication?

- Nuvaring does not protect against HIV infection (AIDS) and other sexually transmitted diseases (STDs).
- Cigarette smoking increases your risk of serious heart side ef-fects when you use birth control. This risk increases even more if you are over the age of 35 and if you smoke 15 or more

cigarettes a day. If you use birth control medications, including Nuvaring, you are strongly advised not to smoke.
- Do not use a diaphragm as a back-up form of birth control with Nuvaring, because it interferes with the correct placement and position of the diaphragm.
- Go for an annual check-up while on Nuvaring so your doctor can evaluate how you are doing, especially if you have high blood pressure or high cholesterol.
- If you have developed serious depression during or prior to therapy, stop using Nuvaring at once and speak to your doctor to determine if the depression is related to the medication.

Who should not take this medication?
Do not use Nuvaring if you have not yet had your period.

Do not use Nuvaring if you have any of the following conditions: pregnancy or suspected pregnancy; a history of blood clots in your legs, lungs, or eyes; heart valve or heart rhythm disorders associated with blood clot formation; chest pain; a history of heart attack or stroke; severe high blood pressure; diabetes with complications of the kidneys, eyes, nerves, or blood vessels; obesity; headaches with neurological symptoms; have or have had breast cancer or cancer of the lining of the uterus, cervix, or vagina; unexplained vaginal bleeding (unless diagnosed by your doctor); jaundice (yellowing of the skin or whites of the eyes) during pregnancy or during past use of birth control medications of any kind; liver tumors or active liver disease; need for a long period of bed rest following major surgery; or an allergic reaction to any of the components of Nuvaring.

Women older than 65 years should not use Nuvaring.

Do not use Nuvaring if you smoke, especially if you smoke more than 15 cigarettes per day and/or are over the age of 35.

What should I tell my doctor before I take the first dose of this medication?
Tell your doctor about all prescription, over-the-counter, and herbal medications you are taking before beginning treatment with

Nuvaring. Also, talk to your doctor about your complete medical history, especially if you have any of the following conditions: a family history of breast cancer; an abnormal breast x-ray or abnormal mammogram; diabetes; high blood pressure; other breast disorders; high cholesterol or triglycerides; headaches or seizures; depression; gallbladder, liver, heart, or kidney disease; irregular menstrual periods; major surgery; severe constipation, or a history of toxic shock syndrome (potentially fatal disease caused by bacteria).

What is the usual dosage?

Please see general statement regarding dosage on page xii.

Adults: Nuvaring is inserted in the vagina once a month. It stays in the vagina continuously for three weeks. It must be removed exactly 21 days after insertion. A new ring is inserted precisely seven days later.

If you were previously on another birth control medication or method, your doctor will tell you when to start using Nuvaring.

How should I take this medication?

- Start Nuvaring on the first day of your cycle (the first day of your period). You may start it on Days 2-5 as well. This medication does not work immediately, so make sure to use other forms of birth control (such as condoms) during the first seven days of Nuvaring use.
- Please review the Patient Information that came with your Nuvaring prescription for detailed instructions on the proper way to insert and remove the ring.
- After removing the ring, place the used ring in the foil pouch it came in and dispose of it in the garbage, away from children and pets. Do not discard it in the toilet.
- Your menstrual period will usually start 2-3 days after the ring is removed and may not have finished before it is time to insert the next ring. For continued pregnancy protection, you need to insert the new ring exactly 1 week after the old one was removed, even if your period has not stopped.

What should I avoid while taking this medication?

Do not smoke or breastfeed while using Nuvaring.

What are possible food and drug interactions associated with this medication?

If Nuvaring is taken with certain other drugs, the effects of either could be increased, decreased, or altered. It is especially important to check with your doctor before combining Nuvaring with the following: acetaminophen, antibiotics (such as ampicillin and tetracycline), antifungals, atorvastatin, certain herbal products (such as St. John's wort), clofibrate, cyclosporine, HIV medications known as protease inhibitors (such as ritonavir and indinavir), morphine, phenylbutazone, prednisolone, rifadin, seizure medications, temazepam, theophylline, or vitamin C.

What are the possible side effects of this medication?

Please see general statement regarding side effects on page xiii.

> **Side effects may include:** abdominal (stomach) cramps, allergic rash, bloating, blood clots, breakthrough bleeding and spotting, breast secretions, change in menstrual flow, changes in the breast such as tenderness or enlargement, dark pigmentation of the skin, depression, headaches, heart attack, high blood pressure, intolerance to contact lenses, missed periods, nausea, problems with the ring, sinus inflammation, swelling, temporary infertility after discontinuing Nuvaring, upper respiratory tract (lung) infections, vaginal inflammation or discharge, vision problems, vomiting, weight gain or loss, yeast infections

Can I receive this medication if I am pregnant or breastfeeding?

Do not use Nuvaring during pregnancy or breastfeeding. Tell your doctor immediately if you are pregnant, plan to become pregnant, or are breastfeeding.

What should I do if I miss a dose of this medication?

In Weeks 1 and 2, if Nuvaring slips out, you will still be protected against pregnancy, provided the ring is replaced within 3 hours.

You can use the old ring (after rinsing it with cool or lukewarm water) or insert a new ring. Remove the ring according to your original schedule. If you are unable to replace the ring within 3 hours, insert it as soon as possible and use an additional method of birth control for seven days.

If the ring slips out during Week 3, contact your doctor or pharmacist for advice.

How should I store this medication?
Store at room temperature. Do not use past four months from the date you received the ring.

Nystatin Suspension
Generic name: Nystatin

What is this medication?
Nystatin suspension is an antifungal medicine that is used to treat fungal infections in the mouth caused by *Candida* species.

What is the most important information I should know about this medication?
• Nystatin can cause irritation or allergic reactions. Contact your doctor immediately if you experience any irritation, rash, facial swelling, or difficulty breathing.

Who should not take this medication?
Do not use nystatin if you are allergic to it or any of its ingredients.

What should I tell my doctor before I take the first dose of this medication?
Tell your doctor about all prescription, over-the-counter, and herbal medications you are taking before beginning treatment with nystatin. Also, talk to your doctor about your complete medical history, especially if you are pregnant, plan to become pregnant, or are breastfeeding.

What is the usual dosage?

Please see general statement regarding dosage on page xii.

Adults and children: The recommended dose is 4-6 milliliters (mL) four times a day.

Infants: The recommended dose is 2 mL four times a day.

How should I take this medication?

- Use nystatin exactly as prescribed by your doctor. Please review the instructions that came with your prescription on how to properly use your medication.
- Shake nystatin suspension well before use.
- Place one-half of your dose of nystatin suspension in each side of your mouth. Retain the suspension in your mouth as long as possible before swallowing. For infants and young children, you can use a dropper to place one-half of your child's dose in each side of their mouth.

What should I avoid while taking this medication?

Do not feed your infant or young child for 5-10 minutes after administration of nystatin.

Do not stop taking nystatin without asking your doctor.

What are possible food and drug interactions associated with this medication?

No significant interactions have been reported with nystatin at this time. However, always tell your doctor about any medicines you take, including over-the-counter medications, vitamins, and herbal supplements.

What are the possible side effects of this medication?

Please see general statement regarding side effects on page xiii.

Side effects may include: airway narrowing, allergic reactions, diarrhea, facial swelling, irritation, muscle pain, nausea, rapid heartbeat, rash, stomach upset, vomiting

Can I receive this medication if I am pregnant or breastfeeding?

The effects of nystatin during pregnancy and breastfeeding are unknown. Tell your doctor immediately if you are pregnant, plan to become pregnant, or are breastfeeding.

What should I do if I miss a dose of this medication?

If you miss a dose of nystatin, take it as soon as you remember. However, if it is almost time for your next dose, skip the one you missed and return to your regular dosing schedule. Do not take two doses at once.

How should I store this medication?

Store at room temperature. Do not freeze.

Nystatin Tablet

Generic name: Nystatin

What is this medication?

Nystatin tablet is an antifungal medicine that is used to treat certain fungal infections in the stomach and intestines caused by *Candida* species.

What is the most important information I should know about this medication?

• Nystatin can cause irritation or allergic reactions. Contact your doctor immediately if you experience any irritation, rash, facial swelling, or difficulty breathing.

Who should not take this medication?

Do not use nystatin if you are allergic to it or any of its ingredients.

What should I tell my doctor before I take the first dose of this medication?

Tell your doctor about all prescription, over-the-counter, and herbal medications you are taking before beginning treatment with nystatin. Also, talk to your doctor about your complete medical history, especially if you are pregnant, plan to become pregnant, or are breastfeeding.

What is the usual dosage?
Please see general statement regarding dosage on page xii.

Adults: The recommended dose is 4-6 tablets three times a day.

How should I take this medication?
• Take nystatin exactly as prescribed by your doctor.

What should I avoid while taking this medication?
Do not stop taking nystatin without asking your doctor.

What are possible food and drug interactions associated with this medication?
No significant interactions have been reported with nystatin at this time. However, always tell your doctor about any medicines you take, including over-the-counter medications, vitamins, and herbal supplements.

What are the possible side effects of this medication?
Please see general statement regarding side effects on page xiii.

Side effects may include: airway narrowing, allergic reactions, diarrhea, facial swelling, irritation, muscle pain, nausea, rapid heartbeat, rash, stomach upset, vomiting

---

Can I receive this medication if I am pregnant or breastfeeding?
The effects of nystatin during pregnancy and breastfeeding are unknown. Tell your doctor immediately if you are pregnant, plan to become pregnant, or are breastfeeding.

What should I do if I miss a dose of this medication?
If you miss a dose of nystatin, take it as soon as you remember. However, if it is almost time for your next dose, skip the one you

missed and return to your regular dosing schedule. Do not take two doses at once.

How should I store this medication?
Store at room temperature.

Nystatin Topical
Generic name: Nystatin

What is this medication?
Nystatin is a topical medicine (applied directly on the skin) that is used to treat certain fungal infections of the skin caused by *Candida* species. Nystatin is available in a cream, ointment, or powder.

What is the most important information I should know about this medication?
• Nystatin is for external use only. Do not use it in your eyes, mouth, or vagina.
• Nystatin can cause irritation or allergic reactions when it is applied. Tell your doctor immediately if this occurs.

Who should not take this medication?
Do not use nystatin if you are allergic to it or any of its ingredients.

What should I tell my doctor before I take the first dose of this medication?
Tell your doctor about all prescription, over-the-counter, and herbal medications you are taking before beginning treatment with nystatin. Also, talk to your doctor about your complete medical history.

What is the usual dosage?
Please see general statement regarding dosage on page xii.

Nystatin Cream or Ointment
Adults and children: Apply to the affected area(s) 2 times a day or as prescribed by your doctor.

Nystatin Powder
Adults and children: Apply to the affected area(s) 2-3 times a day.

How should I take this medication?
• Apply nystatin exactly as prescribed by your doctor. Even if symptoms improve, do not interrupt or stop using nystatin until your doctor tells you to stop. If your fungal infection is on your feet, the powder should be dusted on your feet, as well as in all footwear.

What should I avoid while taking this medication?
Do not use nystatin in your eyes, mouth, or vagina.

What are possible food and drug interactions associated with this medication?
No significant interactions have been reported with nystatin at this time. However, always tell your doctor about any medicines you take, including over-the-counter medications, vitamins, and herbal supplements.

What are the possible side effects of this medication?
Please see general statement regarding side effects on page xiii.

> **Side effects may include:** allergic reactions, burning, eczema (an inflammation or irritation of the skin), itching, pain on application, rash

Can I receive this medication if I am pregnant or breastfeeding?
The effects of nystatin during pregnancy and breastfeeding are unknown. Tell your doctor immediately if you are pregnant, plan to become pregnant, or are breastfeeding.

What should I do if I miss a dose of this medication?
If you miss a dose of nystatin, apply it as soon as you remember. However, if it is almost time for your next dose, skip the one you missed and return to your regular dosing schedule. Do not apply two doses at once.

How should I store this medication?

Store at room temperature. Keep nystatin powder away from excessive heat. Do not freeze nystatin cream.

Nystatin: *see Nystatin Suspension, page 715*

Nystatin: *see Nystatin Tablet, page 717*

Nystatin: *see Nystatin Topical, page 719*

Nystatin/Triamcinolone Acetonide: *see Nystatin and Triamcinolone, page 721*

Nystatin and Triamcinolone

Generic name: Nystatin/Triamcinolone Acetonide

What is this medication?

Nystatin and triamcinolone is a topical medicine (applied directly on the skin) that is used to treat certain fungal infections of the skin caused by *Candida* species. Nystatin and triamcinolone is available in a cream and ointment.

What is the most important information I should know about this medication?

- Nystatin and triamcinolone is for external use only. Do not use it in your eyes.
- Nystatin and triamcinolone can have a greater effect on children because they are more likely to absorb large amounts of the medicine through the skin. Long-term use can affect the growth and development of children. Talk to your doctor if you think your child is not growing at a normal rate after using this medication for a long period of time.
- Do not use nystatin and triamcinolone for any other condition other than that for which your doctor has prescribed.
- Nystatin and triamcinolone can cause irritation or allergic reactions when it is applied. Tell your doctor right away if this occurs.

Who should not take this medication?

Do not use nystatin and triamcinolone if you are allergic to it or any of its ingredients.

What should I tell my doctor before I take the first dose of this medication?

Tell your doctor about all prescription, over-the-counter, and herbal medications you are taking before beginning treatment with nystatin and triamcinolone. Also, talk to your doctor about your complete medical history.

What is the usual dosage?

Please see general statement regarding dosage on page xii.

Adults: Apply to the affected area(s) twice a day.

How should I take this medication?

- Apply nystatin and triamcinolone exactly as prescribed by your doctor.
- Apply nystatin and triamcinolone twice a day, once in the morning and once in the evening.

What should I avoid while taking this medication?

Do not use nystatin and triamcinolone in your eyes.

Do not bandage, cover, or wrap the treated skin area unless directed by your doctor to do so. In addition, children should not wear tight-fitting diapers or plastic pants if the diaper area is being treated.

What are possible food and drug interactions associated with this medication?

No significant interactions have been reported with nystatin and triamcinolone at this time. However, always tell your doctor about any medicines you take, including over-the-counter medications, vitamins, and herbal supplements.

What are the possible side effects of this medication?

Please see general statement regarding side effects on page xiii.

Side effects may include: abnormal hair growth, acne (pimples), burning, dryness, infections, inflamed hair follicles, irritation, itching, loss of skin color, skin inflammation, stretch marks, sweat rash, thinning of skin layers

Can I receive this medication if I am pregnant or breastfeeding?

The effects of nystatin and triamcinolone during pregnancy and breastfeeding are unknown. Tell your doctor immediately if you are pregnant, plan to become pregnant, or are breastfeeding.

What should I do if I miss a dose of this medication?

If you miss a dose of nystatin and triamcinolone, apply it as soon as you remember. However, if it is almost time for your next dose, skip the one you missed and return to your regular dosing schedule. Do not apply two doses at once.

How should I store this medication?

Store at room temperature. Do not freeze.

Ocuflox

Generic name: Ofloxacin

What is this medication?

Ocuflox is an antibiotic known as a quinolone that is available as eye drops. Ocuflox is used to treat pink eye and ulcers of the cornea (clear tissue over the pupil of your eye).

What is the most important information I should know about this medication?

- Ocuflox is for use only in your eyes.
- Ocuflox can cause a serious allergic reaction. Stop using Ocuflox and call your doctor right away if you develop difficulty breathing, hives, itching, rash, or swelling of your face, tongue, or throat.
- If you use Ocuflox for a long period of time, it can cause infections, including fungal infections.

Who should not take this medication?

Do not use Ocuflox if you are allergic to it, any of its ingredients, or other quinolone antibiotics (such as levofloxacin or moxifloxacin).

What should I tell my doctor before I take the first dose of this medication?

Tell your doctor about all prescription, over-the-counter, and herbal medications you are taking before beginning treatment with Ocuflox. Also, talk to your doctor about your complete medical history, especially if you are allergic to quinolone antibiotics, or are pregnant, plan to become pregnant, or are breastfeeding.

What is the usual dosage?

Please see general statement regarding dosage on page xii.

Pink Eye
Adults and children ≥1 year: Apply 1-2 drops in the affected eye(s) every 2-4 hours for the first 2 days, then apply 1-2 drops every 6 hours for the next 5 days.

Corneal Ulcers
Adults and children ≥1 year: Your doctor will prescribe the appropriate dose for you.

How should I take this medication?

- Apply Ocuflox exactly as prescribed by your doctor.
- Please review the instructions that came with your prescription on how to properly use your eye drops.

What should I avoid while taking this medication?

Do not touch the applicator tip to your eyes, fingers, or any other surface as this can contaminate Ocuflox.

What are possible food and drug interactions associated with this medication?

If Ocuflox is used with certain other drugs, the effects of either could be increased, decreased, or altered. It is especially important to check with your doctor before combining Ocuflox with the following: blood thinners (such as warfarin), caffeine, cyclosporine, or theophylline.

What are the possible side effects of this medication?
Please see general statement regarding side effects on page xiii.

Side effects may include: blurred vision, dry eye, eye burning or discomfort, eye pain, feeling like something is in your eye, itching, redness, sensitivity to light, stinging, swelling of your eye or face, tearing

Can I receive this medication if I am pregnant or breastfeeding?
The effects of Ocuflox during pregnancy and breastfeeding are unknown. Do not breastfeed while you are using Ocuflox. Tell your doctor immediately if you are pregnant, plan to become pregnant, or are breastfeeding.

What should I do if I miss a dose of this medication?
If you miss a dose of Ocuflox, apply it as soon as you remember. However, if it is almost time for your next dose, skip the one you missed and return to your regular dosing schedule. Do not apply two doses at once.

How should I store this medication?
Store at room temperature.

Ofloxacin: *see Ocuflox, page 723*

Olanzapine: *see Zyprexa, page 1162*

Olmesartan Medoxomil: *see Benicar, page 133*

Olopatadine HCl: *see Pataday, page 764*

Olopatadine HCl: *see Patanol, page 766*

Omega-3-Acid Ethyl Esters: *see Lovaza, page 590*

Omeprazole: *see Prilosec, page 827*

Omnicef
Generic name: Cefdinir

What is this medication?

Omnicef is an antibiotic used to treat certain bacterial infections of the respiratory (lung) tract, sinuses, throat, tonsils, skin, or ear. Omnicef is also used to treat bronchitis (inflammation of the air passages within the lungs). Omnicef may also be used to treat other bacterial infections, as determined by your doctor. Omnicef is available in capsules or oral suspension.

What is the most important information I should know about this medication?

- Do not take Omnicef if you are allergic to it, any of its ingredients, or similar antibiotics (such as cefazolin or cefotetan). If you are allergic to penicillin antibiotics, it is possible for you to have an allergic reaction to this medication. Tell your doctor right away if you take Omnicef and feel signs of an allergic reaction (such as a rash, swelling, or difficulty breathing).
- Omnicef can cause diarrhea or colitis (inflammation of the colon). This can occur a couple of months after taking the last dose of Omnicef. Tell your doctor right away if you have diarrhea or colitis.
- Take Omnicef as prescribed by your doctor for the full course of treatment, even if symptoms improve earlier. Do not skip doses. Complete the full course of Omnicef. Skipping doses or not completing the full course of Omnicef can decrease its effectiveness and can lead to the growth of bacteria that are resistant to the effects of Omnicef.
- Omnicef suspension contains sugar. Tell your doctor if you have diabetes.

Who should not take this medication?
Do not take Omnicef if you are allergic to it, any of its ingredients, or similar antibiotics.

Do not take Omnicef to treat viral infections, such as the common cold.

What should I tell my doctor before I take the first dose of this medication?
Tell your doctor about all prescription, over-the-counter, and herbal medications you are taking before beginning treatment with Omnicef. Also, talk to your doctor about your complete medical history, especially if you have allergies, a history of colitis, diabetes, or kidney problems.

What is the usual dosage?
Please see general statement regarding dosage on page xii.

Respiratory Tract or Skin Infections
Adults and adolescents ≥13 years: The recommended dose is 300 milligrams (mg) every 12 hours for 10 days.

Bronchitis, Sinus, Throat, or Tonsil Infections
Adults and adolescents ≥13 years: The recommended dose is 300 mg every 12 hours or 600 mg once a day. Based on your condition, your doctor will determine the appropriate duration of treatment.

Ear, Sinus, Throat, or Skin Infections
Children 6 months to 12 years: Your doctor will prescribe the appropriate dose for your child, based on their weight and type of infection.

How should I take this medication?
- Take Omnicef exactly as prescribed by your doctor. You can take Omnicef with or without food.
- Shake Omnicef oral suspension well before each use.
- Antacids containing aluminum or magnesium, or iron-containing supplements or multivitamins can interfere with the effects

of Omnicef. Also, the combination of iron and Omnicef can give your stool a reddish color. This is not a cause for concern. You can take Omnicef at least 2 hours before or after taking these products.

What should I avoid while taking this medication?
Do not skip any doses, or stop taking Omnicef even if you begin to feel better, until you finish your prescribed treatment.

What are possible food and drug interactions associated with this medication?
If Omnicef is taken with certain other drugs, the effects of either could be increased, decreased, or altered. It is especially important to check with your doctor before combining Omnicef with any of the following: antacids, iron-containing supplements or multivitamins, or probenecid.

What are the possible side effects of this medication?
Please see general statement regarding side effects on page xiii.

Side effects may include: abdominal pain, diarrhea, headache, nausea, rash, vaginal infection or inflammation

Can I receive this medication if I am pregnant or breastfeeding?
The effects of Omnicef during pregnancy and breastfeeding are unknown. Tell your doctor immediately if you are pregnant, plan to become pregnant, or are breastfeeding.

What should I do if I miss a dose of this medication?
If you miss a dose of Omnicef, take it as soon as you remember. However, if it is almost time for your next dose, skip the one you missed and return to your regular dosing schedule. Do not take two doses at once.

How should I store this medication?
Store at room temperature.

After mixing Omnicef oral suspension, discard the unused portion after 14 days.

Ondansetron HCI: *see Zofran, page 1146*

Onglyza

Generic name: Saxagliptin

What is this medication?

Onglyza is a medicine that is used with diet and exercise to control high blood sugar in adults with type 2 diabetes by helping the body increase the level of insulin after meals.

What is the most important information I should know about this medication?

- If you experience periods of stress to your body, such as fever, trauma, infection, or surgery, contact your doctor right away, as your medication needs may change.
- It is important to adhere to dietary instructions and regular physical activity while taking Onglyza. It is also important to periodically monitor your blood sugar levels and have A1C testing. This is to monitor how well you are responding to treatment.
- You should be aware of the symptoms of low blood sugar (hypoglycemia). Symptoms include shaking, sweating, rapid heartbeat, vision changes, hunger, headache, and mood changes. The risk of hypoglycemia may be greater if you are taking other diabetes medications, such as glyburide.

Who should not take this medication?

Patients who have type 1 diabetes or diabetic ketoacidosis (a life-threatening medical emergency caused by insufficient insulin) should not take Onglyza.

What should I tell my doctor before I take the first dose of this medication?

Tell your doctor about all prescription, over-the-counter, and herbal medications you are taking before beginning treatment with Onglyza. Also, talk to your doctor about your complete medical history, especially if you have a history or risk of diabetic ketoacidosis, kidney problems, or type 1 diabetes.

What is the usual dosage?

Please see general statement regarding dosage on page xii.

Adults: The recommended dose is 2.5 milligrams (mg) or 5 mg once a day. Your doctor may prescribe 2.5 mg once a day if you have kidney disease.

How should I take this medication?

• Take Onglyza exactly as prescribed. Onglyza can be taken with or without food.

What should I avoid while taking this medication?

Do not change the dose of Onglyza without talking to your doctor.

What are possible food and drug interactions associated with this medication?

If Onglyza is taken with certain other drugs, the effects of either could be increased, decreased, or altered. It is especially important to check with your doctor before combining Onglyza with the following: atazanavir, clarithromycin, other diabetes medications called sulfonylureas (such as glimepiride, glipizide, glyburide) or thiazolidinediones (such as pioglitazone), indinavir, insulin, itraconazole, ketoconazole, nefazodone, nelfinavir, ritonavir, saquinavir, and telithromycin.

What are the possible side effects of this medication?

Please see general statement regarding side effects on page xiii.

Side effects may include: upper respiratory tract infection, urinary tract infection, headache, low blood sugar, swelling or fluid retention of extremities, allergic reactions

an I receive this medication if I am pregnant or reastfeeding?

The effects of Onglyza during pregnancy and breastfeeding are unknown. Tell your doctor immediately if you are pregnant, plan to become pregnant, or are breastfeeding.

What should I do if I miss a dose of this medication?

If you miss a dose of Onglyza, take the missed dose as soon as you remember. However, if it is almost time for your next dose, skip the one you missed and return to your regular dosing schedule. Do not take two doses at once.

ow should I store this medication?

Store at room temperature.

Optivar
eneric name: Azelastine HCl

What is this medication?

Optivar is an eye drop medicine used to treat eye itchiness associated with allergic conjunctivitis ("pink eye").

What is the most important information I should know bout this medication?

- Optivar is for use in your eyes only. Do not use Optivar in your mouth.
- Do not wear contact lenses if your eyes are red. Also, Optivar should not be used to treat contact lens-related irritation. Optivar contains a preservative, benzalkonium chloride, which can be absorbed by soft contact lenses. If you wear soft contact lenses and your eyes are not red, wait at least 10 minutes after applying Optivar before you insert your contact lenses.

ho should not take this medication?

Do not use Optivar if you are allergic to it or any of its ingredients.

What should I tell my doctor before I take the first dose of this medication?

Tell your doctor about all prescription, over-the-counter, and herba medications you are taking before beginning treatment with Opti var. Also, talk to your doctor about your complete medical history

What is the usual dosage?

Please see general statement regarding dosage on page xii.

Adults and children ≥3 years: Apply 1 drop into the affecte eye(s) twice a day.

How should I take this medication?

• Apply Optivar exactly as prescribed by your doctor. Keep th bottle tightly closed when you are not using it.

What should I avoid while taking this medication?

Do not use Optivar for injection or in your mouth.

Do not allow the dropper tip of the bottle to contact your eyelids o any other surrounding area, as this can contaminate Optivar.

Do not wear contact lenses if your eyes are red.

What are possible food and drug interactions associate with this medication?

No significant interactions have been reported with Optivar at thi time. However, always tell your doctor about any medicines yo take, including over-the-counter medications, vitamins, and herba supplements.

What are the possible side effects of this medication?

Please see general statement regarding side effects on page xiii.

Side effects may include: asthma, bitter taste, blurred vision, burning or stinging of the eyes, eye pain, fatigue, flu-like symptoms, headache, itching, runny and stuffy nose, shortness of breath, sore throat

Can I receive this medication if I am pregnant or breastfeeding?

The effects of Optivar during pregnancy and breastfeeding are unknown. Tell your doctor immediately if you are pregnant, plan to become pregnant, or are breastfeeding.

What should I do if I miss a dose of this medication?

If you miss a dose of Optivar, apply it as soon as you remember. However, if it is almost time for your next dose, skip the one you missed and return to your regular dosing schedule. Do not apply two doses at once.

How should I store this medication?

Store at room temperature or in the refrigerator.

Ortho-Cyclen

Generic name: Ethinyl Estradiol/Norgestimate

What is this medication?

Ortho-Cyclen is a birth control pill used to prevent pregnancy.

What is the most important information I should know about this medication?

- Cigarette smoking increases the risk of serious heart-related side effects (such as blood clots, stroke, and heart attack) from use of birth control pills, such as Ortho-Cyclen. The risk increases with age (especially if you are >35 years old and smoke cigarettes). Do not smoke while you are taking birth control pills.
- Use of birth control pills is associated with increased risk of heart attack, clotting disorders, stroke, liver tumors, and gallbladder disease. These risks increase in people with a history of high blood pressure, high cholesterol, obesity, diabetes, clotting disorders, heart attack, stroke, chest pain, cancer of the breast or sex organs, or liver tumors.
- Birth control pills may increase your cholesterol levels. Women with high cholesterol should be monitored closely.

- Ortho-Cyclen does not protect against HIV infection (AIDS) and other sexually transmitted diseases.
- You can experience breakthrough bleeding or spotting while you are taking birth control pills, especially during the first 3 months of use. You may also have irregular periods. If you have missed more than two periods in a row, take a pregnancy test to determine if you are pregnant. Do not use Ortho-Cyclen if you are pregnant.

Who should not take this medication?

Do not use Ortho-Cyclen if you are allergic to it or any of its ingredients.

Do not use Ortho-Cyclen if you are >35 years old and smoke cigarettes.

Do not use Ortho-Cyclen if you have a history of heart attack or stroke; heart disease; blood clots in your legs, lungs, or eyes; chest pain (angina); diabetes with kidney, eye, nerve, or blood vessel damage; history of breast cancer; cancer of the lining of the uterus, cervix, or vagina; unexplained vaginal bleeding; yellowing of your skin or the whites of your eyes during pregnancy or during previous use of oral birth control pills; liver tumors; high blood pressure uncontrolled by medication; certain types of headaches; or if you plan to have surgery with prolonged bed rest. Do not take Ortho-Cyclen if you think you may be pregnant or if you have not had your first period.

What should I tell my doctor before I take the first dose of this medication?

Tell your doctor about all prescription, over-the-counter, and herbal medications you are taking before beginning treatment with Ortho-Cyclen. Tell your doctor if you have ever had any of the health conditions listed above. Also, talk to your doctor about your complete medical history, especially if you have or have had breast nodules; fibrocystic disease of the breast (lumpy and painful breasts); an abnormal breast x-ray or mammogram; diabetes; high cholesterol or triglycerides; high blood pressure; migraines or other headaches; seizures; depression; gallbladder, liver, heart, or kidney dis ease; history of irregular menstrual periods; wear contact lenses; smoke cigarettes; plan to have surgery with prolonged bed rest; or if you are pregnant, plan to become pregnant, or are breastfeeding.

What is the usual dosage?

Please see general statement regarding dosage on page xii.

Adults: Each blue "active" pill of Ortho-Cyclen contains 0.25 milligrams (mg) of norgestimate and 0.035 mg of ethinyl estradiol. Each green "reminder" pill contains inactive ingredients.

Sunday Start: Take the first blue "active" pill of the first pack on the Sunday after your period begins, even if you are still bleeding. If your period begins on a Sunday, start the pack that same day. Take one blue "active" pill a day for 21 days followed by one green "reminder" pill a day for 7 days. After all 28 pills have been taken, start a new course the next day (Sunday).

Day 1 Start: Take the first blue "active" pill of the first pack during the first 24 hours of your period. Take one blue "active" pill a day from the 1st day through the 21st day of the menstrual cycle (counting the day your period starts as Day 1) followed by one green "reminder" pill a day for 7 days. Take the pills without interruption for 28 days. After all 28 tablets have been taken, start a new course the next day.

How should I take this medication?

- Before you start taking Ortho-Cyclen, be sure to read the directions. Take Ortho-Cyclen once a day at the same time every day until the pack is empty. When you finish a pack, start the next pack on the day after your last green "reminder" pill. Do not wait any days between packs. If you are switching from another birth control pill, start Ortho-Cyclen on the same day that a new pack of the previous pills should have been started.
- For the first cycle of a *Sunday Start* regimen, use another method of birth control (such as condoms or spermicide) as a backup method if you have sex anytime from the Sunday you start your first pack until you have been taking the pills for 7 days. You will not need to use a back-up method of birth control for the first cycle of a Day 1 regimen, since you are starting the pill at the beginning of your period.

What should I avoid while taking this medication?

Do not smoke cigarettes or become pregnant while you are taking Ortho-Cyclen. Do not skip pills, even if you are spotting or bleeding between monthly periods, feel sick to your stomach (nausea), or if you do not have sex very often.

What are possible food and drug interactions associated with this medication?

If Ortho-Cyclen is taken with certain other drugs, the effects of either could be increased, decreased, or altered. It is especially important to check with your doctor before combining Ortho-Cyclen with the following: acetaminophen, antibiotics, anti-HIV medicines (such as ritonavir), atorvastatin, bosentan, clofibric acid, cyclosporine, griseofulvin, itraconazole, ketoconazole, morphine, prednisolone, rifampin, salicylic acid, seizure medications (such as carbamazepine, felbamate, lamotrigine, oxcarbazepine, phenobarbital, phenytoin, or topiramate), St. John's wort, temazepam, theophylline, or vitamin C.

What are the possible side effects of this medication?

Please see general statement regarding side effects on page xiii.

> **Side effects may include:** abdominal cramps and bloating, absence of a period, allergic reactions, blotchy darkening of the skin (especially on your face), breakthrough bleeding or spotting, breast tenderness, change in your appetite, change in your vision or inability to wear your contact lenses, depression, dizziness, gallbladder disease, headache, high blood pressure, loss of scalp hair, nausea, nervousness, rash, vaginal infections, vomiting, water retention causing swelling of your fingers or ankles, weight gain

Can I receive this medication if I am pregnant or breastfeeding?

Do not take Ortho-Cyclen if you are pregnant or breastfeeding. Tell your doctor immediately if you are pregnant, plan to become pregnant, or are breastfeeding.

What should I do if I miss a dose of this medication?

If you miss one blue "active" pill, take it as soon as you remember. Take the next pill at your regular time. This means you can take two pills in one day. You do not need a back-up birth control method if you have sex.

If you miss two pills or more, consult the patient information that accompanied your prescription or call your pharmacist for advice.

How should I store this medication?

Store at room temperature. Protect from light.

Ortho Evra

Generic name: Ethinyl Estradiol/Norelgestromin

What is this medication?

Ortho Evra is a birth control patch containing the hormones estrogen and progestin. It is used to prevent pregnancy.

What is the most important information I should know about this medication?

- Do not use Ortho Evra if you smoke cigarettes and are >35 years. Cigarette smoking increases your risk of serious side effects on your heart and blood vessels, including heart attack, blood clots, or stroke. This risk increases with age, especially if you are >35 years, and if you smoke ≥15 cigarettes a day.
- Hormones from Ortho Evra get into your bloodstream and are processed by your body differently than hormones from birth control pills. You will be exposed to about 60% more estrogen if you use Ortho Evra than if you use typical birth control pills containing 35 micrograms of estrogen. Your risk of blood clots in your legs and/or lungs can be increased with Ortho Evra use compared with the use of birth control pills.
- Tell your doctor immediately if you experience breast lumps; coughing of blood; crushing chest pain or tightness in your chest; loss of vision; severe pain in your stomach area; severe problems with sleeping, weakness, lack of energy, fatigue, or

change in mood; shortness of breath; sudden severe headache or vomiting, dizziness, or fainting; yellowing of your skin or whites of your eyes with frequent fever, fatigue, loss of appetite dark-colored urine, or light-colored bowel movements.

- If you use Ortho Evra and need elective surgery, need to stay in bed for a prolonged illness or injury, or have recently delivered a baby, you can be at risk of developing blood clots. Talk to your doctor about stopping Ortho Evra 4 weeks before surgery, and not using it for 2 weeks after surgery or during bedrest. Do not use Ortho Evra soon after delivering a baby. Wait for at least 4 weeks after delivery if you are not breastfeeding. If you are breastfeeding, you should wait until you have weaned your child before using Ortho Evra.
- Ortho Evra can increase your risk of developing strokes, angina (chest pain), heart attacks, gallbladder disease, noncancerous but dangerous liver tumors, and breast cancer.
- There may be times when you may not menstruate regularly during your patch-free week. If you used Ortho Evra correctly and miss one menstrual period, continue using your birth control patches for the next cycle but be sure to tell your doctor before doing so. If you have not used Ortho Evra as instructed and missed a menstrual period, or if you missed two menstrual periods in a row, you could be pregnant. Tell your doctor immediately, to determine if you are pregnant. Stop using Ortho Evra if you are pregnant.
- Ortho Evra may be less effective if you weigh >198 pounds. If you weight >198 pounds, talk to your doctor about which form of birth control may be best for you.
- Ortho Evra does not protect you against HIV infection (AIDS) or any other sexually transmitted disease.

Who should not take this medication?

Do not use Ortho Evra if you are allergic to it, any of its ingredients, or to similar products.

Do not use Ortho Evra if you have a history of heart attack or stroke, blood clots in your legs, lungs, or eyes; an inherited problem that makes your blood clot more than usual; chest pain, disease of heart valves with complications, or severe high blood pressure;

known or suspected breast cancer or cancer of the lining of the uterus, cervix, or vagina; unexplained vaginal bleeding; hepatitis or yellowing of your skin or whites of your eyes during pregnancy or during previous use of hormonal birth control; liver tumor; known or suspected pregnancy, diabetes with complications of the kidneys, eyes, nerves, or blood vessels; headaches with nerve symptoms; use of oral birth control pills; need for a prolonged period of bedrest following major surgery.

What should I tell my doctor before I take the first dose of this medication?

Tell your doctor about all prescription, over-the-counter, and herbal medications you are taking before beginning treatment with Ortho Evra. Also, talk to your doctor about your complete medical history, especially if you have liver, heart, gallbladder, or kidney disease; high blood pressure; high cholesterol; clotting disorders; a history of cancer; diabetes; seizures; depression, migraines or other headaches; irregular menstrual periods; vision problems; or if you smoke.

Tell your doctor if you are scheduled for any laboratory tests because Ortho Evra can affect certain blood tests.

What is the usual dosage?

Please see general statement regarding dosage on page xii.

Adults and adolescents ≥16 years: Ortho Evra uses a 28-day (four-week) cycle. Apply a new patch once a week for 3 weeks (21 total days). Week Four is patch-free. Your menstrual period should start during this patch-free week.

How should I take this medication?

- Use Ortho Evra exactly as prescribed by your doctor. Do not apply extra doses or use the patch more often without asking your doctor.
- If this is the first time you are using Ortho Evra, wait until the day you get your menstrual period and apply your first patch during the first 24 hours of your period. The day you apply your first

patch will be Day 1. Your "Patch Change Day" will be on this day every week.

- You may also choose a Sunday start. Apply your first patch on the first Sunday after your period starts. You must use a back-up birth control method (such as a condom, spermicide, or diaphragm for the first week of your cycle).
- Please review the instructions that came with your prescription on how to properly use your birth control patches.

What should I avoid while taking this medication?

Do not use Ortho Evra if you smoke cigarettes and are >35 years.

Do not use Ortho Evra if you are pregnant.

What are possible food and drug interactions associated with this medication?

If Ortho Evra is used with certain other drugs, the effects of either could be increased, decreased, or altered. It is especially important to check with your doctor before combining Ortho Evra with the following: acetaminophen, antibiotics (such as amoxicillin or erythromycin), ascorbic acid, aspirin, atorvastatin, barbiturates (such as butalbital or phenobarbital), bosentan, carbamazepine, cyclosporine, felbamate, fluconazole, grapefruit juice, griseofulvin, itraconazole, ketoconazole, lamotrigine, morphine, oxcarbazepine, phenytoin, prednisolone, rifampin, rosuvastatin, St. John's wort, temazepam, theophylline, topiramate, or voriconazole.

What are the possible side effects of this medication?

Please see general statement regarding side effects on page xiii.

Side effects may include: acne (pimples), blood clots, breast pain, diarrhea, dizziness, fatigue, headache, heart attack, increased appetite, irregular uterine bleeding, itching, liver problems, migraine, mood disorders, nausea, stomach pain, vaginal yeast infection, vomiting, weight gain

Can I receive this medication if I am pregnant or breastfeeding?

Do not use Ortho Evra if you are pregnant or breastfeeding. Tell your doctor immediately if you are pregnant, plan to become pregnant, or are breastfeeding.

What should I do if I miss a dose of this medication?

If your patch becomes loose or has fallen off for less than 1 day, try to stick it back on or apply a new patch immediately. No back-up birth control method is needed. Your "Patch Change Day" will remain the same. If your patch has been loose or falls off for more than 1 day, or you are not sure for how long. You may become pregnant. Start a new four-week cycle immediately by putting on a new patch. You now have a new Day 1 and a new "Patch Change Day". You must use a back-up birth control for the first week of your new cycle.

How should I store this medication?

Store at room temperature.

Ortho Tri-Cyclen

Generic name: Ethinyl Estradiol/Norgestimate

What is this medication?

Ortho Tri-Cyclen is a birth control pill used to prevent pregnancy. Ortho Tri-Cylcen is also used to treat moderate acne in women ≥15 years who are able to and wish to use Ortho Tri-Cyclen for birth control.

What is the most important information I should know about this medication?

- Cigarette smoking increases the risk of serious heart-related side effects (such as blood clots, stroke, and heart attack) from use of birth control pills, such as Ortho Tri-Cyclen. The risk increases with age (especially if you are >35 years old and smoke). Do not smoke while you are taking birth control pills.

- Use of birth control pills is associated with increased risk of heart attack, clotting disorders, stroke, liver tumors, and gallbladder disease. These risks increase in people with a history of high blood pressure, high cholesterol, obesity, diabetes, clotting disorders, heart attack, stroke, chest pain, cancer of the breast or sex organs, or liver tumors.
- Birth control pills may increase your cholesterol levels. Women with high cholesterol should be monitored closely.
- Ortho Tri-Cyclen does not protect against HIV infection (AIDS) and other sexually transmitted diseases.
- You can experience breakthrough bleeding or spotting while you are taking birth control pills, especially during the first 3 months of use. You may also have irregular periods. If you have missed more than two periods in a row, take a pregnancy test to determine if you are pregnant. Do not use Ortho Tri-Cyclen if you are pregnant.

Who should not take this medication?

Do not use Ortho Tri-Cyclen if you are >35 years old and smoke cigarettes.

Do not use Ortho Tri-Cyclen if you have a history of heart attack or stroke; heart disease; blood clots in your legs, lungs, or eyes; chest pain (angina); diabetes with kidney, eye, nerve or blood vessel damage; history of breast cancer; cancer of the lining of the uterus, cervix, or vagina; unexplained vaginal bleeding; yellowing of your skin or the whites of your eyes during pregnancy or during previous use of oral birth control pills; liver tumors; high blood pressure uncontrolled by medication; certain types of headaches; are allergic to any of the ingredients in Ortho Tri-Cyclen; or if you plan to have surgery with prolonged bed rest. Do not take Ortho Tri-Cyclen if you think you may be pregnant or if you have not had your first period.

What should I tell my doctor before I take the first dose of this medication?

Tell your doctor about all prescription, over-the-counter, and herbal medications you are taking before beginning treatment with Ortho Tri-Cyclen. Tell your doctor if you have ever had any of the health conditions listed above. Also, talk to your doctor about your complete medical history, especially if you have or have had breast nodules; fibrocystic disease of the breast (lumpy and painful breasts); an abnormal breast x-ray or mammogram; diabetes; high cholesterol or triglycerides; high blood pressure; migraines or other headaches; seizures; depression; gallbladder, liver, heart, or kidney disease; history of irregular menstrual periods; wear contact lenses; smoke; plan to have surgery with prolonged bed rest; or if you are pregnant, plan to become pregnant, or are breastfeeding.

What is the usual dosage?
Please see general statement regarding dosage on page xii.

Birth Control and Acne
Adults: Each white "active" pill of Ortho Tri-Cyclen contains 0.18 milligrams (mg) of norgestimate and 0.035 mg of ethinyl estradiol. Each light blue "active" pill contains 0.215 milligrams (mg) of norgestimate and 0.035 mg of ethinyl estradiol. Each blue "active" pill contains 0.25 milligrams (mg) of norgestimate and 0.035 mg of ethinyl estradiol. Each green "reminder" pill contains inactive ingredients.

Sunday Start: Take the first white "active" pill of the first pack on the Sunday after your period begins, even if you are still bleeding. If your period begins on a Sunday, start the pack that same day. Take the white, light blue, and blue (in this order) "active" pills once a day for 21 days followed by one green "reminder" pill a day for 7 days. After all 28 pills have been taken, start a new course the next day (Sunday).

Day 1 Start: Take the first white "active" pill of the first pack during the first 24 hours of your period. Take the white, light blue, and blue (in this order) "active" pill once a day from the 1st day through the 21st day of the menstrual cycle (counting the day your period starts as Day 1) followed by one green "reminder" pill a day for 7 days. Take the pills without interruption for 28 days. After all 28 tablets have been taken, start a new course the next day.

How should I take this medication?

- Before you start taking Ortho Tri-Cyclen, be sure to read the directions. Take Ortho Tri-Cyclen once a day at the same time every day until the pack is empty. When you finish a pack, start the next pack on the day after your last green "reminder" pill. Do not wait any days between packs. If you are switching from another birth control pill, start Ortho Tri-Cyclen on the same day that a new pack of the previous pills should have been started.
- For the first cycle of a *Sunday Start* regimen, use another method of birth control (such as condoms or spermicide) as a backup method if you have sex anytime from the Sunday you start your first pack until you have been taking the pills for 7 days. You will not need to use a back-up method of birth control for the first cycle of a Day 1 regimen, since you are starting the pill at the beginning of your period.

What should I avoid while taking this medication?

Do not smoke or become pregnant while you are taking Ortho Tri-Cyclen. Do not skip pills, even if you are spotting or bleeding between monthly periods, feel sick to your stomach (nausea), or if you do not have sex very often.

What are possible food and drug interactions associated with this medication?

If Ortho Tri-Cyclen is taken with certain other drugs, the effects of either could be increased, decreased, or altered. It is especially important to check with your doctor before combining Ortho Tri-Cyclen with the following: acetaminophen, antibiotics, anti-HIV medicines (such as ritonavir), atorvastatin, bosentan, clofibric acid, cyclosporine, griseofulvin, itraconazole, ketoconazole, morphine, prednisolone, rifampin, salicylic acid, seizure medications (such as carbamazepine, felbamate, lamotrigine, oxcarbazepine, phenobarbital, phenytoin, or topiramate), St. John's wort, temazepam, theophylline, or vitamin C.

What are the possible side effects of this medication?

Please see general statement regarding side effects on page xiii.

Side effects may include: abdominal cramps and bloating, absence of a period, allergic reactions, blotchy darkening of the skin (especially on your face), breakthrough bleeding or spotting, breast tenderness, change in your appetite, change in your vision or inability to wear your contact lenses, depression, dizziness, gallbladder disease, headache, high blood pressure, loss of scalp hair, nausea, nervousness, rash, vaginal infections, vomiting, water retention causing swelling of the fingers or ankles, weight gain

---

Can I receive this medication if I am pregnant or breastfeeding?

Do not take Ortho Tri-Cyclen if you are pregnant or breastfeeding. Tell your doctor immediately if you are pregnant, plan to become pregnant, or are breastfeeding.

What should I do if I miss a dose of this medication?

If you miss one white, light blue, or blue "active" pill, take it as soon as you remember. Take the next pill at your regular time. This means you can take two pills in one day. You do not need a back-up birth control method if you have sex.

If you miss two or more pills, consult the patient information that accompanied your prescription or call your pharmacist for advice.

How should I store this medication?

Store at room temperature. Protect from light.

Ortho Tri-Cyclen Lo

Generic name: Ethinyl Estradiol/Norgestimate

What is this medication?

Ortho Tri-Cyclen Lo is a birth control pill used to prevent pregnancy. Ortho Tri-Cyclen Lo contains the hormones norgestimate and ethinyl estradiol.

What is the most important information I should know about this medication?

- Cigarette smoking can increase your risk of serious side effects on your heart and blood vessels, including heart attack, blood clots, or stroke. This risk increases with age, especially if you are >35 years and if you smoke ≥15 cigarettes a day. Do not smoke if you are taking Ortho Tri-Cyclen Lo.
- Ortho Tri-Cyclen Lo can increase your risk of heart attack, clotting disorders, stroke, gallbladder disease, or liver tumors. These risks increase if you have high blood pressure, diabetes, high cholesterol, tendency to form blood clots, or obesity. Tell your doctor right away if you experience sharp chest pain, coughing of blood, sudden shortness of breath, pain in your calfs, sudden severe headache or vomiting, dizziness or fainting, disturbances of vision or speech, weakness or numbness in your arms or legs, loss of vision, abdominal (stomach) pain or tenderness, or jaundice (yellowing of your skin or whites of your eyes) accompanied by fever, fatigue, loss of appetite, dark-colored urine, or light-colored bowel movements.
- Ortho Tri-Cyclen Lo can increase your risk of developing cancer of your breasts or reproductive organs. Ask your doctor to show you how to examine your breasts. Tell your doctor right away if you notice breast lumps.
- You can experience breakthrough bleeding or spotting while you are taking birth control pills, especially during the first 3 months of use. You may also have irregular periods. If you have missed more than two periods in a row, use a pregnancy test to determine if you are pregnant. Do not use Ortho Tri-Cyclen Lo if you are pregnant.
- Ortho Tri-Cyclen Lo is intended to prevent pregnancy. It does not protect against HIV infection (AIDS) and other sexually transmitted diseases.

Who should not take this medication?

Do not take Ortho Tri-Cyclen Lo if you are allergic to it or any of its ingredients.

Do not take Ortho Tri-Cyclen Lo if you have had a heart attack or stroke; blood clots in your legs, lungs, or eyes; known or suspected breast cancer, cancer of the lining of your uterus, cervix or vagina, or certain hormonally sensitive cancers; liver disease, including liver tumors; chest pain; unexplained vaginal bleeding; jaundice during pregnancy or during previous use of the pill; known or suspected pregnancy; heart disorders; diabetes; migraine headaches; uncontrolled high blood pressure; or if you are going to have surgery or will be on bedrest.

What should I tell my doctor before I take the first dose of this medication?

Tell your doctor about all prescription, over-the-counter, and herbal medications you are taking before beginning treatment with Ortho Tri-Cyclen Lo. Also, talk to your doctor about your complete medical history, especially if you or a family member has ever had breast nodules or any disease of the breast; certain hormonally sensitive cancers; diabetes; high triglycerides or cholesterol; high blood pressure; a tendency to form blood clots; migraines or other headaches; seizures; depression; gallbladder, heart, liver, or kidney disease; or a history of scanty or irregular menstrual periods. Also, tell your doctor if you are going to have surgery or will be on bedrest.

What is the usual dosage?

Please see general statement regarding dosage on page xii.

Adults and adolescents ≥16 years: Ortho Tri-Cyclen Lo may be started in one of two ways: on the Sunday after your period begins or during the first 24 hours of your period, as outlined below.
Sunday Start: Take the first white tablet on the Sunday after your period begins, even if you are still bleeding. Take one white, light blue, or dark blue tablet a day for 21 days, followed by one dark green tablet a day for 7 days. After taking all 28 tablets, start a new course the next day (Sunday).
Day 1 Start: Take the first white tablet during the first 24 hours of your period. Take one white, light blue, or dark blue tablet a day for 21 days, followed by one dark green tablet a day for 7 days. After taking all 28 tablets, start a new course the next day.

How should I take this medication?

- Before you start taking Ortho Tri-Cyclen Lo, be sure to read the directions. Take Ortho Tri-Cyclen Lo once a day, at the same time every day in the order directed on the package.
- For the *Sunday Start*, use another method of birth control (such as a condom or spermicide) as a back-up method if you have sex anytime from the Sunday you start your first pack until the next Sunday (7 days). This also applies if you start Ortho Tri-Cyclen Lo after having been pregnant and you have not had a period since your pregnancy.
- You will not need to use a back-up method of birth control for the *Day 1 Start* because you are starting the pill at the beginning of your period. However, if you start Ortho Tri-Cyclen Lo later than the first day of your period, you should use another method of birth control as a back-up method until you have taken 7 white pills.
- Please follow the instructions on the patient handout that comes with your prescription.

What should I avoid while taking this medication?

Do not smoke cigarettes or become pregnant while you are taking Ortho Tri-Cyclen Lo.

Do not skip pills even if you are spotting or bleeding between monthly periods, feel sick to your stomach (nausea), or if you do not have sex very often.

What are possible food and drug interactions associated with this medication?

If Ortho Tri-Cyclen Lo is taken with certain other drugs, the effects of either could be increased, decreased, or altered. It is especially important to check with your doctor before combining Ortho Tri-Cyclen Lo with the following: bosentan, certain anti-HIV medications (such as ritonavir), certain antibiotics (such as ampicillin, penicillin, rifampin, tetracycline, or troleandomycin), seizure medications (such as carbamazepine, lamotrigine, phenobarbital, phenylbutazone, phenytoin, or topiramate), or St. John's wort.

What are the possible side effects of this medication?
Please see general statement regarding side effects on page xiii.

Side effects may include: allergic reactions, breast tenderness, change in your appetite, change in your vision, depression, dizziness, edema (swelling), headache, inability to wear your contact lenses, irregular vaginal bleeding or spotting, loss of scalp hair, nausea, nervousness, rash, spotty darkening of your skin

Can I receive this medication if I am pregnant or breastfeeding?
Do not take Ortho Tri-Cyclen Lo if you are pregnant or breastfeeding. Tell your doctor immediately if you are pregnant, plan to become pregnant, or are breastfeeding.

What should I do if I miss a dose of this medication?
If you miss one white, light blue, or dark blue pill, take it as soon as you remember. Take the next pill at your regular time. This means you can take two pills in one day. You do not need a back-up birth control method if you have sex. If you miss two white, light blue, or dark blue pills or more, consult the patient information that accompanied your prescription, or call your pharmacist or doctor for advice.

How should I store this medication?
Store at room temperature. Protect from light.

Oxcarbazepine: *see Trileptal, page 1023*

Oxecta
Generic name: Oxycodone HCl

What is this medication?
Oxecta is a narcotic pain medicine that contains oxycodone. Oxecta is used for the management of sudden and long-term moderate to severe pain.

Oxecta is a federally controlled substance because it has abuse potential.

What is the most important information I should know about this medication?

- Oxecta has the potential to become habit-forming and can cause severe side effects, including severe breathing problems and even death, if not taken according to your doctor's directions. Tell your doctor if the medicine is not relieving your pain effectively.
- Prevent theft, misuse, or abuse by keeping Oxecta in a safe place to protect it from being stolen. Oxecta can be a target for people who misuse or abuse prescription medicines or street drugs. Also, do not give Oxecta to anyone else, even if they have the same symptoms you have because it can harm them or even cause death.

Who should not take this medication?

Do not take Oxecta if you are allergic to it, any of its ingredients, or if you have severe asthma or lung problems.

Do not take Oxecta if you have paralytic ileus (impairment of the small intestine).

What should I tell my doctor before I take the first dose of this medication?

Tell your doctor about all prescription, over-the-counter, and herbal medications you are taking before beginning treatment with Oxecta. Also, talk to your doctor about your complete medical history, especially if you have trouble breathing or lung problems, head injury, liver or kidney disease, thyroid problems, seizures, alcoholism, adrenal gland problems, hallucinations or other severe mental problems, and past or present substance abuse or drug addiction problems.

What is the usual dosage?

Please see general statement regarding dosage on page xii.

Adults: The recommended starting dose is 5-15 milligrams (mg) taken every 4 to 6 hours as needed for pain.

Your doctor will adjust the dose for you based on your physical condition, the type of painkillers you have been taking, and your tolerance for narcotics.

How should I take this medication?
- Take Oxecta exactly as directed by your doctor. Do not adjust the dose or stop using Oxecta without consulting your doctor.
- Take each Oxecta tablet with enough water to ensure you swallow it immediately after placing it in your mouth. You have to swallow Oxecta tablets whole; never crush or chew them. Do not pre-soak, lick, or otherwise wet the tablet prior to placing it in your mouth.
- Contact your doctor if you have to stop taking this medication. Your doctor can provide you a dose schedule to gradually discontinue the medication, if necessary.
- Dispose all unused tablets by flushing them down the toilet.

What should I avoid while taking this medication?
Do not drink alcohol or take other medications that will make you sleepy while you are taking Oxecta. They can increase the drowsiness and dizziness caused by Oxecta and could be dangerous.

Do not drive, operate machinery, or perform other hazardous activities while you are taking Oxecta.

What are possible food and drug interactions associated with this medication?
If Oxecta is taken with certain other drugs, the effects of either could be increased, decreased, or altered. Oxecta may interact with numerous medications. Therefore, it is very important that you tell your doctor about any other medications you are taking.

What are the possible side effects of this medication?
Please see general statement regarding side effects on page xiii.

> **Side effects may include:** constipation, dizziness, drowsiness, headache, insomnia, itching, nausea, weakness, vomiting

Can I receive this medication if I am pregnant or breastfeeding?

The effects of Oxecta during pregnancy are unknown. Oxecta can be found in your breast milk if you use it while breastfeeding. Tell your doctor immediately if you are pregnant, plan to become pregnant, or are breastfeeding.

What should I do if I miss a dose of this medication?

If you miss a dose of Oxecta, take it as soon as you remember. However, if it is almost time for your next dose, skip the one you missed and return to your regular dosing schedule. Do not take two doses at once.

How should I store this medication?

Store at room temperature. Protect from moisture.

Oxybutynin

Generic name: Oxybutynin Chloride

What is this medication?

Oxybutynin is a medicine used to treat symptoms of overactive bladder. Symptoms of overactive bladder include frequent urination, urgency (increased need to urinate), urge incontinence (inability to control urination) and dysuria (painful urination). Oxybutynin is available in tablets and a syrup.

What is the most important information I should know about this medication?

- Oxybutynin can cause angioedema (a condition involving swelling of the face, extremities, eyes, lips, and tongue). Stop taking this medication and tell your doctor immediately if you experience these symptoms or have difficulty breathing.

- Heat prostration (fever and heat stroke due to decreased sweating) can occur while you are taking oxybutynin. You may become overheated in a warm environment.
- Oxybutynin can cause dizziness or blurred vision. These effects may become worse if you take oxybutynin with alcohol or certain medicines.
- Oxybutynin can aggravate the symptoms of overactive thyroid, heart disease or congestive heart failure, irregular or rapid heartbeat, or high blood pressure.
- Oxybutynin can also aggravate enlarged prostate, hiatal hernia (protrusion of part of the stomach through the diaphragm) or myasthenia gravis (a disease characterized by long-lasting fatigue and muscle weakness or loss of muscle control).

Who should not take this medication?

Do not take oxybutynin if you are allergic to it or any of its ingredients.

Do not take oxybutynin if you are not able to empty your bladder or have delayed or slow emptying of your stomach (gastric retention).

Do not take oxybutynin if you have glaucoma (high pressure in the eyes) not controlled by medicine.

What should I tell my doctor before I take the first dose of this medication?

Tell your doctor about all prescription, over-the-counter, and herbal medications you are taking before beginning treatment with oxybutynin. Also, talk to your doctor about your complete medical history, especially if you have nervous disorders or had liver, kidney, or digestive problems.

What is the usual dosage?

Please see general statement regarding dosage on page xii.

Tablets:

Adults: The usual dose is one 5-milligram (mg) tablet taken two to three times a day. The maximum recommended daily dose is one 5-mg tablet four times a day. If you are elderly, your doctor may adjust your dose.

Children ≥5 years: The usual dose is one 5-mg tablet two times a day. The maximum recommended daily dose is one 5-mg tablet three times a day.

Syrup:
Adults: The usual dose is one teaspoonful of syrup taken two to three times a day. The maximum recommended daily dose is one teaspoonful of syrup four times a day. If you are elderly, your doctor may adjust your dose.

Children ≥5 years: The usual dose is one teaspoonful of syrup two times a day. The maximum recommended daily dose is one teaspoonful of syrup three times a day.

How should I take this medication?
• Take oxybutynin as prescribed by your doctor.

What should I avoid while taking this medication?
Avoid becoming overheated in hot weather or during activity.

What are possible food and drug interactions associated with this medication?
If oxybutynin is taken with certain other drugs, the effects of either could be increased, decreased, or altered. It is especially important to check with your doctor before combining oxybutynin with the following: antibiotics (clarithromycin or erythromycin); antifungal medicines (such as ketoconazole, itraconazole, or miconazole); ipratropium or tolterodine; medicines used to prevent bone loss (such as alendronate or ibandronate).

What are the possible side effects of this medication?
Please see general statement regarding side effects on page xiii.

Side effects may include: blurred vision, constipation, decreased sweating, dizziness, drowsiness, dry mouth, headache, inability to urinate, nausea, trouble falling or staying asleep, weakness

---

Can I receive this medication if I am pregnant or breastfeeding?

The effects of oxybutynin during pregnancy and breastfeeding are unknown. Tell your doctor immediately if you are pregnant, plan to become pregnant, or are breastfeeding.

What should I do if I miss a dose of this medication?

If you miss a dose of oxybutynin, take it as soon as you remember. However, if it is almost time for your next dose, skip the one you missed and return to your regular dosing schedule. Do not take two doses at once.

How should I store this medication?

Store at room temperature.

Oxybutynin Chloride: *see Oxybutynin, page 752*

Oxycodone HCI: *see Oxecta, page 749*

Oxycodone HCI: *see Oxycodone Immediate-Release, page 755*

Oxycodone HCI: *see Oxycontin, page 758*

Oxycodone HCI: *see Roxicodone, page 911*

Oxycodone Immediate-Release

Generic name: Oxycodone HCI

What is this medication?

Oxycodone is a narcotic pain medicine used for the relief of moderate to moderately severe pain.

Oxycodone is a federally controlled substance because it has abuse potential.

What is the most important information I should know about this medication?

- Oxycodone has abuse potential. Mental and physical dependence can occur with the use of oxycodone when it is used improperly for long periods of time.
- Oxycodone can cause serious breathing problems that can become life-threatening, especially when it is used in the wrong way for long periods of time. Tell your doctor if you have any lung or breathing problems (such as asthma); your doctor will monitor you.
- Oxycodone can reduce your blood pressure. This is more likely to happen if you have certain heart problems, or are taking other medications that can reduce your blood pressure.
- Oxycodone can impair your mental and physical abilities. Do not drive or operate machinery until you know how oxycodone affects you. Also, do not drink alcohol or take other medications that can affect your brain (such as medications that make you drowsy and narcotic painkillers) while using oxycodone.

Who should not take this medication?

Do not take oxycodone if you are allergic to it, any of its ingredients, or if you are having an asthma attack, have severe asthma, trouble breathing, or lung problems.

Do not take oxycodone if you have paralytic ileus (impairment of the small intestines).

What should I tell my doctor before I take the first dose of this medication?

Tell your doctor about all prescription, over-the-counter, and herbal medications you are taking before beginning treatment with oxycodone. Also, talk to your doctor about your allergies and complete medical history, especially if you have breathing problems; brain problems, head injury, or seizures; abdominal problems; pancreatitis (inflammation of the pancreas); severe liver or kidney problems; hypothyroidism (an underactive thyroid gland); adrenal gland problems; urinary blockage; alcoholism; history of or a present drug abuse or addiction problem; or a family history of drug abuse or addiction problem.

What is the usual dosage?
Please see general statement regarding dosage on page xii.

Adults: The recommended dose is 5 milligrams (mg) every 6 hours as needed for pain. Your doctor will adjust the dose for you based on the severity of your pain and your response to this medication.

How should I take this medication?
• Take oxycodone exactly as prescribed by your doctor.

What should I avoid while taking this medication?
Do not drive or operate machinery until you know how oxycodone affects you.

Do not drink alcohol while you are taking oxycodone.

What are possible food and drug interactions associated with this medication?
If oxycodone is taken with certain other drugs, the effects of either could be increased, decreased, or altered. It is especially important to check with your doctor before combining oxycodone with the following: alcohol, certain antipsychotics (such as clozapine or fluphenazine), or certain painkillers (such as buprenorphine, butorphanol, nalbuphine, or pentazocine), or other medications that slow down your brain function (such as alprazolam, diazepam, or phenobarbital).

What are the possible side effects of this medication?
Please see general statement regarding side effects on page xiii.

Side effects may include: constipation, dizziness, drowsiness, euphoria (a feeling of happiness and well-being), itchiness, light-headedness, nausea, rash, vomiting

Can I receive this medication if I am pregnant or breastfeeding?
The effects of oxycodone during pregnancy are unknown. Oxycodone can be found in your breast milk if you take it while

breastfeeding. Do not take oxycodone while you are breastfeeding. Tell your doctor immediately if you are pregnant, plan to become pregnant, or are breastfeeding.

What should I do if I miss a dose of this medication?
Oxycodone should be given only as needed.

How should I store this medication?
Store at room temperature. Protect from light and moisture.

Oxycontin
Generic name: Oxycodone HCl

What is this medication?
Oxycontin is a pain medicine that contains the narcotic painkiller oxycodone. Oxycontin is used to treat moderate to severe around-the-clock pain.

Oxycontin is a federally controlled substance because it has abuse potential.

What is the most important information I should know about this medication?
- Oxycontin has abuse potential. Mental and physical dependence can occur with the use of Oxycontin when it is used improperly.
- Oxycontin can cause serious breathing problems that can become life-threatening, especially when it is used in the wrong way.
- Oxycontin can cause low blood pressure. You can experience dizziness, lightheadedness, or fainting. To prevent this, carefully get up from a sitting or lying position. Sit or lie down at the first sign of any of these symptoms.
- Oxycontin can cause allergic reactions or anaphylaxis (a serious and rapid allergic reaction that may result in death if not immediately treated). Stop taking Oxycontin and tell your doctor immediately if you develop a rash, difficulty breathing, or swelling of your face, mouth, or throat.

Who should not take this medication?

Do not take Oxycontin if you are allergic to it or any of its ingredients.

Do not take Oxycontin if you have severe asthma, trouble breathing, or other lung problems.

Do not take Oxycontin if you have paralytic ileus (bowel blockage) or narrowing of the stomach or small intestine.

What should I tell my doctor before I take the first dose of this medication?

Tell your doctor about all prescription, over-the-counter, and herbal medications you are taking before beginning treatment with Oxycontin. Also, talk to your doctor about your complete medical history, especially if you have trouble breathing or lung problems, head injury, liver or kidney disease, thyroid problems, seizures, problems urinating, pancreas or gallbladder problems, mental health problems, or a history of alcohol or drug abuse.

What is the usual dosage?

Please see general statement regarding dosage on page xii.

Adults: The recommended starting dose is 10 milligrams every 12 hours. Your doctor will adjust your dose based on your condition, previous treatment with painkillers, and your tolerance for narcotics.

If you are elderly or have liver impairment, your doctor will adjust your dose appropriately.

How should I take this medication?

- Take Oxycontin exactly as prescribed by your doctor. Do not change your dose or stop taking Oxycontin without first talking to your doctor.
- Take Oxycontin one tablet at a time. Take each dose every 12 hours at the same time every day. Take each tablet with enough water to immediately swallow it.
- Swallow Oxycontin tablets whole. Do not cut, break, chew, crush, dissolve, or inject them.

- Do not pre-soak, lick, or otherwise wet the Oxycontin tablet before placing it in your mouth.

What should I avoid while taking this medication?

Do not drink alcohol or take other medications that contain alcohol while you are taking Oxycontin.

Do not drive or operate heavy machinery until you know how Oxycontin affects you.

Do not share Oxycontin with others.

What are possible food and drug interactions associated with this medication?

If Oxycontin is taken with certain other drugs, the effects of either could be increased, decreased, or altered. It is especially important to check with your doctor before combining Oxycontin with the following: alcohol, anticholinergics (such as ipratropium or oxybutynin), anti-HIV medications (such as ritonavir), butorphanol, carbamazepine, certain antibiotics (such as erythromycin), certain antidepressants (such as fluoxetine), certain antifungals (such as ketoconazole), certain heart medicines (such as quinidine), diuretics (water pills), general anesthetics, muscle relaxants (such as tubocurarine), nalbuphine, pentazocine, phenothiazines (such as chlorpromazine or mesoridazine), phenytoin, rifampin, sedative-hypnotics (such as alprazolam or diazepam), tranquilizers (such as chlordiazepoxide).

What are the possible side effects of this medication?

Please see general statement regarding side effects on page xiii.

> **Side effects may include:** abdominal pain, constipation, dizziness, headache, nausea, sleepiness, tiredness, vomiting

Can I receive this medication if I am pregnant or breastfeeding?

The effects of Oxycontin during pregnancy are unknown. Oxycontin can be found in your breast milk if you take it while breastfeeding.

Do not breastfeed while you are taking Oxycontin. Tell your doctor immediately if you are pregnant, plan to become pregnant, or are breastfeeding.

What should I do if I miss a dose of this medication?

If you miss a dose of Oxycontin, take it as soon as you remember and then take your next dose 12 hours later. However, if it is almost time for your next dose, skip the one you missed and return to your regular dosing schedule. Do not take more than one dose in 12 hours.

How should I store this medication?

Store at room temperature.

Paliperidone: *see Invega, page 478*

Pamelor

Generic name: Nortriptyline HCl

What is this medication?

Pamelor is a medicine used to treat the symptoms of depression. Pamelor is available in capsules and oral solution.

What is the most important information I should know about this medication?

- Pamelor can increase suicidal thoughts or actions in some children, teenagers, and young adults within the first few months of treatment.
- Depression and other serious mental illnesses are the most important causes of suicidal thoughts and actions. You may have a particularly high risk of having suicidal thoughts or actions if you have (or have a family history of) bipolar illness (also called manic-depressive illness).
- Pay close attention to any changes, especially sudden changes, in mood, behaviors, thoughts, or feelings. Tell your doctor right

away if you develop any changes. This is very important when Pamelor is started or when the dose is changed.

- Keep all follow-up visits with your doctor as scheduled. Call your doctor between visits as needed, especially if you have concerns about symptoms.

Who should not take this medication?

Do not use Pamelor if you are allergic to it, any of its ingredients, or to similar medicines.

Do not take Pamelor in combination with monoamine oxidase inhibitors (MAOIs), a class of drugs used to treat depression and other psychiatric conditions. You must wait at least 14 days after stopping an MAOI before starting Pamelor.

Do not take Pamelor if you have recently had a heart attack.

What should I tell my doctor before I take the first dose of this medication?

Tell your doctor about all prescription, over-the-counter, and herbal medications you are taking before beginning treatment with Pamelor. Also, talk to your doctor about your complete medical history, especially if you have a history of bipolar disorder or suicidal thoughts or actions; have liver, kidney, or heart problems; have glaucoma or difficulty urinating; have a history of seizures; have hyperthyroidism (an overactive thyroid gland); or are pregnant, plan to become pregnant, or are breastfeeding.

What is the usual dosage?

Please see general statement regarding dosage on page xii.

Adults: The recommended starting dose is 25 milligrams (mg) 3 to 4 times a day. Alternatively, you can take the total daily dose once a day. Your doctor will prescribe the appropriate dose for you and will increase your dose as needed, until the desired effect is achieved.

Elderly and adolescent patients: The recommended dose is 30-50 mg, taken in divided doses or once a day.

How should I take this medication?
• Take Pamelor exactly as prescribed by your doctor. You can take Pamelor once a day or in divided doses.

What should I avoid while taking this medication?
Do not drive a car or operate dangerous machinery until you know how Pamelor affects you. Pamelor can impair your mental and physical abilities.

Do not drink alcohol or take other medications that can make you sleepy while you are taking Pamelor.

Do not excessively expose yourself to sunlight while you are taking Pamelor.

What are possible food and drug interactions associated with this medication?
If Pamelor is taken with certain other drugs, the effects of either could be increased, decreased, or altered. It is especially important to check with your doctor before combining Pamelor with the following: alcohol, blood pressure medications (such as guanethidine), certain antidepressants (such as fluoxetine, paroxetine, or sertraline), cimetidine, chlorpropamide, flecainide, MAOIs, propafenone, quinidine, reserpine, or thyroid medications.

What are the possible side effects of this medication?
Please see general statement regarding side effects on page xiii.

Side effects may include: blurred vision, changes in blood pressure, changes in blood sugar levels, confusion, constipation, diarrhea, dizziness, drowsiness, dry mouth, enlargement of breasts, fever, flushing, hair loss, headache, itching, light sensitivity, loss of appetite, loss of muscle coordination, nausea, numbness or tingling in your hands or feet, rapid or irregular heartbeat, rash, seizures, swelling, taste disturbances, tiredness, trouble urinating, vomiting, weakness, weight changes

Can I receive this medication if I am pregnant or breastfeeding?

The effects of Pamelor during pregnancy and breastfeeding are unknown. Tell your doctor immediately if you are pregnant, plan to become pregnant, or are breastfeeding.

What should I do if I miss a dose of this medication?

If you miss a dose of Pamelor, take the missed dose as soon as you remember. However, if it is almost time for your next dose, skip the one you missed and return to your regular dosing schedule. Do not take two doses at once.

How should I store this medication?

Store at room temperature.

Pantoprazole Sodium: *see Protonix, page 862*

Paroxetine HCl: *see Paxil, page 768*

Paroxetine Mesylate: *see Pexeva, page 783*

Pataday

Generic name: Olopatadine HCl

What is this medication?

Pataday is an eye drop medicine used to treat eye itching associated with allergic conjunctivitis ("pink eye").

What is the most important information I should know about this medication?

- Pataday is for use in your eyes only. Do not use Pataday in your mouth.
- Do not wear contact lenses if your eyes are red. Also, Pataday should not be used to treat contact lens-related irritation. Pataday contains a preservative, benzalkonium chloride, which can be absorbed by soft contact lenses. If you wear soft contact

lenses and your eyes are not red, wait at least 10 minutes after applying Pataday before you insert your contact lenses.

Who should not take this medication?
Do not use Pataday if you are allergic to it or any of its ingredients.

What should I tell my doctor before I take the first dose of this medication?
Tell your doctor about all prescription, over-the-counter, and herbal medications you are taking before beginning treatment with Pataday. Also, talk to your doctor about your complete medical history.

What is the usual dosage?
Please see general statement regarding dosage on page xii.

Adults and children ≥2 years: Apply 1 drop into the affected eye(s) once a day.

How should I take this medication?
• Apply Pataday exactly as prescribed by your doctor. Keep the bottle tightly closed when you are not using it.

What should I avoid while taking this medication?
Do not use Pataday for injection or in your mouth.

Do not allow the dropper tip of the bottle to contact your eyelids or any other surrounding area, as this can contaminate Pataday.

Do not wear contact lenses if your eyes are red.

What are possible food and drug interactions associated with this medication?
No significant interactions have been reported with Pataday at this time. However, always tell your doctor about any medicines you take, including over-the-counter medications, vitamins, and herbal supplements.

What are the possible side effects of this medication?
Please see general statement regarding side effects on page xiii.

> **Side effects may include:** allergic reactions, back pain, blurred vision, burning or stinging, change in taste, cold symptoms, conjunctivitis, dry eye, eye itching or pain, "flu-like" symptoms, foreign body sensation in your eyes, headache, increased cough, infection, nausea, red eye, runny nose, sore throat, swelling of your eye lids, weakness

Can I receive this medication if I am pregnant or breastfeeding?

The effects of Pataday during pregnancy and breastfeeding are unknown. Tell your doctor immediately if you are pregnant, plan to become pregnant, or are breastfeeding.

What should I do if I miss a dose of this medication?

If you miss a dose of Pataday, apply it as soon as you remember. However, if it is almost time for your next dose, skip the one you missed and return to your regular dosing schedule. Do not apply two doses at once.

How should I store this medication?

Store at room temperature or in the refrigerator.

Patanol

Generic name: Olopatadine HCl

What is this medication?

Patanol is an eye drop medicine used to treat signs and symptoms of allergic conjunctivitis ("pink eye").

What is the most important information I should know about this medication?

• Patanol is for use in your eyes only. Do not use Patanol in your mouth.
• Do not wear contact lenses if your eyes are red. Also, Patanol should not be used to treat contact lens-related irritation. Patanol contains a preservative, benzalkonium chloride, which can be absorbed by soft contact lenses. If you wear soft contact

lenses and your eyes are not red, wait at least 10 minutes after applying Patanol before you insert your contact lenses.

Who should not take this medication?
Do not use Patanol if you are allergic to it or any of its ingredients.

What should I tell my doctor before I take the first dose of this medication?
Tell your doctor about all prescription, over-the-counter, and herbal medications you are taking before beginning treatment with Patanol. Also, talk to your doctor about your complete medical history.

What is the usual dosage?
Please see general statement regarding dosage on page xii.

Adults and children ≥3 years: Apply 1 drop into the affected eye(s) twice a day, 6-8 hours apart.

How should I take this medication?
• Apply Patanol exactly as prescribed by your doctor. Keep the bottle tightly closed when you are not using it.

What should I avoid while taking this medication?
Do not use Patanol for injection or in your mouth.

Do not allow the dropper tip of the bottle to contact your eyelids or any other surrounding area, as this can contaminate Patanol.

Do not wear contact lenses if your eyes are red.

What are possible food and drug interactions associated with this medication?
No significant interactions have been reported with Patanol at this time. However, always tell your doctor about any medicines you take, including over-the-counter medications, vitamins, and herbal supplements.

What are the possible side effects of this medication?
Please see general statement regarding side effects on page xiii.

Side effects may include: allergic reactions, blurred vision, burning or stinging, change in taste, cold-like symptoms, dry eye, feeling like something is in your eyes, headache, inflammation of the cornea (the clear tissue over the pupil of your eye), itching, nausea, red eyes, runny and stuffy nose, sore throat, swelling of your eye lids, weakness

Can I receive this medication if I am pregnant or breastfeeding?

The effects of Patanol during pregnancy and breastfeeding are unknown. Tell your doctor immediately if you are pregnant, plan to become pregnant, or are breastfeeding.

What should I do if I miss a dose of this medication?

If you miss a dose of Patanol, apply it as soon as you remember. However, if it is almost time for your next dose, skip the one you missed and return to your regular dosing schedule. Do not apply two doses at once.

How should I store this medication?

Store at room temperature or in the refrigerator.

Paxil

Generic name: Paroxetine HCl

What is this medication?

Paxil is an antidepressant medicine known as a selective serotonin reuptake inhibitor (SSRI). It is used to treat major depressive disorder, obsessive compulsive disorder, panic disorder, social anxiety disorder, generalized anxiety disorder, and post-traumatic stress disorder. Paxil is available in tablets and an oral solution.

What is the most important information I should know about this medication?

- Paxil can increase the risk of suicidal thoughts and behavior in children, adolescents, and young adults. Your doctor will monitor you closely for clinical worsening, suicidal or unusual behavior after you start taking Paxil or start a new dose of Paxil. Tell your doctor right away if you experience anxiety, hostility, sleeplessness, restlessness, impulsive or dangerous behavior, or thoughts about suicide or dying; or if you have new symptoms or seem to be feeling worse.

- Paxil can cause serotonin syndrome (a potentially life-threatening drug reaction that causes the body to have too much serotonin, a chemical produced by the nerve cells) or neuroleptic malignant syndrome (a brain disorder) when you take it alone or in combination with other medicines. You can experience mental status changes, an increase in your heart rate and temperature, lack of coordination, overactive reflexes, muscle rigidity, nausea, vomiting, or diarrhea. Tell your doctor right away if you experience any of these signs or symptoms.

- Paxil can cause severe allergic reactions. Stop taking this medication and tell your doctor immediately if you develop a rash, trouble breathing, or swelling of your face, tongue, eyes, or mouth.

- Your risk of abnormal bleeding or bruising can increase if you take Paxil, especially if you also take blood thinners (such as warfarin), nonsteroidal anti-inflammatory drugs (NSAIDs) (such as ibuprofen or naproxen), or aspirin.

- You can experience manic episodes while you are taking Paxil. Tell your doctor if you experience greatly increased energy, severe trouble sleeping, racing thoughts, reckless behavior, unusually grand ideas, excessive happiness or irritability, or talking more or faster than usual.

- Paxil can cause seizures or changes in your appetite or weight. Your doctor will monitor you for these effects during treatment.

- Paxil can decrease your blood sodium levels, especially if you are elderly. Tell your doctor if you have a headache, weakness, an unsteady feeling, confusion, problems concentrating or thinking, or memory problems while you are taking Paxil.

- Do not stop taking Paxil without first talking to your doctor. Stopping Paxil suddenly can cause serious symptoms, including anxiety, irritability, changes in your mood, feeling restless, changes in your sleep habits, headache, sweating, nausea, dizziness, electric shock-like sensations, shaking, or confusion.

Who should not take this medication?

Do not take Paxil if you are allergic to it or any of its ingredients.

Do not take Paxil while you are taking other medicines known as monoamine oxidase inhibitors (MAOIs) (such as linezolid, methylene blue, or phenelzine), a class of medications used to treat depression and other conditions. Do not take Paxil if you are taking pimozide or thioridazine.

Do not take Paxil if you are taking medicines called Paxil CR or Pexeva, since these medicines contain the same active ingredient.

What should I tell my doctor before I take the first dose of this medication?

Tell your doctor about all prescription, over-the-counter, and herbal medications you are taking before beginning treatment with Paxil. Also, talk to your doctor about your complete medical history, especially if you have high blood pressure; heart, liver, or kidney problems; history of stroke; glaucoma (high pressure in the eye); bleeding problems; seizures; mania or bipolar disorder; or low sodium levels in your blood. Also, tell your doctor if you are pregnant, plan to become pregnant, or are breastfeeding.

What is the usual dosage?

Please see general statement regarding dosage on page xii.

Major Depressive Disorder, Obsessive-Compulsive Disorder, Social Anxiety Disorder, Generalized Anxiety Disorder, and Post-Traumatic Stress Disorder

Adults: The recommended starting dose is 20 milligrams (mg) once a day.

Panic Disorder

Adults: The recommended starting dose is 10 mg once a day.

Your doctor will increase your dose as needed until the desired effect is achieved.

If you are elderly or have liver impairment, your doctor will adjust your dose appropriately.

How should I take this medication?
- Take Paxil exactly as prescribed by your doctor. Take Paxil once a day, in the morning. Take it with or without food.
- Swallow Paxil tablets whole. Do not crush or chew it.
- Shake the Paxil oral solution well before you take the medicine.

What should I avoid while taking this medication?
Do not drive, operate heavy machinery, or engage in other danger-ous activities until you know how Paxil affects you.

Do not drink alcohol while you are taking Paxil.

Do not stop taking Paxil suddenly without first talking to your doc-tor, as this can cause serious side effects.

Do not take Paxil and MAOIs together or within 14 days of each other. Combining these medicines with Paxil can cause serious and even life-threatening reactions.

What are possible food and drug interactions associated with this medication?
If Paxil is taken with certain other drugs, the effects of either could be increased, decreased, or altered. Paxil may interact with numer-ous medications. Therefore, it is very important that you tell your doctor about any other medications you are taking.

What are the possible side effects of this medication?
Please see general statement regarding side effects on page xiii.

Side effects may include: constipation, dizziness, dry mouth, feeling anxious, infections, loss of appetite, nausea, sexual prob-lems, shaking, sleepiness, sweating, trouble sleeping, weakness, yawning

Can I receive this medication if I am pregnant or breastfeeding?

Do not take Paxil if you are pregnant. Paxil can be found in your breast milk if you take it while breastfeeding. Tell your doctor immediately if you are pregnant, plan to become pregnant, or are breastfeeding.

What should I do if I miss a dose of this medication?

If you miss a dose of Paxil, take it as soon as you remember. However, if it is almost time for your next dose, skip the one you missed and return to your regular dosing schedule. Do not take two doses at once.

How should I store this medication?

Store at room temperature.

Penicillin V Potassium: see Penicillin VK, page 772

Penicillin VK

Generic name: Penicillin V Potassium

What is this medication?

Penicillin VK is an antibiotic used to treat certain bacterial infections of the throat, heart, middle ear, skin, and respiratory (lung) tract; and gum disease. It may also be used to treat or prevent other bacterial infections, as determined by your doctor. Penicillin VK is available in tablets and powder for oral solution.

What is the most important information I should know about this medication?

- Do not take penicillin VK if you are allergic to it, any of its ingredients, or similar antibiotics (such as amoxicillin, cefazolin, cefaclor, or cefotetan). Tell your doctor right away if you take penicillin VK and feel signs of an allergic reaction (such as a rash, swelling, or difficulty breathing).

- Penicillin VK can cause diarrhea or colitis (inflammation of the colon). This can occur a couple of months after taking the last dose of penicillin VK. Tell your doctor right away if you have diarrhea or colitis.
- Use penicillin VK as prescribed by your doctor for the full course of treatment, even if symptoms improve earlier. Do not skip doses. Skipping doses or not completing the full course of penicillin VK can decrease its effectiveness and can lead to the growth of bacteria that are resistant to the effects of penicillin VK.

Who should not take this medication?

Do not take penicillin VK if you are allergic to it, any of its ingredients, or similar antibiotics.

Do not take penicillin VK to treat viral infections, such as the common cold.

What should I tell my doctor before I take the first dose of this medication?

Tell your doctor about all prescription, over-the-counter, and herbal medications you are taking before beginning treatment with penicillin VK. Also, talk to your doctor about your complete medical history, especially if you have allergies, asthma, kidney disease, diarrhea, or stomach problems.

What is the usual dosage?

Please see general statement regarding dosage on page xii.

Adults and children ≥12 years: Your doctor will prescribe the appropriate dose and duration of treatment for you based on the type of your infection.

How should I take this medication?

- Take penicillin VK exactly as prescribed by your doctor. Take penicillin VK on a full or empty stomach.
- If your doctor has prescribed penicillin VK oral solution, ask your pharmacist for a medicine dropper or medicine cup to help you measure the correct amount of the solution. Do not use a household teaspoon. Shake the solution well before each use.

What should I avoid while taking this medication?

Do not take penicillin VK with medicines that can cause kidney injury or damage.

What are possible food and drug interactions associated with this medication?

No significant interactions have been reported with penicillin VK at this time. However, always tell your doctor about any medicines you take, including over-the-counter medications, vitamins, and herbal supplements.

What are the possible side effects of this medication?

Please see general statement regarding side effects on page xiii.

Side effects may include: allergic reactions, black hairy tongue, diarrhea, fever, hives, nausea, skin rash, stomach upset or pain, swelling in your throat, vomiting

---

Can I receive this medication if I am pregnant or breastfeeding?

The effects of penicillin VK during pregnancy and breastfeeding are unknown. Tell your doctor immediately if you are pregnant, plan to become pregnant, or are breastfeeding.

What should I do if I miss a dose of this medication?

If you miss a dose of penicillin VK, take it as soon as you remember. However, if it is almost time for your next dose, skip the one you missed and return to your regular dosing schedule. Do not take two doses at once.

How should I store this medication?

Store at room temperature.

After mixing, store penicillin VK oral solution in the refrigerator. Discard the unused portion after 14 days.

Pepcid
Generic name: Famotidine

What is this medication?
Pepcid is a medicine used to treat ulcers in the intestines, stomach, or esophagus (tube that connects your mouth and stomach). It is also used to treat gastroesophageal reflux disease (GERD) or heartburn, or to reduce stomach acid in certain diseases where the stomach secretes too much acid (hypersecretory conditions), such as Zollinger-Ellison syndrome.

Pepcid belongs to a class of medicines called histamine H_2 blockers. It works by decreasing the amount of acid secreted into your stomach. Pepcid is available in tablets or suspension.

What is the most important information I should know about this medication?
- Pepcid can be used for up to 8 or 12 weeks, depending on the type of ulcer. The ulcer can heal within 4 weeks of therapy.
- Tell your doctor if you have kidney impairment. If you take Pepcid and have kidney problems, you can experience seizures or other effects on your nervous system, or irregular heartbeat.

Who should not take this medication?
Do not take Pepcid if you are allergic to it, any of its ingredients, or other similar medications.

What should I tell my doctor before I take the first dose of this medication?
Tell your doctor about all prescription, over-the-counter, and herbal medications you are taking before beginning treatment with Pepcid. Also, talk to your doctor about your complete medical history, especially if you have kidney or stomach problems, or seizures.

What is the usual dosage?
Please see general statement regarding dosage on page xii.

Pepcid oral suspension may be substituted for Pepcid tablets for any of the indications below. Each milliliter (mL) of Pepcid oral suspension contains 8 milligrams (mg) of famotidine.

Active Duodenal Ulcer (ulcer in the upper intestine) or Active Stomach Ulcer
Adults: The recommended dose is 40 mg or one teaspoonful once a day at bedtime.

Children: Your doctor will prescribe the appropriate dose for your child, based on their weight.

Maintenance of a Healed Duodenal Ulcer
Adults: The recommended dose is 20 mg or half a teaspoonful once a day at bedtime.

GERD
Adults: The recommended dose is 20 mg or half a teaspoonful twice a day.

Children: Your doctor will prescribe the appropriate dose for your child, based on their weight.

Hypersecretory Conditions
Adults: The recommended dose is 20 mg or half a teaspoonful every 6 hours.

If you have kidney impairment, your doctor will adjust your dose appropriately.

How should I take this medication?
- Take Pepcid exactly as prescribed by your doctor. Take Pepcid by mouth, with or without food. You can take antacids while you are taking Pepcid if needed.
- Shake Pepcid suspension well for 5 to 10 seconds before each use. Discard any unused oral suspension after 30 days.

What should I avoid while taking this medication?

Do not change your dose or take more often without talking to your doctor.

What are possible food and drug interactions associated with this medication?

No significant interactions have been reported with Pepcid at this time. However, always tell your doctor about any medicines you take, including over-the-counter medications, vitamins, and herbal supplements.

What are the possible side effects of this medication?

Please see general statement regarding side effects on page xiii.

> **Side effects may include:** agitation, anxiety, confusion, constipation, depression, diarrhea, dizziness, dry mouth, fever, headache, muscle cramps or pain, nausea, rash, seizures, tiredness, trouble sleeping, vomiting, weakness

Can I receive this medication if I am pregnant or breastfeeding?

The effects of Pepcid during pregnancy are unknown. Pepcid can be found in your breast milk if you take it while breastfeeding. Tell your doctor immediately if you are pregnant, plan to become pregnant, or are breastfeeding.

What should I do if I miss a dose of this medication?

If you miss a dose of Pepcid, take it as soon as you remember. However, if it is almost time for your next dose, skip the one you missed and return to your regular dosing schedule. Do not take two doses at once.

How should I store this medication?

Store at room temperature. Protect the suspension from freezing.

Percocet
Generic name: Acetaminophen/Oxycodone HCl

What is this medication?
Percocet is a pain medicine that contains the narcotic painkiller oxycodone and the non-narcotic painkiller acetaminophen. Percocet is used to relieve moderate to moderately severe pain.

What is the most important information I should know about this medication?
- Percocet has abuse potential. Mental and physical dependence can occur with the use of Percocet when it is used improperly.
- Percocet can cause serious breathing problems that can become life-threatening, especially when it is used in the wrong way. Tell your doctor if you have any lung or breathing problems; your doctor will monitor you.
- Percocet contains acetaminophen, which can cause severe liver injury. Do not take more than 4000 milligrams (mg) of acetaminophen per day or take other products containing acetaminophen. The risk of liver injury can be higher if you have underlying liver disease or drink alcohol while you are taking Percocet.
- Percocet can cause allergic reactions or anaphylaxis (a serious and rapid allergic reaction that may result in death if not immediately treated). Stop taking Percocet and tell your doctor immediately if you develop a rash, difficulty breathing, or swelling of your face, mouth, or throat.
- Percocet can impair your mental or physical abilities. Do not drive or operate machinery until you know how Percocet affects you.
- Keep Percocet in a secure place out of the reach of children. In the case of accidental ingestion, get emergency medical care immediately.

Who should not take this medication?
Do not take Percocet if you are allergic to it, any of its ingredients, or other narcotic painkillers.

Do not take Percocet if you have paralytic ileus (impairment of the small intestines), severe lung problems, or severe asthma.

What should I tell my doctor before I take the first dose of this medication?

Tell your doctor about all prescription, over-the-counter, and herbal medication you are taking before beginning treatment with Percocet. Also, talk to your doctor about your complete medical history, especially if you have ever had kidney or liver disease, hypothyroidism (an underactive thyroid gland), adrenal gland problems, heart disease, seizures, gallbladder problems, severe diarrhea, paralytic ileus, difficulty urinating, an enlarged prostate, stomach problems (such as an ulcer), a history of substance abuse or dependence, mental disorders (such as depression) or suicidal thoughts, low blood pressure, if you are taking medications to lower your blood pressure, or if you have experienced a head injury.

What is the usual dosage?

Please see general statement regarding dosage on page xii.

Percocet 2.5 mg/325 mg Tablets
Adults: The usual dose is 1-2 tablets every 6 hours.

All Other Percocet Strengths
Adults: The usual dose is 1 tablet every 6 hours as needed for pain.

How should I take this medication?

- Take Percocet exactly as prescribed by your doctor. Do not adjust your dose or discontinue Percocet without speaking to your doctor. Attempts to taper (gradually reduce the dose) or discontinue the medication should be made at specific intervals, through the guidance of your doctor.

What should I avoid while taking this medication?

Do not take Percocet with alcohol, other narcotic painkillers, tranquilizers (such as alprazolam or lorazepam), sedatives (such as diphenhydramine or phenobarbital), or other central nervous system (CNS) depressants unless under the recommendation and guidance of your doctor.

Percocet can impair your mental and physical ability to perform potentially hazardous tasks (such as driving or operating heavy machinery). Do not participate in any activities that require full alertness until you know how Percocet effects you.

Do not share Percocet with others; it may be habit-forming. Therefore, it should be used only by the person it was prescribed for.

Dispose all unused tablets by flushing them down the toilet.

What are possible food and drug interactions associated with this medication?

If Percocet is taken with certain other drugs, the effects of either could be increased, decreased, or altered. It is especially important to check with your doctor before combining Percocet with the following: alcohol; birth control pills; certain painkillers; diuretics (water pills) (such as furosemide); CNS depressants (such as alprazolam, diazepam, or phenobarbital); lamotrigine; probenecid; propranolol; sedative-hypnotics; or zidovudine.

What are the possible side effects of this medication?

Please see general statement regarding side effects on page xiii.

> **Side effects may include:** constipation, difficulty breathing, dizziness, exaggerated feelings of well-being, high blood pressure, itching, lightheadedness, low blood pressure, nausea, sedation, skin rash, upset stomach, urinary retention (inability to urinate normally), vomiting

Can I receive this medication if I am pregnant or breastfeeding?

The effects of Percocet during pregnancy are unknown. Percocet can be found in your breast milk if you take it while breastfeeding. Do not take Percocet while you are breastfeeding. Tell your doctor immediately if you are pregnant, plan to become pregnant, or are breastfeeding.

What should I do if I miss a dose of this medication?
Percocet should be taken only as needed.

How should I store this medication?
Store at room temperature. Protect from heat, moisture, and light.

Peridex
Generic name: Chlorhexidine Gluconate

What is this medication?
Peridex is a medicine used to treat gingivitis (gum disease).

What is the most important information I should know about this medication?
- Peridex is used only for gingivitis. Tell your doctor or dentist if you also have periodontitis (disease of the tissue that supports and attaches the teeth). Your doctor or dentist may need to give you additional treatment.
- Peridex can cause staining inside the mouth, such as on the tooth surfaces and the tongue. These stains have no adverse effect on your gums, and usually can be cleaned by your dentist. Brush and floss your teeth every day. Peridex can also cause an excess of tartar build-up on your teeth.
- Some people can experience a change in taste while using Peridex. This usually goes away with continued use of Peridex. You can use Peridex after meals to avoid taste interference.

Who should not take this medication?
Do not use Peridex if you are allergic to it or any of its ingredients.

What should I tell my doctor before I take the first dose of this medication?
Tell your doctor about all prescription, over-the-counter, and herbal medications you are taking before beginning treatment with Peridex. Also, talk to your doctor about your complete medical history, especially if you have fillings or other dental work on your front teeth, or if you have periodontitis.

What is the usual dosage?
Please see general statement regarding dosage on page xii.

Adults: The recommended dose is 15 milliliters (mL) twice a day.

How should I take this medication?
• Take Peridex as directed by your doctor. Rinse for 30 seconds every morning and evening after brushing your teeth. Do not swallow Peridex. You should spit out Peridex after rinsing.

What should I avoid while taking this medication?
Do not rinse with water or other mouthwashes, brush your teeth, or eat right after using Peridex.

What are possible food and drug interactions associated with this medication?
No significant interactions have been reported with Peridex at this time. However, always tell your doctor about any medicines you take, including over-the-counter medications, vitamins, and herbal supplements.

What are the possible side effects of this medication?
Please see general statement regarding side effects on page xiii.

Side effects may include: allergic reactions, change in taste, mouth irritation, staining of teeth and other mouth surfaces, tartar formation

Can I receive this medication if I am pregnant or breastfeeding?
The effects of Peridex during pregnancy and breastfeeding are unknown. Tell your doctor immediately if you are pregnant, plan to become pregnant, or are breastfeeding.

What should I do if I miss a dose of this medication?
If you miss a dose of Peridex, use it as soon as you remember. However, if it is almost time for your next dose, skip the one you

missed and return to your regular dosing schedule. Do not take two doses at once.

How should I store this medication?
Store at room temperature. Do not freeze.

Pexeva
Generic name: Paroxetine Mesylate

What is this medication?
Pexeva is an antidepressant medicine known as a selective serotonin reuptake inhibitor (SSRI). It is used to treat major depressive disorder, obsessive compulsive disorder, panic disorder, and generalized anxiety disorder.

What is the most important information I should know about this medication?
- Pexeva can increase the risk of suicidal thoughts and behavior in children, adolescents, and young adults. Your doctor will monitor you closely for clinical worsening, suicidal or unusual behavior after you start taking Pexeva or start a new dose of Pexeva. Tell your doctor right away if you experience anxiety, hostility, sleeplessness, restlessness, impulsive or dangerous behavior, or thoughts about suicide or dying; or if you have new symptoms or seem to be feeling worse.
- Pexeva can cause serotonin syndrome (a potentially life-threatening drug reaction that causes the body to have too much serotonin, a chemical produced by the nerve cells) or neuroleptic malignant syndrome (a brain disorder) when you take it alone or in combination with other medicines. You can experience mental status changes, an increase in your heart rate and temperature, lack of coordination, overactive reflexes, muscle rigidity, nausea, vomiting, or diarrhea. Tell your doctor right away if you experience any of these signs or symptoms.
- Pexeva can cause severe allergic reactions. Stop taking this medication and tell your doctor immediately if you develop a

rash, trouble breathing, or swelling of your face, tongue, eyes, or mouth.

- Your risk of abnormal bleeding or bruising can increase if you take Pexeva, especially if you also take blood thinners (such as warfarin), nonsteroidal anti-inflammatory drugs (NSAIDs) (such as ibuprofen or naproxen), or aspirin.
- You can experience manic episodes while you are taking Pexeva. Tell your doctor if you experience greatly increased energy, severe trouble sleeping, racing thoughts, reckless behavior, unusually grand ideas, excessive happiness or irritability, or talking more or faster than usual.
- Pexeva can cause seizures or changes in your appetite or weight. Your doctor will monitor you for these effects during treatment.
- Pexeva can decrease your blood sodium levels, especially if you are elderly. Tell your doctor if you have a headache, weakness, an unsteady feeling, confusion, problems concentrating or thinking, or memory problems while you are taking Pexeva.
- Do not stop taking Pexeva without first talking to your doctor. Stopping Pexeva suddenly can cause serious symptoms, including anxiety, irritability, changes in your mood, feeling restless, changes in your sleep habits, headache, sweating, nausea, dizziness, electric shock-like sensations, shaking, or confusion.

Who should not take this medication?
Do not take Pexeva if you are allergic to it or any of its ingredients.

Do not take Pexeva while you are taking other medicines known as monoamine oxidase inhibitors (MAOIs) (such as phenelzine), a class of medications used to treat depression and other conditions.

Do not take Pexeva if you are taking pimozide or thioridazine.

Do not take Pexeva if you are taking medicines called Paxil or Paxil CR, since these medicines contain the same active ingredient.

What should I tell my doctor before I take the first dose of this medication?
Tell your doctor about all prescription, over-the-counter, and herbal medications you are taking before beginning treatment with

Pexeva. Also, talk to your doctor about your complete medical history, especially if you have high blood pressure; heart, liver, or kidney problems; history of stroke; glaucoma (high pressure in the eye); bleeding problems; seizures; mania or bipolar disorder; or low blood sodium levels. Also, tell your doctor if you are pregnant, plan to become pregnant, or are breastfeeding.

What is the usual dosage?
Please see general statement regarding dosage on page xii.

Major Depressive Disorder, Obsessive-Compulsive Disorder, and Generalized Anxiety Disorder
Adults: The recommended starting dose is 20 milligrams (mg) once a day.

Panic Disorder
Adults: The recommended starting dose is 10 mg once a day.

Your doctor will increase your dose as needed until the desired effect is achieved.

If you are elderly or have liver impairment, your doctor will adjust your dose appropriately.

How should I take this medication?
- Take Pexeva exactly as prescribed by your doctor. Take Pexeva once a day, in the morning.
- Take Pexeva tablet with or without food.
- Swallow Pexeva whole. Do not crush or chew it.

What should I avoid while taking this medication?
Do not drive, operate heavy machinery, or engage in other dangerous activities until you know how Pexeva affects you.

Do not drink alcohol while you are taking Pexeva.

Do not stop taking Pexeva suddenly without first talking to your doctor, as this can cause serious side effects.

Do not take Pexeva and MAOIs together or within 14 days of each other. Combining these medicines with Pexeva can cause serious and even life-threatening reactions.

What are possible food and drug interactions associated with this medication?

If Pexeva is taken with certain other drugs, the effects of either could be increased, decreased, or altered. Pexeva may interact with numerous medications. Therefore, it is very important that you tell your doctor about any other medications you are taking.

What are the possible side effects of this medication?

Please see general statement regarding side effects on page xiii.

Side effects may include: constipation, dizziness, dry mouth, feeling anxious, infections, loss of appetite, nausea, sexual problems, shaking, sleepiness, sweating, trouble sleeping, weakness, yawning

---

Can I receive this medication if I am pregnant or breastfeeding?

Do not take Pexeva if you are pregnant. Pexeva can be found in your breast milk if you take it while breastfeeding. Tell your doctor immediately if you are pregnant, plan to become pregnant, or are breastfeeding.

What should I do if I miss a dose of this medication?

If you miss a dose of Pexeva, take it as soon as you remember. However, if it is almost time for your next dose, skip the one you missed and return to your regular dosing schedule. Do not take two doses at once.

How should I store this medication?

Store at room temperature. Protect from humidity.

Phenazopyridine

Generic name: Phenazopyridine HCl

What is this medication?

Phenazopyridine is a medicine used to relieve urinary pain, burning, irritation, and increased need to urinate caused by infection, trauma, surgery, catheters, or other procedures in the urinary tract.

What is the most important information I should know about this medication?

- Phenazopyridine produces a reddish-orange color in the urine and may stain fabric and contact lenses.
- Tell your doctor if you experience yellowing of your skin or the whites of your eyes. This can mean that your kidneys are not eliminating the medication as they should.

Who should not take this medication?

Do not take phenazopyridine if you are allergic to it or any of its ingredients.

Do not take phenazopyridine if you have kidney disease.

What should I tell my doctor before I take the first dose of this medication?

Tell your doctor about all prescription, over-the-counter, and herbal medications you are taking before beginning treatment with phenazopyridine. Also, talk to your doctor about your complete medical history, especially if you have kidney disease.

What is the usual dosage?

Please see general statement regarding dosage on page xii.

Adults: The usual dose is two 100-milligram (mg) tablets or one 200-mg tablet three times a day after meals.

How should I take this medication?

- Take phenazopyridine exactly as prescribed by your doctor. Take it after meals.

What should I avoid while taking this medication?

Do not take phenazopyridine for more than 2 days if you are also
taking an antibiotic to treat a urinary tract infection.

What are possible food and drug interactions associated with this medication?

No significant interactions have been reported with phenazopyridine at this time. However, always tell your doctor about any medicines you take, including over-the-counter medications, vitamins,
and herbal supplements.

What are the possible side effects of this medication?

Please see general statement regarding side effects on page xiii.

> **Side effects may include:** allergic reactions, headache, itching,
> rash, upset stomach

Can I receive this medication if I am pregnant or breastfeeding?

The effects of phenazopyridine during pregnancy and breastfeeding are unknown. Tell your doctor immediately if you are pregnant,
plan to become pregnant, or are breastfeeding.

What should I do if I miss a dose of this medication?

If you miss a dose of phenazopyridine, take it as soon as you remember. However, if it is almost time for your next dose, skip the
one you missed and return to your regular dosing schedule. Do not
take two doses at once.

How should I store this medication?

Store at room temperature.

Phenazopyridine HCl: *see Phenazopyridine, page 787*

Phenobarbital

Generic name: Phenobarbital

What is this medication?

Phenobarbital is a medicine known as a barbiturate used for sedation. It is also used to treat certain types of seizures.

What is the most important information I should know about this medication?

- Phenobarbital can be habit-forming. You can become tolerant
  and need more of this medicine to achieve the same effect. You
  can become physically and psychologically dependent with continued use. Do not increase the dose of the medicine without
  first talking to your doctor. If you have a history of drug abuse,
  tell your doctor before taking phenobarbital.
- Phenobarbital can impair your mental and/or physical abilities
  required to perform hazardous tasks, such as driving a car or
  operating machinery.
- Phenobarbital can cause excitement, depression, or confusion in
  elderly or ill individuals. It usually causes excitement in children.

Who should not take this medication?

Do not take phenobarbital if you are allergic to it, any of its ingredients, or to other barbiturates.

Also, do not take phenobarbital if you have a history of porphyria
(a blood disorder), severe liver impairment, or respiratory (lung)
disease.

What should I tell my doctor before I take the first dose of this medication?

Tell your doctor about all prescription, over-the-counter, and herbal
medications you are taking before beginning treatment with phenobarbital. Also, talk to your doctor about your complete medical
history, especially if you have a history of kidney or liver problems,
drug abuse, acute (sudden) or chronic (long-term) pain, or adrenal
gland problems. Tell your doctor if you are pregnant, plan to become pregnant, or are breastfeeding.

What is the usual dosage?

Please see general statement regarding dosage on page xii.

Your doctor will prescribe the appropriate dose based on your age, weight, and condition. The dose of phenobarbital is individualized for each patient according to their needs.

Sedation
Adults: The usual dose is 30-120 milligrams (mg) a day in 2 or 3 divided doses. Your doctor will prescribe the appropriate dose for you based on your condition and will increase your dose as appropriate.

Seizures
Adults: The usual dose is 60-200 mg a day. Your doctor will prescribe the appropriate dose for you based on your condition and will increase your dose as appropriate.

Children: Your doctor will prescribe the appropriate dose for your child, based on their weight.

If you are elderly, ill, or have kidney or liver impairment, your doctor will adjust your dose appropriately.

How should I take this medication?
• Take phenobarbital exactly as prescribed by your doctor.
• Do not stop taking phenobarbital without first talking to your doctor, especially if you are using this medication for seizures. Do not take extra doses or take more often without asking your doctor.

What should I avoid while taking this medication?
Do not drive or operate machinery until you know how phenobarbital affects you.

Do not drink alcohol while you are taking phenobarbital.

Do not take other medications that can cause dizziness or drowsiness while you are taking phenobarbital.

What are possible food and drug interactions associated with this medication?

If phenobarbital is taken with certain other drugs, the effects of either could be increased, decreased, or altered. It is especially important to check with your doctor before combining phenobarbital with the following: alcohol, antidepressants known as monoamine oxidase inhibitors (MAOIs) (such as phenelzine or tranylcypromine), antihistamines (such as diphenhydramine or doxylamine), blood thinners (such as warfarin), corticosteroids (such as prednisone), doxycycline, griseofulvin, birth control pills, phenytoin, steroidal hormones (such as progesterone or estrone), tranquilizers (such as alprazolam or diazepam), or valproic acid.

What are the possible side effects of this medication?

Please see general statement regarding side effects on page xiii.

> **Side effects may include:** allergic reactions, drowsiness, headache, fatigue, nausea, oversedation, sleepiness, slowed or delayed breathing, dizziness, vomiting

Can I receive this medication if I am pregnant or breastfeeding?

Phenobarbital can harm your unborn baby if you take it during pregnancy. Phenobarbital can be found in your breast milk if you take it while breastfeeding. Do not breastfeed while you are taking phenobarbital. Tell your doctor immediately if you are pregnant, plan to become pregnant, or are breastfeeding.

What should I do if I miss a dose of this medication?

If you miss a dose of phenobarbital, take it as soon as you remember. However, if it is almost time for your next dose, skip the one you missed and return to your regular dosing schedule. Do not take two doses at once.

How should I store this medication?

Store at room temperature.

Phenobarbital: see Phenobarbital, page 789

Phentermine HCl: see Adipex-P, page 31

Phenytoin Sodium: see Dilantin, page 320

Pioglitazone HCl: see Actos, page 22

Plaquenil

Generic name: Hydroxychloroquine Sulfate

What is this medication?

Plaquenil is a medicine used to treat an infection called malaria. This medication is also used to treat lupus erythematosus (disease that affects the immune system) and rheumatoid arthritis.

What is the most important information I should know about this medication?

- Plaquenil can have a greater effect on children. Your child can experience fatal effects if he/she accidentally takes Plaquenil, even in relatively small doses. Keep this medication out of the reach of children.
- Do not take Plaquenil during pregnancy, except if you are taking it for the treatment or prevention of malaria. Your doctor will weigh the benefit of using Plaquenil during pregnancy against the risk.
- Plaquenil can exacerbate psoriasis or porphyria. Tell your doctor if you have psoriasis (immune disorder that affects the skin) or porphyria (a blood disorder that interferes with how your body produces heme, which is the oxygen-carrying component of your red blood cells) before you start taking this medication.
- Take Plaquenil with caution if you have active liver disease, have a history of alcohol abuse, or are taking medications that can affect your liver. Your doctor will monitor your liver while you are taking Plaquenil.
- Your doctor will monitor you for blood problems while you are taking Plaquenil. Tell your doctor if you have glucose-

6-phosphate dehydrogenase (G6PD) deficiency (lack of an enzyme responsible for the breakdown of red blood cells) before you start taking Plaquenil.

- Plaquenil can cause eye or vision problems, especially with long-term or high doses of Plaquenil. Stop taking Plaquenil and tell your doctor right away if you experience vision disturbances. Plaquenil can cause severe muscle weakness if you take it for a long time. Your doctor will perform periodic physical exams, including testing of your knee and ankle reflexes to detect muscular weakness. Stop taking Plaquenil and tell your doctor right away if you experience weakness.

- Plaquenil can cause skin rash or inflammation. Use Plaquenil carefully when you take it with any medication that can cause this skin reaction. Tell your doctor if you develop skin rash or inflammation while you are taking Plaquenil.

Who should not take this medication?

Do not take Plaquenil if you are allergic to it, any of its ingredients, or similar medications.

Do not take Plaquenil if you experienced eye or vision changes while taking Plaquenil or similar medications.

Plaquenil should not be used for long-term therapy in children.

What should I tell my doctor before I take the first dose of this medication?

Tell your doctor about all prescription, over-the-counter, and herbal medications you are taking before beginning treatment with Plaquenil. Also, talk to your doctor about your complete medical history, especially if you have a history of alcohol abuse, nervous system problems, stomach or intestinal problems, eye damage or visual changes, G6PD deficiency, kidney or liver problems, psoriasis, or porphyria.

What is the usual dosage?

Please see general statement regarding dosage on page xii.

Malaria Prevention
Adults: The usual dose is 400 milligrams (mg) once a week, on exactly the same day of each week.

Children: Your doctor will prescribe the appropriate dose for your child, based on their weight.

Malaria (Acute Attack)
Adults: The usual starting dose is 800 mg, followed by 400 mg in 6 to 8 hours and then 400 mg for two more days. Alternatively, your doctor can prescribe a single dose of 800 mg.

Children: Your doctor will prescribe the appropriate dose for your child, based on their weight.

Lupus Erythematosus
Adults: The usual starting dose is 400 mg once or twice a day.

Rheumatoid Arthritis
Adults: The usual starting dose is 400-600 mg a day, taken with a meal or a glass of milk.

How should I take this medication?
- Take Plaquenil exactly as prescribed by your doctor. Take Plaquenil for the full course of treatment.
- If you are taking Plaquenil for rheumatoid arthritis, take each dose with a meal or glass of milk.
- If you are taking Plaquenil as preventive therapy, you can start 2 weeks before exposure. If this is not possible, your doctor will have you take a starting dose of 800 mg, which may be divided into 2 doses taken 6 hours apart. You should continue treatment for 8 weeks after leaving the area where malaria occurs.

What should I avoid while taking this medication?
Do not drink alcohol while taking Plaquenil.

What are possible food and drug interactions associated with this medication?

If Plaquenil is taken with certain other drugs, the effects of either could be increased, decreased, or altered. It is especially important to check with your doctor before combining Plaquenil with alcohol or any medication that can affect your liver.

What are the possible side effects of this medication?

Please see general statement regarding side effects on page xiii.

Side effects may include: abdominal cramps, bleaching of hair, diarrhea, dizziness, emotional changes, eye toxicity or vision defects, hair loss, headache, inflammation of your skin, irritability, itching, lightening of hair, loss of appetite, muscle pain or weakness, nausea, nervousness, nightmares, rash, sensitivity to light, vomiting, weight loss

Can I receive this medication if I am pregnant or breastfeeding?

The effects of Plaquenil during pregnancy and breastfeeding are unknown. Do not take Plaquenil during pregnancy, except when it is used to treat malaria. Tell your doctor immediately if you are pregnant, plan to become pregnant, or are breastfeeding.

What should I do if I miss a dose of this medication?

If you miss a dose of Plaquenil, take it as soon as you remember. However, if it is almost time for your next dose, skip the one you missed and return to your regular dosing schedule. Do not take two doses at once.

How should I store this medication?

Store at room temperature.

Plavix

Generic name: Clopidogrel Bisulfate

What is this medication?

Plavix is a blood thinner used to treat people with acute (sudden) coronary syndrome (angina or heart attack). It is also used in people who have recently had a heart attack, stroke, or disease of the peripheral arteries (arteries outside the brain and heart). This medicine has been shown to reduce your chance of these events occurring again.

What is the most important information I should know about this medication?

- Plavix increases the risk of bleeding. You may bruise or bleed more easily while taking Plavix, and it may take longer than usual to stop bleeding. However, prolonged or excessive bleeding, or bloody stools or urine, is not normal; contact your doctor right away if this occurs. Taking Plavix with aspirin may increase the risk of bleeding in people with a history of recent stroke. Tell your doctor if you plan to have surgery, and make your surgeon or dentist aware that you are taking Plavix.
- Plavix can cause thrombotic thrombocytopenic purpura (TTP). TTP is a rare but serious condition in which blood clots form in your blood vessels, potentially blocking the blood supply to the organs. TTP feels like the flu, with symptoms such as fever, tiredness, and aching joints. Seek medical help immediately if you experience extreme skin paleness, purple skin patches, or yellowing of your skin or whites of your eyes.

Who should not take this medication?

Do not take Plavix if you are allergic to it or any of its ingredients.

Plavix should not be used if you have active bleeding (such as stomach ulcer or brain bleeding).

What should I tell my doctor before I take the first dose of this medication?

Tell your doctor about all prescription, over-the-counter, and herbal medications you are taking before beginning treatment with Plavix.

Also, talk to your doctor about your complete medical history, especially if you have a stomach ulcer or any other type of internal bleeding, if you have kidney problems, or if you will be having surgery or dental work. It is recommended that you stop taking Plavix 5 days before the scheduled surgery.

What is the usual dosage?
Please see general statement regarding dosage on page xii.

Acute Coronary Syndrome
Adults: The recommended daily dose is a single starting dose of 300 milligrams (mg) followed by 75 mg once a day. Aspirin (75-325 mg once a day) should be started and continued in combination with Plavix.

Recent Heart Attack, Stroke, or Peripheral Arterial Disease
Adults: The recommended daily dose is 75 mg once a day.

How should I take this medication?
- Take Plavix exactly as prescribed by your doctor.
- You can take Plavix with or without food.
- Do not stop taking Plavix without first talking to your doctor.

What should I avoid while taking this medication?
Do not take aspirin or aspirin-containing products while you are taking Plavix unless approved by your doctor.

What are possible food and drug interactions associated with this medication?
If Plavix is taken with certain other drugs, the effects of either could be increased, decreased, or altered. It is especially important to check with your doctor before combining Plavix with the following: nonsteroidal anti-inflammatory drugs (such as ibuprofen or naproxen), omeprazole, or warfarin.

What are the possible side effects of this medication?
Please see general statement regarding side effects on page xiii.

Side effects may include: bleeding or bruising easily

Can I receive this medication if I am pregnant or breastfeeding?

The effects of Plavix during pregnancy are unknown. Plavix may pass into your breast milk. Tell your doctor if you are pregnant, plan to become pregnant, or are breastfeeding.

What should I do if I miss a dose of this medication?

If you miss a dose of Plavix, take it as soon as you remember. However, if it is almost time for your next dose, skip the dose you missed and return to your regular dosing schedule. Do not take two doses at once.

How should I store this medication?

Store at room temperature.

Pletal

Generic name: Cilostazol

What is this medication?

Pletal is a medicine used to reduce symptoms of intermittent claudication (disease that causes narrowing and hardening of the arteries that supply blood flow to the legs and feet).

What is the most important information I should know about this medication?

• Although rare, Pletal can cause decreased platelets (type of blood cells that form clots to help stop bleeding) and white blood cells in your blood. Your doctor will monitor your blood counts while you are on Pletal.

Who should not take this medication?

Do not take Pletal if you are allergic to it, any of its ingredients, or if you have congestive heart failure (a condition in which the heart cannot pump enough blood throughout the body), any blood disorders, are currently bleeding, or have a history of bleeding, stomach ulcers, or bleeding in the brain.

What should I tell my doctor before I take the first dose of this medication?

Tell your doctor about all prescription, over-the-counter, and herbal medications you are taking before beginning treatment with Pletal. Also, talk to your doctor about your complete medical history, especially if you have congestive heart failure, a bleeding or blood disorder, stomach ulcers, bleeding in your brain, kidney or liver impairment, are pregnant, plan to become pregnant, or are breastfeeding.

What is the usual dosage?

Please see general statement regarding dosage on page xii.

Adults: The recommended dose is 100 milligrams (mg) twice a day. If you are taking other certain medications, your doctor might prescribe a lower dose for you.

How should I take this medication?

• Take Pletal exactly as prescribed by your doctor. Take Pletal twice a day at least half an hour before or two hours after breakfast and dinner.

What should I avoid while taking this medication?

Do not stop taking Pletal or change the way you take it without talking to your doctor.

What are possible food and drug interactions associated with this medication?

If Pletal is taken with certain other drugs, the effects of either could be increased, decreased, or altered. Pletal may interact with numerous medications. Therefore, it is very important that you tell your doctor about any other medications you are taking.

What are the possible side effects of this medication?

Please see general statement regarding side effects on page xiii.

> **Side effects may include:** abdominal pain, abnormal stools or heartbeats, back pain, chills, cough, diarrhea, dizziness, fever, gas, headache, increased heart rate, infection, muscle pain, nausea, shortness of breath, stuffy nose, swelling, throat inflammation, upset stomach

Can I receive this medication if I am pregnant or breastfeeding?

The effects of Pletal during pregnancy and breastfeeding are unknown. Tell your doctor immediately if you are pregnant, plan to become pregnant, or are breastfeeding.

What should I do if I miss a dose of this medication?

If you miss a dose of Pletal, take it as soon as you remember. However, if it is almost time for your next dose, skip the one you missed and return to your regular dosing schedule. Do not take two doses at once.

How should I store this medication?

Store at room temperature.

Polyethylene Glycol 3350: *see Miralax, page 641*

Potassium Chloride: *see K-Dur, page 499*

Potassium Chloride: *see Micro-K, page 635*

Pradaxa

Generic name: Dabigatran etexilate Mesylate

What is this medication?

Pradaxa is a blood thinner medicine used to reduce the risk of stroke and blood clots in people who have a heart condition called atrial fibrillation (an irregular, fast heartbeat).

What is the most important information I should know about this medication?

- Pradaxa can cause bleeding that can be serious, and sometimes lead to death. The risk of bleeding is increased because Pradaxa lessens the ability of your blood to clot. You may bruise more easily or it may take longer for your body to stop bleeding while you are taking Pradaxa.
- There is a higher risk of bleeding in those who are >75 years old, have kidney problems, stomach or intestine bleeding that is recent or keeps coming back, or stomach ulcers. There is also a higher risk of bleeding in those who take other medicines that increase the risk of bleeding.
- Call your doctor or get medical help right away if you have any unexpected bleeding or bleeding that lasts a long time (such as unusual bleeding from the gums, nose bleeds, or heavier than normal menstrual or vaginal bleeding) or severe or uncontrolled bleeding.
- Also, call your doctor or get medical help right away if you have pink or brown urine, red or black stools (looks like tar), bruises that happen without a known cause or get larger, or if you cough up or vomit blood (or your vomit looks like "coffee grounds").
- Also, call your doctor or get medical help right away if you have unexpected pain, swelling, joint pain, or headaches, or feel dizzy or weak.
- Pradaxa may need to be stopped, if possible, for one or more days before any surgery or medical or dental procedure. If you need to stop taking Pradaxa for any reason, talk to the doctor who prescribed Pradaxa for you to find out when you should stop taking it. Your doctor will tell you when to start taking Pradaxa again after your surgery or procedure.

Who should not take this medication?

Do not take Pradaxa if you currently have certain types of abnormal bleeding or have had a serious allergic reaction to Pradaxa.

What should I tell my doctor before I take the first dose of this medication?

Tell your doctor about all prescription, over-the-counter, and herbal medications you are taking before beginning treatment with

Pradaxa. Also, talk to your doctor about your complete medical history, especially if you have kidney problems, have ever had bleeding problems or stomach ulcers, or have any other medical condition.

Also, talk to your doctor if you are pregnant, plan to become pregnant, are breastfeeding or plan to breastfeed, or plan to have any surgery or a medical or dental procedure.

What is the usual dosage?
Please see general statement regarding dosage on page xii.

Adults: The recommended dose is 150 milligrams twice a day.

If you have kidney problems, your doctor may prescribe a lower dose.

How should I take this medication?
- Take Pradaxa exactly as prescribed by your doctor. Do not take Pradaxa more often than your doctor tells you to.
- Take Pradaxa with or without food. Swallow Pradaxa capsules whole. Do not break, chew, or empty the pellets from the capsule.

What should I avoid while taking this medication?
Your doctor will decide how long you should take Pradaxa. Do not stop taking Pradaxa without first talking to your doctor. Stopping Pradaxa may increase your risk of stroke.

Do not run out of Pradaxa. Refill your prescription before you run out.

What are possible food and drug interactions associated with this medication?
If Pradaxa is taken with certain other drugs, the effects of either could be increased, decreased, or altered. It is especially important to check with your doctor before combining Pradaxa with the following: rifampin or medicines that increase your risk of bleeding (including aspirin or aspirin-containing products, long-term use of

non-steroidal anti-inflammatory drugs [NSAIDs], warfarin, heparin, clopidogrel, or prasugrel).

What are the possible side effects of this medication?
Please see general statement regarding side effects on page xiii.

> **Side effects may include:** allergic reactions (such as hives, itching, or rash), indigestion, upset stomach, burning, stomach pain
>
> Tell your doctor or get medical help right away if you get any of the following symptoms of a serious allergic reaction with Pradaxa: chest pain or chest tightness, swelling of your face or tongue, trouble breathing or wheezing, or feeling dizzy or faint.

Can I receive this medication if I am pregnant or breastfeeding?
The effects of Pradaxa during pregnancy and breastfeeding are unknown. Tell your doctor immediately if you are pregnant, plan to become pregnant, are breastfeeding, or plan to breastfeed.

What should I do if I miss a dose of this medication?
If you miss a dose of Pradaxa, take it as soon as you remember. However, if your next dose is less than 6 hours away, skip the missed dose. Do not take two doses at once.

How should I store this medication?
Store at room temperature. Store in the original package to keep medication dry. Do not put medication in pill boxes or pill organizers.

After opening the bottle, use within 4 months. Safely throw away any unused medication after 4 months.

Pramipexole Dihydrochloride: *see Mirapex, page 643*

Prasugrel: *see Effient, page 359*

Pravachol
Generic name: Pravastatin Sodium

What is this medication?
Pravachol belongs to a class of medicines called "statins," which are used to lower your cholesterol when a low-fat diet is not enough. Pravachol lowers your total cholesterol and the "bad" low-density lipoprotein (LDL) cholesterol, thereby helping to slow the hardening of your arteries, and lower your risk of a heart attack or stroke, death from coronary heart disease (narrowing of small blood vessels that supply blood and oxygen to the heart), or the need for procedures to restore the blood flow back to the heart or to another part of the body.

What is the most important information I should know about this medication?
- Taking Pravachol is not a substitute for following a healthy low-fat and low-cholesterol diet and exercising to lower your cholesterol.
- Do not take Pravachol if you are pregnant, think you may be pregnant, plan to become pregnant, or are breastfeeding.
- Pravachol can cause muscle pain, tenderness, weakness, fatigue, loss of appetite, right upper abdominal discomfort, dark urine, or yellowing of your skin or whites of your eyes. Call your doctor right away if you notice any of these symptoms.

Who should not take this medication?
Do not take Pravachol if you are allergic to it or any of its ingredients, or if you currently have liver disease. Also, do not take Pravachol if you are pregnant, plan to become pregnant, or are breastfeeding.

What should I tell my doctor before I take the first dose of this medication?
Tell your doctor about all prescription, over-the-counter, and herbal medications you are taking before beginning treatment with Pravachol. Also, talk to your doctor about your complete medical history, especially if you drink excessive amounts of alcohol or you have liver, kidney, thyroid, or heart problems; or muscle aches or

weakness. Tell your doctor if you are pregnant, plan to become pregnant, or are breastfeeding.

What is the usual dosage?

Please see general statement regarding dosage on page xii.

Adults and adolescents 14-18 years: The recommended starting dose is 40 milligrams (mg) once a day. Your doctor will check your blood cholesterol levels during treatment with Pravachol and will change your dose based on the results.

Children 8-13 years: The recommended dose is 20 mg once a day. Your doctor will check your blood cholesterol levels during treatment with Pravachol and will change your dose based on the results.

If you have kidney impairment or you are taking other medications, your doctor will adjust your dose appropriately.

How should I take this medication?

- Your doctor will likely start you on a low-cholesterol diet before giving you Pravachol. Stay on this diet while you are taking Pravachol.
- Take Pravachol at any time of the day, with or without food.
- If you take other cholesterol-lowering medicines known as bile acid resins (such as cholestyramine or colestipol), take Pravachol either 1 hour or more before or 4 hours after you take the resin.

What should I avoid while taking this medication?

Do not become pregnant or breastfeed while you are taking Pravachol.

What are possible food and drug interactions associated with this medication?

If Pravachol is taken with certain other drugs, the effects of either could be increased, decreased, or altered. It is especially important to check with your doctor before combining Pravachol with the following: alcohol, cholesterol-lowering medicines known as fibrates (such as fenofibrate or gemfibrozil), clarithromycin, colchicine, cyclosporine, or niacin.

What are the possible side effects of this medication?
Please see general statement regarding side effects on page xiii.

> **Side effects may include:** chest pain, diarrhea, dizziness, fatigue, gas, headache, inflammation of the lining of your nose, muscle pain, nausea, rash, upper respiratory infections, vomiting

Can I receive this medication if I am pregnant or breastfeeding?
Do not take Pravachol during pregnancy or breastfeeding. Tell your doctor immediately if you are pregnant, plan to become pregnant, or are breastfeeding.

What should I do if I miss a dose of this medication?
If you miss a dose of Pravachol, take it as soon as you remember. However, if it is almost time for your next dose, skip the one you missed and return to your regular dosing schedule. Do not take two doses at once.

How should I store this medication?
Store at room temperature. Protect from light.

Pravastatin Sodium: *see Pravachol, page 804*

Prednisolone
Generic name: Prednisolone

What is this medication?
Prednisolone is a synthetic corticosteroid medicine. Prednisolone is used when your adrenal glands do not make enough hormones that help your body respond to stress or regulate your blood pressure and water and salt intake. Prednisolone can also be used for

conditions affecting many different parts of your body, including your skin, stomach or intestines, blood, eyes, lungs, or glands. In addition, this medication can be used to treat severe allergies, arthritis, lupus, or certain cancers.

What is the most important information I should know about this medication?

- Prednisolone can cause increased blood pressure, holding onto salt and water in your body, or decreased blood potassium levels. Your doctor will check your blood pressure and electrolyte levels (chemicals that are important for the cells in your body to function, such as sodium and potassium) while you are using prednisolone.
- Prednisolone can mask some signs of infection, making it difficult for your doctor to diagnose it. Also, prednisolone can lower your resistance to infections and make them harder to treat. Tell your doctor if you develop fever or other signs of infection.
- Do not expose yourself to chickenpox or measles while you are using prednisolone. This can be very serious and even fatal in children and adults who have not had chickenpox or measles. Also, prednisolone can reactivate an inactive case of tuberculosis (a bacterial infection that affects the lungs).
- Cataracts (clouding of the eye's lens), glaucoma (high pressure in the eye), other eye problems, or eye infections can occur while you are using prednisolone.

Who should not take this medication?

Do not take prednisolone if you are allergic to it or any of its ingredients, or if you have a fungal infection.

What should I tell my doctor before I take the first dose of this medication?

Tell your doctor about all prescription, over-the-counter, and herbal medications you are taking before beginning treatment with prednisolone. Also, talk to your doctor about your complete medical history, especially if you have any infections, cataracts, glaucoma, certain eye infections, tuberculosis, heart problems, high blood pressure, kidney or liver disease, thyroid problems, psychiatric conditions, ulcerative colitis (inflammatory disease of the large intestine), other intestinal problems, stomach ulcers, osteoporosis (thin, weak bones), myasthenia gravis (a disease characterized by long-lasting fatigue and muscle weakness), diabetes, or stress (such as trauma, surgery, or severe illness).

What is the usual dosage?
Please see general statement regarding dosage on page xii.

Adults and children: The doctor will prescribe the appropriate dose for you or your child based on your condition or response. Attempts to taper or discontinue the medication should be made at specific intervals, with the guidance of your doctor.

How should I take this medication?
- Take prednisolone exactly as prescribed by your doctor. Do not take extra doses or take more often without asking your doctor. Take prednisolone syrup by mouth only.
- Tell your doctor if you are anticipating stress (such as trauma, surgery, or severe illness). Your doctor may need to adjust your dose of prednisolone before, during, and after any stressful situation.

What should I avoid while taking this medication?
Do not miss your scheduled follow-up appointments with your doctor. It is important to check your progress.

Do not receive certain vaccines or other immunization procedures during treatment with prednisolone without first talking to your doctor.

Do not discontinue the use of prednisolone suddenly or without the guidance of your doctor.

What are possible food and drug interactions associated with this medication?
No significant interactions have been reported with prednisolone at this time. However, always tell your doctor about any medicines you take, including over-the-counter medications, vitamins, and herbal supplements.

What are the possible side effects of this medication?
Please see general statement regarding side effects on page xiii.

Side effects may include: decrease in blood potassium levels, dizziness, eye problems, headache, high blood sugar levels, impaired wound healing, increase in blood pressure, intestinal or stomach problems, muscle weakness, osteoporosis, seizures, sweating, swelling

Can I receive this medication if I am pregnant or breastfeeding?
The effects of prednisolone during pregnancy and breastfeeding are unknown. Tell your doctor immediately if you are pregnant, plan to become pregnant, or are breastfeeding.

What should I do if I miss a dose of this medication?
If you miss a dose of prednisolone, take it as soon as you remember. However, if it is almost time for your next dose, skip the one you missed and return to your regular dosing schedule. Do not take two doses at once.

How should I store this medication?
Store at room temperature. Do not refrigerate.

Prednisolone: see Prednisolone, page 806

Prednisone
Generic name: Prednisone

What is this medication?
Prednisone, a steroid drug, is used to reduce inflammation and alleviate symptoms in a variety of disorders, including rheumatoid arthritis and severe cases of asthma. It may be given to treat adrenal cortex insufficiency (lack of sufficient adrenal hormone in the body).

What is the most important information I should know about this medication?

- Prednisone may lower your resistance to infections and make them harder to treat. Prednisone may also mask some of the signs of an infection, making it difficult for your doctor to diagnose it.
- Do not get a smallpox vaccination or any other immunization while you are taking prednisone.
- Also avoid exposure to chickenpox or measles, which can be very serious and even fatal in both children and adults taking prednisone.
- Prednisone may reactivate an inactive case of tuberculosis (TB).

Who should not take this medication?

Do not take prednisone if you have ever had an allergic reaction to it or have a fungal infection.

What should I tell my doctor before I take the first dose of this medication?

Tell your doctor about all prescription, over-the-counter, and herbal medications you are taking before beginning treatment with prednisone. Also, talk to your doctor about your complete medical history, especially if you have kidney disease, liver disease, high blood pressure, heart disease, eye herpes, ulcerative colitis (inflammation of the bowel), diverticulitis (inflammation in the large intestines that results in pouches), stomach ulcers, hypothyroidism (low thyroid levels), a psychiatric condition, osteoporosis (thin, weak bones), myasthenia gravis (loss of muscular control), or type 2 diabetes (high blood sugar).

What is the usual dosage?

Please see general statement regarding dosage on page xii.

Adults: Dosage is determined by the condition being treated and your response to the drug. Typical starting doses can range from 5 milligrams (mg) to 60 mg a day. Once you respond to the drug, your doctor will lower the dose gradually to the minimum effective amount.

Children: Dosage is determined by the condition being treated and their response to the drug.

How should I take this medication?

- Take prednisone exactly as prescribed, and with food to avoid stomach upset.
- If you are on alternate-day therapy or have been prescribed a single daily dose, take prednisone in the morning with breakfast, before 9 a.m. If you have been prescribed several doses per day, take them at evenly spaced intervals around the clock.
- For large doses, taking an antacid in between meals may prevent stomach ulcers.
- If you have been taking prednisone for a period of time, you may need an increased dosage of the medication before, during, and after any stressful situation. Always consult your doctor if you are anticipating stress and think you may need a temporary dosage increase.

What should I avoid while taking this medication?

Avoid alcohol. Alcohol and prednisone may damage the stomach.

Avoid sources of infection; your immune system may be weakened while taking prednisone. Wash your hands frequently and keep them away from your mouth and eyes.

Do not receive immunizations during treatment with prednisone without first talking to your doctor.

Avoid abrupt withdrawal of prednisone. Speak to your doctor before stopping it. Signs of withdrawal include muscle pain, joint pain, and feeling ill.

What are possible food and drug interactions associated with this medication?

If prednisone is taken with certain other drugs, the effects of either could be increased, decreased, or altered. It is especially important to check with your doctor before combining prednisone with the following: amphotericin B, anticholinesterase agents (such as neostigmine, pyridostigmine), aspirin and other nonsteroidal anti-inflammatory agents (NSAIDs), barbiturates, blood thinners (such as warfarin), bupropion, carbamazepine, cholestyramine, cyclosporine, digitalis, estrogen drugs, fluoroquinolones (such as ciprofloxacin, levofloxacin), indinavir, insulin, isoniazid, itraconazole, ketoconazole, macrolide antibiotics (such as erythromycin), birth control pills, oral diabetes medication, phenobarbital, phenytoin, potent diuretics, quetiapine, rifampin, ritonavir, thalidomide, troleandomycin, and vaccines.

What are the possible side effects of this medication?

Please see general statement regarding side effects on page xiii.

> **Side effects may include:** euphoria, insomnia, mood changes, personality changes, psychotic behavior, severe depression, or worsening of any existing emotional instability
>
> At a high dosage, prednisone may cause fluid retention and high blood pressure.

Can I receive this medication if I am pregnant or breastfeeding?

The effects of prednisone during pregnancy and breastfeeding are unknown. Tell your doctor immediately if you are pregnant, plan to become pregnant, or are breastfeeding.

What should I do if I miss a dose of this medication?

Take the missed dose as soon as you remember. If it is almost time for your next dose, skip the missed dose and take the medicine at the next regularly scheduled time. Do not take two doses at once.

How should I store this medication?

Store at room temperature.

Prednisone: *see Prednisone, page 809*

Pregabalin: *see Lyrica, page 600*

Premarin

Generic name: Conjugated Estrogens

What is this medication?

Premarin is a medicine that contains a mixture of estrogen hormones. Premarin is used to treat moderate to severe symptoms of menopause, such as hot flashes or severe dryness, itching, and burning in or around your vagina. Also, Premarin is used to treat certain conditions in which a young woman's ovaries do not produce enough estrogens naturally, certain prostate cancers in men, certain breast cancers in selected women and men, and to reduce your chances of getting postmenopausal osteoporosis (thin, weak bones).

What is the most important information I should know about this medication?

- Estrogens increase your risk of developing cancer of the uterus. Tell your doctor immediately if you experience any unusual vaginal bleeding while you are using Premarin.
- Do not take Premarin to prevent heart disease, heart attacks, strokes, or dementia (an illness involving loss of memory, judgment, and confusion). Using Premarin can increase your chances of getting heart attacks, strokes, breast cancer, or blood clots.
- Premarin can also increase your risk of dementia, gallbladder disease, ovarian cancer, visual abnormalities, high blood pressure, pancreatitis (inflammation of your pancreas), or thyroid problems. Talk regularly with your doctor about whether you still need treatment with Premarin.
- You can lower your chances of serious side effects with Premarin by having a breast exam and mammogram (breast x-ray) every year, unless directed by your doctor to have it more often. See your doctor right away if you get vaginal bleeding while you are taking Premarin. Also, ask your doctor for ways to lower your chances of getting heart disease, especially if you have high blood pressure, high cholesterol, or diabetes, if you are overweight, or if you use tobacco.

Who should not take this medication?

Do not take Premarin if you are allergic to it or any of its ingredients.

Do not take Premarin if you are pregnant or think you may be pregnant.

Do not take Premarin if you have a history of stroke or heart attack, blood clots, liver problems, unusual vaginal bleeding, or certain cancers, including cancer of your breast or uterus.

What should I tell my doctor before I take the first dose of this medication?

Tell your doctor about all prescription, over-the-counter, and herbal medications you are taking before beginning treatment with Premarin. Also, talk to your doctor about your complete medical history, especially if you are pregnant or breastfeeding, or have any unusual vaginal bleeding, asthma, seizures, diabetes, migraine headaches, endometriosis (a common gynecological disorder that may result in sores and pain), porphyria (a blood disorder that interferes with how your body produces heme, which is the oxygen-carrying component of your red blood cells), lupus (disease that affects the immune system), high blood calcium levels, or problems with your heart, liver, thyroid, or kidneys. Also, tell your doctor if you are going to have surgery or will be on bedrest.

What is the usual dosage?
Please see general statement regarding dosage on page xii.

Your doctor might prescribe different doses than those listed below based on your condition and will adjust your dose according to your individual response to the medication.

Treatment of Menopausal Symptoms and Prevention of Osteoporosis
Adults: The recommended starting dose is 0.3 milligrams (mg) once a day.

Attempts to taper or discontinue the medication should be made at specific intervals, through the guidance of your doctor.

Treatment of Low Estrogen Levels
Adults: Your doctor will prescribe the appropriate dose for you.

Treatment of Breast Cancer
Adults: The recommended dose is 10 mg three times a day for at least 3 months.

Treatment of Androgen-Dependent Prostate Cancer
Adults: The recommended dose is 1.25-2.5 mg three times a day.

How should I take this medication?
- Take Premarin exactly as prescribed by your doctor.
- Talk to your doctor regularly (every 3-6 months) about the dose you are taking and whether you still need treatment with Premarin.

What should I avoid while taking this medication?
Do not take Premarin for conditions for which it was not prescribed.

Grapefruit juice can increase your risk of side effects with Premarin. Talk to your doctor before including grapefruit or grapefruit juice in your diet while you are taking Premarin.

What are possible food and drug interactions associated with this medication?
If Premarin is taken with certain other drugs, the effects of either could be increased, decreased, or altered. It is especially important to check with your doctor before combining Premarin with the following: carbamazepine, clarithromycin, erythromycin, grapefruit juice, itraconazole, ketoconazole, phenobarbital, rifampin, ritonavir, or St. John's wort.

What are the possible side effects of this medication?
Please see general statement regarding side effects on page xiii.

Side effects may include: abdominal (stomach) pain, bloating, breast pain, fluid retention, hair loss, headache, high blood pressure, high blood sugar, irregular vaginal bleeding or spotting, liver problems, nausea, spotty darkening of your skin, vaginal yeast infections, vomiting

If you experience symptoms of breast lumps, changes in your speech, changes in your vision, chest pain, dizziness and faintness, pain in your legs, severe headaches, shortness of breath, unusual vaginal bleeding, vomiting, or yellowing of your skin or whites of your eyes, contact your doctor right away.

Can I receive this medication if I am pregnant or breastfeeding?

Do not take Premarin if you are pregnant. Premarin can be found in your breast milk if you take it while breastfeeding. Tell your doctor immediately if you are pregnant, plan to become pregnant, or are breastfeeding.

What should I do if I miss a dose of this medication?

If you miss a dose of Premarin, take it as soon as you remember. However, if it is almost time for your next dose, skip the one you missed and return to your regular dosing schedule. Do not take two doses at once.

How should I store this medication?

Store at room temperature.

Premphase

Generic name: Conjugated Estrogens/Medroxyprogesterone Acetate

What is this medication?

Premphase is a medicine containing two kinds of hormones, estrogen and progestin. It is used to treat moderate to severe symptoms of menopause (such as hot flashes and changes in or around your vagina). Premphase also helps to reduce your chances of getting postmenopausal osteoporosis (thin, weak bones).

What is the most important information I should know about this medication?

- Estrogens increase your risk of developing cancer of the uterus. Tell your doctor immediately if you experience any unusual vaginal bleeding while you are taking Premphase.
- Do not take Premphase to prevent heart disease, heart attacks, strokes, or dementia (an illness involving loss of memory, judgment, and confusion). Taking Premphase can increase your chances of getting heart attacks, strokes, breast cancer, or blood clots.
- Premphase can also increase your risk of dementia, gallbladder disease, ovarian cancer, visual abnormalities, high blood pressure, pancreatitis (inflammation of your pancreas), or thyroid problems. Talk to your doctor regularly (every 3-6 months) about the dose you are taking and whether you still need treatment with Premphase.
- You can lower your chances of serious side effects with Premphase by having a pelvic exam, breast exam, and mammogram (breast x-ray) every year, unless directed by your doctor to have it more often.
- See your doctor immediately if you get vaginal bleeding while you are taking Premphase.
- Also, ask your doctor for ways to lower your chances of getting heart disease, especially if you have high blood pressure, high cholesterol, or diabetes, if you are overweight, or if you use tobacco.

Who should not take this medication?

Do not take Premphase if you are allergic to it or any of its ingredients. Do not take Premphase if you are pregnant or think you may be pregnant.

Do not take Premphase if you have had your uterus removed, have a history of stroke or heart attack, blood clots, liver problems, unusual vaginal bleeding or other bleeding disorders, or certain cancers, including cancer of your breast or uterus.

What should I tell my doctor before I take the first dose of this medication?

Tell your doctor about all prescription, over-the-counter, and herbal medications you are taking before beginning treatment with Premphase. Also, talk to your doctor about your complete medical history, especially if you are pregnant or breastfeeding, or have any unusual vaginal bleeding. Tell your doctor if you have asthma, seizures, diabetes, migraine headaches, endometriosis (a common gynecological disorder that may result in sores and pain), lupus (disease that affects the immune system), high blood calcium levels, or problems with your heart, liver, thyroid, or kidneys. Also, tell your doctor if you are going to have surgery or will be on bed rest.

What is the usual dosage?

Please see general statement regarding dosage on page xii.

Adults: The recommended dose is 1 maroon tablet on days 1-14, followed by 1 light-blue tablet on days 15-28.

How should I take this medication?

- Take Premphase exactly as prescribed by your doctor.
- Take this medication at the same time each day.

What should I avoid while taking this medication?

Do not smoke while you are taking Premphase. If you smoke, your chances of getting heart disease can increase.

Grapefruit juice can increase your risk of side effects with Premphase. Talk to your doctor before including grapefruit or grapefruit juice in your diet while you are taking Premphase.

What are possible food and drug interactions associated with this medication?

If Premphase is taken with certain other drugs, the effects of either could be increased, decreased, or altered. It is especially important to check with your doctor before combining Premphase with the following: aminoglutethimide, antibiotics (such as clarithromycin, erythromycin, or rifampin), antifungals (such as itraconazole or ketoconazole), grapefruit juice, ritonavir, seizure medications (such as carbamazepine or phenobarbital), or St. John's wort.

What are the possible side effects of this medication?
Please see general statement regarding side effects on page xiii.

> **Side effects may include:** abdominal pain, bloating, breast pain, fluid retention, hair loss, headache, irregular vaginal bleeding or spotting, nausea, vomiting
>
> If you experience symptoms of breast lumps; changes in your speech or vision; chest pain; pain in your legs; severe headaches; shortness of breath; swollen lips, tongue, or face; or unusual vaginal bleeding; contact your doctor immediately.

Can I receive this medication if I am pregnant or breastfeeding?
Do not take Premphase if you are pregnant or breastfeeding. The hormones in Premphase can be found in your breast milk if you take it while you are breastfeeding. Tell your doctor immediately if you are pregnant, plan to become pregnant, or are breastfeeding.

What should I do if I miss a dose of this medication?
If you miss a dose of Premphase, take it as soon as you remember. However, if it is almost time for your next dose, skip the one you missed and return to your regular dosing schedule. Do not take two doses at once.

How should I store this medication?
Store at room temperature.

Prempro
Generic name: Conjugated Estrogens/Medroxyprogesterone Acetate

What is this medication?
Prempro is a medicine containing the hormones, estrogen and progestin. It is used to treat moderate to severe symptoms of menopause, such as hot flashes and changes in or around your vagina. Prempro also helps to reduce your chances of getting postmenopausal osteoporosis (thin, weak bones).

What is the most important information I should know about this medication?
- Estrogens increase your risk of developing cancer of the uterus. Tell your doctor immediately if you experience any unusual vaginal bleeding while you are taking Prempro.
- Do not take Prempro to prevent heart disease, heart attacks, strokes, or dementia. Taking Prempro can increase your chances of getting heart attacks, strokes, breast cancer, or blood clots.
- Prempro can also increase your risk of dementia, gallbladder disease, ovarian cancer, visual abnormalities, high blood pressure, pancreatitis (inflammation of the pancreas), or thyroid problems. Talk regularly with your doctor about whether you still need treatment with Prempro.
- You can lower your chances of serious side effects with Prempro by having a pelvic exam, breast exam, and mammogram (breast x-ray) every year, unless directed by your doctor to have it more often. See your doctor immediately if you get vaginal bleeding while you are taking Prempro. Also, ask your doctor for ways to lower your chances of getting heart disease, especially if you have high blood pressure, high cholesterol, or diabetes, if you are overweight, or if you use tobacco.

Who should not take this medication?
Do not take Prempro if you are allergic to it or any of its ingredients, or if you are pregnant or think you may be pregnant.

Do not take Prempro if you have had your uterus removed, have a history of stroke or heart attack, blood clots, liver problems, unusual vaginal bleeding or other bleeding disorders, or certain cancers, including cancer of your breast or uterus.

What should I tell my doctor before I take the first dose of this medication?

Tell your doctor about all prescription, over-the-counter, and herbal medications you are taking before beginning treatment with Prempro. Also, talk to your doctor about your complete medical history, especially if you are pregnant or breastfeeding, or have any unusual vaginal bleeding, asthma, seizures, diabetes, migraine headaches, endometriosis (a common gynecological disorder that may result in sores and pain), lupus (disease that affects the immune system), high blood calcium levels, or problems with your heart, liver, thyroid, or kidneys. Also, tell your doctor if you are going to have surgery or will be on bed rest.

What is the usual dosage?

Please see general statement regarding dosage on page xii.

Adults: The recommended dose is 1 tablet once a day.

How should I take this medication?

- Take Prempro exactly as prescribed by your doctor. Take this medication at the same time each day. Talk to your doctor regularly (every 3-6 months) about the dose you are taking and whether you still need treatment with Prempro.

What should I avoid while taking this medication?

Do not smoke while you are taking Prempro. If you smoke, your chances of getting heart disease can increase.

Grapefruit juice can increase your risk of side effects with Prempro. Talk to your doctor before including grapefruit or grapefruit juice in your diet while you are taking Prempro.

What are possible food and drug interactions associated with this medication?

If Prempro is taken with certain other drugs, the effects of either could be increased, decreased, or altered. It is especially important to check with your doctor before combining Prempro with the following: aminoglutethimide, antibiotics (such as clarithromycin, erythromycin, or rifampin), antifungals (such as itraconazole or ketoconazole), grapefruit juice, ritonavir, seizure medications (such as carbamazepine or phenobarbital), or St. John's wort.

What are the possible side effects of this medication?
Please see general statement regarding side effects on page xiii.

Side effects may include: abdominal pain, breast pain, fluid retention, hair loss, headache, irregular vaginal bleeding or spotting, nausea, vomiting

If you experience symptoms of breast lumps, changes in your speech, changes in your vision, chest pain, dizziness and faintness, pain in your legs, severe headaches, shortness of breath, unusual vaginal bleeding, vomiting, or yellowing of your skin or whites of your eyes, contact your doctor immediately.

Can I receive this medication if I am pregnant or breastfeeding?
Do not take Prempro if you are pregnant or breastfeeding. The hormones in Prempro can be found in your breast milk if you take it while you are breastfeeding. Tell your doctor immediately if you are pregnant, plan to become pregnant, or are breastfeeding.

What should I do if I miss a dose of this medication?
If you miss a dose of Prempro, take it as soon as you remember. However, if it is almost time for your next dose, skip the one you missed and return to your regular dosing schedule. Do not take two doses at once.

How should I store this medication?
Store at room temperature.

Prevacid

Generic name: Lansoprazole

What is this medication?

Prevacid is a medicine called a proton pump inhibitor (PPI). It reduces the amount of acid in your stomach. Prevacid is used in adults for the short-term treatment of stomach and duodenal ulcers (ulcer in the upper intestine), gastroesophageal reflux disease, and erosive esophagitis (inflammation of the esophagus [tube that connects your mouth and stomach] due to excess acid).

Prevacid is also used to prevent a relapse of duodenal ulcer or esophagitis; to reduce the risk of stomach ulcers in people on continuous therapy with nonsteroidal anti-inflammatory drugs (NSAIDs) (such as ibuprofen or naproxen); for long-term treatment of conditions where your stomach makes too much acid, such as Zollinger-Ellison syndrome; and with other medicines to eliminate the bacteria that often causes ulcers (known as *Helicobacter pylori*).

In addition, Prevacid is used for the short-term treatment of gastroesophageal reflux disease and erosive esophagitis in children and adolescents.

What is the most important information I should know about this medication?

- Prevacid can cause low magnesium levels in your body. Tell your doctor immediately if you have seizures, dizziness, abnormal or fast heartbeat, jitteriness, jerking movements or shaking, muscle weakness, spasms of your hands and feet, cramps or muscle aches, or spasm of your voice box.
- Tell your doctor if you experience any symptoms of a serious allergic reaction with Prevacid (such as rash, face swelling, throat tightness, or difficulty breathing).
- People who are taking multiple daily doses of Prevacid for a long period of time may have an increased risk of fractures of the hip, wrist, or spine.
- If you have a condition known as phenylketonuria (an inability to process phenylalanine, a protein in your body), be aware

that Prevacid SoluTab orally disintegrating tablets contain phenylalanine.

Who should not take this medication?

Do not take Prevacid if you are allergic to it or any of its ingredients.

What should I tell my doctor before I take the first dose of this medication?

Tell your doctor about all prescription, over-the-counter, and herbal medications you are taking before beginning treatment with Prevacid. Also, talk to your doctor about your complete medical history, especially if you have low magnesium levels, liver problems, or phenylketonuria. Tell your doctor if you are pregnant, plan to become pregnant, or are breastfeeding.

What is the usual dosage?

Please see general statement regarding dosage on page xii.

Erosive Esophagitis

Adults: The recommended dose is 30 milligrams (mg) once a day for up to 8 weeks. Depending on your response, your doctor may suggest another 8 weeks of treatment. To prevent a relapse, your doctor may suggest taking 15 mg once a day.

Adolescents 12-17 years: The recommended dose is 30 mg once a day for up to 8 weeks.

Children 1-11 years: Depending on your child's weight, the recommended dose is 15 mg or 30 mg once a day for up to 12 weeks. If your child's symptoms do not improve after 2 or more weeks, your doctor may increase the dose as needed.

Gastroesophageal Reflux Disease

Adults and adolescents 12-17 years: The recommended dose is 15 mg once a day for up to 8 weeks.

Children 1-11 years: Depending on your child's weight, the recommended dose is 15 mg or 30 mg once a day for up to 12 weeks. If your child's symptoms do not improve after 2 or more weeks, your doctor may increase the dose as needed.

Prevention of Duodenal Ulcer Due to *H. pylori* Infection
Adults: This treatment involves taking two or three different medications. The usual dose for the dual therapy is: Prevacid 30 mg three times a day for 14 days and amoxicillin 1000 mg three times a day for 14 days. The usual dose for the triple therapy is: Prevacid 30 mg twice a day for 10 or 14 days, amoxicillin 1000 mg twice a day for 10 or 14 days, and clarithromycin 500 mg twice a day for 10 or 14 days.

Treatment or Prevention of Duodenal Ulcer
Adults: The recommended dose is 15 mg once a day for 4 weeks. Your doctor may suggest continuing treatment to prevent a relapse.

Treatment or Prevention of Stomach Ulcer Due to NSAIDs
Adults: The recommended dose to treat symptoms is 30 mg once a day for 8 weeks. The recommended dose to help prevent a recurrence is 15 mg once a day for up to 12 weeks.

Short-Term Treatment of Stomach Ulcer
Adults: The recommended dose is 30 mg once a day for up to 8 weeks.

Treatment of Excess Stomach Acid (Such as Zollinger-Ellison Syndrome)
Adults: The recommended dose is 60 mg once a day. Your doctor might prescribe a different dose or duration based on your condition.

How should I take this medication?
- Take Prevacid before meals. Swallow the delayed-release capsules whole.
- If you are taking the orally disintegrating Prevacid SoluTabs, place the tablet on your tongue and let it dissolve, with or without water.

PDR® Pocket Guide to Prescription Drugs

• Please review the instructions that came with your prescription on how to properly take Prevacid.

What should I avoid while taking this medication?
Do not crush, chew, cut, or break the capsules or tablets. This will damage them and the medicine will not work.

If you are unable to swallow Prevacid, your doctor will give you instructions on how to take the medication.

What are possible food and drug interactions associated with this medication?
If Prevacid is taken with certain other drugs, the effects of either could be increased, decreased, or altered. It is especially important to check with your doctor before combining Prevacid with the following: ampicillin, atazanavir, digoxin, ketoconazole, methotrexate, products that contain iron, sucralfate, tacrolimus, theophylline, or warfarin.

What are the possible side effects of this medication?
Please see general statement regarding side effects on page xiii.

> **Side effects may include:** constipation, diarrhea, dizziness, headache, nausea, stomach pain

Can I receive this medication if I am pregnant or breastfeeding?
The effects of Prevacid during pregnancy and breastfeeding are unknown. Tell your doctor immediately if you are pregnant, plan to become pregnant, or are breastfeeding.

What should I do if I miss a dose of this medication?
If you miss a dose of Prevacid, take it as soon as you remember. However, if it is almost time for your next dose, skip the one you missed and return to your regular dosing schedule. Do not take two doses at once.

How should I store this medication?
Store at room temperature.

Prilosec
Generic name: Omeprazole

What is this medication?

Prilosec is a medicine called a proton pump inhibitor (PPI). It reduces the amount of acid in your stomach. Prilosec is used in adults for the short-term treatment of stomach and duodenal ulcers (ulcer in the upper intestine), gastroesophageal reflux disease (GERD), and erosive esophagitis (inflammation of the esophagus [tube that connects your mouth and stomach] due to excess acid).

Prilosec is also used to prevent a relapse of esophagitis; for long-term treatment of conditions where the stomach makes too much acid, such as Zollinger-Ellison syndrome; and with other medicines to eliminate the bacteria that often cause ulcers (known as *Helicobacter pylori*).

In addition, Prilosec is used for the short-term treatment of GERD and erosive esophagitis in children and adolescents. Prilosec is available as capsules or an oral suspension.

Prilosec OTC, an over-the-counter product, is only used to treat frequent heartburn (occurring 2 or more days a week).

What is the most important information I should know about this medication?

- Prilosec can cause low magnesium levels in your body. Tell your doctor immediately if you have seizures, dizziness, abnormal or fast heartbeat, jitteriness, jerking movements or shaking, muscle weakness, spasms of your hands and feet, cramps or muscle aches, or spasm of your voice box.
- Tell your doctor if you experience any symptoms of a serious allergic reaction with Prilosec (such as rash, face swelling, throat tightness, or difficulty breathing).
- People who are taking multiple daily doses of Prilosec for a long period of time may have an increased risk of fractures of the hip, wrist, or spine.

Who should not take this medication?

Do not take Prilosec if you are allergic to it, any of its ingredients, or to any other PPI.

What should I tell my doctor before I take the first dose of this medication?

Tell your doctor about all prescription, over-the-counter, and herbal medications you are taking before beginning treatment with Prilosec. Also, talk to your doctor about your complete medical history, especially if you have low magnesium levels, liver problems, or if you are pregnant, plan to become pregnant, or are breastfeeding.

What is the usual dosage?

Please see general statement regarding dosage on page xii.

Erosive Esophagitis

Adults: The recommended dose is 20 milligrams (mg) once a day for 4-8 weeks. Depending on your response, your doctor may suggest another 4 weeks of treatment. To prevent a relapse, your doctor may suggest taking 20 mg once a day.

Children and adolescents 1-16 years: Depending on your child's weight, the recommended dose is 5 mg, 10 mg, or 20 mg once a day.

GERD

Adults: The recommended dose is 20 mg once a day for up to 4 weeks.

Children and adolescents 1-16 years: Depending on your child's weight, the recommended dose is 5 mg, 10 mg, or 20 mg once a day.

Prevention of Duodenal Ulcer Due to *H. pylori* Infection

Adults: This treatment involves taking two or three different medications. The usual dose for the dual therapy is: Prilosec 40 mg three times a day for 14 days and clarithromycin 500 mg three times a day for 14 days. The usual dose for the triple therapy is: Prilosec 20 mg twice a day for 10 days, amoxicillin 1000 mg twice a day for 10 days, and clarithromycin 500 mg twice a day for 10 days.

Treatment of Duodenal Ulcer
Adults: The recommended dose is 20 mg once a day for 4 weeks.

Short-Term Treatment of Stomach Ulcer
Adults: The recommended dose is 40 mg once a day for 4-8 weeks.

Treatment of Excess Stomach Acid (Such as Zollinger-Ellison Syndrome)
Adults: The recommended starting dose is 60 mg once a day. Your doctor might prescribe a different dose or duration based on your condition.

If you have liver impairment, your doctor will adjust your dose appropriately.

How should I take this medication?
- Take Prilosec exactly as prescribed by your doctor. Take it at least 1 hour before a meal.
- Swallow Prilosec capsules whole. If you have trouble with this, open the capsule and empty the contents into a tablespoon of applesauce. Swallow the applesauce mixture right away. Do not chew the mixture or store it for later use.
- To prepare Prilosec oral suspension, empty the contents of the 2.5-mg packet into a container with one teaspoon of water or empty the contents of the 10-mg packet into a container with one tablespoon of water. Stir contents together and allow 2-3 minutes for the mixture to thicken. Drink the mixture within 30 minutes. Any remaining medicine should be mixed with more water, stirred, and taken right away.
- Please review the instructions that came with your prescription on how to properly take Prilosec.

What should I avoid while taking this medication?
Do not crush or chew the capsules. This will damage them and the medicine will not work.

Do not change your dose or stop taking Prilosec without first talk-ing to your doctor.

What are possible food and drug interactions associated with this medication?

If Prilosec is taken with certain other drugs, the effects of either could be increased, decreased, or altered. It is especially impor-tant to check with your doctor before combining Prilosec with the following: ampicillin, atazanavir, cilostazol, clopidrogrel, diazepam, digoxin, disulfiram, erlotinib, iron-containing products, ketocon-azole, methotrexate, nelfinavir, phenytoin, rifampin, saquinavir, St. John's wort, tacrolimus, voriconazole, or warfarin.

What are the possible side effects of this medication?

Please see general statement regarding side effects on page xiii.

Side effects may include: diarrhea, fever, gas, headache, nau-sea, stomach pain, upper respiratory tract infection, vomiting

---

Can I receive this medication if I am pregnant or breastfeeding?

The effects of Prilosec during pregnancy are unknown. Prilosec can be found in your breast milk if you take it during breastfeeding. Do not breastfeed while you are taking Prilosec. Tell your doctor immediately if you are pregnant, plan to become pregnant, or are breastfeeding.

What should I do if I miss a dose of this medication?

If you miss a dose of Prilosec, take it as soon as you remember. However, if it is almost time for your next dose, skip the one you missed and return to your regular dosing schedule. Do not take two doses at once.

How should I store this medication?

Store at room temperature. Protect from light and moisture.

Prinivil

Generic name: Lisinopril

What is this medication?

Prinivil is a medicine known as an angiotensin-converting enzyme (ACE) inhibitor. Prinivil is used alone or in combination with other medications to treat high blood pressure or heart failure. Also, it is used after a heart attack to improve survival in some people.

What is the most important information I should know about this medication?

- Prinivil can cause a rare but serious allergic reaction leading to extreme swelling of your face, lips, tongue, throat, or gut (causing severe abdominal pain). You may have an increased risk of experiencing these symptoms if you have ever had an allergy to ACE inhibitor-type medicines or if you are African American. If you experience any of these symptoms, seek emergency medical attention immediately.

- Tell your doctor if you experience lightheadedness, especially during the first few weeks of Prinivil therapy. If you faint, stop taking Prinivil and tell your doctor immediately.

- Vomiting, diarrhea, fever, exercise, hot weather, alcohol, excessive perspiration, and dehydration may lead to an excessive fall in your blood pressure. Tell your doctor if you experience any of these.

- Prinivil may decrease your blood neutrophil (type of blood cells that fight infections) levels, especially if you have a collagen vascular disease (such as lupus [disease that affects the immune system]) or kidney disease.

- Promptly report any signs of infection (such as sore throat or fever) to your doctor.

- Prinivil may not work as well in African Americans, who may also have a higher risk of side effects. Contact your doctor if your symptoms do not improve or if they become worse.

Who should not take this medication?

Do not take Prinivil if you are allergic to it or any of its ingredients.

Do not take Prinivil if you have a history of angioedema (a condition involving swelling of the face, extremities, eyes, lips, and tongue) related to previous treatment with similar medicines. Also do not take Prinivil if you have a history of certain types of angioedema (such as hereditary or idiopathic).

What should I tell my doctor before I take the first dose of this medication?

Tell your doctor about all prescription, over-the-counter, and herbal medications you are taking before beginning treatment with Prinivil. Also, talk to your doctor about your complete medical history, especially if you have liver problems, kidney disease, or diabetes. Tell your doctor if you have bone marrow problems or any blood disease, any disease that affects the immune system (such as lupus or scleroderma), collagen vascular disease, narrowing or hardening of the arteries of your brain or heart, chest pain, or if you have ever had an allergy or sensitivity to ACE inhibitors such as Prinivil.

What is the usual dosage?

Please see general statement regarding dosage on page xii.

High Blood Pressure
Adults: The usual starting dose is 10 milligrams (mg) once a day. Your doctor will adjust your dose based on your previous blood pressure medication and will increase your dose as needed, until the desired effect is achieved.

Children ≥6 years: Your doctor will prescribe the appropriate dose for your child, based on their weight.

Heart Failure
Adults: The usual starting dose is 5 mg once a day. Your doctor may give you a higher dose depending on your needs.

Heart Attack
Adults: The usual starting dose is 5 mg, then increased to 10 mg once a day for 6 weeks. Your doctor will prescribe the appropriate dose for you based on your condition.

If you have kidney impairment, your doctor will adjust your dose appropriately.

How should I take this medication?

- Take Prinivil at the same time every day. Continue to take Prinivil even if you feel well.
- Do not take extra doses or take more often without asking your doctor.

What should I avoid while taking this medication?

Do not become pregnant or breastfeed while you are taking Prinivil.

Do not drive or operate heavy machinery until you know how Prinivil affects you.

Do not take salt substitutes or supplements containing potassium without consulting your doctor.

Do not stand or sit up quickly when you take Prinivil, especially in the morning. Sit or lie down at the first sign of dizziness, lightheadedness, or fainting.

What are possible food and drug interactions associated with this medication?

If Prinivil is taken with certain other drugs, the effects of either could be increased, decreased, or altered. It is especially important to check with your doctor before combining Prinivil with the following: amiloride, dextran, diuretics (water pills) (such as furosemide, hydrochlorothiazide, spironolactone, or triamterene), lithium, nonsteroidal anti-inflammatory medications (such as ibuprofen or naproxen), potassium supplements, or salt substitutes containing potassium.

What are the possible side effects of this medication?

Please see general statement regarding side effects on page xiii.

Side effects may include: chest pain, cough, diarrhea, dizziness, fatigue, headache, low blood pressure, rash, upper respiratory infection

Can I receive this medication if I am pregnant or breastfeeding?

Do not take Prinivil if you are pregnant or breastfeeding. Prinivil can harm your unborn baby. Tell your doctor immediately if you are pregnant, plan to become pregnant, or are breastfeeding.

What should I do if I miss a dose of this medication?

If you miss a dose of Prinivil, take it as soon as you remember. However, if it is almost time for your next dose, skip the one you missed and return to your regular dosing schedule. Do not take two doses at once.

How should I store this medication?

Store at room temperature.

Prinzide

Generic name: Hydrochlorothiazide/Lisinopril

What is this medication?

Prinzide is a combination medicine used to treat high blood pressure. Prinzide contains two medicines: lisinopril (an angiotensin-converting enzyme [ACE] inhibitor) and hydrochlorothiazide (a diuretic [water pill]).

What is the most important information I should know about this medication?

- Prinzide can cause a rare but serious allergic reaction leading to extreme swelling of your face, lips, tongue, throat, or gut (causing severe abdominal pain). You may have an increased risk of experiencing these symptoms if you have ever had an allergy to angiotensin-converting enzyme (ACE) inhibitor-type medicines or if you are African American. If you experience any of these symptoms, seek emergency medical attention immediately.
- Tell your doctor if you experience lightheadedness, especially during the first few days of Prinzide therapy. If you faint, stop taking Prinzide and tell your doctor immediately.

- Vomiting, diarrhea, fever, exercise, hot weather, drinking alcohol, excessive perspiration, and dehydration may lead to an excessive fall in your blood pressure. Tell your doctor if you experience any of these. Make sure to drink plenty of fluids when you are taking Prinzide.
- Prinzide may decrease your blood neutrophil (type of blood cells that fight infection) levels, especially if you have a collagen vascular disease (such as lupus [disease that affects the immune system]) or kidney disease.
- Promptly report any signs of infection (such as sore throat or fever) to your doctor.
- Prinzide is not recommended in people with severe kidney problems.
- Prinzide can raise your blood sugar. High blood sugar may make you feel confused, drowsy, or thirsty. It can also make you flush, breathe faster, or have a fruit-like breath odor. If these symptoms occur, tell your doctor right away.
- Prinzide may not work as well in African Americans and may increase the risk of side effects. Contact your doctor if your symptoms do not improve or if they become worse.

Who should not take this medication?

Do not take Prinzide if you are allergic to it or any of its ingredients.

Do not take Prinzide if you are unable to produce urine. Do not take Prinzide if you have a history of angioedema (a condition involving swelling of the face, extremities, eyes, lips, and tongue) related to previous treatment with similar medicines. Also, do not take Prinzide if you have a history of certain types of angioedema (such as hereditary or idiopathic).

What should I tell my doctor before I take the first dose of this medication?

Tell your doctor about all prescription, over-the-counter, and herbal medications you are taking before beginning treatment with Prinzide. Also, talk to your doctor about your complete medical history, especially if you have diabetes, or liver or kidney problems. Tell your doctor if you have bone marrow suppression, heart disease, skin disease, severe immune system problems, lupus, or asthma, or are on a sodium-restricted diet. Also, tell your doctor if you have ever had an allergy or sensitivity to ACE inhibitors or .sulfonamide-type medications.

What is the usual dosage?
Please see general statement regarding dosage on page xii.

Adults: The usual dose is 10/12.5 (10 milligrams [mg] of lisinopril and 12.5 mg of hydrochlorothiazide) or 20/12.5 (20 mg of lisinopril and 12.5 mg of hydrochlorothiazide) once a day. Your doctor may give you a higher dose depending on your needs.

How should I take this medication?
• Take Prinzide at the same time every day with or without food. Continue to use Prinzide even if you feel well.
• Do not take extra doses or take more often without asking your doctor.

What should I avoid while taking this medication?
Do not become pregnant or breastfeed while you are taking Prinzide.

Do not drive or operate heavy machinery until you know how Prinzide affects you.

Do not become dehydrated. Drink adequate fluids while you are taking Prinzide.

Do not take salt substitutes or supplements containing potassium without consulting your doctor.

Do not stand or sit up quickly when taking Prinzide, especially in the morning. Sit or lie down at the first sign of dizziness, lightheadedness, or fainting.

What are possible food and drug interactions associated with this medication?
If Prinzide is taken with certain other drugs, the effects of either could be increased, decreased, or altered. It is especially important

to check with your doctor before combining Prinzide with the following: certain diuretics (such as amiloride, spironolactone, or triamterene), cholestyramine, colestipol, corticosteroids, insulin and oral antidiabetic medicines, lithium, norepinephrine, nonsteroidal anti-inflammatory drugs (such as ibuprofen or naproxen), potassium supplements, salt substitutes containing potassium, or skeletal muscle relaxants.

What are the possible side effects of this medication?
Please see general statement regarding side effects on page xiii.

> **Side effects may include:** cough, diarrhea, dizziness, headache, fatigue, low blood pressure (especially when rising from a seated position), muscle cramps, nausea, tiredness, upper respiratory infection

Can I receive this medication if I am pregnant or breastfeeding?
Do not take Prinzide if you are pregnant or breastfeeding. Prinzide can harm your unborn baby. It can be found in your breast milk if you take it while breastfeeding. Tell your doctor immediately if you are pregnant, plan to become pregnant, or are breastfeeding.

What should I do if I miss a dose of this medication?
If you miss a dose of Prinzide, take it as soon as you remember. However, if it is almost time for your next dose, skip the one you missed and return to your regular dosing schedule. Do not take two doses at once.

How should I store this medication?
Store at room temperature.

Pristiq
Generic name: Desvenlafaxine

What is this medication?
Pristiq belongs to the class of medications called serotonin-norepinephrine reuptake inhibitors (SNRIs). Pristiq is used to treat major
depressive disorder.

What is the most important information I should know about this medication?
- Pristiq can increase suicidal thoughts or actions in some children, teenagers, and young adults when the medicine is first
started.
- Depression and other serious mental illnesses are the most serious causes of suicidal thoughts and actions. People with bipolar
disorder, or who have a family history of bipolar disorder (also
called manic-depressive illness) are at a greater risk. Contact
your doctor immediately if you experience any changes in your
mood, behavior, thoughts, or feelings. This is very important
when an antidepressant medicine is first started or when the
dose is changed.
- Pristiq can cause a severe, possibly life-threatening condition
called serotonin syndrome (a drug reaction that causes the body
to have too much serotonin, a chemical produced by the nerve
cells) or neuroleptic malignant syndrome (a life-threatening
brain disorder). Contact your doctor immediately if you experience agitation, hallucinations, coma, fast heartbeat, changes in
your blood pressure, increased body temperature, lack of coordination, overactive reflexes, nausea, vomiting, or diarrhea.
- Pristiq can cause an increase in your blood pressure. Check your
blood pressure regularly, especially if you already have high
blood pressure.
- Do not suddenly stop taking Pristiq without talking to your doctor first, as this can cause serious side effects.
- Pristiq can cause mydriasis (prolonged dilation of the pupils of
your eye). Notify your doctor if you have a history of glaucoma
(high pressure in your eye).
- Pristiq can cause low blood sodium levels. Contact your doctor
immediately if you experience headache, difficulty concentrating,

confusion, weakness, unsteadiness, hallucinations, falls, or seizures.

- Pristiq can cause seizures to develop, especially if you have a history of seizures.
- Pristiq can increase your risk of bleeding. Do not take Pristiq with aspirin, nonsteroidal anti-inflammatory drugs (NSAIDs) (such as ibuprofen), or blood-thinners (such as warfarin).
- Pristiq can increase your cholesterol. Your doctor may measure your cholesterol levels if you will be on long-term treatment with Pristiq.

Who should not take this medication?

Do not take Pristiq if you are allergic to it, any of its ingredients, or to venlafaxine hydrochloride, the active ingredient in Effexor and Effexor XR.

Also, never take Pristiq while you are taking other medicines known as monoamine oxidase inhibitors (MAOIs) (such as phenelzine), a class of medications used to treat depression and other conditions.

What should I tell my doctor before I take the first dose of this medication?

Tell your doctor about all prescription, over-the-counter, and herbal medication you are taking before beginning treatment with Pristiq. Also, talk to your doctor about your complete medical history, especially if you have high blood pressure; heart, liver, or kidney problems; high cholesterol or high triglycerides; history of stroke; glaucoma; bleeding problems; seizures; mania or bipolar disorder; or low sodium levels in your blood. Also, tell your doctor if you are pregnant, plan to become pregnant, or are breastfeeding.

What is the usual dosage?

Please see general statement regarding dosage on page xii.

Adults: The recommended dose is 50 milligrams once a day.

If you have kidney or liver impairment, your doctor will adjust your dose appropriately.

How should I take this medication?

- Take Pristiq with or without food at about the same time every day.
- Swallow the tablets whole with water. Do not crush, cut, chew, or dissolve them.
- When you take Pristiq, you may see something in your stool that looks like a tablet. This is the empty shell from the tablet after the medicine has been absorbed in your body.

What should I avoid while taking this medication?

Do not drive or operate dangerous machinery until you know how Pristiq affects you.

Pristiq may cause you to feel drowsy or less alert and may affect your judgment.

Do not drink alcohol while you are taking Pristiq, as it can worsen these side effects.

Do not stop taking Pristiq suddenly without talking to your doctor first, as this can cause serious side effects.

Pristiq can increase your risk of bleeding. Do not take aspirin, NSAIDs, or blood thinners while you are taking Pristiq.

Do not take Pristiq and MAOIs together or within 14 days of each other. Wait at least 7 days after stopping Pristiq before starting an MAOI. Combining these medicines with Pristiq can cause serious and even fatal reactions.

Do not take Pristiq with other medicines that contain venlafaxine.

What are possible food and drug interactions associated with this medication?

If Pristiq is taken with certain drugs, the effects of either could be increased, decreased, or altered. It is important to check with your doctor before combining Pristiq with the following: alcohol, antipsychotic medications, aspirin, certain antidepressants (such as amitriptyline or desipramine), certain migraine products, ketoconazole, linezolid, lithium, MAOIs, metoclopramide, midazolam, NSAIDs, other SNRIs, silbutramine, St. John's wort, tramadol, tryptophan, or warfarin.

What are the possible side effects of this medication?
Please see general statement regarding side effects on page xiii.

Side effects may include: abnormal ejaculation, anxiety, constipation, decreased sexual desire, diarrhea, dilated pupils, dizziness, drowsiness, dry mouth, headache, loss of appetite, nausea, sweating, tremor, trouble sleeping, vomiting

Can I receive this medication if I am pregnant or breastfeeding?
The effects of Pristiq during pregnancy are unknown. Pristiq can be found in your breast milk if you take it while breastfeeding. Tell your doctor immediately if you are pregnant, plan to become pregnant, or are breastfeeding.

What should I do if I miss a dose of this medication?
If you miss a dose of Pristiq, take it as soon as you remember. However, if it is almost time for your next dose, skip the one you missed and return to your regular dosing schedule. Do not take two doses at once.

How should I store this medication?
Store at room temperature.

Proair HFA
Generic name: Albuterol Sulfate

What is this medication?
Proair HFA is an inhaled medicine used to prevent and treat airway narrowing associated with certain breathing problems (such as asthma). Proair HFA is also used to prevent exercise-induced airway narrowing.

What is the most important information I should know about this medication?

- Do not use Proair HFA more frequently than your doctor recommends. Increasing the number of doses can be dangerous and may actually make symptoms of asthma worse. If the dose your doctor recommends does not provide relief of your symptoms, or if your symptoms become worse, tell your doctor right away.
- You can have an immediate, serious allergic reaction to the first dose of Proair HFA, with hives, rash, and swelling of your mouth, throat, lips, or tongue. This medication can cause life-threatening breathing problems, especially with the first dose from a new canister. If you experience an allergic reaction or trouble breathing, call your doctor right away.

Who should not take this medication?

Do not use Proair HFA if you are allergic to it or any of its ingredients.

What should I tell my doctor before I take the first dose of this medication?

Tell your doctor about all prescription, over-the-counter, and herbal medications you are taking before beginning treatment with Proair HFA. Also, talk to your doctor about your complete medical history, especially if you have a heart condition, seizure disorder, high blood pressure, arrhythmia (life-threatening irregular heartbeat), overactive thyroid gland, low blood potassium levels, or diabetes.

What is the usual dosage?

Please see general statement regarding dosage on page xii.

Prevention or Treatment of Airway Narrowing

Adults and children ≥4 years: The usual dose is 2 inhalations every 4-6 hours. Your or your child's doctor will adjust your dose appropriately.

Exercise-Induced Airway Narrowing

Adults and children ≥4 years: The usual dose is 2 inhalations 15-30 minutes before exercise.

How should I take this medication?

- Use Proair HFA exactly as prescribed by your doctor. Shake the inhaler well before each use.
- You must prime the inhaler if you are using it for the first time and when it has not been used for more than 2 weeks. To do this, press the pump 3 times into the air, away from your face.
- Breathe out fully through your mouth, then place the mouthpiece into your mouth and close your lips around it. While breathing in deeply and slowly through your mouth, press down on the top of the metal canister. Hold your breath for 10 seconds if possible.
- If your doctor has prescribed more than one inhalation, wait one minute between inhalations. Clean the mouthpiece without the metal canister at least once a week.
- Please review the instructions that came with your prescription on how to properly use Proair HFA.

What should I avoid while taking this medication?

Do not spray Proair HFA into your eyes.

Do not inhale extra doses or stop using Proair HFA without talking to your doctor.

Do not clean the metal canister or allow it to become wet.

What are possible food and drug interactions associated with this medication?

If Proair HFA is used with certain other drugs, the effects of either could be increased, decreased, or altered. It is especially important to check with your doctor before combining Proair HFA with the following: blood pressure/heart medications known as beta-blockers (such as metoprolol or propranolol), certain antidepressants (such as amitriptyline or phenelzine), certain diuretics (water pills) (such as furosemide or hydrochlorothiazide), digoxin, or medicines similar to Proair HFA (such as terbutaline and epinephrine).

What are the possible side effects of this medication?

Please see general statement regarding side effects on page xiii.

> **Side effects may include:** chest pain, dizziness, fast heart rate, fluttery or throbbing heartbeat, headache, nervousness, runny nose, shakiness, sore throat

Can I receive this medication if I am pregnant or breastfeeding?

The effects of Proair HFA during pregnancy and breastfeeding are unknown. Do not breastfeed while you are using Proair HFA. Tell your doctor immediately if you are pregnant, plan to become pregnant, or are breastfeeding.

What should I do if I miss a dose of this medication?

If you miss a dose of Proair HFA, take it as soon as you remember. However, if it is almost time for your next dose, skip the one you missed and return to your regular dosing schedule. Do not take two doses at once.

How should I store this medication?

Store at room temperature. Protect from heat, open flame, or direct sunlight.

Procardia XL

Generic name: Nifedipine

What is this medication?

Procardia XL is a medicine known as a calcium channel blocker, which is used alone or in combination with other medications to treat angina (chest pain) or high blood pressure.

What is the most important information I should know about this medication?

• While on Procardia XL, your blood pressure can become lower than normal or your heart rate can increase. Tell your doctor about any dizziness, feeling faint, or lightheadedness you experience while taking Procardia XL.

- If you experience chest pain that gets worse, or that does not
  go away during treatment with Procardia XL, get medical help
  right away.

Who should not take this medication?
Do not take Procardia XL if you are allergic to it or any of its
ingredients.

What should I tell my doctor before I take the first dose of this medication?
Tell your doctor about all prescription, over-the-counter, and herbal
medications you are taking before beginning treatment with Procardia XL. Also, talk to your doctor about your complete medical
history, especially if you have any other heart or blood vessel conditions, stomach or intestinal problems, liver disease, or are pregnant, plan to become pregnant, or are breastfeeding.

What is the usual dosage?
Please see general statement regarding dosage on page xii.

Adults: The recommended starting dose is 30 or 60 milligrams
once a day. Your doctor will prescribe the appropriate dose for
you and will increase your dose as needed, until the desired effect
is achieved.

How should I take this medication?
- Take Procardia XL exactly as prescribed by your doctor.
- Take Procardia XL once a day. Take this medication at the same
  time each day. Take Procardia XL with or without food.
- Swallow Procardia XL tablets whole. Do not chew, divide, or
  crush the tablets.
- Do not change your dose or stop taking this medication abruptly
  without first talking to your doctor.
- Do not be concerned if something that looks like a tablet appears
  in your stool. This is normal and means that the medication has
  been released, and the shell that contained the medication has
  been eliminated from your body.

What should I avoid while taking this medication?

Do not miss any of your follow-up appointments with your doctor to check your blood pressure while on treatment with Procardia XL.

What are possible food and drug interactions associated with this medication?

If Procardia XL is taken with certain other drugs, the effects of either could be increased, decreased, or altered. It is especially important to check with your doctor before combining Procardia XL with the following: blood pressure/heart medications known as beta-blockers (such as metoprolol), blood thinners (such as warfarin), cimetidine, or digoxin.

What are the possible side effects of this medication?

Please see general statement regarding side effects on page xiii.

> **Side effects may include:** constipation, dizziness, flushing, giddiness, headache, heartburn, heat sensation, lightheadedness, nausea, swelling, tiredness, weakness

Can I receive this medication if I am pregnant or breastfeeding?

The effects of Procardia XL during pregnancy and breastfeeding are unknown. Tell your doctor immediately if you are pregnant, plan to become pregnant, or are breastfeeding.

What should I do if I miss a dose of this medication?

If you miss a dose of Procardia XL, take it as soon as you remember. However, if it is almost time for your next dose, skip the one you missed and return to your regular dosing schedule. Do not take two doses at once.

How should I store this medication?

Store at room temperature. Protect from moisture and humidity.

Promethazine DM

Generic name: Dextromethorphan HBr/Promethazine HCl

What is this medication?

Promethazine DM is a medicine used to treat cough and upper respiratory symptoms you can have with allergies or a cold. Promethazine DM contains two medicines: promethazine (an antihistamine) and dextromethorphan (a cough suppressant).

What is the most important information I should know about this medication?

- This medication can cause drowsiness or dizziness and impair mental and/or physical abilities required for hazardous tasks, such as driving a car or operating machinery.
- Promethazine DM can cause serious and possibly life-threatening respiratory depression (decreased rate of breathing) or increase your risk for a seizure. Tell your doctor if you have any breathing problems (such as chronic obstructive pulmonary disease [narrowing of the lungs that makes it hard to breath] or sleep apnea [you stop breathing temporarily during sleep]) or a history of seizures.
- Promethazine DM can cause neuroleptic malignant syndrome (a life-threatening brain disorder). Tell your doctor if you experience a fever, stiff muscles, changes in your mental status, fast or irregular heartbeat, changes in your blood pressure, or excessive sweating.
- Tell your doctor if you experience any uncontrollable muscle movements.

Who should not take this medication?

Do not take Promethazine DM if you are allergic to it or any of its ingredients. Also, do not take Promethazine DM to treat certain breathing problems (such as asthma).

Do not take Promethazine DM while you are taking other medicines known as monoamine oxidase inhibitors (MAOIs) (such as phenelzine or tranylcypromine), a class of medications used to treat depression and other conditions.

Do not give Promethazine DM to children <2 years due to an increased risk of respiratory depression.

What should I tell my doctor before I take the first dose of this medication?

Tell your doctor about all prescription, over-the-counter, and herbal medications you are taking before beginning treatment with Promethazine DM. Also, talk to your doctor about your complete medical history, especially if you have narrow-angle glaucoma (high pressure in your eye); bone marrow disorders; heart disease; enlarged prostate; or bladder, liver, or stomach problems (such as stomach ulcers).

Tell your doctor if your child has certain skin conditions (such as eczema).

What is the usual dosage?
Please see general statement regarding dosage on page xii.

Adults: The usual dose is 1 teaspoon (5 milliliters [mL]) every 4-6 hours. Do not take more than 6 teaspoons (30 mL) in 24 hours.

Children 6-12 years: The usual dose is 1/2 to 1 teaspoon (2.5-5 mL) every 4-6 hours. Do not take more than 4 teaspoons (20 mL) in 24 hours.

Children 2-6 years: The usual dose is 1/4 to 1/2 teaspoon (1.25-2.5 mL) every 4-6 hours. Do not take more than 2 teaspoons (10 mL) in 24 hours.

How should I take this medication?
• Take Promethazine DM exactly as prescribed by your doctor.

What should I avoid while taking this medication?
Do not drive or operate machinery until you know how Promethazine DM affects you.

Supervise your child while bike riding or engaging in other possibly dangerous activities until you know how Promethazine DM affects your child.

Do not expose yourself to excessive amounts of sunlight.

What are possible food and drug interactions associated with this medication?

If Promethazine DM is taken with certain other drugs, the effects of either could be increased, decreased, or altered. It is especially important to check with your doctor before combining it with the following: alcohol, anticholinergics (such as atropine or ipratropium), barbiturates (such as phenobarbital), certain antidepressants (such as amitriptyline or imipramine), epinephrine, general anesthetics, narcotic painkillers (such as hydrocodone or oxycodone), phenothiazines (such as chlorpromazine), sedatives, or tranquilizers (such as chlordiazepoxide).

What are the possible side effects of this medication?

Please see general statement regarding side effects on page xiii.

> **Side effects may include:** blurred vision, confusion, dizziness, drowsiness, dry mouth, increased or decreased blood pressure, nausea, skin reactions, stomach problems, vomiting

Can I receive this medication if I am pregnant or breastfeeding?

The effects of Promethazine DM during pregnancy and breastfeeding are unknown. Tell your doctor immediately if you are pregnant, plan to become pregnant, or are breastfeeding.

What should I do if I miss a dose of this medication?

If you miss a dose of Promethazine DM, take it as soon as you remember. However, if it is almost time for your next dose, skip the one you missed and return to your regular dosing schedule. Do not take two doses at once.

How should I store this medication?
Store at room temperature. Protect from light.

Promethazine HCl: see Promethazine hydrochloride, page 850

Promethazine hydrochloride
Generic name: Promethazine HCl

What is this medication?
Promethazine is an antihistamine used to treat the symptoms of seasonal and year-round allergies, non-allergic runny nose, conjunctivitis ("pink eye") due to inhalant allergens and foods, or allergic skin reactions. In addition, promethazine is used to prevent or control pain or nausea and vomiting during and after surgery and for the treatment and prevention of motion sickness. It is also used to help produce light sleep. Promethazine is available as a tablet, syrup, and suppository.

What is the most important information I should know about this medication?
- Promethazine can cause drowsiness and impair mental or physical abilities. Do not drive or operate machinery until you know how promethazine affects you. Do not drink alcohol or take certain medicines that can cause drowsiness (such as sedatives and tranquilizers) without speaking to your doctor.
- Promethazine should not be used in children under 2 years of age. Serious and sometimes fatal breathing problems can occur when promethazine is used by children in this age group.
- Neuroleptic malignant syndrome (NMS) (a life-threatening brain disorder) can occur if you take promethazine. Tell your doctor immediately if you develop a fever, stiff muscles, fast or irregular heartbeat, or sweating.
- Promethazine should be used with caution if you have a seizure disorder, are taking other medications that can increase your risk for seizures, have a breathing problem or lung disease, or have bone marrow depression.

Who should not take this medication?

Do not take promethazine if you are allergic to it or any of its ingredients. Also, do not take promethazine for the treatment of lower respiratory (lung) tract symptoms, including asthma. Children under 2 years of age should not take promethazine.

What should I tell my doctor before I take the first dose of this medication?

Tell your doctor about all prescription, over-the-counter, and herbal medications you are taking before beginning treatment with promethazine. Also, talk to your doctor about your complete medical history, especially if you have central nervous system (CNS) problems, bone marrow depression, asthma or lung disease, glaucoma (high pressure in the eye), stomach or intestinal disorders, urinary problems caused by enlargement of your prostate gland or blockage of your bladder, heart problems, liver problems, Reye's syndrome (a potentially fatal disease of the brain and liver that most commonly occurs in children after a viral infection, such as chickenpox), alcoholism, are pregnant, plan to become pregnant, or are breastfeeding.

What is the usual dosage?

Please see general statement regarding dosage on page xii.

Adults and children ≥2 years: Your doctor will prescribe the appropriate dose for you based on your age and condition.

How should I take this medication?

- Take promethazine exactly as prescribed by your doctor.
- Promethazine tablets and syrup are taken by mouth. Promethazine syrup should be taken using an accurate measuring device. Your pharmacist can provide an accurate device and instructions for measuring the correct dose.
- Promethazine suppositories are for rectal use only.

What should I avoid while taking this medication?

Do not drive or operate machinery until you know how promethazine affects you.

Do not drink alcohol or take certain medicines that can cause drowsiness without consulting your doctor.

Limit your exposure to sunlight; promethazine can make you become more sensitive to the sun.

What are possible food and drug interactions associated with this medication?

If promethazine is taken with certain other drugs, the effects of either could be increased, decreased, or altered. It is especially important to check with your doctor before combining promethazine with the following: alcohol, anticholinergics (such as atropine or ipratropium), certain medicines that can cause drowsiness (such as alprazolam, diazepam, or oxycodone), epinephrine, or monoamine oxidase inhibitors (MAOIs), such as phenelzine, a class of drugs used to treat depression and other psychiatric conditions.

What are the possible side effects of this medication?

Please see general statement regarding side effects on page xiii.

Side effects may include: allergic reactions, blurred vision, breathing difficulty, changes in your blood pressure or heartbeat, confusion, disorientation, dizziness, drowsiness, dry mouth, excitability, faintness, hallucinations, involuntary muscle movements, nausea, NMS, rash, seizures, sensitivity to light, sleepiness, vomiting, yellowing of your skin or whites of your eyes

If you experience symptoms of NMS, contact your doctor immediately.

Can I receive this medication if I am pregnant or breastfeeding?

The effects of promethazine during pregnancy and breastfeeding are unknown. Tell your doctor immediately if you are pregnant, plan to become pregnant, or are breastfeeding.

What should I do if I miss a dose of this medication?

If you miss a dose of promethazine, take it as soon as you remember. However, if it is almost time for your next dose, skip the one you missed and return to your regular dosing schedule. Do not take two doses at once.

For certain conditions, promethazine should be given under special circumstances determined by your doctor or given only as needed.

How should I store this medication?

Store tablets or syrup at room temperature, and store suppositories in the refrigerator. Protect from light.

Promethazine with codeine

Generic name: Codeine Phosphate/Promethazine HCl

What is this medication?

Promethazine with codeine is a medicine used to treat cough and upper respiratory symptoms you can have with allergies or a cold. Promethazine is an antihistamine and codeine is a narcotic cough suppressant.

What is the most important information I should know about this medication?

- Promethazine with codeine has abuse potential. Mental and physical dependence can occur with the use of promethazine with codeine when it is used improperly.
- Promethazine with codeine can cause drowsiness and impair mental and/or physical abilities required for hazardous tasks, such as driving a car or operating machinery.
- Promethazine with codeine can cause serious and possibly life-threatening respiratory depression (decreased rate of breathing) or increase your risk for a seizure. Tell your doctor if you have any breathing problems (such as chronic obstructive pulmonary disease [narrowing of the lungs that makes it hard to breath], sleep apnea [you stop breathing temporarily during sleep]), or a history of seizures.

- Promethazine with codeine can cause neuroleptic malignant syndrome (a life-threatening brain disorder). Tell your doctor if you experience a fever, stiff muscles, changes in your mental status, fast or irregular heartbeat, changes in your blood pressure, or excessive sweating.
- Tell your doctor if you experience any uncontrollable muscle movements.
- Promethazine with codeine can cause lightheadedness or fainting, especially when you stand up from a lying or sitting position.

Who should not take this medication?

Do not take promethazine with codeine if you are allergic to it or any of its ingredients. Also, do not take promethazine with codeine to treat certain breathing problems (such as asthma).

Do not give promethazine with codeine to children <6 years due to an increased risk of respiratory depression.

What should I tell my doctor before I take the first dose of this medication?

Tell your doctor about all prescription, over-the-counter, and herbal medications you are taking before beginning treatment with promethazine with codeine. Also, talk to your doctor about your complete medical history, especially if you have narrow-angle glaucoma (high pressure in your eye); bone marrow disorders; heart disease; underactive thyroid gland; Addison's disease (adrenal gland failure); ulcerative colitis (inflammatory disease of the large intestine); enlarged prostate; or bladder, liver, kidney, or stomach problems (such as stomach ulcers).

Tell your doctor if your child has certain skin conditions (such as eczema).

What is the usual dosage?

Please see general statement regarding dosage on page xii.

Adults and children ≥12 years: The usual dose is 1 teaspoon (5 milliliters [mL]) every 4-6 hours. Do not take more than 30 mL in 24 hours.

Children 6-12 years: The usual dose is 1/2 to 1 teaspoon (2.5-5 mL) every 4-6 hours. Do not take more than 30 mL in 24 hours.

How should I take this medication?

- Take promethazine with codeine exactly as prescribed by your doctor.
- Use an appropriate measuring device to take the medicine. Your pharmacist can give you an appropriate device and show you how to measure the correct dose.

What should I avoid while taking this medication?

Do not increase your dose if your cough does not go away. Call your doctor if your cough does not improve within 5 days.

Do not drive or operate machinery until you know how promethazine with codeine affects you. Also, supervise your child while bike riding or engaging in other possibly dangerous activities until you know how promethazine with codeine affects him/her.

Do not expose yourself to excessive amounts of sunlight.

What are possible food and drug interactions associated with this medication?

If promethazine with codeine is taken with certain other drugs, the effects of either could be increased, decreased, or altered. It is especially important to check with your doctor before combining promethazine with codeine with the following: alcohol, anticholinergics (such as atropine or ipratropium), barbiturates (such as phenobarbital), certain antidepressants (such as amitriptyline or phenelzine), epinephrine, general anesthetics, narcotic painkillers (such as hydrocodone or oxycodone), phenothiazines (such as chlorpromazine), sedatives, or tranquilizers (such as chlordiazepoxide).

What are the possible side effects of this medication?

Please see general statement regarding side effects on page xiii.

Side effects may include: blurred vision, confusion, constipation, dizziness, drowsiness, dry mouth, flushing of your face, fluttery or throbbing heartbeat, inability to urinate normally, increased or decreased blood pressure, itching, lightheadedness, nausea, skin reactions, stomach problems, sweating, vomiting

Can I receive this medication if I am pregnant or breastfeeding?

The effects of promethazine with codeine during pregnancy are unknown. Promethazine with codeine can be found in your breast milk if you take it while breastfeeding. Tell your doctor immediately if you are pregnant, plan to become pregnant, or are breastfeeding.

What should I do if I miss a dose of this medication?

If you miss a dose of promethazine with codeine, take it as soon as you remember. However, if it is almost time for your next dose, skip the one you missed and return to your regular dosing schedule. Do not take two doses at once.

How should I store this medication?

Store at room temperature.

Propecia

Generic name: Finasteride

What is this medication?

Propecia is a medication used to treat baldness in men with mild to moderate hair loss on the top of the head and the front of the midscalp area (male-pattern baldness).

What is the most important information I should know about this medication?

• Women should not handle crushed or broken Propecia tablets when they are pregnant or maybe pregnant.
• Propecia lowers readings of the prostate specific antigen (PSA) screening test for prostate cancer. If you're scheduled to have

your PSA level checked, make sure the doctor knows you are taking Propecia.
- Promptly report any changes in your breasts such as lumps, pain, or nipple discharge to your doctor.

Who should not take this medication?
Do not take Propecia if you are allergic to it or any of its ingredients. Women and children should not take Propecia.

What should I tell my doctor before I take the first dose of this medication?
Tell your doctor about all prescription, over-the-counter, and herbal medications you are taking before beginning treatment with Propecia. Also, talk to your doctor about your complete medical history, especially if you have liver or prostate problems.

What is the usual dosage?
Please see general statement regarding dosage on page xii.

Adult men: The recommended dosage is a single 1 milligram (mg) tablet once a day.

How should I take this medication?
- Take Propecia regularly once a day, with or without food. Do not take more than one tablet a day. Propecia will not work faster or better if you take it more often.

What should I avoid while taking this medication?
Women who are pregnant or maybe pregnant should avoid handling crushed or broken Propecia tablets.

What are possible food and drug interactions associated with this medication?
No significant interactions have been reported with Propecia at this time. However, always tell your doctor about any medicines you take, including over-the-counter drugs, vitamins, and herbal supplements.

What are the possible side effects of this medication?
Please see general statement regarding side effects on page xiii.

> **Side effects may include:** allergic reactions (such as rash, itching, hives, or swelling of the lips and face), breast changes, decreased sex drive, decreased amount of semen or problems with ejaculation, impotence, testicular pain

Can I receive this medication if I am pregnant or breastfeeding?
This medication is not used in women. Avoid touching crushed or broken Propecia tablets if you are pregnant, plan to become pregnant, or are breastfeeding. This drug may cause severe deformities in your unborn child.

What should I do if I miss a dose of this medication?
Take it as soon as you remember. If it is almost time for your next dose, skip the dose you missed and go back to your regular schedule. Do not take two doses at once.

How should I store this medication?
Store at room temperature.

Propranolol
Generic name: Propranolol HCl

What is this medication?
Propranolol is a medicine known as a beta-blocker, which is used to treat high blood pressure, chest pain, atrial fibrillation (an irregular, fast heartbeat), or tremors. It is also used after a heart attack to lower the risk of death or to prevent common migraine headaches. In addition, propranolol is used to improve symptoms associated with hypertrophic subaortic stenosis (a heart condition characterized by heart muscle thickening). It is also used with other medicines to control blood pressure and reduce symptoms associated with pheochromocytoma (tumor of the adrenal gland).

What is the most important information I should know about this medication?

- Do not stop taking propranolol without talking to your doctor. Stopping this medication suddenly can cause harmful effects. Your doctor should gradually reduce your dose when stopping treatment with this medication.
- Propranolol can worsen heart failure, cause breathing problems, or hide symptoms of low blood sugar levels if you have diabetes. Tell your doctor if you experience trouble breathing while you are taking propranolol. If you have diabetes, monitor your blood sugar frequently, especially when you first start taking propranolol.
- Propranolol can cause serious allergic reactions. Tell your doctor if you develop any skin reactions.

Who should not take this medication?

Do not take propranolol if you are allergic to it or any of its ingredients. In addition, do not take propranolol if you have asthma, a slow heart rate, heart block, or severe blood circulation disorders.

What should I tell my doctor before I take the first dose of this medication?

Tell your doctor about all prescription, over-the-counter, and herbal medications you are taking before beginning treatment with propranolol. Also, talk to your doctor about your complete medical history, especially if you have any allergies; heart problems or heart failure; a history of heart attack; breathing problems (such as asthma, chronic bronchitis [long-term inflammation of the lungs], or emphysema [lung disease that causes shortness of breath]); diabetes; glaucoma (high pressure in the eye); kidney, liver, or thyroid problems; Wolff-Parkinson-White syndrome (a type of heart condition); or are planning to have a major surgery.

Tell your doctor if you have a history of severe allergic reactions to any allergens, because propranolol may decrease the effectiveness of epinephrine used to treat the reaction.

What is the usual dosage?

Please see general statement regarding dosage on page xii.

High Blood Pressure
Adults: The usual starting dose is 40 milligrams (mg) twice a day, either alone or in combination with other blood pressure-lowering medicines. Your doctor will increase your dose as needed until the desired effect is achieved.

Atrial Fibrillation
Adults: The recommended dose is 10-30 mg three or four times a day before meals and at bedtime.

Tremors
Adults: The usual starting dose is 40 mg twice a day. Your doctor will increase your dose as needed until the desired effect is achieved.

Migraine
Adults: The usual starting dose is 80 mg a day in divided doses. Your doctor will increase your dose as needed until the desired effect is achieved.

Hypertrophic Subaortic Stenosis
Adults: The usual dose is 20-40 mg three or four times a day before meals and at bedtime.

Chest pain, Heart Attack, Pheochromocytoma
Adults: Your doctor will prescribe the appropriate dose for you based on your condition.

How should I take this medication?
• Take propranolol exactly as prescribed by your doctor.

What should I avoid while taking this medication?
Do not stop taking propranolol without first talking to your doctor.

What are possible food and drug interactions associated with this medication?
If propranolol is taken with certain other drugs, the effects of either could be increased, decreased, or altered. Propranolol may interact

with numerous medications. Therefore, it is very important that you tell your doctor about any other medications you are taking.

What are the possible side effects of this medication?
Please see general statement regarding side effects on page xiii.

> **Side effects may include:** abdominal cramping, allergic reactions, depression, difficulty breathing, fever, hallucinations, lightheadedness, low blood pressure, male impotence, memory loss, nausea, rash, skin reactions, slower heartbeat, sore throat, tiredness, vivid dreams, vomiting, weakness

Can I receive this medication if I am pregnant or breastfeeding?
The effects of propranolol during pregnancy are unknown. Propranolol can be found in your breast milk if you take it while breastfeeding. Tell your doctor immediately if you are pregnant, plan to become pregnant, or are breastfeeding.

What should I do if I miss a dose of this medication?
If you miss a dose of propranolol, take it as soon as you remember. However, if it is almost time for your next dose, skip the one you missed and return to your regular dosing schedule. Do not take two doses at once.

How should I store this medication?
Store at room temperature. Protect from light.

Propranolol HCl: *see Inderal LA, page 466*

Propranolol HCl: *see Propranolol, page 858*

Protonix

Generic name: Pantoprazole Sodium

What is this medication?

Protonix is a medicine called a proton pump inhibitor (PPI). It reduces the amount of acid in your stomach. Protonix is used in adults for the short-term treatment of erosive esophagitis (inflammation of the esophagus [tube that connects your mouth and stomach] due to excess acid) caused by gastroesophageal reflux disease (GERD), to maintain healing of erosive esophagitis, and to help prevent the return of heartburn symptoms caused by GERD. Protonix is available in tablets and an oral suspension.

Protonix is also used for long-term treatment of conditions where your stomach makes too much acid, such as Zollinger-Ellison syndrome.

In addition, Protonix is used for the short-term treatment of erosive esophagitis caused by GERD in children and adolescents 5-16 years old.

What is the most important information I should know about this medication?

- Protonix can cause low magnesium levels in your body. Tell your doctor immediately if you have seizures, dizziness, abnormal or fast heartbeat, jitteriness, jerking movements or shaking, muscle weakness, spasms of your hands and feet, cramps or muscle aches, or spasm of your voice box.
- Tell your doctor if you experience any symptoms of a serious allergic reaction with Protonix (such as rash, face swelling, throat tightness, or difficulty breathing).
- People who are taking multiple daily doses of Protonix for a long period of time may have an increased risk of fractures of the hip, wrist, or spine.
- Long-term use with Protonix may cause weakening of your stomach lining and low vitamin B12 levels.

Who should not take this medication?

Do not take Protonix if you are allergic to it, any of its ingredients, or any other PPI.

What should I tell my doctor before I take the first dose of this medication?

Tell your doctor about all prescription, over-the-counter, and herbal medications you are taking before beginning treatment with Protonix. Also, talk to your doctor about your complete medical history, especially if you have low magnesium levels. Tell your doctor if you are pregnant, plan to become pregnant, or are breastfeeding.

What is the usual dosage?

Please see general statement regarding dosage on page xii.

Short-Term Treatment of Erosive Esophagitis Associated with GERD

Adults: The recommended dose is 40 milligrams (mg) once a day for up to 8 weeks. Depending on your response, your doctor may suggest another 8 weeks of treatment.

Children ≥5 years: Depending on your child's weight, the recommended dose is 20 mg or 40 mg once a day for up to 8 weeks.

Maintenance of Healing of Erosive Esophagitis

Adults: The recommended dose is 40 mg once a day.

Treatment of Excess Stomach Acid (Such as Zollinger-Ellison Syndrome)

Adults: The recommended dose is 40 mg twice a day. Your doctor might prescribe a different dose or duration based on your condition.

How should I take this medication?

- Take Protonix exactly as prescribed by your doctor. Swallow the tablets whole, with or without food. If you are unable to swallow a 40-mg tablet, take two 20-mg tablets instead.
- Take the oral suspension in applesauce or apple juice 30 minutes before to a meal.

- To take with applesauce, open the packet and sprinkle the granules on 1 teaspoonful of applesauce. Swallow within 10 minutes of preparation. Take sips of water to make sure the granules are washed down into the stomach. Repeat water sips as necessary.
- To take in apple juice, open the packet and empty the granules into a small cup or teaspoon with 1 teaspoonful of apple juice. Stir for 5 seconds and swallow immediately. Rinse the container once or twice with apple juice to remove any remaining granules and swallow immediately to be sure you receive the entire dose.

What should I avoid while taking this medication?

Do not split, chew, or crush the tablets. This will damage them and the medicine will not work.

Do not take the oral suspension in or with water, other liquids, or other foods.

Do not crush or chew the granules for oral suspension.

Do not divide the oral suspension packet to make a smaller dose.

What are possible food and drug interactions associated with this medication?

If Protonix is taken with certain other drugs, the effects of either could be increased, decreased, or altered. It is especially important to check with your doctor before combining Protonix with the following: ampicillin, atazanavir, digoxin, iron supplements, ketoconazole, methotrexate, nelfinavir, or warfarin.

What are the possible side effects of this medication?

Please see general statement regarding side effects on page xiii.

> **Side effects may include:** diarrhea, dizziness, fever, gas, headache, nausea, pain in your joints, rash, stomach pain, upper respiratory infection, vomiting

Can I receive this medication if I am pregnant or breastfeeding?

The effects of Protonix during pregnancy are unknown. Protonix can be found in your breast milk if you take it while breastfeeding. Tell your doctor immediately if you are pregnant, plan to become pregnant, or are breastfeeding.

What should I do if I miss a dose of this medication?

If you miss a dose of Protonix, take it as soon as you remember. However, if it is almost time for your next dose, skip the one you missed and return to your regular dosing schedule. Do not take two doses at once.

How should I store this medication?

Store at room temperature.

Proventil HFA

Generic name: Albuterol Sulfate

What is this medication?

Proventil HFA is an inhaled medicine used to prevent and treat airway narrowing associated with certain breathing problems (such as asthma). Proventil HFA is also used to prevent exercise-induced airway narrowing.

What is the most important information I should know about this medication?

- Do not use Proventil HFA more frequently than your doctor recommends. Increasing the number of doses can be dangerous and may actually make symptoms of asthma worse. If the dose your doctor recommends does not provide relief of your symptoms, or if your symptoms become worse, tell your doctor right away.
- You can have an immediate, serious allergic reaction to the first dose of Proventil HFA, with hives, rash, and swelling of your mouth, throat, lips, or tongue. This medication can cause life-threatening breathing problems, especially with the first dose

from a new canister. If you experience an allergic reaction or trouble breathing, call your doctor right away.

Who should not take this medication?
Do not use Proventil HFA if you are allergic to it or any of its ingredients.

What should I tell my doctor before I take the first dose of this medication?
Tell your doctor about all prescription, over-the-counter, and herbal medications you are taking before beginning treatment with Proventil HFA. Also, talk to your doctor about your complete medical history, especially if you have a heart condition, seizure disorder, high blood pressure, arrhythmia (life-threatening irregular heartbeat), overactive thyroid gland, low blood potassium levels, or diabetes.

What is the usual dosage?
Please see general statement regarding dosage on page xii.

Prevention or Treatment of Airway Narrowing
Adults and children ≥4 years: The usual dose is 2 inhalations every 4-6 hours. Your or your child's doctor will adjust your dose appropriately.

Exercise-Induced Airway Narrowing
Adults and children ≥4 years: The usual dose is 2 inhalations 15-30 minutes before exercise.

How should I take this medication?
• Use Proventil HFA exactly as prescribed by your doctor. Shake the inhaler well before each use.
• You must prime the inhaler if you are using it for the first time and when it has not been used for more than 2 weeks. To do this, press the pump 4 times into the air, away from your face.
• Breathe out fully through your mouth, then place the mouthpiece into your mouth and close your lips around it. While breathing in deeply and slowly through your mouth, press down on the

top of the metal canister. Hold your breath for 10 seconds if possible.

- If your doctor has prescribed more than one inhalation, wait one minute between inhalations. Clean the mouthpiece without the metal canister at least once a week.
- Please review the instructions that came with your prescription on how to properly use Proventil HFA.

What should I avoid while taking this medication?

Do not spray Proventil HFA into your eyes.

Do not inhale extra doses or stop using Proventil HFA without talking to your doctor.

Do not clean the metal canister or allow it to become wet.

What are possible food and drug interactions associated with this medication?

If Proventil HFA is used with certain other drugs, the effects of either could be increased, decreased, or altered. It is especially important to check with your doctor before combining Proventil HFA with the following: blood pressure/heart medications known as beta-blockers (such as metoprolol or propranolol), certain antidepressants (such as amitriptyline or phenelzine), certain diuretics (water pills) (such as furosemide or hydrochlorothiazide), digoxin, or medicines similar to Proventil HFA (such as terbutaline and epinephrine).

What are the possible side effects of this medication?

Please see general statement regarding side effects on page xiii.

Side effects may include: allergic reactions, back pain, breathing problems, feeling or tasting the medicine when you inhale it, fever, inflammation of the lining of your nose, nausea, nervousness, rapid heart rate, shaking, upper respiratory tract infection, urinary tract infection, vomiting

Can I receive this medication if I am pregnant or breastfeeding?

The effects of Proventil HFA during pregnancy and breastfeeding are unknown. Do not breastfeed while you are using Proventil HFA. Tell your doctor immediately if you are pregnant, plan to become pregnant, or are breastfeeding.

What should I do if I miss a dose of this medication?

If you miss a dose of Proventil HFA, take it as soon as you remember. However, if it is almost time for your next dose, skip the one you missed and return to your regular dosing schedule. Do not take two doses at once.

How should I store this medication?

Store at room temperature. Protect from heat or open flame.

Provera

Generic name: Medroxyprogesterone Acetate

What is this medication?

Provera is a medicine that contains a progestin hormone. It is used to treat menstrual periods that have stopped and abnormal uterine bleeding when these conditions are due to an imbalance of hormones. Provera is also used to reduce the risk of uterine cancer in women who are being treated with estrogen.

What is the most important information I should know about this medication?

- Do not use Provera to prevent heart disease, heart attacks, or strokes. Using Provera can increase your chances of getting heart attacks, strokes, breast cancer, or blood clots. It may also increase your risk of dementia.
- If you have high blood pressure, high cholesterol, diabetes, are overweight, or if you smoke, you can have a higher chance of getting heart disease while on Provera.
- You should have a pelvic exam, breast exam, and mammogram (breast x-ray) every year unless your doctor tells you otherwise.

If members of your family have had breast cancer or if you have ever had breast lumps or an abnormal mammogram, you may need to have breast exams more often.

- Estrogens increase your risk of developing endometrial (inner lining of the uterus) cancer. Tell your doctor immediately if you have any unusual vaginal bleeding while you are taking Provera. Vaginal bleeding after menopause may be a warning sign of endometrial cancer.
- Talk regularly with your doctor about whether you still need treatment with Provera.

Who should not take this medication?

Do not take Provera if you are allergic to it or any of its ingredients. Also, do not take Provera if you have undiagnosed vaginal bleeding, currently have or have had certain cancers, liver problems, blood clots, or a stroke or heart attack in the past year.

What should I tell my doctor before I take the first dose of this medication?

Tell your doctor about all prescription, over-the-counter, and herbal medications you are taking before beginning treatment with Provera. Also, talk to your doctor about your complete medical history, especially if you have asthma; diabetes; seizures; migraine headaches; endometriosis (a common gynecological disorder that may result in sores and pain); lupus (disease that affects the immune system); problems with your heart, liver, thyroid, or kidneys; or if you have high calcium levels in your blood.

What is the usual dosage?

Please see general statement regarding dosage on page xii.

To Restore Menstrual Periods

Adults: The usual dose is 5 or 10 milligrams (mg) once a day for 5-10 days.

Abnormal Uterine Bleeding Due to Hormonal Imbalance

Adults: The usual dose is 5 or 10 mg once a day for 5-10 days, beginning on the 16th or 21st day of your menstrual cycle.

<u>**To Accompany Estrogen Replacement Therapy to Reduce Risk**</u>
<u>**of Endometrial Cancer**</u>
Adults: The usual dose is 5 or 10 mg once a day for 12-14 consecutive days per month, either beginning on the 1st or 16th day of your menstrual cycle.

How should I take this medication?

- Take Provera exactly as prescribed by your doctor. Do not take extra doses or take more often without asking your doctor. Start at the lowest dose and talk to your doctor about how well that dose is working for you. You and your doctor should talk regularly (every 3-6 months) about your response to Provera and whether you still need treatment.

What should I avoid while taking this medication?

Do not become pregnant or breastfeed while you are taking Provera.

Do not use Provera as a test for pregnancy.

Do not take Provera for conditions for which it was not prescribed. Do not give Provera to other people, even if they have the same symptoms you have. It may harm them.

What are possible food and drug interactions associated with this medication?

No significant interactions have been reported with Provera at this time. However, always tell your doctor about any medicines you take, including over-the-counter medications, vitamins, and herbal supplements.

What are the possible side effects of this medication?

Please see general statement regarding side effects on page xiii.

Side effects may include: absence of menstrual periods, acne (pimples), bloating, blood clots, breakthrough bleeding, breast milk secretion, breast tenderness, changes in vision, depression, difficulty sleeping, dizziness, fever, hair growth, hair loss, headaches, inflamed veins, irregular periods, itching, nervousness, rash, sleepiness, spotting (minor vaginal bleeding), stomach pain, swelling, tiredness, vaginal secretions, weight gain

These are not all the possible side effects of Provera. For more information, ask your doctor or pharmacist.

Can I receive this medication if I am pregnant or breastfeeding?

Provera may cause harm to your unborn baby if you take it while pregnant. Do not breastfeed while you are taking Provera. Tell your doctor immediately if you are pregnant, plan to become pregnant, or are breastfeeding.

What should I do if I miss a dose of this medication?

If you miss a dose of Provera, take it as soon as you remember. However, if it is almost time for your next dose, skip the one you missed and return to your regular dosing schedule. Do not take two doses at once.

How should I store this medication?

Store at room temperature.

Prozac

Generic name: Fluoxetine HCl

What is this medication?

Prozac is an antidepressant medicine known as a selective serotonin reuptake inhibitor (SSRI). It is used to treat major depressive disorder, obsessive compulsive disorder, bulimia (eating disorder), and panic disorder. Prozac is also used with an antipsychotic medicine called olanzapine to treat depressive episodes associated with bipolar disorder and treatment-resistant depression (depression that has not improved with two separate treatments of different antidepressant medicines).

What is the most important information I should know about this medication?

- Prozac can increase the risk of suicidal thoughts and behavior in children, adolescents, and young adults. Your doctor will monitor you closely for clinical worsening, suicidal or unusual behavior after you start taking Prozac or start a new dose of Prozac. Tell your doctor right away if you experience anxiety, hostility, sleeplessness, restlessness, impulsive or dangerous behavior, or thoughts about suicide or dying; or if you have new symptoms or seem to be feeling worse.

- Prozac can cause serotonin syndrome (a potentially life-threatening drug reaction that causes the body to have too much serotonin, a chemical produced by the nerve cells) or neuroleptic malignant syndrome (a brain disorder) when you take it alone or in combination with other medicines. You can experience mental status changes, an increase in your heart rate and temperature, lack of coordination, overactive reflexes, muscle rigidity, nausea, vomiting, or diarrhea. Tell your doctor right away if you experience any of these signs or symptoms.

- Prozac can cause severe allergic reactions. Tell your doctor right away if you develop a rash, trouble breathing, or swelling of your face, tongue, eyes, or mouth.

- Your risk of abnormal bleeding or bruising can increase if you take Prozac, especially if you also take blood thinners (such as warfarin), nonsteroidal anti-inflammatory drugs (NSAIDs) (such as ibuprofen or naproxen), or aspirin.

- You can experience manic episodes while you are taking Prozac. Tell your doctor if you experience greatly increased energy, severe trouble sleeping, racing thoughts, reckless behavior, unusually grand ideas, excessive happiness or irritability, or talking more or faster than usual.

- Prozac can cause seizures or changes in your appetite or weight. Your doctor will monitor you for these effects during treatment.

- Prozac can decrease your blood sodium levels, especially if you are elderly. Tell your doctor if you have a headache, weakness, an unsteady feeling, confusion, problems concentrating or thinking, or memory problems while you are taking Prozac.

- Prozac can affect your blood sugar levels. If you are a diabetic, make sure you check your blood sugar levels regularly.
- Do not stop taking Prozac without first talking to your doctor. Stopping Prozac suddenly can cause serious symptoms, including anxiety, irritability, changes in your mood, feeling restless, changes in your sleep habits, headache, sweating, nausea, dizziness, electric shock-like sensations, shaking, or confusion.

Who should not take this medication?

Do not take Prozac if you are allergic to it or any of its ingredients.

Do not take Prozac while you are taking other medicines known as monoamine oxidase inhibitors (MAOIs) (such as phenelzine), a class of medications used to treat depression and other conditions. Do not take Prozac if you are taking pimozide or thioridazine.

Do not take Prozac if you are taking medications called Symbyax, Sarafem, or Prozac Weekly since these medicines contain the same active ingredient.

What should I tell my doctor before I take the first dose of this medication?

Tell your doctor about all prescription, over-the-counter, and herbal medications you are taking before beginning treatment with Prozac. Also, talk to your doctor about your complete medical history, especially if you have high blood pressure; heart, liver, or kidney problems; history of stroke; glaucoma (high pressure in the eye); diabetes; bleeding problems; seizures; mania or bipolar disorder; or low blood sodium levels. Also, tell your doctor if you are pregnant, plan to become pregnant, or are breastfeeding.

What is the usual dosage?

Please see general statement regarding dosage on page xii.

Major Depressive Disorder

Adults: The usual starting dose is 20 milligrams (mg) once a day, in the morning.

Children and adolescents 8-18 years: The usual starting dose is 10 or 20 mg once a day.

Obsessive-Compulsive Disorder
Adults: The usual starting dose is 20 mg once a day, in the morning.

Children and adolescents 7-18 years: The usual starting dose is 10 mg once a day.

Bulimia
Adults: The usual dose is 60 mg once a day, in the morning.

Panic Disorder
Adults: The usual starting dose is 10 mg once a day.

Depressive Episodes Associated with Bipolar Disorder and Treatment-Resistant Depression
Adults: The usual starting dose is 20 mg of Prozac once a day and 5 mg of olanzapine once a day, in the evening.

Your doctor will increase your dose as needed until the desired effect is achieved.

If you are elderly or have liver impairment, your doctor will adjust your dose appropriately.

How should I take this medication?
- Take Prozac exactly as prescribed by your doctor. Take Prozac once a day, in the morning or in the evening as directed. Take it with or without food.

What should I avoid while taking this medication?
Do not drive, operate heavy machinery, or engage in other dangerous activities until you know how Prozac affects you.

Do not drink alcohol while you are taking Prozac.

Do not stop taking Prozac suddenly without first talking to your doctor, as this can cause serious side effects.

Do not take Prozac and MAOIs together or within 14 days of each other. Wait at least 5 weeks after stopping Prozac before starting an MAOI. Combining these medicines with Prozac can cause serious and even fatal reactions.

What are possible food and drug interactions associated with this medication?

If Prozac is taken with certain other drugs, the effects of either could be increased, decreased, or altered. Prozac may interact with numerous medications. Therefore, it is very important that you tell your doctor about any other medications you are taking.

What are the possible side effects of this medication?

Please see general statement regarding side effects on page xiii.

Side effects may include: diarrhea; dry mouth; feeling anxious, fatigued, nervous, or tired; "flu-like" symptoms; hot flashes; loss of appetite; nausea; rash; sexual problems; shaking; sinus infection or sore throat; sweating; trouble sleeping; unusual dreams; upset stomach; vomiting; weakness; yawning

Can I receive this medication if I am pregnant or breastfeeding?

The effects of Prozac during pregnancy are unknown. Prozac can be found in your breast milk if you take it while breastfeeding. Do not breastfeed while you are taking Prozac. Tell your doctor immediately if you are pregnant, plan to become pregnant, or are breastfeeding.

What should I do if I miss a dose of this medication?

If you miss a dose of Prozac, take it as soon as you remember. However, if it is almost time for your next dose, skip the one you missed and return to your regular dosing schedule. Do not take two doses at once.

How should I store this medication?

Store at room temperature.

Quetiapine Fumarate: *see Seroquel, page 920*

Quetiapine Fumarate: *see Seroquel XR, page 924*

Quinapril HCl: *see Accupril, page 8*

Qvar

Generic name: Beclomethasone Dipropionate

What is this medication?

Qvar is an inhaled corticosteroid medicine used for the long-term treatment of asthma. It also helps to prevent symptoms of asthma.

What is the most important information I should know about this medication?

- Qvar does not treat the symptoms of a sudden asthma attack. Always have a short-acting rescue inhaler (such as albuterol) to treat sudden symptoms. If you do not have a short-acting inhaler, tell your doctor to have one prescribed for you. Tell your doctor immediately if an asthma attack does not respond to the rescue inhaler or if you require more doses than usual.
- If you use Qvar, you can have a higher risk of getting an infection. If you have not had or not been vaccinated against chickenpox or measles, stay away from people who are infected while you are using Qvar. Tell your doctor immediately if you are exposed to these diseases.
- Qvar can cause slowed or delayed growth in children. Check your child's growth regularly during treatment with Qvar.
- It may take 1-4 weeks after starting Qvar for your asthma symptoms to improve. Tell your doctor if your symptoms do not improve or get worse.

• Do not stop using Qvar or change your dose, even if your symptoms get better. Your doctor will change your medicine as needed.

Who should not take this medication?

Do not take Qvar if you are allergic to it or any of its ingredients. Do not use Qvar to treat a sudden severe asthma attack.

What should I tell my doctor before I take the first dose of this medication?

Tell your doctor about all prescription, over-the-counter, and herbal medications you are taking before beginning treatment with Qvar. Also, talk to your doctor about your complete medical history, especially if you have or had chickenpox or measles, or have recently been near anyone with chickenpox or measles; have tuberculosis (a bacterial infection that affects the lungs), or any type of infection; or have cataracts or glaucoma. Tell your doctor if you take a corticosteroid medicine, or medicines that suppress your immune system (such as cyclosporine or tacrolimus).

What is the usual dosage?

Please see general statement regarding dosage on page xii.

Adults and adolescents ≥12 years: Your doctor will prescribe the appropriate dose for you based on your previous asthma medication.

Children 4-11 years: The recommended starting dose is 40 micrograms twice a day.

How should I take this medication?

• Use Qvar exactly as prescribed by your doctor. You do not need to shake the inhaler before use.
• If you are using the inhaler for the first time or have not used it for more than 10 days, you must prime it. To do this, take the cap off the mouthpiece, then spray the inhaler two times into the air, away from your eyes and face.
• Breathe out as fully as you comfortably can, then place the mouthpiece into your mouth and close your lips around it,

keeping your tongue below it. While breathing in deeply and slowly, press down on the can with your finger. When you have finished breathing in, hold your breath for 5-10 seconds if possible.
• Rinse your mouth with water after treatment.
• Please be sure to review the instructions that came with your prescription on how to properly use Qvar.

What should I avoid while taking this medication?
Do not spray Qvar in your eyes.

Do not wash or put any part of your inhaler in water.

Discard the canister after the date calculated by your doctor or pharmacist.

Do not use the mouthpiece with any other inhaler. Qvar canister should only be used with the Qvar mouthpiece.

What are possible food and drug interactions associated with this medication?
No significant interactions have been reported with Qvar at this time. However, always tell your doctor about any medicines you take, including over-the-counter medications, vitamins, and herbal supplements.

What are the possible side effects of this medication?
Please see general statement regarding side effects on page xiii.

Side effects may include: back pain; cough; headache; increased asthma symptoms; inflammation of your nose, sinuses, or throat; nausea; upper respiratory tract infection; voice problems

---

Can I receive this medication if I am pregnant or breastfeeding?
The effects of Qvar during pregnancy are unknown. Qvar can be found in your breast milk if you use it while breastfeeding. Tell your

doctor immediately if you are pregnant, plan to become pregnant, or are breastfeeding.

What should I do if I miss a dose of this medication?
If you miss a dose of Qvar, take it as soon as you remember. However, if it is almost time for your next dose, skip the one you missed and return to your regular dosing schedule. Do not take two doses at once.

How should I store this medication?
Store at room temperature. Do not store near heat or open flame.

Rabeprazole Sodium: see Aciphex, page 12

Raloxifene HCl: see Evista, page 378

Ramipril: see Altace, page 55

Ranitidine HCl: see Zantac, page 1124

Remeron
Generic name: Mirtazapine

What is this medication?
Remeron is an antidepressant medication. It is used to treat major depressive disorder (MDD).

What is the most important information I should know about this medication?
- Remeron can increase the risk of suicidal thoughts and behavior in children, adolescents, and young adults. Your doctor will monitor you closely for clinical worsening, suicidality, or unusual behavior after you start taking Remeron or a new dose. Tell your doctor immediately if you experience anxiety, hostility, sleeplessness, restlessness, impulsive or dangerous behavior,

or thoughts about suicide or dying; or if you have new symptoms or seem to be feeling worse.

- You can experience manic episodes while you are taking Remeron. Tell your doctor if you experience greatly increased energy, severe trouble sleeping, racing thoughts, reckless behavior, unusually grand ideas, excessive happiness or irritability, or talking more or faster than usual.

- Remeron can lower your white blood cells called neutrophils (type of blood cells that fight infections). Tell your doctor if you develop fever, chills, sore throat, mouth or nose sores, or other "flu-like" symptoms.

- Remeron can cause serotonin syndrome (a potentially life-threatening drug reaction that causes the body to have too much serotonin, a chemical produced by the nerve cells) or neuroleptic malignant syndrome (a brain disorder) when you take it alone or in combination with other medicines. You can experience agitation, hallucinations, coma or other mental status changes; coordination problems or muscle twitching (overactive reflexes); racing heartbeat, high or low blood pressure; sweating or fever; nausea, vomiting, or diarrhea; or muscle rigidity. Tell your doctor right away if you experience any of these signs or symptoms.

- Remeron can cause seizures or changes in your appetite or weight. Your doctor will monitor you for these effects during treatment. Also, Remeron can decrease your blood sodium levels, especially if you are elderly. Tell your doctor if you have a headache, weakness, feeling unsteady, confusion, problems concentrating or thinking, or memory problems while you are taking Remeron.

- Remeron can cause severe allergic reactions or severe skin reactions. Stop taking this medication and tell your doctor immediately if you develop a rash, trouble breathing, or swelling of your face, tongue, eyes, or mouth.

- Do not stop taking Remeron without first talking to your doctor. Stopping Remeron suddenly can cause serious symptoms, including dizziness, abnormal dreams, agitation, anxiety, fatigue, confusion, headache, shaking, tingling sensation, nausea, vomiting, or sweating.

Who should not take this medication?

Do not take Remeron if you are allergic to it or any of its ingredients.

Do not take Remeron if you are taking monoamine oxidase inhibitors (MAOIs), a class of drugs used to treat depression and other psychiatric conditions, or if you stopped taking an MAOI in the last 14 days.

What should I tell my doctor before I take the first dose of this medication?

Tell your doctor about all prescription, over-the-counter, and herbal medications you are taking before beginning treatment with Remeron. Also, talk to your doctor about your complete medical history, especially if you have liver or kidney disease, heart problems, seizures or convulsions, bipolar disorder or mania, a tendency to get dizzy or faint, or if you are pregnant, plan to become pregnant, or are breastfeeding.

What is the usual dosage?

Please see general statement regarding dosage on page xii.

Adults: The recommended starting dose is 15 milligrams once a day. Your doctor may increase your dose as appropriate.

If you are elderly or have kidney or liver impairment, your doctor will adjust your dose appropriately.

How should I take this medication?

• Take Remeron exactly as prescribed by your doctor. Do not change the dose or stop taking this medication abruptly without first talking to your doctor.
• Take Remeron as a single dose at the same time each day, preferably in the evening before you sleep. You can take Remeron with or without food.

What should I avoid while taking this medication?

Do not drive, operate heavy machinery, or do other dangerous activities until you know how Remeron affects you. Remeron can cause dizziness or may affect your ability to make decisions, think clearly, or react quickly.

Do not drink alcohol or take other medications that make you sleepy or dizzy while taking Remeron.

What are possible food and drug interactions associated with this medication?
If Remeron is taken with certain other drugs, the effects of either could be increased, decreased, or altered. It is especially important to check with your doctor before combining Remeron with the following: alcohol, carbamazepine, cimetidine, diazepam, erythromycin, ketoconazole, linezolid, lithium, MAOIs, nefazodone, phenytoin, rifampicin, serotonin reuptake inhibitors, St. John's wort, tramadol, triptans, tryptophan, venlafaxine, and warfarin.

What are the possible side effects of this medication?
Please see general statement regarding side effects on page xiii.

> **Side effects may include:** abnormal dreams, abnormal thinking, confusion, constipation, dizziness, drowsiness, dry mouth, "flu-like" symptoms, increased appetite, nausea, sleepiness, weight gain, weakness

Can I receive this medication if I am pregnant or breastfeeding?
The effects of Remeron during pregnancy and breastfeeding are unknown. Tell your doctor immediately if you are pregnant, plan to become pregnant, or are breastfeeding.

What should I do if I miss a dose of this medication?
If you miss a dose of Remeron, take it as soon as you remember. However, if it is almost time for your next dose, skip the one you missed and return to your regular dosing schedule. Do not take two doses at once.

How should I store this medication?
Store at room temperature. Keep away from light.

Requip

Generic name: Ropinirole HCl

What is this medication?

Requip is a medicine used to treat the symptoms of Parkinson's disease. Requip is also used to treat moderate to severe primary restless legs syndrome (RLS) (urge to move one's body to stop uncomfortable or odd sensations). Requip is available in tablets and extended-release tablets (Requip XL).

Requip XL is used to treat the symptoms of Parkinson's disease. It is not used for the treatment of RLS.

What is the most important information I should know about this medication?

• Requip can cause sleepiness or falling asleep during the day without warning while you are doing everyday activities (such as talking, eating, or driving a car). Tell your doctor if you experience any of these symptoms. Do not drive a car, operate machinery, or do anything that might put you at risk of getting hurt until you know how Requip affects you.

• Requip can cause changes in your blood pressure. If you faint, feel dizzy, nauseated, or sweaty when you stand up from sitting or lying down, this can mean that your blood pressure is decreased. This effect usually happens when you start Requip treatment or when the dose is increased. Do not get up too fast from sitting or after lying down, especially if you have been sitting or lying down for a long period of time.

• Requip can cause or worsen mental or psychotic problems, or cause unusual behavior. Tell your doctor if you experience hallucinations (seeing or hearing things that are not real), confusion, excessive suspicion, aggressive behavior, agitation, delusional beliefs (believing things that are not real), disorganized thinking, feeling of depression, new or increased gambling urges, increased sexual urges, or other intense urges.

• Requip can also cause or worsen dyskinesias (sudden uncontrolled movements), especially if you are taking levodopa. Tell your doctor if you are taking levodopa before taking Requip.

Who should not take this medication?

Do not take Requip if you are allergic to it or any of its ingredients.

What should I tell my doctor before I take the first dose of this medication?

Tell your doctor about all prescription, over-the-counter, and herbal medications you are taking before beginning treatment with Requip. Also, talk to your doctor about your complete medical history, especially if you have a past history of heart disease, have daytime sleepiness from a sleep disorder, have high or low blood pressure, are pregnant, plan to become pregnant, are breastfeeding, or if you smoke or drink alcohol.

What is the usual dosage?

Please see general statement regarding dosage on page xii.

Parkinson's Disease

Adults: The recommended starting dose of Requip is 0.25 milligrams (mg) three times a day. The recommended starting dose of Requip XL is 2 mg once a day. Your doctor will prescribe the appropriate dose for you and will increase your dose as needed, until the desired effect is achieved.

Restless Legs Syndrome

Adults: The recommended starting dose of Requip is 0.25 mg once a day, 1 to 3 hours before bedtime. Your doctor will prescribe the appropriate dose for you and will increase your dose as needed, until the desired effect is achieved.

How should I take this medication?

- Take Requip or Requip XL exactly as prescribed by your doctor. Do not suddenly stop taking Requip or Requip XL without talking to your doctor.
- Take Requip XL tablets at or around the same time each day. Swallow Requip XL tablets whole. Do not chew, crush, or split the tablets.
- You can take Requip or Requip XL with or without food. If you feel nausea, taking the tablets with food can help.

What should I avoid while taking this medication?

Do not drink alcohol or take medications that will make you drowsy while you are taking Requip.

Do not drive, operate machinery, or work at heights until you know how Requip affects you.

What are possible food and drug interactions associated with this medication?

If Requip is taken with certain other drugs, the effects of either could be increased, decreased, or altered. It is especially important to check with your doctor before combining Requip with the following: alcohol, certain antipsychotics (such as butyrophenones, phenothiazines, or thioxanthenes), ciprofloxacin, estrogens, levodopa, metoclopramide, or other medications that cause drowsiness.

What are the possible side effects of this medication?

Please see general statement regarding side effects on page xiii.

Side effects may include: changes in blood pressure, dizziness, fainting, falling asleep during normal activities, hallucinations, headache, leg swelling, nausea, sleepiness, sweating, tiredness, uncontrolled sudden movements, upset stomach, vomiting

Can I receive this medication if I am pregnant or breastfeeding?

The effects of Requip during pregnancy are unknown. Requip can be found in your breast milk if you take it while breastfeeding. Tell your doctor immediately if you are pregnant, plan to become pregnant, or are breastfeeding.

What should I do if I miss a dose of this medication?

If you miss a dose of Requip, take it as soon as you remember. However, if it is almost time for your next dose, skip the one you missed and return to your regular dosing schedule. Do not take two doses at once.

How should I store this medication?

Store at room temperature. Protect from direct sunlight.

Restasis

Generic name: Cyclosporine

What is this medication?

Restasis is an eye drop medicine used to increase tear production for dry eyes caused by eye inflammation.

What is the most important information I should know about this medication?

- Restasis is for use in your eyes only.
- Restasis is not used to treat eye dryness that is related to an infection. Tell your doctor if you have ever had herpes in either eye.

Who should not take this medication?

Do not use Restasis if you are allergic to it or any of its ingredients.

Do not use Restasis if you currently have an eye infection.

What should I tell my doctor before I take the first dose of this medication?

Tell your doctor about all prescription, over-the-counter, and herbal medications you are taking before beginning treatment with Restasis. Also, talk to your doctor about your complete medical history, especially if you have an eye infection.

What is the usual dosage?

Please see general statement regarding dosage on page xii.

Adults: Apply 1 drop into the affected eye(s) twice a day, about 12 hours apart.

How should I take this medication?

- Apply Restasis exactly as prescribed by your doctor.

- Turn each individual, single-use vial upside down a few times before use to mix the solution (it should look white with no streaks). After opening the vial, insert Restasis drops into one or both eyes right away.
- Throw away the remaining contents in each vial after using it. You can use artificial tears during treatment with Restasis. If you use artificial tears, use it at least 15 minutes before or after using Restasis.
- Restasis contains a preservative that may be absorbed by your contact lenses. Remove your contact lenses prior to the administration of Restasis and reinsert them after 15 minutes.

What should I avoid while taking this medication?

Do not allow the tip of the vial to touch your eye or any surface, as this can contaminate Restasis.

What are possible food and drug interactions associated with this medication?

No significant interactions have been reported with Restasis at this time. However, always tell your doctor about any medicines you take, including over-the-counter medications, vitamins, and herbal supplements.

What are the possible side effects of this medication?

Please see general statement regarding side effects on page xiii.

> **Side effects may include:** burning in your eye, eye discharge, eye pain, foreign body sensation, itching and stinging of your eye, red eye, visual disturbances or blurring, watery eyes

Can I receive this medication if I am pregnant or breastfeeding?

The effects of Restasis during pregnancy and breastfeeding are unknown. Tell your doctor immediately if you are pregnant, plan to become pregnant, or are breastfeeding.

What should I do if I miss a dose of this medication?

If you miss a dose of Restasis, apply it as soon as you remember. However, if it is almost time for your next dose, skip the one you missed and return to your regular dosing schedule. Do not apply two doses at once.

How should I store this medication?

Store at room temperature.

Restoril

Generic name: Temazepam

What is this medication?

Restoril is a medicine used for the short-term treatment of a sleep problem called insomnia.

Restoril is a federally controlled substance because it has abuse potential.

What is the most important information I should know about this medication?

- Restoril has abuse potential and can cause dependence. Mental and physical dependence can occur with the use of Restoril when it is used improperly for long periods of time. Keep Restoril in a safe place to prevent misuse and abuse. Selling or giving away Restoril can harm others, and is against the law. Tell your doctor if you have ever abused or have been dependent on alcohol, prescription medicines, or street drugs.
- Tell your doctor if your insomnia worsens or is not better within 7-10 days. This may mean that there is another condition causing your sleep problem.
- Restoril can cause a serious allergic reaction. Get emergency medical help right away if you develop swelling of your tongue or throat, difficulty breathing, or nausea and vomiting.
- Restoril can cause you to get up out of bed while not being fully awake and engage in activities that you do not know you are doing (such as driving a car ["sleep-driving"], making and eating

food, talking on the phone, having sex, or sleep-walking). Tell
your doctor right away if you find out that you have done any of
these activities after taking Restoril.
- Restoril can also cause you to have abnormal thoughts or behavior, memory loss, or anxiety. Tell your doctor if you experience more outgoing or aggressive behavior than normal, confusion, agitation, hallucinations, worsening of your depression, or
suicidal thought or actions.

Who should not take this medication?
Do not take Restoril if you are allergic to it or any of its ingredients.

Do not take Restoril if you are pregnant or plan to become pregnant.

What should I tell my doctor before I take the first dose of this medication?
Tell your doctor about all prescription, over-the-counter, and herbal
medications you are taking before beginning treatment with Restoril. Also, talk to your doctor about your complete medical history,
especially if you have a history of depression, mental illness, or
suicidal thoughts; have a history of drug or alcohol abuse or addiction; have kidney or liver disease; have lung disease or breathing problems; or are pregnant, plan to become pregnant, or are
breastfeeding.

What is the usual dosage?
Please see general statement regarding dosage on page xii.

   Adults: The recommended dose is 15 milligrams right before you
   get in bed. Your doctor may give you a lower or higher dose based
   on your condition.

If you are elderly, your doctor will adjust your dose appropriately.

How should I take this medication?
- Take Restoril exactly as prescribed by your doctor. Take it right
before you go to bed.
- Do not take Restoril unless you are able to get a full night's sleep.

What should I avoid while taking this medication?
Do not stop taking Restoril without first talking to your doctor.

Do not drive or engage in other dangerous activities after taking Restoril until you feel fully awake.

What are possible food and drug interactions associated with this medication?
If Restoril is taken with certain other drugs, the effects of either could be increased, decreased, or altered. It is especially important to check with your doctor before combing Restoril with other medicines that can make you sleepy.

What are the possible side effects of this medication?
Please see general statement regarding side effects on page xiii.

> **Side effects may include:** dizziness, drowsiness, "hangover" feeling the next day, headache, nausea, nervousness, tiredness

Can I receive this medication if I am pregnant or breastfeeding?
Do not take Restoril if you are pregnant. Restoril can harm your unborn baby. The effects of Restoril during breastfeeding are unknown. Tell your doctor immediately if you are pregnant, plan to become pregnant, or are breastfeeding.

What should I do if I miss a dose of this medication?
Restoril should be taken under special circumstances. If you miss your scheduled dose, contact your doctor or pharmacist for advice.

How should I store this medication?
Store at room temperature.

Retin-A

Generic name: Tretinoin

What is this medication?

Retin-A is a topical medicine (applied directly on the skin) used to treat acne. It is available in a gel, cream, and solution.

What is the most important information I should know about this medication?

- Retin-A is for external use only. Do not use it in your eyes, mouth, or corners of your nose.
- Limit sun exposure while you are using Retin-A. If you have a sunburn, wait until it fully recovers before you start this medicine. Use sunscreen products (at least SPF 15) and wear protective clothing over treated areas when you cannot avoid being exposed to the sun. Weather extremes, such as wind and cold, can irritate your skin and should also be avoided while using this medicine.
- During the early weeks of treatment, a worsening of your condition can occur due to the action of Retin-A on deep, previously unseen lesions. Acne usually improves after 6-12 weeks of treatment. If it gets worse, do not stop using Retin-A, but tell your doctor.

Who should not take this medication?

Do not use Retin-A if you are allergic to it or any of its ingredients.

What should I tell my doctor before I take the first dose of this medication?

Tell your doctor about all prescription, over-the-counter, and herbal medications you are taking before beginning treatment with Retin-A, especially if you have any allergies, sunburn, or other skin disorders such as eczema (an inflammation or irritation of the skin).

What is the usual dosage?

Please see general statement regarding dosage on page xii.

Adults: Apply to the affected area(s) once a day.

How should I take this medication?

- Apply Retin-A exactly as prescribed by your doctor. Retin-A is usually used in the evening. Cleanse the affected area thoroughly before applying Retin-A. Use enough medication to lightly cover the affected area. Any change in dosage form, strength, or frequency should be closely monitored by your doctor to determine your tolerance and response.
- For Retin-A liquid, you can use a fingertip, gauze pad, or cotton swab to apply it. Do not put too much of the solution on the gauze or cotton so that it does not run into areas where treatment is not intended.

What should I avoid while taking this medication?

Do not use Retin-A in your eyes, mouth, or corners of your nose.

Do not use a harsh soap; avoid frequent washings and harsh scrubbing.

Do not excessively expose your skin to the sun, wind, or cold to prevent further irritation.

Do not expose Retin-A gel to heat or flame.

What are possible food and drug interactions associated with this medication?

If Retin-A is used with certain other drugs, the effects of either could be increased, decreased, or altered. It is important to check with your doctor before combining Retin-A with any other medication.

What are the possible side effects of this medication?

Please see general statement regarding side effects on page xiii.

Side effects may include: allergic reactions, blistering, changes in skin color, crusting or peeling of your skin, redness, sensitivity to sunlight, skin irritation, swelling

Can I receive this medication if I am pregnant or breastfeeding?

The effects of Retin-A during pregnancy and breastfeeding are unknown. Tell your doctor immediately if you are pregnant, plan to become pregnant, or are breastfeeding.

What should I do if I miss a dose of this medication?

If you miss a dose of Retin-A apply it as soon as you remember. However, if it is almost time for your next dose, skip the one you missed and return to your regular dosing schedule. Do not apply two doses at once.

How should I store this medication?

Store at room temperature.

Rhinocort Aqua

Generic name: Budesonide

What is this medication?

Rhinocort Aqua is a medicine used to treat nasal symptoms (such as stuffy and runny nose, itching, or sneezing) of seasonal or year-round allergies. Rhinocort Aqua is available as a nasal spray.

What is the most important information I should know about this medication?

- Rhinocort Aqua is for use in your nose only.
- Rhinocort Aqua can cause infections in your nose and throat, form a hole in the wall between your nostrils, or impair wound healing. Do not use Rhinocort Aqua if you have a sore in your nose, have had nasal surgery, or a recent nasal injury until healing has occurred.
- Cataracts (clouding of the eye's lens), glaucoma (high pressure in the eye), or other eye problems can occur while you are using Rhinocort Aqua. Tell your doctor if you experience a change in your vision.
- If you use Rhinocort Aqua, you can have a higher risk of getting an infection. Do not expose yourself to chickenpox or measles

while you are using Rhinocort Aqua. This can be very serious and even fatal in children and adults who have not had chicken-pox or measles.

- Use Rhinocort Aqua with caution if you have active or inactive tuberculosis (a bacterial infection that affects the lungs), or un-treated fungal, bacterial, or viral infections.
- Rhinocort Aqua can cause slowed or delayed growth in children. Check your child's growth regularly during treatment with Rhi-nocort Aqua.
- A decrease in nasal symptoms may occur 10 hours after start-ing treatment with Rhinocort Aqua. The full benefit of Rhinocort Aqua may not be achieved until you have used it for several days. Tell your doctor if your symptoms do not improve within that time, or if your condition worsens.

Who should not take this medication?

Do not use Rhinocort Aqua if you are allergic to it or any of its ingredients.

What should I tell my doctor before I take the first dose of this medication?

Tell your doctor about all prescription, over-the-counter, and herbal medications you are taking before beginning treatment with Rhi-nocort Aqua. Also, talk to your doctor about your complete medi-cal history, especially if you recently had nasal sores, surgery, or injury; have eye or vision problems; have any infections or had exposure to chickenpox or measles; liver problems; or if you have asthma or other medical conditions that require long-term steroid treatment.

What is the usual dosage?

Please see general statement regarding dosage on page xii.

Adults and children ≥6 years: The recommended starting dose is 1 spray in each nostril once a day. Your doctor will increase your dose as needed, until the desired effect is achieved.

How should I take this medication?

- Use Rhinocort Aqua exactly as prescribed by your doctor. Shake the bottle gently before each use.
- You must prime the nasal spray unit if you are using it for the first time. To do this, press the pump eight times. Also, you must prime the pump by pressing one time or until you see a fine mist if it has not been used for 2 days in a row or longer.
- Gently blow your nose to clear your nostrils. Close one nostril and tilt your head forward slightly when you spray Rhinocort Aqua into each of your nostrils. Gently breathe in through your nostril and while breathing in press down on the applicator to release a spray.
- Please review the instructions that came with your prescription on how to properly use Rhinocort Aqua.

What should I avoid while taking this medication?

Do not spray Rhinocort Aqua into your eyes.

Do not apply extra doses or stop using Rhinocort Aqua without talking to your doctor.

What are possible food and drug interactions associated with this medication?

If Rhinocort Aqua is used with certain other drugs, the effects of either could be increased, decreased, or altered. It is especially important to check with your doctor before combining Rhinocort Aqua with atazanavir, clarithromycin, indinavir, itraconazole, ketoconazole, nefazodone, nelfinavir, ritonavir, saquinavir, or telithromycin.

What are the possible side effects of this medication?

Please see general statement regarding side effects on page xiii.

Side effects may include: cough, difficulty breathing (such as chest tightening or wheezing), irritation of your nose, nose bleeds, sore throat

Can I receive this medication if I am pregnant or breastfeeding?

The effects of Rhinocort Aqua during pregnancy and breastfeeding are unknown. Tell your doctor immediately if you are pregnant, plan to become pregnant, or are breastfeeding.

What should I do if I miss a dose of this medication?

If you miss a dose of Rhinocort Aqua, apply it as soon as you remember. However, if it is almost time for your next dose, skip the one you missed and return to your regular dosing schedule. Do not apply two doses at once.

How should I store this medication?

Store at room temperature in an upright position. Protect from light and do not freeze.

Rilpivirine: see Edurant, page 352

Risedronate Sodium: see Actonel, page 14

Risperdal

Generic name: Risperidone

What is this medication?

Risperdal is a medication used to treat schizophrenia. It is also used for the short-term treatment of mania associated with bipolar disorder and irritability associated with autistic disorders in children and adolescents. Risperdal is available in tablets, oral solution, and oral desintegrating tablets (Risperdal M-Tab).

What is the most important information I should know about this medication?

• Risperdal can increase your risk of death when it is used to treat mental problems caused by dementia (an illness involving loss of memory and judgment, or confusion) in elderly patients.

Risperdal is not approved to treat mental problems caused by dementia.

- Risperdal can cause tardive dyskinesia (abnormal muscle movements, including tremor, shuffling, and uncontrolled, involuntary movements). Elderly women appear to be at a higher risk for this condition. Tell your doctor immediately if you begin to have any involuntary muscle movements. You may need to discontinue Risperdal therapy.

- Risperdal can mask signs and symptoms of medication overdose and of conditions such as intestinal obstruction, brain tumor, and Reye's syndrome (a potentially fatal disease of the brain and liver that most commonly occurs in children after a viral infection, such as chickenpox). Risperdal can also cause difficulty when swallowing, which in turn can cause a type of pneumonia.

- Risperdal can cause neuroleptic malignant syndrome (NMS) (a life-threatening brain disorder) marked by muscle stiffness or rigidity, fast heartbeat or irregular pulse, increased sweating, high fever, and blood pressure irregularities. Tell your doctor immediately if you experience any of these symptoms.

- Risperdal can increase your risk of developing high blood sugar. See your doctor immediately if you develop signs of high blood sugar, including dry mouth, unusual thirst, increased urination, or fatigue. If you have diabetes or have a high risk of developing it, see your doctor regularly for blood sugar testing.

- Risperdal can affect the production of disease-fighting white blood cells. Tell your doctor immediately if you have a fever or infection.

- Risperdal can cause dizziness, lightheadedness, or fainting. Alcohol, hot weather, exercise, or fever may increase these effects. To prevent them, sit up or stand slowly, especially in the morning. Sit or lie down at the first sign of any of these effects. These effects may be more prominent when you first start taking Risperdal.

- Risperdal can impair your judgment, thinking, or motor skills. Do not drive or perform other possibly unsafe tasks until you know how Risperdal affects you.

- Risperdal can increase the amount of prolactin in your blood (a hormone which can affect lactation, menstruation, and fertility).

If high prolactin levels develop, you can experience enlarged breasts, missed menstrual periods, decreased sexual ability, or nipple discharge. Tell your doctor immediately if you have any of these symptoms.

- Risperdal can rarely cause a prolonged, painful erection. This could happen even when you are not having sex. If this is not treated right away, it could lead to permanent sexual problems such as impotence. Tell your doctor immediately if this happens.
- In rare instances, Risperdal can cause seizures. It is important to tell your doctor if you have a history of seizures.

Who should not take this medication?
Do not take Risperdal if you are allergic to it or any of its ingredients.

Risperdal must not be used in elderly patients and in those with dementia due to an increased risk of death.

Do not take the Risperdal M-Tab formulation if you have phenyl-ketonuria (an inability to process phenylalanine, a protein in your body).

What should I tell my doctor before I take the first dose of this medication?
Tell your doctor about all prescription, over-the-counter, and herbal medications you are taking before beginning treatment with Risperdal. Also, talk to your doctor about your complete medical history, especially if you have breast cancer, liver, kidney or heart disease, high or low blood pressure, heart rhythm problems, a history of heart attack or stroke, seizures, alcohol or substance abuse or dependence, diabetes or elevated blood sugar, Alzheimer's disease or dementia, stomach or bowel problems, history of neuroleptic malignant syndrome, a history of suicidal thoughts, phenylketon-uria, Parkinson's disease, trouble swallowing, or a low white blood cell count.

What is the usual dosage?
Please see general statement regarding dosage on page xii.

Irritability Associated with Autistic Disorder
Children and adolescents 5-16 years: Your doctor will prescribe the appropriate dose for your child.

Bipolar Mania (Short-Term Treatment of Acute Episodes)
Adults: The recommended starting dose is 2-3 milligrams (mg) a day, given as a single dose. Your doctor will adjust your dose as necessary to achieve the optimal effect.

Children and adolescents 10-17 years: The recommended starting dose is 0.5 mg a day, given as a single dose. Your doctor will adjust your dose as necessary to achieve the optimal effect.

Schizophrenia
Adults: The recommended starting dose is 2 mg a day, given once a day, or divided in half, and taken twice a day. Your doctor will adjust your dose as necessary to achieve the optimal effect.

Adolescents 13-17 years: The recommended starting dose is 0.5 mg a day, given as a single dose. Your doctor will adjust your dose as necessary to the achieve optimal effect.

How should I take this medication?
- Take Risperdal exactly as prescribed by your doctor. Do not take extra doses or take more often without asking your doctor.
- You can take Risperdal with or without food. Take Risperdal on a regular schedule to get the most benefit from it. Taking Risperdal at the same time each day will help you remember to take it.
- Continue to take Risperdal even if you feel well. Do not miss any doses.
- Risperdal oral solution comes with a calibrated pipette to use for measuring. The oral solution can be taken with water, coffee, orange juice, and low-fat milk, but not with cola drinks or tea.
- Risperdal M-Tab comes in 0.5 mg, 1 mg, 2 mg, 3 mg, and 4 mg strengths. Remove the tablets from the blister unit with dry hands and immediately place it on the tongue. The tablets are

designed to quickly dissolve in your mouth, and can be swallowed with liquid if needed. Do not chew or divide the tablets.

What should I avoid while taking this medication?

Risperdal can make you sleepy. Avoid driving or operating dangerous machinery and do not participate in any activities that require full alertness until you know how Risperdal affects you.

Do not drink alcohol while you are taking Risperdal.

Check with your doctor before taking medicines that may cause drowsiness (such as sleep aids or muscle relaxers) while you are using Risperdal; it may add to their effects.

What are possible food and drug interactions associated with this medication?

If Risperdal is taken with certain other drugs, the effects of either could be increased, decreased, or altered. It is especially important to check with your doctor before combining Risperdal with the following: blood pressure medicines, bromocriptine mesylate, carbamazepine, cimetidine, clozapine, fluoxetine, levodopa, paroxetine, phenobarbital, phenytoin, quinidine, ranitidine, rifampin, or valproic acid.

What are the possible side effects of this medication?

Please see general statement regarding side effects on page xiii.

> **Side effects may include:** abdominal (stomach) pain, anxiety, constipation, cough, difficulty sleeping, dizziness, drooling, dry mouth, fatigue, headache, increased appetite, nasal congestion, nausea, rash, sedation, stuffy nose, tremor, vomiting

Can I receive this medication if I am pregnant or breastfeeding?

The effects of Risperdal during pregnancy are unknown. Risperdal is excreted in breast milk; do not breastfeed while you are taking Risperdal. Tell your doctor immediately if you are pregnant, plan to become pregnant, or are breastfeeding.

What should I do if I miss a dose of this medication?

If you miss a dose of Risperdal, take it as soon as you remember. However, if it is almost time for your next dose, skip the one you missed and return to your regular dosing schedule. Do not take two doses at once.

How should I store this medication?

Store at room temperature. Protect the tablets from light and moisture. Protect the oral solution from light and freezing.

Risperdal Consta

Generic name: Risperidone

What is this medication?

Risperdal Consta is a medicine used to treat schizophrenia. It is also used to treat bipolar disorder alone or in combination with lithium or valproate. Risperdal Consta is administered intramuscularly (injected into the muscle).

What is the most important information I should know about this medication?

- Risperdal Consta can increase the risk of stroke in elderly patients. Risperdal Consta is not approved to treat psychosis in the elderly with dementia (an illness involving loss of memory, judgement, and confusion).
- Risperdal Consta can cause neuroleptic malignant syndrome (NMS) (a life-threatening brain disorder) marked by muscle stiffness or rigidity, fast heartbeat or irregular pulse, increased sweating, high fever, and blood pressure irregularities. Tell your doctor immediately if you experience any of these symptoms.
- Risperdal Consta can cause tardive dyskinesia (abnormal muscle movements, including tremor, shuffling, and uncontrolled, involuntary movements). Elderly women may be at a higher risk for this condition. Tell your doctor immediately if you begin to have any involuntary muscle movements.
- Risperdal Consta can increase your risk of developing high blood sugar and diabetes. See your doctor immediately if you

develop signs of high blood sugar, including dry mouth, unusual thirst, increased urination, or fatigue. If you have diabetes or have a high risk of developing it, see your doctor regularly for blood sugar testing.

- Risperdal Consta can increase the amount of prolactin in your blood (a hormone that can affect lactation, menstruation, and fertility). If high prolactin levels develop, you can experience enlarged breasts, missed menstrual periods, decreased sexual ability, or nipple discharge. Tell your doctor immediately if you have any of these symptoms.

- Risperdal Consta can cause dizziness, lightheadedness, or fainting. To prevent this, sit up or stand slowly, especially in the morning. Sit or lie down at the first sign of any of these effects. These effects may be more prominent when you first start taking Risperdal Consta.

- Risperdal Consta can affect the production of disease-fighting white blood cells. Tell your doctor immediately if you have a fever or infection.

- In rare instances, Risperdal Consta can cause seizures. Tell your doctor if you have a history of seizures.

- Risperdal Consta can rarely cause a prolonged, painful erection. This could happen even when you are not having sex. If this is not treated right away, it could lead to permanent sexual problems (such as impotence). Tell your doctor immediately if this happens.

- Risperdal Consta can mask signs and symptoms of medication overdose and of conditions such as intestinal obstruction, brain tumor, and Reye's syndrome (a potentially fatal disease of the brain and liver that most commonly occurs in children after a viral infection, such as chickenpox). Risperdal Consta can also cause difficulty when swallowing, which in turn can cause a type of pneumonia.

Who should not take this medication?

Your doctor will not administer Risperdal Consta to you if you are allergic to it or any of its ingredients.

What should I tell my doctor before I take the first dose of this medication?

Tell your doctor about all prescription, over-the-counter, and herbal medications you are taking before beginning treatment with Risperdal Consta. Also, talk to your doctor about your complete medical history, especially if you have breast cancer; liver, kidney, or heart disease; high or low blood pressure; heart rhythm problems; a history of heart attack or stroke; seizures; alcohol or substance abuse or dependence; diabetes or elevated blood sugar; Alzheimer's disease or dementia; stomach or bowel problems; history of neuroleptic malignant syndrome; a history of suicidal thoughts; Parkinson's disease; trouble swallowing; or a low white blood cell count.

What is the usual dosage?

Please see general statement regarding dosage on page xii.

Adults: The recommended dose is 25 milligrams by intramuscular injection every 2 weeks. Your doctor will increase your dose as needed, until the desired effect is achieved.

If you have kidney or liver impairment, your doctor will adjust your dose appropriately.

How should I take this medication?

• Your doctor will administer Risperdal Consta to you.

What should I avoid while taking this medication?

Do not drink alcohol while you are receiving Risperdal Consta.

Do not drive or operate dangerous machinery until you know how Risperdal Consta affects you.

Do not miss your follow-up appointments with your doctor.

What are possible food and drug interactions associated with this medication?

If Risperdal Consta is used with certain other drugs, the effects of either could be increased, decreased, or altered. It is especially important to check with your doctor before combining Risperdal

Consta with the following: alcohol, blood pressure medicines, carbamazepine, cimetidine, clozapine, dopamine, fluoxetine, levodopa, paroxetine, phenobarbital, phenytoin, ranitidine, rifampin, topiramate, or valproate.

What are the possible side effects of this medication?
Please see general statement regarding side effects on page xiii.

> **Side effects may include:** constipation, dizziness, dry mouth, fatigue, headache, movement disorder, muscle rigidity or stiffness, pain in extremity, restlessness, sedation, shaking, slow movement, upset stomach, weight gain

Can I receive this medication if I am pregnant or breastfeeding?
The effects of Risperdal Consta during pregnancy are unknown. Risperdal Consta can be found in your breast milk if you receive it while breastfeeding. Do not breastfeed while you are receiving Risperdal Consta and for at least 12 weeks after your last injection. Tell your doctor immediately if you are pregnant, plan to become pregnant, or are breastfeeding.

What should I do if I miss a dose of this medication?
Risperdal Consta should be given under special circumstances determined by your doctor. If you miss your scheduled dose, contact your doctor or pharmacist for advice.

How should I store this medication?
Store in the refrigerator. Protect from light.

Risperidone: *see Risperdal, page 896*

Risperidone: *see Risperdal Consta, page 901*

Ritalin

Generic name: Methylphenidate HCl

What is this medication?

Ritalin is a medicine used to treat attention-deficit hyperactivity disorder (ADHD). This medicine can help to increase attention and decrease impulsiveness and hyperactivity in people with ADHD. Ritalin is also used to treat narcolepsy (a sleep disorder characterized by excessive daytime sleepiness). Ritalin is also available as extended-release forms (releases medicine into your body throughout the day) called Ritalin SR tablets and Ritalin LA capsules.

What is the most important information I should know about this medication?

- Ritalin has a high potential for abuse. Taking Ritalin for long periods of time may lead to extreme emotional and physical dependence. Your doctor will monitor your response and make sure you receive the correct dose. Tell your doctor if you have a history of drug or alcohol abuse.
- Ritalin can cause serious heart-related and mental problems, stroke and heart attacks in adults, and increased blood pressure and heart rate. It can also cause new or worsening behavior and thought problems, bipolar illness, and aggressive or hostile behavior.
- In addition, new symptoms (such as hearing voices, believing things that are not true, or manic symptoms) can occur. Call your doctor immediately if you or your child experiences chest pain, shortness of breath, fainting, or new mental problems while taking Ritalin.
- The doctor will check your child's height and weight while he/she is taking Ritalin. If your child is not growing in height or gaining weight as expected, the doctor may stop this medicine.
- Ritalin can cause eyesight changes or blurred vision. If this occurs, tell your doctor.

Who should not take this medication?

Do not take Ritalin if you are allergic to it or any of its ingredients. Do not take Ritalin if you are very anxious, tense, or agitated.

Do not take Ritalin if you have glaucoma (high pressure in the eye), tics (repeated movements or sounds that cannot be controlled), or Tourette's syndrome or a family history of Tourette's (a brain disorder characterized by involuntary movements and vocalizations called tics).

Also, do not take Ritalin if you are taking antidepressant medications known as monoamine oxidase inhibitors (MAOIs) (such as phenelzine or tranylcypromine) or have taken them within the past 14 days.

What should I tell my doctor before I take the first dose of this medication?

Tell your doctor about all prescription, over-the-counter, and herbal medications you are taking before beginning treatment with Ritalin. Also, talk to your doctor about your complete medical history, including heart problems, heart defects, high blood pressure, or a family history of these problems. Tell your doctor if you have a history of mental problems or a family history of psychosis, mania, bipolar disorder, or depression; tics or Tourette's syndrome; or seizures or an abnormal brain wave test (EEG).

What is the usual dosage?
Please see general statement regarding dosage on page xii.

ADHD and Narcolepsy

Ritalin Tablets
Adults: The average dose is 20-30 milligrams (mg) a day, divided into 2 or 3 times a day.

Children ≥6 years: The usual starting dose is 5 mg twice a day (before breakfast and lunch).

Ritalin SR Tablets
Adults and children ≥6 years: These tablets continue working for 8 hours. Your doctor will decide if they should be used in place of the regular tablets.

ADHD

Ritalin LA Capsules
Adults and children ≥6 years: The recommended starting dose is 20 mg once a day in the morning.

Your doctor will adjust your dose as needed, until the desired effect is achieved.

How should I take this medication?
- Take Ritalin exactly as prescribed by your doctor. Take Ritalin and Ritalin SR 30-45 minutes before a meal.
- If you have trouble sleeping, take Ritalin tablets before 6 pm.
- Swallow Ritalin SR tablets and Ritalin LA capsules whole with water or other liquids. Do not chew or crush them.
- If you cannot swallow Ritalin LA capsules, open it and sprinkle the medicine over a spoonful of applesauce. Swallow the applesauce and medicine mixture right away without chewing. Drink water or another liquid after you swallow the mixture.

What should I avoid while taking this medication?
Do not start any new medicine while you are taking Ritalin without first talking to your doctor.

What are possible food and drug interactions associated with this medication?
If Ritalin is taken with certain other drugs, the effects of either could be increased, decreased, or altered. It is especially important to check with your doctor before combining Ritalin with the following: antacids, antipsychotics (such as haloperidol), blood thinners (such as warfarin), blood pressure medications, certain antidepressants (such as clomipramine, desipramine, or imipramine), MAOIs, or seizure medications (such as phenobarbital, phenytoin, or primidone).

What are the possible side effects of this medication?
Please see general statement regarding side effects on page xiii.

> **Side effects may include:** decreased appetite, headache, nausea, nervousness, stomach ache, trouble sleeping

Can I receive this medication if I am pregnant or breastfeeding?
The effects of Ritalin during pregnancy and breastfeeding are unknown. Tell your doctor immediately if you are pregnant, plan to become pregnant, or are breastfeeding.

What should I do if I miss a dose of this medication?
If you miss a dose of Ritalin, take it as soon as you remember. However, if it is almost time for your next dose, skip the one you missed and return to your regular dosing schedule. Do not take two doses at once.

How should I store this medication?
Store at room temperature. Protect Ritalin and Ritalin SR from light and moisture.

Ritonavir: see Norvir, page 701

Rivaroxaban: see Xarelto, page 1106

Robaxin
Generic name: Methocarbamol

What is this medication?
Robaxin is a muscle relaxant used in combination with rest, physical therapy, and other measures, for the relief of discomfort associated with sudden painful musculoskeletal conditions. Robaxin is available as 500-milligram (mg) tablets and 750-mg tablets called Robaxin-750.

What is the most important information I should know about this medication?

- Robaxin can impair your mental and/or physical abilities. Do not drive a car or operate machinery until you know how Robaxin affects you.
- The effects of Robaxin can be enhanced if you take it with alcohol or other medicines that impair your mental and/or physical abilities (such as alprazolam, haloperidol, or oxycodone).

Who should not take this medication?

Do not take Robaxin if you are allergic to it or any of its ingredients.

What should I tell my doctor before I take the first dose of this medication?

Tell your doctor about all prescription, over-the-counter, and herbal medications you are taking before beginning treatment with Robaxin. Also, talk to your doctor about your complete medical history, especially if you have kidney or liver disease, myasthenia gravis (a disease characterized by long-lasting fatigue and muscle weakness), or are pregnant, plan to become pregnant, or are breastfeeding.

What is the usual dosage?

Please see general statement regarding dosage on page xii.

Robaxin Tablets
Adults ≥16 years: The recommended starting dose is 3 tablets four times a day.

Robaxin-750 Tablets
Adults ≥16 years: The recommended starting dose is 2 tablets four times a day.

How should I take this medication?

- Take Robaxin exactly as prescribed by your doctor.

What should I avoid while taking this medication?

Do not drive or operate dangerous machinery until you know how Robaxin affects you.

What are possible food and drug interactions associated with this medication?

If Robaxin is taken with certain other drugs, the effects of either could be increased, decreased, or altered. It is especially important to check with your doctor before combining Robaxin with the following: alcohol, other medicines that impair your mental and/or physical abilities, or pyridostigmine.

What are the possible side effects of this medication?

Please see general statement regarding side effects on page xiii.

> **Side effects may include:** allergic reactions, blurred vision, dizziness, drowsiness, fever, headache, low blood pressure, low white blood cell count, nausea, slow heart rate, stuffy nose, upset stomach, vomiting

Can I receive this medication if I am pregnant or breastfeeding?

The effects of Robaxin during pregnancy and breastfeeding are unknown. Tell your doctor immediately if you are pregnant, plan to become pregnant, or are breastfeeding.

What should I do if I miss a dose of this medication?

If you miss a dose of Robaxin, take it as soon as you remember. However, if it is almost time for your next dose, skip the one you missed and return to your regular dosing schedule. Do not take two doses at once.

How should I store this medication?

Store at room temperature.

Roflumilast: *see Daliresp, page 294*

Ropinirole HCl: *see Requip, page 883*

Rosuvastatin Calcium: *see Crestor, page 282*

Roxicodone
Generic name: Oxycodone HCl

What is this medication?
Roxicodone is a pain medicine that contains the narcotic painkiller oxycodone. Roxicodone is used to treat moderate to severe pain.

Roxicodone is a federally controlled substance because it has abuse potential.

What is the most important information I should know about this medication?
- Roxicodone has abuse potential. Mental and physical dependence can occur with the use of Roxicodone when it is used improperly.
- Roxicodone can cause serious breathing problems that can become life-threatening, especially when it is used in the wrong way.
- Roxicodone can cause low blood pressure. You can experience dizziness, lightheadedness, or fainting. To prevent this, carefully get up from a sitting or lying position. Sit or lie down at the first sign of any of these symptoms.

Who should not take this medication?
Do not take Roxicodone if you are allergic to it or any of its ingredients.

Do not take Roxicodone if you have severe asthma, trouble breathing, or other lung problems.

Do not take Roxicodone if you have paralytic ileus (bowel blockage).

What should I tell my doctor before I take the first dose of this medication?
Tell your doctor about all prescription, over-the-counter, and herbal medications you are taking before beginning treatment with Roxicodone. Also, talk to your doctor about your complete medical history, especially if you have trouble breathing or lung problems; head injury; liver or kidney disease; thyroid problems; Addison's

disease (adrenal gland failure); seizures; enlarged prostate or problems urinating; pancreas, gallbladder, or mental health problems; or a history of alcohol or drug abuse.

What is the usual dosage?

Please see general statement regarding dosage on page xii.

Adults: The recommended starting dose is 5-15 milligrams every 4-6 hours as needed for pain. Your doctor will adjust your dose based on your condition, previous treatment with painkillers, and your tolerance for narcotics.

If you have liver or kidney impairment, your doctor will adjust your dose appropriately.

How should I take this medication?

• Take Roxicodone exactly as prescribed by your doctor. Do not change your dose or stop taking Roxicodone without first talking to your doctor.

What should I avoid while taking this medication?

Do not drink alcohol or take sleeping pills or tranquilizers while you are taking Roxicodone.

Do not drive or operate heavy machinery until you know how Roxicodone affects you.

Do not share Roxicodone with others.

What are possible food and drug interactions associated with this medication?

If Roxicodone is taken with certain other drugs, the effects of either could be increased, decreased, or altered. It is especially important to check with your doctor before combining Roxicodone with the following: alcohol, antidepressant medications known as monoamine oxidase inhibitors (MAOIs) (such as phenelzine or tranylcypromine), butorphanol, buprenorphine, general anesthetics, muscle relaxants (such as tubocurarine), nalbuphine, pentazocine, phenothiazines (such as chlorpromazine or mesoridazine), sedative-hypnotics (such as alprazolam or diazepam), or tranquilizers (such as chlordiazepoxide).

What are the possible side effects of this medication?
Please see general statement regarding side effects on page xiii.

> **Side effects may include:** constipation, headache, itching, nausea, vomiting

Can I receive this medication if I am pregnant or breastfeeding?
The effects of Roxicodone during pregnancy are unknown. Roxicodone can be found in your breast milk if you take it while breastfeeding. Do not breastfeed while you are taking Roxicodone. Tell your doctor immediately if you are pregnant, plan to become pregnant, or are breastfeeding.

What should I do if I miss a dose of this medication?
If you miss a dose of Roxicodone, take it as soon as you remember. However, if it is almost time for your next dose, skip the one you missed and return to your regular dosing schedule. Do not take two doses at once.

How should I store this medication?
Store at room temperature. Protect from moisture.

Ruxolitinib: *see Jakafi, page 486*

Rybix ODT
Generic name: Tramadol HCl

What is this medication?
Rybix ODT (orally disintegrating tablets) is an opioid (narcotic) painkiller that is used to treat moderate to moderately severe pain.

What is the most important information I should know about this medication?

- Rybix ODT can cause seizures. The risk is greater if you have a history of seizures, are suffering from alcohol or drug withdrawal (abrupt discontinuation or a decrease in the dose of medicines, recreational drugs, or alcohol you take), or nervous system infections. Your risk of seizures may increase if you are taking monoamine oxidase inhibitors (MAOIs), a class of medicines used to treat depression and other psychiatric conditions (such as phenelzine); antidepressant/psychiatric medicines in classes known as selective serotonin reuptake inhibitors (SSRIs) (such as fluoxetine and paroxetine), selective norepinephrine reuptake inhibitors (SNRIs) (such as venlafaxine), or tricyclic antidepressants (TCAs) (such as amitriptyline); certain migraine products (such as sumatriptan); or other opioids.
- You can develop a serotonin syndrome (a potentially life-threatening drug reaction that causes the body to have too much serotonin, a chemical produced by the nerve cells) when you are using Rybix ODT, especially if you take it in combination with MAOIs, SSRIs, SNRIs, certain migraine products, or certain antidepressants. Symptoms can include hallucinations, increase in your heart rate, fever, incoordination, and/or stomach problems. Contact your doctor immediately if you develop any of these signs or symptoms.
- Anaphylactoid reactions (a serious and rapid allergic reaction that may result in death if not immediately treated) can occur. Contact your doctor or get emergency help immediately if you experience difficulty breathing; swelling of the throat, tongue, or mouth; or hives.
- Taking Rybix ODT can also lead to abuse, addiction, and dependence.

Who should not take this medication?

Do not take Rybix ODT if you have attempted suicide or are addiction prone. Do not take Rybix ODT if you are allergic to it or any of it ingredients, or to other opioids.

What should I tell my doctor before I take the first dose of this medication?

Tell your doctor about all prescription, over-the-counter, and herbal medications you are taking before beginning treatment with Rybix ODT. Also, talk to your doctor about your complete medical history, especially if you have a history of seizures, difficulty breathing, depression, head injury, phenylketonuria (an inability to process phenylalanine, a protein in your body), kidney or liver disease, attempted suicide, or are addicted or allergic to opioids.

What is the usual dosage?

Please see general statement regarding dosage on page xii.

Adults ≥17 years: Your doctor will prescribe the appropriate dose for you and will increase your dose as needed, until the desired effect is achieved.

If you are >75 years old, or have kidney or liver disease, your doctor will adjust your dose appropriately.

How should I take this medication?

- Take Rybix ODT exactly as prescribed by your doctor. Place Rybix ODT tablet on your tongue until it completely disintegrates, and then swallow it with or without water. To open the blister pack, peel back the foil on the blister. Do not push the tablet through the foil. Do not chew, break, or split the tablet.

What should I avoid while taking this medication?

Do not drive a car or operate dangerous machinery while you are using this medication.

Do not drink alcohol while you are taking this medication.

Do not adjust your dose or stop taking Rybix ODT suddenly without first talking to your doctor.

What are possible food and drug interactions associated with this medication?

If Rybix ODT is taken with certain other drugs, the effects of either could be increased, decreased, or altered. It is especially important to check with your doctor before combining Rybix ODT with the following: alcohol, antidepressants (including MAOIs, SSRIs, SNRIs, or TCAs), antipsychotics (such as haloperidol), carbamazepine, certain migraine products, cyclobenzaprine, digoxin, erythromycin, ketoconazole, linezolid, lithium, phenothiazines (such as promethazine), quinidine, rifampin, sleep aids (such as temazepam), St. John's wort, tranquilizers (such as alprazolam), or warfarin.

What are the possible side effects of this medication?

Please see general statement regarding side effects on page xiii.

Side effects may include: constipation, diarrhea, dizziness, drowsiness, dry mouth, headache, itching, nausea, sweating, vomiting, weakness

Can I receive this medication if I am pregnant or breastfeeding?

The effects of Rybix ODT during pregnancy and breastfeeding are unknown. Tell your doctor immediately if you are pregnant, plan to become pregnant, or are breastfeeding.

What should I do if I miss a dose of this medication?

Rybix ODT should be given under special circumstances determined by your doctor (or given only as needed). If you miss your scheduled dose, contact your doctor or pharmacist for advice.

How should I store this medication?

Store at room temperature.

Ryzolt

Generic name: Tramadol HCl

What is this medication?

Ryzolt is an opioid painkiller that is used to treat moderate to moderately severe long-term pain that requires treatment for an extended period.

What is the most important information I should know about this medication?

- Ryzolt can cause seizures. The risk is greater if you have a history of seizures, are suffering from alcohol or drug withdrawal (abrupt discontinuation or a decrease in the dose of medicines, recreational drugs, or alcohol you take), or nervous system infections. Your risk of seizures may also be increased if you are taking monoamine oxidase inhibitors (MAOIs), a class of medicines used to treat depression and other psychiatric conditions (such as phenelzine); antidepressant/psychiatric medicines in classes known as selective serotonin reuptake inhibitors (SSRIs) (such as fluoxetine or paroxetine), selective norepinephrine reuptake inhibitors (SNRIs) (such as venlafaxine), or tricyclic antidepressants (TCAs) (such as amitriptyline); certain migraine products (such as sumatriptan); or other opioids.

- You can develop a serotonin syndrome (a potentially life-threatening drug reaction that causes the body to have too much serotonin, a chemical produced by the nerve cells) when you are using Ryzolt, especially if you take it in combination with MAOIs, SSRIs, SNRIs, certain migraine products, or certain antidepressants. Symptoms can include hallucinations, increase in your heart rate, fever, incoordination, and/or stomach problems. Contact your doctor immediately if you develop any of these signs or symptoms.

- Anaphylactoid reactions (a serious and rapid allergic reaction that may result in death if not immediately treated) can occur. Contact your doctor or get emergency help immediately if you experience difficulty breathing; swelling of the throat, tongue, or mouth; or hives.

- Taking Ryzolt can also lead to abuse, addiction, and dependence.

Who should not take this medication?

Do not take Ryzolt if you have attempted suicide or are addiction prone. Do not take Ryzolt if you are allergic to it or any of its ingredients, or to other opioids.

What should I tell my doctor before I take the first dose of this medication?

Tell your doctor about all prescription, over-the-counter, and herbal medications you are taking before beginning treatment with Ryzolt. Also, talk to your doctor about your complete medical history, especially if you have a history of seizures, asthma, difficulty breathing, depression, head injury, kidney or liver disease, attempted suicide, or are addicted or allergic to opioids.

What is the usual dosage?

Please see general statement regarding dosage on page xii.

Adults ≥17 years: Your doctor will prescribe the appropriate dose for you and will increase your dose as needed, until the desired effect is achieved.

How should I take this medication?

• Take Ryzolt exactly as prescribed by your doctor. Swallow the tablet whole with liquid. Do not chew, break, or split the tablet.

What should I avoid while taking this medication?

Do not drive a car or operate dangerous machinery while using Ryzolt.

Do not drink alcohol while using Ryzolt.

Do not adjust your dose or stop taking Ryzolt suddenly without first talking to your doctor.

What are possible food and drug interactions associated with this medication?

If Ryzolt is taken with certain other drugs, the effects of either could be increased, decreased, or altered. It is especially important to check with your doctor before combining Ryzolt with the following: alcohol, antidepressants (including MAOIs, SSRIs, SNRIs, or TCAs), antipsychotics (such as haloperidol), carbamazepine, certain migraine products, cyclobenzaprine, digoxin, erythromycin, ketoconazole, linezolid, lithium, phenothiazines (such as promethazine), quinidine, rifampin, sleep aids (such as temazepam), St. John's wort, tranquilizers (such as alprazolam), or warfarin.

What are the possible side effects of this medication?

Please see general statement regarding side effects on page xiii.

> **Side effects may include:** constipation, diarrhea, dizziness, drowsiness, dry mouth, headache, itching, nausea, sweating, vomiting, weakness

Can I receive this medication if I am pregnant or breastfeeding?

The effects of Ryzolt during pregnancy and breastfeeding are unknown. Tell your doctor immediately if you are pregnant, plan to become pregnant, or are breastfeeding.

What should I do if I miss a dose of this medication?

If you miss a dose of Ryzolt, take it as soon as you remember. However, if it is almost time for your next dose, skip the one you missed and return to your regular dosing schedule. Do not take two doses at once.

How should I store this medication?

Store at room temperature.

Saxagliptin: *see Onglyza, page 729*

Seroquel

Generic name: Quetiapine Fumarate

What is this medication?

Seroquel is a medicine used to treat schizophrenia. This medicine is also used alone or in combination with lithium or divalproex to treat manic or depressive episodes associated with bipolar disorder.

What is the most important information I should know about this medication?

- Seroquel can increase the risk of suicidal thoughts and behavior in children, adolescents, and young adults. Your doctor will monitor you closely for clinical worsening, suicidal or unusual behaviour after you start taking Seroquel or a new dose of Seroquel. Tell your doctor immediately if you experience anxiety, hostility, sleeplessness, restlessness, impulsive or dangerous behavior, or thoughts about suicide or dying; or if you have new symptoms or seem to be feeling worse.
- Seroquel can cause neuroleptic malignant syndrome (NMS) (a life-threatening brain disorder). NMS is a medical emergency. Tell your doctor immediately if you experience high fever, muscle rigidity, confusion, fast or irregular heartbeat, changes in your blood pressure, or increased sweating.
- Seroquel can cause an increase in your blood sugar levels or diabetes. Tell your doctor if you experience excessive thirst, an increase in urination, an increase in appetite, or weakness. If you have diabetes or are at risk for diabetes, monitor your blood sugar regularly, as determined by your doctor.
- Seroquel can cause tardive dyskinesia (abnormal muscle movements, including tremor, shuffling and uncontrolled, involuntary movements). Tell your doctor if you experience uncontrollable muscle movements.
- Seroquel can cause a sudden decrease in your blood pressure with dizziness, rapid heartbeat, and faintness. Tell your doctor if you have heart problems, brain disorders (such as stroke), or other conditions that can cause low blood pressure.

- Seroquel can cause high blood pressure in children and adolescents. Your doctor will check your child's blood pressure before starting Seroquel and during treatment.
- Seroquel can lower the ability of your body to fight infections. Tell your doctor if you develop signs of an infection (such as a fever, sore throat, rash, or chills).
- Seroquel can also cause hyperprolactinemia (an increase in a hormone called prolactin, which can affect lactation, menstruation, and fertility). Tell your doctor immediately if you experience missed menstrual periods, leakage of milk from your breasts, development of the breasts in men, or problems with erections.
- Seroquel can cause a type of abnormal heartbeat that can be dangerous and life-threatening. Do not take Seroquel with other medications that can cause this irregular heartbeat (such as amiodarone, chlorpromazine, levomethadyl acetate, methadone, pentamidine, procainamide, quinidine, sotalol, thioridazine, or ziprazidone) or certain antibiotics (such as gatifloxacin or moxifloxacin).
- Seroquel can cause a prolonged, painful erection. If this is not treated right away, it could lead to permanent sexual problems (such as impotence). Tell your doctor right away if this happens.

Who should not take this medication?

Do not take Seroquel if you are allergic to it or any of its ingredients.

Seroquel is not approved for treating psychosis in the elderly with dementia (an illness involving loss of memory, judgment, and confusion).

What should I tell my doctor before I take the first dose of this medication?

Tell your doctor about all prescription, over-the-counter, and herbal medications you are taking before beginning treatment with Seroquel. Also, talk to your doctor about your complete medical history, especially if you have past or current heart or liver problems, high cholesterol, low or high blood pressure, cataracts, seizures, abnormal thyroid tests, high prolactin levels, diabetes, or a history of low white blood cell counts.

What is the usual dosage?
Please see general statement regarding dosage on page xii.

Schizophrenia
Adults and adolescents 13-17 years: The recommended starting dose is 25 milligrams (mg) twice a day.

Bipolar Mania (alone or in combination with lithium or divalproex)
Adults: The recommended starting dose is 50 mg twice a day.

Children 10-17 years: The recommended starting dose is 25 mg twice a day.

Bipolar Depression
Adults: The recommend starting dose is 50 mg once a day at bedtime.

Your doctor will increase your dose as needed, until the desired effect is achieved.

If you are elderly or have hepatic impairment, your doctor will adjust your dose appropriately.

How should I take this medication?
- Take Seroquel exactly as prescribed by your doctor. Do not change your dose without first talking to your doctor.
- Take Seroquel with or without food.

What should I avoid while taking this medication?
Do not drink alcohol while you are taking Seroquel.

Do not drive, operate machinery, or engage in other dangerous activities until you know how Seroquel affects you.

Do not expose yourself to extreme heat or dehydration while you are taking Seroquel.

What are possible food and drug interactions associated with this medication?

If Seroquel is taken with certain other drugs, the effects of either could be increased, decreased, or altered. It is especially important to check with your doctor before combining Seroquel with the following: alcohol, anti-HIV medications (such as indinavir or ritonavir), barbiturates (such as phenobarbital), carbamazepine, cimetidine, divalproex, dopamine, erythromycin, fluconazole, itraconazole, ketoconazole, levodopa, lorazepam, phenytoin, rifampin, corticosteroids (such as dexamethasone or prednisone), thioridazine, or valproate.

What are the possible side effects of this medication?

Please see general statement regarding side effects on page xiii.

> **Side effects may include:** abdominal pain, abnormal liver tests, constipation, difficulty swallowing, dizziness, drowsiness, dry mouth, fatigue, increased appetite, increased blood cholesterol and triglyceride levels, nausea, rapid heart rate, sluggishness, sore throat, sudden drop in your blood pressure upon standing, upset stomach, vomiting, weakness, weight gain

Can I receive this medication if I am pregnant or breastfeeding?

The effects of Seroquel during pregnancy are unknown. Seroquel can be found in your breast milk if you take it while breastfeeding. Do not breastfeed while you are taking Seroquel. Tell your doctor immediately if you are pregnant, plan to become pregnant, or are breastfeeding.

What should I do if I miss a dose of this medication?

If you miss a dose of Seroquel, take it as soon as you remember. However, if it is almost time for your next dose, skip the one you missed and return to your regular dosing schedule. Do not take two doses at once.

How should I store this medication?

Store at room temperature.

Seroquel XR
Generic name: Quetiapine Fumarate

What is this medication?
Seroquel XR is a medicine used to treat schizophrenia. This medication can also be used to treat manic or depressive episodes associated with bipolar disorder alone or in combination with lithium or divalproex. Also, Seroquel XR is used to treat major depressive disorder in addition to other antidepressants.

What is the most important information I should know about this medication?
- Seroquel XR can be life-threatening when used in elderly people with mental problems caused by dementia (an illness involving loss of memory, judgment, and confusion). Seroquel XR is not approved to treat mental problems caused by dementia.
- Seroquel XR can increase the risk of suicidal thoughts and behavior in children, adolescents, and young adults. Your doctor will monitor you closely for clinical worsening, suicidality, or unusual behavior after you start taking Seroquel XR or a new dose. Tell your doctor right away if you experience anxiety, hostility, sleeplessness, restlessness, impulsive or dangerous behavior, or thoughts about suicide or dying; or if you have new symptoms or seem to be feeling worse.
- In rare cases, Seroquel XR can cause neuroleptic malignant syndrome (NMS) (a life-threatening brain disorder). NMS is a medical emergency, get medical help right away. Tell your doctor right away if you experience high fever, muscle rigidity, confusion, fast or irregular heartbeat, changes in your blood pressure, or increased sweating.
- Seroquel XR can cause tardive dyskinesia (abnormal muscle movements, including tremor, shuffling and uncontrolled, involuntary movements). Tell your doctor if you experience uncontrollable muscle movements.
- Seroquel XR can cause an increase in your blood sugar levels or diabetes. Tell your doctor if you experience excessive thirst, an increase in urination, an increase in appetite, or weakness. If you have diabetes or are at risk for diabetes, monitor your blood sugar regularly, as determined by your doctor. Also, you

can experience an increase in your blood cholesterol levels or weight gain while you are taking Seroquel XR. Monitor your weight regularly.

- Seroquel XR can cause sudden decrease in your blood pressure with dizziness, rapid heartbeat, and faintness. However, Seroquel XR can cause high blood pressure in children and adolescents.
- Seroquel XR can also cause hyperprolactinemia (an increase in a hormone called prolactin, which can affect lactation, menstruation, and fertility). Tell your doctor right away if you experience missed menstrual periods, leakage of milk from your breasts, development of the breasts in men, or problems with erections.
- Seroquel XR can cause a type of abnormal heartbeat that can be dangerous and life-threatening. Do not take Seroquel XR with other medications that can cause this irregular heartbeat (such as amiodarone, chlorpromazine, or thioridazine) or certain antibiotics (such as gatifloxacin or moxifloxacin).
- Seroquel XR can lower the ability of your body to fight infections. Tell your doctor if you notice any signs of infection such as a fever, sore throat, rash, or chills.
- Seroquel XR can also cause seizures, problems with your body temperature regulation, difficulty swallowing, or impairment of your judgment, thinking, or motor skills.
- Seroquel XR can cause a prolonged, painful erection. If this is not treated right away, it could lead to permanent sexual problems (such as impotence). Tell your doctor right away if this happens.

Who should not take this medication?
Do not take Seroquel XR if you are allergic to it or any of its ingredients.

Seroquel XR is not approved to treat mental problems caused by dementia in the elderly.

What should I tell my doctor before I take the first dose of this medication?
Tell your doctor about all prescription, over-the-counter, and herbal medications you are taking before beginning treatment with

Seroquel XR. Also, talk to your doctor about your complete medical history, especially if you or your family member has diabetes; high cholesterol; high or low blood pressure; low white blood cell count; cataracts; seizures; high prolactin levels; heart, liver, or thyroid problems; or are pregnant, plan to become pregnant, or are breastfeeding.

What is the usual dosage?
Please see general statement regarding dosage on page xii.

Schizophrenia
Adults: The recommended starting dose is 300 milligrams (mg) a day. Your doctor will increase your dose as needed, until the desired effect is achieved.

Bipolar Mania
Adults: The recommended starting dose is 300 mg once a day on Day 1, 600 mg on Day 2, and 400-800 mg on Day 3. Your doctor will increase your dose as needed, until the desired effect is achieved.

Bipolar Depression
Adults: The recommended starting dose is 50 mg once a day on Day 1, 100 mg on Day 2; 200 mg on Day 3; and 300 mg on Day 4. Your doctor will increase your dose as needed, until the desired effect is achieved.

Major Depressive Disorder
Adults: The recommended starting dose is 50 mg once a day on Day 1 and 2, then 150 mg a day on Day 3 and 4. Your doctor will increase your dose as needed, until the desired effect is achieved.

If you have hepatic impairment, your doctor will adjust your dose appropriately.

How should I take this medication?
• Take Seroquel XR exactly as prescribed by your doctor. Do not take extra doses or take more often without asking your doctor.

- Take Seroquel XR every day, preferably in the evening. Take Seroquel XR with a light meal or without food. Swallow Seroquel XR tablets whole. Do not split, chew, or crush the tablet.
- If you feel you need to stop Seroquel XR, talk to your doctor first.

What should I avoid while taking this medication?

Do not drink alcohol while you are taking Seroquel XR.

Do not drive or operate machinery until you know how Seroquel XR affects you.

Do not expose yourself to extreme heat or dehydration while you are taking Seroquel XR.

What are possible food and drug interactions associated with this medication?

If Seroquel XR is taken with certain other drugs, the effects of either could be increased, decreased, or altered. It is especially important to check with your doctor before combining Seroquel XR with the following: alcohol, anti-HIV medications (such as indinavir or ritonavir), barbiturates (such as phenobarbital), carbamazepine, cimetidine, corticosteroids (such as dexamethasone or prednisone), divalproex, erythromycin, fluconazole, itraconazole, ketoconazole, levodopa, lorazepam, phenytoin, rifampin, thioridazine, or valproate.

What are the possible side effects of this medication?

Please see general statement regarding side effects on page xiii.

Side effects may include: abdominal (stomach) pain, constipation, difficulty swallowing, disturbance in your speech and language, dizziness, drowsiness, dry mouth, increased appetite, stuffy nose, sudden drop in your blood pressure upon standing, tiredness, upset stomach, vomiting, weakness, weight gain

---

Can I receive this medication if I am pregnant or breastfeeding?

The effects of Seroquel XR during pregnancy are unknown. Seroquel XR can be found in your breast milk if you take it while breastfeeding. Do not breastfeed while you are taking Seroquel XR. Tell your doctor immediately if you are pregnant, plan to become pregnant, or are breastfeeding.

What should I do if I miss a dose of this medication?

If you miss a dose of Seroquel XR, take it as soon as you remember. However, if it is almost time for your next dose, skip the one you missed and return to your regular dosing schedule. Do not take two doses at once.

How should I store this medication?

Store at room temperature.

Sertraline HCl: *see Zoloft, page 1148*

Sildenafil Citrate: *see Viagra, page 1064*

Simvastatin: *see Zocor, page 1143*

Simvastatin/Sitagliptin: *see Juvisync, page 496*

Sinemet

Generic name: Carbidopa/Levodopa

What is this medication?

Sinemet is a medicine used to treat the symptoms of Parkinson's disease. Sinemet contains two medicines, carbidopa and levodopa.

What is the most important information I should know about this medication?

- The period of desired effect after each dose may begin to shorten and you may notice more pronounced symptoms; this is called a "wearing-off" effect. Tell your doctor if this "wearing-off" effect is troublesome.

- Sinemet can cause mental disturbances. Contact your doctor right away if you become depressed or experience any thoughts of suicide.
- Occasionally, dark color (red, brown, or black) can appear in your saliva, urine, or sweat after taking Sinemet. Although the color is not a cause for concern, it may stain your clothing.
- Sinemet can cause involuntary movements. Tell your doctor if you notice any of these, as a lower dose may be required.
- Do not change your dose or abruptly discontinue your treatment without first talking to your doctor. A condition that resembles neuroleptic malignant syndrome (a life-threatening brain disorder) can occur if you abruptly stop taking this medication.

Who should not take this medication?

Do not take Sinemet if you are allergic to it or any of its ingredients.

Do not take Sinemet if you are taking a nonselective monoamine oxidase inhibitor (MAOI), a class of medications used to treat depression and other psychiatric conditions (such as phenelzine or tranylcypromine).

Do not take Sinemet if you have narrow-angle glaucoma (high pressure in the eye), or if you have undiagnosed skin lesions or a history of melanoma (skin cancer).

What should I tell my doctor before I take the first dose of this medication?

Tell your doctor about all prescription, over-the-counter, and herbal medications you are taking before beginning treatment with Sinemet. Also, talk to your doctor about your complete medical history, especially if you have severe heart problems, a history of heart attacks, irregular heartbeat, psychosis, skin cancer, stomach ulcers, asthma, lung disorders, kidney or liver impairment, endocrine (hormonal) diseases, or are pregnant, plan to become pregnant, or are breastfeeding.

What is the usual dosage?

Please see general statement regarding dosage on page xii.

Adults: The recommended starting dose is 25-100 milligrams three times a day. Your doctor will prescribe the appropriate dose for you, depending on the severity of your condition and other medications you have previously taken. Your doctor will increase your dose as needed, until the desired effect is achieved.

How should I take this medication?

- Take Sinemet exactly as prescribed by your doctor. Take Sinemet at regular intervals every day after meals.
- If you have been taking levodopa alone, you should stop taking it for at least 12 hours before starting to take Sinemet.

What should I avoid while taking this medication?

Do not change your diet to foods that are high in protein because this may reduce the absorption of Sinemet.

Do not drive or operate machines until you know how Sinemet affects you.

What are possible food and drug interactions associated with this medication?

If Sinemet is taken with certain other drugs, the effects of either could be increased, decreased, or altered. It is especially important to check with your doctor before combining Sinemet with the following: certain antidepressants (such as amitriptyline), dopamine blockers (such as chlorpromazine or haloperidol), iron supplements, isoniazid, MAOIs, metoclopramide, multivitamins with iron, papaverine, phenytoin, or risperidone.

What are the possible side effects of this medication?

Please see general statement regarding side effects on page xiii.

Side effects may include: abdominal (stomach) pain, agitation, allergic reactions, back pain, blurred vision, chest pain, confusion, constipation, cough, dark saliva, dark sweat, diarrhea, dizziness, dream abnormalities, drowsiness, dry mouth, fatigue, flushing skin, hallucinations (seeing things when they aren't really there), headache, heart attack, high or low blood pressure, hot flashes, irregular heartbeat, leg pain, muscle cramps, rash, shoulder pain, sweating, taste alterations, urinary tract infections, vomiting, weakness, weight gain or loss

Can I receive this medication if I am pregnant or breastfeeding?

The effects of Sinemet during pregnancy and breastfeeding are unknown. Tell your doctor immediately if you are pregnant, plan to become pregnant, or are breastfeeding.

What should I do if I miss a dose of this medication?

If you miss a dose of Sinemet, take the missed dose as soon as you remember. However, if it is almost time for your next dose, skip the one you missed and return to your regular dosing schedule. Do not take two doses at once.

How should I store this medication?

Store at room temperature.

Sinemet CR

Generic name: Carbidopa/Levodopa

What is this medication?

Sinemet CR is a medicine used to treat the symptoms of Parkinson's disease. Sinemet CR contains two medicines, carbidopa and levodopa.

What is the most important information I should know about this medication?

- Sinemet CR can cause mental disturbances. Contact your doctor right away if you become depressed or experience any thoughts of suicide.
- Occasionally, dark color (red, brown, or black) can appear in your saliva, urine, or sweat after taking Sinemet CR. Although the color is not a cause for concern, it may stain your clothing.
- Sinemet CR can cause involuntary movements. Tell your doctor if you notice any of these, as a lower dose may be required.
- Do not change your dose or abruptly discontinue your treatment without first talking to your doctor. A condition that resembles neuroleptic malignant syndrome (a life-threatening brain disorder) can occur if you abruptly stop taking this medication.

Who should not take this medication?

Do not take Sinemet CR if you are allergic to it or any of its ingredients.

Do not take Sinemet CR or if you are taking a nonselective monoamine oxidase inhibitor (MAOI) (such as phenelzine), a class of medications used to treat depression and other psychiatric conditions.

Do not take Sinemet CR if you have narrow-angle glaucoma (high pressure in the eye), or if you have undiagnosed skin lesions or a history of melanoma (skin cancer).

What should I tell my doctor before I take the first dose of this medication?

Tell your doctor about all prescription, over-the-counter, and herbal medications you are taking before beginning treatment with Sinemet CR. Also, talk to your doctor about your complete medical history, especially if you have severe heart problems, a history of heart attacks, irregular heartbeat, psychosis, skin cancer, stomach ulcers, asthma, lung disorders, kidney or liver impairment, endocrine (hormonal) diseases, or are pregnant, plan to become pregnant, or are breastfeeding.

What is the usual dosage?
Please see general statement regarding dosage on page xii.

Adults: The recommended starting dose is 50-200 milligrams twice a day. Your doctor will prescribe the appropriate dose for you, depending on the severity of your condition and other medications you have previously taken. Your doctor will increase your dose as needed, until the desired effect is achieved.

How should I take this medication?
- Take Sinemet CR exactly as prescribed by your doctor.
- Take Sinemet CR at regular intervals every day after meals. Swallow Sinemet CR tablets whole. Do not chew or crush the tablets.
- If you have been taking levodopa alone, you should stop taking it for at least 12 hours before starting to take Sinemet CR.

What should I avoid while taking this medication?
Do not change your diet to foods that are high in protein because this may reduce the absorption of Sinemet CR.

Do not drive or operate machines until you know how Sinemet CR affects you.

What are possible food and drug interactions associated with this medication?
If Sinemet CR is taken with certain other drugs, the effects of either could be increased, decreased, or altered. It is especially important to check with your doctor before combining Sinemet CR with the following: certain antidepressants (such as amitriptyline), dopamine blockers (such as chlorpromazine or haloperidol), iron supplements, isoniazid, MAOIs, metoclopramide, multivitamins with iron, papaverine, phenytoin, or risperidone.

What are the possible side effects of this medication?
Please see general statement regarding side effects on page xiii.

Side effects may include: abdominal (stomach) pain, back pain, blurred vision, confusion, depression, diarrhea, dizziness, dream abnormalities, dry mouth, hallucinations (seeing things when they are not really there), headache, high or low blood pressure, hot flashes, impaired movement, nausea, rash, shortness of breath, sweating, taste alterations, urinary tract infections, vomiting, weakness, weight gain or loss

Can I receive this medication if I am pregnant or breastfeeding?

The effects of Sinemet CR during pregnancy and breastfeeding are unknown. Tell your doctor immediately if you are pregnant, plan to become pregnant, or are breastfeeding.

What should I do if I miss a dose of this medication?

If you miss a dose of Sinemet CR, take the missed dose as soon as you remember. However, if it is almost time for your next dose, skip the one you missed and return to your regular dosing schedule. Do not take two doses at once.

How should I store this medication?

Store at room temperature.

Singulair

Generic name: Montelukast Sodium

What is this medication?

Singulair is a medicine used for the long-term treatment and prevention of asthma. It is also used to prevent exercise-induced breathing problems. In addition, Singulair is used to relieve nasal symptoms (such as stuffy and runny nose, itching, or sneezing) of seasonal or year-round allergies. Singulair is available as chewable tablets, oral granules, and tablets.

What is the most important information I should know about this medication?

- Singulair does not treat the symptoms of a sudden asthma attack. Always have a short-acting rescue inhaler (such as albuterol) to treat sudden symptoms. If you do not have a short-acting inhaler, tell your doctor to have one prescribed for you. Tell your doctor immediately if an asthma attack does not respond to the rescue inhaler or if you require more doses than usual.
- Singulair can cause changes in your behavior and mood. Tell your doctor right away if you or your child experience hallucinations, disorientation, agitation, anxiousness, irritability, restlessness, bad or vivid dreams, depression, sleep walking, tremor, trouble sleeping, or suicidal thoughts or actions.
- In rare cases, Singulair can increase certain white blood cells in your body and possibly cause swelling of blood vessels throughout your body. Tell your doctor right away if you or your child develops pins and needles or numbness of your arms or legs, a flu-like illness, rash, or pain and swelling in your sinuses.
- If you have a condition known as phenylketonuria (an inability to process phenylalanine, a protein in your body), be aware that Singulair chewable tablets contain phenylalanine.

Who should not take this medication?

Do not take Singulair if you are allergic to it or any of its ingredients.

What should I tell my doctor before I take the first dose of this medication?

Tell your doctor about all prescription, over-the-counter, and herbal medications you are taking before beginning treatment with Singulair. Also, talk to your doctor about your complete medical history, especially if you are allergic to aspirin, have phenylketonuria, or if you are pregnant, plan to become pregnant, or are breastfeeding.

What is the usual dosage?

Please see general statement regarding dosage on page xii.

Asthma

Adults and adolescents ≥15 years: The usual dose is one 10-milligram (mg) tablet once a day in the evening.

Children 6-14 years: The usual dose is one 5-mg chewable tablet once a day in the evening.

Children 2-5 years: The usual dose is one 4-mg chewable tablet or one packet of 4-mg oral granules once a day in the evening.

Children 12-23 months: The usual dose is one packet of 4-mg oral granules once a day in the evening.

Exercise-Induced Breathing Problems
Adults and children ≥15 years: The usual dose is one 10-mg tablet taken at least 2 hours before exercise.

Children 6-14 years: The usual dose is one 5-mg chewable tablet taken at least 2 hours before exercise.

If you or your child are already taking one tablet a day for your asthma or allergies, do not take another dose before you exercise.

Treatment of Seasonal and Year-Round Allergy Symptoms
Adults and adolescents ≥15 years: The usual dose is one 10-mg tablet once a day.

Children 6-14 years: The usual dose is one 5-mg chewable tablet once a day.

Children 2-5 years: The usual dose is one 4-mg chewable tablet or one packet of 4-mg oral granules once a day.

Treatment of Year-Round Allergy Symptoms
Children 6-23 months: The usual dose is one packet of 4-mg oral granules once a day.

How should I take this medication?
- Take Singulair exactly as prescribed by your doctor. Do not change your dose or stop taking Singulair without first talking to your doctor. Take it with or without food.
- If you or your child have both asthma and allergies, take only one Singulair dose a day in the evening.

- Give your child the Singulair oral granules right in their mouth or dissolve them in 1 teaspoonful of cold or room temperature baby formula or breast milk. Do not mix the oral granules with any other liquid. Your child can drink other liquids after he/she has swallowed the mixture.
- You can also mix the granules with 1 spoonful of cold or room temperature applesauce, mashed carrots, rice, or ice cream.
- Give your child all of the mixture right away. Do not store it for later use.

What should I avoid while taking this medication?

Do not take aspirin or other medicines called nonsteroidal anti-inflammatory drugs (such as ibuprofen) while you are taking Singulair.

What are possible food and drug interactions associated with this medication?

If Singulair is taken with certain other drugs, the effects of either could be increased, decreased, or altered. It is especially important to check with your doctor before combining Singulair with pheno-barbital or rifampin.

What are the possible side effects of this medication?

Please see general statement regarding side effects on page xiii.

Side effects may include: cough, diarrhea, earache or ear infection, fever, flu, headache, runny nose, sinus infection, sore throat, stomach upset, upper respiratory infection

---

Can I receive this medication if I am pregnant or breastfeeding?

The effects of Singulair during pregnancy and breastfeeding are unknown. Tell your doctor immediately if you are pregnant, plan to become pregnant, or are breastfeeding.

What should I do if I miss a dose of this medication?

If you miss a dose of Singulair, take it as soon as you remember. However, if it is almost time for your next dose, skip the one you

missed and return to your regular dosing schedule. Do not take two doses at once.

How should I store this medication?
Store at room temperature. Protect from moisture and light.

Sitagliptin: see Januvia, page 494

Skelaxin
Generic name: Metaxalone

What is this medication?
Skelaxin is a muscle relaxant used in combination with rest, physical therapy, and other measures, for the relief of discomfort associated with sudden painful musculoskeletal conditions.

What is the most important information I should know about this medication?
- Skelaxin can impair your mental and/or physical abilities. Do not drive a car or operate machinery until you know how Skelaxin affects you.
- The effects of Skelaxin can be enhanced if you take it with food. Elderly people are especially susceptible to these effects.

Who should not take this medication?
Do not take Skelaxin if you are allergic to it or any of its ingredients.

Do not take Skelaxin if you have a history of anemia (blood disorder) or severe kidney or liver disease.

What should I tell my doctor before I take the first dose of this medication?
Tell your doctor about all prescription, over-the-counter, and herbal medications you are taking before beginning treatment with Skelaxin. Also, talk to your doctor about your complete medical history,

especially if you have anemia, kidney or liver disease, or are pregnant, plan to become pregnant, or are breastfeeding.

What is the usual dosage?
Please see general statement regarding dosage on page xii.

Adults and children ≥12 years: The recommended dose is one 800-milligram tablet 3-4 times a day.

How should I take this medication?
• Take Skelaxin exactly as prescribed by your doctor.

What should I avoid while taking this medication?
Do not drive or operate dangerous machinery until you know how Skelaxin affects you.

What are possible food and drug interactions associated with this medication?
If Skelaxin is taken with certain other drugs, the effects of either could be increased, decreased, or altered. It is especially important to check with your doctor before combining Skelaxin with the following: alcohol, benzodiazepines (such as alprazolam or lorazepam), certain antidepressants (such as amitriptyline or imipramine), or narcotic painkillers (such as hydrocodone or oxycodone).

What are the possible side effects of this medication?
Please see general statement regarding side effects on page xiii.

Side effects may include: dizziness, drowsiness, headache, irritability, nausea, nervousness, stomach upset, vomiting

Can I receive this medication if I am pregnant or breastfeeding?
The effects of Skelaxin during pregnancy and breastfeeding are unknown. Do not breastfeed while you are taking Skelaxin. Tell your doctor immediately if you are pregnant, plan to become pregnant, or are breastfeeding.

What should I do if I miss a dose of this medication?

If you miss a dose of Skelaxin, take it as soon as you remember. However, if it is almost time for your next dose, skip the one you missed and return to your regular dosing schedule. Do not take two doses at once.

How should I store this medication?

Store at room temperature.

Solifenacin Succinate: *see Vesicare, page 1062*

Soma

Generic name: Carisoprodol

What is this medication?

Soma is a medicine used to relieve the symptoms associated with acute (sudden), painful musculoskeletal conditions, such as muscle strains and spasms.

What is the most important information I should know about this medication?

- Soma can cause you to become drowsy and dizzy. Do not take Soma before engaging in potentially hazardous activities, such as driving.
- Soma can be habit-forming if you take higher doses than those recommended or if you take it over long periods of time.
- Do not stop taking Soma completely at once; you may develop symptoms, such as agitation, anxiety, runny nose, sweating, chills, diarrhea, a rapid heartbeat, high blood pressure, rapid breathing, dilation of your pupils, or tearing.

Who should not take this medication?

Do not take Soma if you are allergic to it or any of its ingredientes, or to meprobamate. Also, do not take Soma if you have porphyria (an inherited blood disorder).

What should I tell my doctor before I take the first dose of this medication?

Tell your doctor about all prescription, over-the-counter, and herbal medications you are taking before beginning treatment with Soma. Also, talk to your doctor about your complete medical history, especially if you have kidney or liver problems, seizures, a history of drug dependence, or if you are pregnant, plan to become pregnant, or are breastfeeding.

What is the usual dosage?

Please see general statement regarding dosage on page xii.

Adults and adolescents ≥16 years: The recommended dose is one 250-milligram (mg) or 350-mg tablet 3 times a day, at bedtime, for 2-3 weeks.

How should I take this medication?

- Take Soma exactly as prescribed by your doctor. You can take it with or without food.

What should I avoid while taking this medication?

Do not take Soma for a longer period than prescribed by your doctor.

Do not drive a car or operate dangerous machinery until you know how Soma affects you.

Do not take Soma with other medications that can make you feel drowsy, including alcohol.

What are possible food and drug interactions associated with this medication?

If Soma is taken with certain other drugs, the effects of either could be increased, decreased, or altered. It is especially important to check with your doctor before combining Soma with the following: alcohol, benzodiazepines (such as alprazolam), certain antidepressants (such as fluoxetine), certain painkillers, or meprobamate.

What are the possible side effects of this medication?
Please see general statement regarding side effects on page xiii.

Side effects may include: agitation, depression, dizziness, drowsiness, facial flushing, fainting, headache, hiccups, inability to fall or stay asleep, irritability, lightheadedness upon standing up, loss of coordination, nausea, rapid heart rate, stomach upset, tremors, vertigo, vomiting

Can I receive this medication if I am pregnant or breastfeeding?
The effects of Soma during pregnancy and breastfeeding are unknown. Soma can be found in your breast milk if you take it while breastfeeding. Tell your doctor immediately if you are pregnant, plan to become pregnant, or are breastfeeding.

What should I do if I miss a dose of this medication?
If you miss a dose of Soma, take it as soon as you remember. However, if it is almost time for your next dose, skip the one you missed and return to your regular dosing schedule. Do not take two doses at once.

How should I store this medication?
Store at room temperature.

Spiriva Handihaler
Generic name: Tiotropium Bromide

What is this medication?
Spiriva Handihaler is a medicine used for long-term, once-a-day treatment to help reduce bronchial spasms (wheezing) associated with chronic obstructive pulmonary disease (COPD), which includes chronic bronchitis and emphysema. It comes as a capsule (not to be swallowed) containing dry powder, which is inhaled through the mouth only using the Handihaler device. When inhaled,

Spiriva opens up narrow air passages, allowing more oxygen to reach the lungs.

What is the most important information I should know about this medication?

- Spiriva Handihaler is not a rescue medicine and should not be used for treating sudden breathing problems.
- An immediate allergic reaction (hives, swelling, or rash) is possible when you first use Spiriva Handihaler. Inhaled medications such as Spiriva can also cause difficulty breathing in some people. If you have an allergic reaction or you start wheezing, stop using Spiriva Handihaler immediately and contact your doctor.

Who should not take this medication?

Do not use Spiriva Handihaler if you have an allergic reaction to it or if you are allergic to atropine or any of its derivatives, such as ipratropium. Also, do not use Spiriva Handihaler if you are allergic to any milk products, such as lactose.

What should I tell my doctor before I take the first dose of this medication?

Tell your doctor about all prescription, over-the-counter, and herbal medications you are taking before beginning treatment with Spiriva Handihaler. Also, talk to your doctor about your complete medical history, especially if you have glaucoma (high pressure in the eye), an enlarged prostate, problems passing urine, kidney problems, or have a serious allergy to milk.

What is the usual dosage?

Please see general statement regarding dosage on page xii.

Adults: The recommended dose is the inhalation of the contents of 1 capsule, taken once a day, with the Handihaler device.

How should I take this medication?

- Spiriva capsules are designed to be used only with the Handihaler inhalation device. The capsules should not be swallowed. Try to use the inhaler at the same time each day.

- Please refer to the Patient Information for detailed instructions on how to properly use this medication.
- When removing a capsule from the blister card, peel back only the foil that is covering the capsule you are about to use. The capsule's effectiveness may be reduced if it is not used immediately after the foil is opened. If you accidentally remove the foil covering of any of the other capsules, you must throw them away.

What should I avoid while taking this medication?

Avoid getting the Spiriva powder into your eyes. It may cause blurred vision.

Spiriva Handihaler can cause dizziness and blurred vision. Be careful when driving a car or operating appliances or other machines.

Spiriva is for oral inhalation only. Do not swallow Spiriva capsules.

What are possible food and drug interactions associated with this medication?

If Spiriva Handihaler is used with certain other drugs, the effects of either could be increased, decreased, or altered. It is especially important to check with your doctor before combining Spiriva Handihaler with the following: benztropine, ipratropium, or tolterodine.

What are the possible side effects of this medication?

Please see general statement regarding side effects on page xiii.

Side effects may include: abdominal pain, chest pain, common cold, constipation, dry mouth, indigestion, infection, muscle pain, nose bleeds, rash, runny nose or nasal inflammation, sinus infection, sore throat, swelling, urinary tract infection, vomiting, yeast infection

---

Can I receive this medication if I am pregnant or breastfeeding?

The effects of Spiriva Handihaler during pregnancy and breastfeeding are unknown. Tell your doctor immediately if you are pregnant, plan to become pregnant, or are breastfeeding.

What should I do if I miss a dose of this medication?

If you miss a dose of Spiriva Handihaler, take it as soon as you remember. However, if it is almost time for your next dose, skip the one you missed and return to your regular dosing schedule. Do not take two doses at once.

How should I store this medication?

Store at room temperature. Do not store capsules in the Handihaler.

Keep capsules away from moisture and extreme temperatures, such as in the refrigerator or in direct sunlight.

Keep the capsules sealed until ready to use.

Spironolactone: *see Aldactone, page 50*

Stendra

Generic name: Avanafil

What is this medication?

Stendra is a medicine used to treat erectile dysfunction in men.

What is the most important information I should know about this medication?

- Stendra can cause your blood pressure to drop suddenly to an unsafe level. This can happen if you take certain medicines for chest pain (such as nitrates). Stendra can cause you to feel dizzy, faint, or have a heart attack or stroke.
- If you need emergency medical care for a heart problem, tell your doctor when you last took Stendra.

- Stop sexual activity and get medical help immediately if you experience chest pain, dizziness, or nausea during sex.

Who should not take this medication?
Do not take Stendra if you are allergic to it or any of its ingredients.

Do not take Stendra if you take nitrates or street drugs called "poppers" (such as amyl nitrate and butyl nitrate).

What should I tell my doctor before I take the first dose of this medication?
Tell your doctor about all prescription, over-the-counter, and herbal medications you are taking before beginning treatment with Stendra. Also, talk to your doctor about your complete medical history, especially if you have high blood pressure not controlled by medication; have low blood pressure; or have a history of stroke or heart problems (such as heart attack, irregular heartbeat, angina, or heart failure); or have had heart surgery within the last 6 months.

Tell your doctor if you have a deformed penis shape or have had an erection that lasted for more than four hours.

Also, tell your doctor if you have problems with your blood cells (such as sickle cell anemia, multiple myeloma, or leukemia); retinitis pigmentosa (a rare genetic eye disease); bleeding, liver, or kidney problems, or are having kidney dialysis; have or have had stomach ulcers; or have had severe vision loss.

What is the usual dosage?
Please see general statement regarding dosage on page xii.

Adults: The starting dose is 100 milligrams (mg) taken as needed 30 minutes before sexual activity. Your doctor may increase the dose to 200 mg or decrease it to 50 mg.

How should I take this medication?
- Take one Stendra tablet about 30 minutes before you will have sexual activity.

• Take it with or without food. Do not take more than one tablet a day.

What should I avoid while taking this medication?

Do not drink too much alcohol when you are taking Stendra (for example, 3 glasses of wine, or 3 shots of whiskey). Drinking too much alcohol can increase your chances of getting a headache or getting dizzy. It can also increase your heart rate or lower your blood pressure.

What are possible food and drug interactions associated with this medication?

If Stendra is taken with certain other drugs, the effects of either could be increased, decreased, or altered. It is especially important to check with your doctor before combining Stendra with the following: nitrates, blood pressure/prostate medications known as alpha blockers (such as alfuzosin, doxazosin, or prazosin), other blood pressure medications, HIV medications called protease inhibitors (such as atazanavir, indinavir, or saquinavir), antifungal medicines (such as ketoconazole or itraconazole), antibiotics (such as clarithromycin, erythromycin, or telithromycin), or other medications for erectile dysfunction.

What are the possible side effects of this medication?

Please see general statement regarding side effects on page xiii.

> **Side effects may include:** back pain, flushing, headache, sore throat, stuffy or runny nose
>
> If you experience an erection that lasts more than four hours, sudden loss of vision in one or both eyes, sudden hearing decrease, hearing loss, ringing in your ears or dizziness, get medical help immediately.

Can I receive this medication if I am pregnant or breastfeeding?

This medication is not used in women.

What should I do if I miss a dose of this medication?
Stendra is not for regular use. Take Stendra about 30 minutes before sexual activity.

Do not take more than one time a day.

How should I store this medication?
Store at room temperature, away from light.

Strattera
Generic name: Atomoxetine HCl

What is this medication?
Strattera is a medicine used to treat attention-deficit hyperactivity disorder (ADHD). Strattera can help increase attention and decrease impulsiveness and hyperactivity in people with ADHD.

What is the most important information I should know about this medication?
- Strattera can increase the risk of suicidal thoughts and behavior in children and teenagers. Tell your child's doctor right away if your child has thoughts about suicide or sudden changes in mood or behavior, especially early during treatment or after a change in dose. Also, tell your child's doctor right away if your child experiences anxiety, agitation, panic attacks, trouble sleeping, irritability, hostility, aggressiveness, impulsivity, restlessness, mania, or depression.
- Strattera can cause severe liver damage. Tell your child's doctor right away if your child has itching, right upper belly pain, dark urine, yellow skin or eyes, or unexplained "flu-like" symptoms.
- Strattera can cause serious heart-related and mental problems, stroke and heart attacks in adults, or increased blood pressure and heart rate. It can also cause new or worsening behavior and thought problems, bipolar illness, or aggressive or hostile behavior.
- In addition, new symptoms (such as hearing voices, believing things that are not true, or manic symptoms) can occur. Tell

your child's doctor right away if your child experiences chest pain, shortness of breath, fainting, or new mental problems while taking Strattera.

• The doctor will check your child's height and weight while he/she is taking Strattera. If your child is not growing in height or gaining weight as expected, the doctor may stop this medicine.

Who should not take this medication?

Do not give Strattera if your child is allergic to it or any of its ingredients.

Do not give Strattera if your child has glaucoma (high pressure in the eye) or pheochromocytoma (tumor of the adrenal gland).

Do not give Strattera if your child is taking antidepressant medications known as monoamine oxidase inhibitors (MAOIs) (such as phenelzine) or took them within the past 14 days.

What should I tell my doctor before I take the first dose of this medication?

Tell your child's doctor about all prescription, over-the-counter, and herbal medications your child is taking before beginning treatment with Strattera. Also, talk to your child's doctor about his/her complete medical history, especially if your child has or you have a family history of suicide thoughts or actions, heart problems, high or low blood pressure, irregular heartbeat, mental problems, bipolar disorder, depression, or liver disease.

What is the usual dosage?

Please see general statement regarding dosage on page xii.

Adolescents and children ≥6 years and ≤70 kilograms (kg): Your doctor will prescribe the appropriate dose for your child, based on their weight.

Adolescents and children ≥6 years and >70 kg: The usual starting dose is 40 milligrams (mg) a day. Your doctor may increase your child's dose as appropriate.

If your child has liver impairment, the doctor will adjust your child's dose appropriately.

How should I take this medication?
- Take Strattera exactly as prescribed by your doctor. Take Strattera once a day in the morning, or twice a day, once in the morning and once in the late afternoon or early evening. Take the dose at the same time each day to help you remember.
- Swallow Strattera capsules whole with water or other liquids. Do not chew, crush, or open the capsules. Your child can take Strattera with or without food.

What should I avoid while taking this medication?
Do not touch a broken Strattera capsule. Wash hands and surfaces that touched an open capsule. If any powder gets in your eyes or your child's eyes, rinse them with water right away and call your doctor.

Do not drive, operate machinery, or perform other hazardous activities until you know how Strattera affects you.

What are possible food and drug interactions associated with this medication?
If Strattera is taken with certain other drugs, the effects of either could be increased, decreased, or altered. It is especially important to check with your child's doctor before combining Strattera with the following: albuterol or similar asthma medications, blood pressure medications (such as dobutamine or dopamine), certain antidepressants (such as desipramine, fluoxetine, or paroxetine), cold or allergy medicines that contain decongestants, MAOIs, midazolam, or quinidine.

What are the possible side effects of this medication?
Please see general statement regarding side effects on page xiii.

Side effects may include: abdominal pain, constipation, dizziness, dry mouth, hot flush, impotence, loss of appetite, menstrual cramps, mood swings, nausea, priapism (painful, prolonged erections), problems urinating, tiredness, trouble sleeping, upset stomach, vomiting

Can I receive this medication if I am pregnant or breastfeeding?

The effects of Strattera during pregnancy and breastfeeding are unknown. Tell your doctor immediately if you are pregnant, plan to become pregnant, or are breastfeeding.

What should I do if I miss a dose of this medication?

If you miss a dose of Strattera, take it as soon as you remember. However, if it is almost time for your next dose, skip the one you missed and return to your regular dosing schedule. Do not take two doses at once.

How should I store this medication?

Store at room temperature.

Suboxone

Generic name: Buprenorphine/Naloxone

What is this medication?

Suboxone is a medicine used for maintenance treatment of opioid dependence.

Suboxone is a federally controlled narcotic with potential for abuse.

What is the most important information I should know about this medication?

- It can be dangerous to mix Suboxone with medications like benzodiazepines, sleeping pills and other tranquilizers, certain antidepressants, other opioid medications, or alcohol, especially when not under the care of a doctor or in doses different from those prescribed by your doctor. Mixing these medications can lead to drowsiness, sedation, unconsciousness, and death, especially if injected. It is important to let your doctor know about all medications and substances you are taking. Your doctor can provide guidance if any of these medications are prescribed for the treatment of other medical conditions you may have.

- Suboxone has potential for abuse and can produce dependence.
- Suboxone can cause drowsiness and slow reaction times. This may occur more often in the first few weeks of treatment or when your dose is being changed, but can also occur if you drink alcohol or take other sedative medicines when you are taking Suboxone. Use caution when you are driving a car or operating machinery.
- Suboxone can cause your blood pressure to drop, making you feel dizzy if you get up too fast from sitting or lying down.
- Follow up with your doctor regularly for blood tests to monitor your liver before and during treatment with Suboxone.

Who should not take this medication?
Do not take Suboxone if you are allergic to it or any of its ingredients.

What should I tell my doctor before I take the first dose of this medication?
Tell your doctor about all prescription, over-the-counter, and herbal medications you are taking before beginning treatment with Suboxone. Also, talk to your doctor about your complete medical history, especially if you have adrenal gland problems, a history of drug or alcohol addiction, head injury, hepatitis or other liver problems, kidney problems, lung disease, problems with your prostate, or thyroid problems.

What is the usual dosage?
Please see general statement regarding dosage on page xii.

Adults: The recommended dose is 16/4 milligrams (mg) once a day. Your doctor will prescribe the appropriate dose for you and will increase or decrease your dose as needed, until the desired effect is achieved.

How should I take this medication?
- Take Suboxone exactly as prescribed by your doctor. Do not take extra doses or take more often without asking your doctor. Do not stop taking Suboxone suddenly.
- Place the prescribed number of tablets under your tongue until they are dissolved completely. You may place all the tablets at once or alternatively.

What should I avoid while taking this medication?
Do not drink alcohol or take antianxiety medications (such as benzodiazepines), other opioid narcotics, general anesthetics, sedative or hypnotic medications, other tranquilizers or any other medication that slows down your brain function.

Do not drive, operate heavy machinery, or perform any other dangerous activities until you know how Suboxone affects you.

Do not inject ("shoot-up") Suboxone tablets. Also, do not chew or swallow the tablets because the medicine will not work as well.

What are possible food and drug interactions associated with this medication?
If Suboxone is taken with certain other drugs, the effects of either could be increased, decreased, or altered. It is especially important to check with your doctor before combining Suboxone with the following: alcohol, antibiotics (such as erythromycin), antifungals (such as ketoconazole), benzodiazepines (such as alprazolam, diazepam, or lorazepam), or HIV medications (such as indinavir, ritonavir, or saquinavir).

What are the possible side effects of this medication?
Please see general statement regarding side effects on page xiii.

Side effects may include: constipation, headache, nausea, pain in the stomach, sweating, vomiting

Stop taking Suboxone immediately and call your doctor if you have: darker urine, difficulty breathing, low blood pressure, pinpoint pupils, sedation, yellowing of your skin or whites of your eyes

---

Can I receive this medication if I am pregnant or breastfeeding?

The effects of Suboxone during pregnancy are unknown. Subox-one can be found in your breast milk if you take it while breastfeeding. It is recommended that you do not breastfeed while you are taking Suboxone. Tell your doctor immediately if you are pregnant, plan to become pregnant, or are breastfeeding.

What should I do if I miss a dose of this medication?

If you miss a dose of Suboxone, take it as soon as you remember. However, if it is almost time for your next dose, skip the one you missed and return to your regular dosing schedule. Do not take two doses at once.

How should I store this medication?

Store at room temperature.

Sucralfate: *see Carafate, page 175*

Sulfamethoxazole/Trimethoprim: *see Bactrim, page 127*

Sumatriptan: *see Imitrex, page 460*

Symbicort

Generic name: Budesonide/Formoterol Fumarate Dihydrate

What is this medication?

Symbicort is a combination medicine used to treat and prevent the symptoms of asthma and airway narrowing associated with chronic obstructive pulmonary disease (COPD), including chronic bronchitis (long-term inflammation of the lungs) and emphysema (lung disease that causes shortness of breath). Symbicort contains two medicines: budesonide (decreases inflammation in the lungs) and formoterol (relaxes muscles in the airways).

What is the most important information I should know about this medication?

- Symbicort can cause an increased risk of death from asthma problems. Tell your doctor if your breathing problems worsen over time while you are using Symbicort. Get emergency medical help if your breathing problems worsen quickly or if you use your rescue inhaler medicine, but it does not relieve your symptoms.
- When your asthma is well controlled, your doctor may tell you to stop using Symbicort. Your doctor will decide if you can stop Symbicort without loss of your asthma control. You will continue using your long-term asthma-control medication.
- Children and adolescents who use Symbicort can have an increased risk of being hospitalized for asthma problems.
- Do not use Symbicort for rapid relief of an asthma attack or acute bronchospasm. Symbicort does not treat the symptoms of a sudden asthma attack. Always have a short-acting rescue inhaler (such as albuterol) to treat sudden symptoms. If you do not have a short-acting inhaler, tell your doctor to have one prescribed for you. Tell your doctor right away if an asthma attack does not respond to the rescue inhaler or if you require more doses than usual.
- Do not stop using Symbicort, even if your symptoms get better. Your doctor will change your medicine as needed.

Who should not take this medication?

Do not use Symbicort if you are allergic to it or any of its ingredients.

Do not use Symbicort to treat sudden severe symptoms of asthma or COPD.

What should I tell my doctor before I take the first dose of this medication?

Tell your doctor about all prescription, over-the-counter, and herbal medications you are taking before beginning treatment with Symbicort. Also, talk to your doctor about your complete medical history, especially if you have heart, thyroid, liver, or immunes system problems; high blood pressure; seizures; diabetes; osteoporosis (thin, weak bones); cataracts or glaucoma (high pressure in the eye); allergies; are exposed to chickenpox or measles, or have recently been near anyone with chickenpox or measles; have or have had tuberculosis or other infections; or are pregnant, plan to become pregnant, or are breastfeeding.

What is the usual dosage?
Please see general statement regarding dosage on page xii.

Asthma
Adults and children ≥12 years: The usual dose is 2 inhalations twice a day (morning and evening, approximately 12 hours apart).

Chronic Obstructive Pulmonary Disease
Adults: The usual dose is 2 inhalations twice a day.

How should I take this medication?
• Use Symbicort exactly as prescribed by your doctor. Do not take extra doses or take more often without asking your doctor.
• Rinse your mouth and spit the water after each dose. Do not swallow the water. This will reduce your chance of getting a fungal infection (thrush) in your mouth.
• Please review the instructions that came with your prescription on how to properly use your inhaler.

What should I avoid while taking this medication?
Do not spray Symbicort in your eyes. If accidental exposure occurs, rinse your eyes with water. Tell your doctor if redness or irritation persists.

Do not expose yourself to chicken pox or measles while you are using Symbicort, especially if you have immune system problems.

Do not give Symbicort to other people, even if they have the same symptoms that you have. It may harm them.

The contents of your Symbicort canister are under pressure. Do not puncture or throw the canister into a fire or incinerator. Do not use or store it near heat or open flame.

What are possible food and drug interactions associated with this medication?

If Symbicort is used with certain other drugs, the effects of either could be increased, decreased, or altered. It is especially important to check with your doctor before combining Symbicort with the following: atazanavir, blood pressure/heart medications known as beta-blockers (such as propranolol), certain antidepressants (such as amitriptyline or nortriptyline), clarithromycin, diuretics (water pills) (such as furosemide), indinavir, itraconazole, ketoconazole, monoamine oxidase inhibitors (MAOIs), a class of medications used to treat depression and other psychiatric conditions (such as phenelzine or tranylcypromine), nefazodone, nelfinavir, ritonavir, saquinavir, or telithromycin.

What are the possible side effects of this medication?

Please see general statement regarding side effects on page xiii.

> **Side effects may include:** allergic reactions, back pain, chest pain, eye problems, fast and irregular heartbeat, flu, headache, increased blood pressure, increased risk of infections, nasal congestion, nervousness, respiratory (lung) tract infections, sinus inflammation, shaking, slowed growth in children, stomach discomfort, throat irritation or pain, thrush, vomiting, wheezing

Can I receive this medication if I am pregnant or breastfeeding?

The effects of Symbicort during pregnancy and breastfeeding are unknown. Budesonide, one of the active ingredients in Symbicort can be found in your breast milk if you take it while breastfeeding. Tell your doctor immediately if you are pregnant, plan to become pregnant, or are breastfeeding.

What should I do if I miss a dose of this medication?

If you miss a dose of Symbicort, take it as soon as you remember. However, if it is almost time for your next dose, skip the one you missed and return to your regular dosing schedule. Do not take two doses at once.

How should I store this medication?

Store at room temperature. Do not store it near heat or flame.

Discard Symbicort when the counter reaches "0" or 3 months after removal from its foil pouch, whichever comes first.

Synthroid

Generic name: Levothyroxine Sodium

What is this medication?

Synthroid is a medicine used to treat hypothyroidism (an underactive thyroid gland). Synthroid is a synthetic hormone that is intended to replace a hormone that is normally produced by your thyroid gland. It is also used to treat or prevent certain other thyroid conditions such as goiter (an enlarged thyroid gland); inflammation of the thyroid gland; thyroid hormone deficiency due to surgery, radiation, or certain medications; or for the management of certain thyroid cancers.

What is the most important information I should know about this medication?

- Do not use Synthroid to treat obesity or weight loss.
- Synthroid is a replacement therapy, so you need to take it every day for life unless your condition is temporary. Improvement in your symptoms can be seen several weeks after you start Synthroid. Continue taking your medication as directed by your doctor. Tell your doctor immediately if you experience rapid or irregular heartbeats, chest pain, shortness of breath, leg cramps, headache, nervousness, irritability, sleeplessness, tremors, change in your appetite, weight gain or loss, vomiting, diarrhea, excessive sweating, heat intolerance, fever, changes in menstrual periods, hives, or skin rash.
- Long-term Synthroid use can weaken bones, especially in women after menopause.
- If you have heart disease, your doctor may need to start you on a lower dose of Synthroid to see how you respond to this medication.

- Also, if you have diabetes, your doctor will determine if the dose of your diabetes medication needs to be adjusted. Your doctor will monitor your blood sugar levels.
- If you are taking an oral blood thinner (such as warfarin), your doctor will monitor your blood clotting status to determine if the dose of your blood thinner needs to be adjusted.
- Tell your doctor or dentist that you are taking Synthroid before having any surgery.
- Synthroid can cause partial hair loss during the first few months of treatment. This is usually temporary.

Who should not take this medication?
Do not take Synthroid if you are allergic to it or any of its ingredients.

Do not take Synthroid if you have an overactive thyroid gland, reduced adrenal function, or had a recent heart attack.

What should I tell my doctor before I take the first dose of this medication?
Tell your doctor about all prescription, over-the-counter, and herbal medications you are taking before beginning treatment with Synthroid. Also, talk to your doctor about your complete medical history, especially if you have anemia, diabetes, heart disease, blood clotting disorders, problems with your pituitary or adrenal glands, or if you are pregnant, plan to become pregnant, or are breastfeeding.

What is the usual dosage?
Please see general statement regarding dosage on page xii.

__Adults and children:__ Your doctor will prescribe the appropriate dose for you or your child based on your age, weight, and condition.

How should I take this medication?
- Take Synthroid exactly as prescribed by your doctor. Take it on an empty stomach, 30 minutes to 1 hour before breakfast.
- Certain foods and supplements can decrease the amount of Synthroid in your body. Do not take Synthroid within 4 hours of taking antacids and iron or calcium supplements.

• If an infant or child cannot swallow whole tablets, crush the tablet and mix it into 1-2 teaspoonfuls of water. Have the child drink the mixture immediately. Do not store it for later use. Soybean infant formula can decrease the amount of Synthroid in your baby's body and should not be used for administering the crushed tablets.

What should I avoid while taking this medication?

Do not stop taking Synthroid or change the amount or how often you take it without talking to your doctor.

What are possible food and drug interactions associated with this medication?

If Synthroid is taken with certain other drugs, the effects of either could be increased, decreased, or altered. Synthroid may interact with numerous medications. Therefore, it is very important that you tell your doctor about any other medications you are taking.

What are the possible side effects of this medication?

Please see general statement regarding side effects on page xiii.

Side effects may include: change in your appetite or menstrual periods, chest pain, diarrhea, excessive sweating, fever, headache, heat intolerance, hives, irritability, leg cramps, nervousness, rapid or irregular heartbeats, shortness of breath, skin rash, sleeplessness, tremors, vomiting, weight gain or loss

---

Can I receive this medication if I am pregnant or breastfeeding?

You can continue to take Synthroid during pregnancy. However, a dose adjustment may be necessary. Small amounts of thyroid hormone are excreted in your breast milk. Tell your doctor immediately if you are pregnant, plan to become pregnant, or are breastfeeding.

What should I do if I miss a dose of this medication?

If you miss a dose of Synthroid, take it as soon as you remember. However, if it is almost time for your next dose, skip the one you

missed and return to your regular dosing schedule. Do not take two doses at once.

How should I store this medication?
Store at room temperature, away from heat, light, and moisture.

Tadalafil: *see Cialis, page 212*

Tamoxifen
Generic name: Tamoxifen Citrate

What is this medication?
Tamoxifen is a medicine used to lower the risk of developing breast cancer in high-risk women and in women who had surgery and radiation for cancer inside the milk ducts. Tamoxifen is also used to treat breast cancer in women after they have finished early treatment (such as surgery, radiation, or chemotherapy). In addition, tamoxifen is used to treat breast cancer in women and men that has spread to other parts of the body.

What is the most important information I should know about this medication?
- Tamoxifen can cause changes in the lining or body of your uterus. These changes may be serious, including cancer of the uterus. Tell your doctor right away if you develop vaginal bleeding or bloody discharge that could be a rusty or brown color, changes in your monthly period (such as the amount or timing of bleeding or increased clotting), or pain or pressure in your pelvis (below your belly button).
- Tamoxifen can also cause noncancerous changes to your uterus. These include endometriosis, fibroids in the uterus, menstrual cycle irregularities, or the absence of menstrual periods.
- Tamoxifen can cause blood clots in your veins or lungs. You may get blood clots up to 2-3 months after you stop taking tamoxifen. Tell your doctor right away if you experience sudden chest

pain, shortness of breath, coughing up blood, or pain, tenderness, or swelling in one or both of your legs.

- Tamoxifen can cause a stroke. Tell your doctor right away if you develop sudden confusion, trouble speaking or understanding, trouble seeing in one or both eyes, trouble walking, dizziness, loss of balance or coordination, severe headaches with no known cause, or weakness, tingling, or numbness in your face, arm, or leg, especially on one side of your body.
- Tamoxifen can cause cataracts or increase the risk of needing cataract surgery. Tell your doctor right away if you experience blurred vision.
- Tamoxifen can cause liver problems, including liver cancer. Tell your doctor right away if you experience a lack of appetite, or yellowing of your skin or whites of your eyes.
- Tamoxifen can harm your unborn baby if you take it during pregnancy. Do not take tamoxifen if you are pregnant. Do not become pregnant for 2 months after you stop taking tamoxifen. If you have not gone through menopause and are sexually active, use an effective non-hormonal birth control (such as condoms, diaphragms with spermicide, or plain intrauterine devices [IUDs]) while you are taking tamoxifen and for 2 months after you stop taking it.
- Have regular gynecology checkups, breast exams, and mammograms. Your doctor will tell you how often. Tell your doctor right away if you have any new breast lumps. Also, tell all of your doctors that you are taking tamoxifen.

Who should not take this medication?
Do not take tamoxifen if you are allergic to it or any of its ingredients.

Do not take tamoxifen if you are taking blood thinners (such as warfarin) or if you have a history of blood clots in your legs or lungs.

What should I tell my doctor before I take the first dose of this medication?
Tell your doctor about all prescription, over-the-counter, and herbal medications you are taking before beginning treatment with tamoxifen. Also, talk to your doctor about your complete medical history,

especially if you have anemia, low blood platelet levels, or are pregnant, plan to become pregnant, or are breastfeeding.

What is the usual dosage?

Please see general statement regarding dosage on page xii.

Risk Reduction in Women with Cancer Inside the Milk Ducts and High-Risk Women

Adults: The recommended dose is 20 milligrams (mg) a day for 5 years.

Treatment of Breast Cancer

Adults: The recommended dose is 20-40 mg a day. If you are taking >20 mg a day, your doctor will prescribe the medicine in two smaller doses, to be taken in the morning and evening.

How should I take this medication?

- Take tamoxifen exactly as prescribed by your doctor. Take it with or without food. It may be easier to remember if you take it at the same time each day.
- Start taking tamoxifen during your menstrual period. If you do not have a regular menstrual period, your doctor will give you a pregnancy test before you start taking tamoxifen.
- Swallow tamoxifen tablets whole, with water or another non-alcoholic drink.
- Take tamoxifen every day for 5 years, unless your doctor tells you otherwise.

What should I avoid while taking this medication?

Do not become pregnant while you are taking tamoxifen or for 2 months after you stop taking it.

Do not breastfeed while you are taking tamoxifen.

What are possible food and drug interactions associated with this medication?

If tamoxifen is taken with certain other drugs, the effects of either could be increased, decreased, or altered. It is especially important to check with your doctor before combining tamoxifen with the following: aminoglutethimide, anastrazole, blood thinners, bromocriptine, letrozole, medroxyprogesterone, phenobarbital, or rifampin.

What are the possible side effects of this medication?
Please see general statement regarding side effects on page xiii.

> **Side effects may include:** hot flashes, vaginal discharge

Can I receive this medication if I am pregnant or breastfeeding?
Do not become pregnant or breastfeed while you are taking tamoxifen. Tell your doctor immediately if you are pregnant, plan to become pregnant, or are breastfeeding.

What should I do if I miss a dose of this medication?
If you miss a dose of tamoxifen, take it as soon as you remember. However, if it is almost time for your next dose, skip the one you missed and return to your regular dosing schedule. Do not take two doses at once.

How should I store this medication?
Store at room temperature.

Tamoxifen Citrate: *see Tamoxifen, page 961*

Tamsulosin HCl: *see Flomax, page 391*

Tapazole
Generic name: Methimazole

What is this medication?
Tapazole is a medicine used to treat hyperthyroidism (an overactive thyroid gland). Tapazole is used to decrease symptoms of hyperthyroidism in preparation for surgery to remove your thyroid

gland or radioactive iodine therapy, or when thyroid surgery is not a treatment option.

What is the most important information I should know about this medication?

- Tapazole can cause agranulocytosis (blood disorder in which white blood cells are not made in adequate numbers or are not made at all). Stop taking this medication and tell your doctor immediately if you experience a fever or sore throat.
- Tapazole can cause severe liver problems. Tell your doctor immediately if you experience a loss of appetite, itchiness, or pain or tenderness in your right upper stomach area. Your doctor will monitor your liver function.
- Your doctor will monitor your blood thyroid hormone levels regularly.

Who should not take this medication?

Do not take Tapazole if you are allergic to it or any of its ingredients.

Do not take Tapazole if you are breastfeeding.

What should I tell my doctor before I take the first dose of this medication?

Tell your doctor about all prescription, over-the-counter, and herbal medications you are taking before beginning treatment with Tapazole. Also, talk to your doctor about your complete medical history, especially if you have liver or blood problems, or are pregnant or breastfeeding.

What is the usual dosage?

Please see general statement regarding dosage on page xii.

Adults: Your doctor will prescribe the appropriate dose for you, based on the severity of your condition.

Children: Your doctor will prescribe the appropriate dose for your child, based on their weight.

How should I take this medication?
• Take Tapazole exactly as prescribed by your doctor.

What should I avoid while taking this medication?
Do not take more Tapazole than prescribed by your doctor. If you take too much of this medication, you can experience nausea, vomiting, pain or tenderness in your upper stomach area, headache, fever, joint pain, itchiness, or swelling.

What are possible food and drug interactions associated with this medication?
If Tapazole is taken with certain other drugs, the effects of either could be increased, decreased, or altered. It is especially important to check with your doctor before combining Tapazole with the following: blood pressure/heart medications known as beta-blockers (such as metoprolol or propranolol), blood thinners (such as warfarin), digoxin, or theophylline.

What are the possible side effects of this medication?
Please see general statement regarding side effects on page xiii.

Side effects may include: drowsiness, fever, headache, itchiness, joint pain, liver inflammation, loss of hair, loss of taste, muscle pain, nausea, pain or tenderness in your upper stomach area, skin rash, sore throat, swelling, tingling, tiredness, vomiting, yellowing of your skin or whites of your eyes

Can I receive this medication if I am pregnant or breastfeeding?
Tapazole can cause harm to your unborn or newborn baby if you use it during pregnancy or breastfeeding. Tapazole can be found in your breast milk and should not be used while breastfeeding. Tell your doctor immediately if you are pregnant, plan to become pregnant, or are breastfeeding.

What should I do if I miss a dose of this medication?
If you miss a dose of Tapazole, take it as soon as you remember. However, if it is almost time for your next dose, skip the one you

missed and return to your regular dosing schedule. Do not take two doses at once.

How should I store this medication?
Store at room temperature.

Tarceva
Generic name: Erlotinib

What is this medication?
Tarceva is a medicine used to treat advanced non-small cell lung cancer (NSCLC) that is located in the lung or that has spread throughout the body (metastatic) but has not progressed after four cycles of chemotherapy.

Tarceva is also used to treat NSCLC that is located in the lung or spread throughout the body if you have not responded to other types of chemotherapy.

Additionally, Tarceva is used in combination with gemcitabine to treat advanced pancreatic cancer that cannot be treated surgically or that has spread throughout the body.

What is the most important information I should know about this medication?
- Tarceva can cause interstitial lung disease (ILD). ILD is a group of lung diseases affecting the tissue and space around the air sacs of your lungs. ILD is a serious and life-threatening condition. Tell your doctor right away if you experience shortness of breath, cough, or a fever.
- Tarceva can cause significant kidney or liver problems. Your doctor will perform periodic blood tests to monitor your kidney and liver function while you are taking Tarceva. It is important to tell your doctor if you have a history of kidney or liver problems.
- You can develop a gastrointestinal perforation (a hole in the stomach or intestine) while you are taking Tarceva. Tell your

doctor right away if you develop serious or ongoing diarrhea, nausea, loss of appetite, or vomiting.

• Tarceva can cause a serious skin disorder. Contact your doctor immediately if you develop a new or worsening skin rash.

• Tarceva can cause serious eye disorders. Contact your doctor if you experience any eye pain or vision problems.

• Smoking may affect how well Tarceva works for you. If you smoke, you should stop smoking before starting treatment with Tarceva. If you continue to smoke, you should talk to your doctor before taking Tarceva.

• Tarceva can cause harm to your unborn baby if you use it during pregnancy. Make sure to use adequate contraception to prevent pregnancy while on therapy with Tarceva and continue to use adequate contraception for at least two weeks after discontinuing Tarceva.

Who should not take this medication?

Do not take Tarceva if you are allergic to it or any of its ingredients.

What should I tell my doctor before I take the first dose of this medication?

Tell your doctor about all prescription, over-the-counter, and herbal medications you are taking before beginning treatment with Tarceva. Also, talk to your doctor about your complete medical history, especially if you have liver, kidney, or stomach problems; ulcers; if you smoke; or are pregnant, plan to become pregnant, or are breastfeeding.

What is the usual dosage?

Please see general statement regarding dosage on page xii.

NSCLC

Adults: The recommended dose is 150 milligrams (mg) a day.

Pancreatic Cancer

Adults: The recommended dose is 100 mg a day. It is taken in combination with gemcitabine. Your doctor will prescribe the appropriate gemcitabine dose for you.

How should I take this medication?
• Take Tarceva at least 1 hour before or 2 hours after eating.

What should I avoid while taking this medication?
Do not smoke while you are taking Tarceva.

Do not eat grapefruit or drink grapefruit juice while on treatment with Tarceva.

What are possible food and drug interactions associated with this medication?
If Tarceva is taken with certain other drugs, the effects of either could be increased, decreased, or altered. It is important to check with your doctor before combining Tarceva with any other medication.

What are the possible side effects of this medication?
Please see general statement regarding side effects on page xiii.

> **Side effects may include:** bone pain, constipation, cough, diarrhea, fatigue, fever, infection, inflammation in your mouth, loss of appetite, muscle pain, nausea, rash, shortness of breath, stomach pain, swelling, vomiting, weight loss

Can I receive this medication if I am pregnant or breastfeeding?
Do not become pregnant while you are taking Tarceva. Make sure to use adequate contraception to prevent pregnancy while on therapy with Tarceva and continue to use adequate contraception for at least two weeks after discontinuing Tarceva. Do not breastfeed while you are taking Tarceva. Tell your doctor immediately if you are pregnant, plan to become pregnant, or are breastfeeding.

What should I do if I miss a dose of this medication?
If you miss a dose of Tarceva, take it as soon as you remember. However, if it is almost time for your next dose, skip the one you missed and return to your regular dosing schedule. Do not take two doses at once.

How should I store this medication?
Store at room temperature.

Tegretol
Generic name: Carbamazepine

What is this medication?
Tegretol is a medicine used to treat tonic-clonic (grand mal), complex partial (psychomotor or temporal lobe) seizures, and certain types of nerve pain (trigeminal and glossopharyngeal neuralgia). It is available in chewable tablets, tablets, extended-release tablets (Tegretol-XR), and a suspension.

What is the most important information I should know about this medication?
- Tegretol can cause rare but serious skin rashes that may be life-threatening. These serious skin reactions are more likely to happen within the first 4 months of treatment, but can occur at later times. These reactions are more likely to be seen in people of Asian descent. If you are of Asian descent, you may need a genetic blood test before you take Tegretol to see if you are at a higher risk for serious skin reactions with this medicine. Tell your doctor right away if you develop skin rash, hives, or sores in your mouth.
- Tegretol can cause rare but serious blood problems. Tell your doctor right away if you experience a fever, sore throat, other infections that come and go or do not go away, easy bruising, red or purple spots on your body, bleeding gums or nose, or severe fatigue or weakness.
- Do not stop taking Tegretol without first talking to your doctor. Stopping Tegretol suddenly can cause serious problems, including seizures that will not stop (status epilepticus).
- Tegretol can cause suicidal thoughts or actions. Tell your doctor right away if you have thoughts about suicide or dying; attempt to commit suicide; have new or worsening depression, anxiety, or irritability; have panic attacks; have trouble sleeping (insomnia); have an extreme increase in activity and talking (mania); are feeling agitated or restless; acting aggressive; being angry

or violent; acting on dangerous impulses; or have other unusual changes in your behavior or mood.

- Tegretol is not a regular pain medicine and should not be used for aches or pains.

Who should not take this medication?

Do not take Tegretol if you are allergic to it, any of its ingredients, or to certain antidepressants (such as fluoxetine).

Do not take Tegretol if you have a history of bone marrow depression, if you are taking nefazodone or have taken a monoamine oxidase inhibitor (MAOI) (such as phenelzine), a class of medications used to treat depression and other psychiatric conditions, in the last 14 days.

What should I tell my doctor before I take the first dose of this medication?

Tell your doctor about all prescription, over-the-counter, and herbal medications you are taking before beginning treatment with Tegretol. Also, talk to your doctor about your complete medical history, especially if you have or have had suicidal thoughts or actions, depression, or mood problems; heart, blood, liver or kidney problems; allergic reactions to medicines; increased pressure in your eye; drink grapefruit juice or eat grapefruit; use birth control; or if you are pregnant, plan to become pregnant, or are breastfeeding.

What is the usual dosage?

Please see general statement regarding dosage on page xii.

Seizures

Adults and children >12 years: The recommended starting dose is 200 milligrams (mg) twice a day for tablets or extended-release tablets. The recommended starting dose is 1 teaspoonful four times a day for suspension. Your doctor will increase your or your child's dose as appropriate.

Children 6-12 years: The recommended starting dose is 100 mg twice a day or 1/2 teaspoonful four times a day. Your doctor will increase your child's dose as appropriate.

Children <6 years: Your doctor will prescribe the appropriate dose for your child, based on their weight.

Nerve Pain
Adults and children >12 years: The recommended starting dose is 100 mg twice a day for tablets or extended-release tablets. The recommended starting dose is 1/2 teaspoonful four times a day for suspension. Your doctor will increase your or your child's dose as appropriate, to achieve freedom from pain.

How should I take this medication?
- Take Tegretol exactly as prescribed by your doctor. Do not change your dose or stop taking this medication abruptly without first talking to your doctor. Take Tegretol with food.
- Swallow Tegretol-XR tablets whole. Do not crush, chew, or break the tablets.
- Shake the Tegretol suspension well before use.

What should I avoid while taking this medication?
Do not drink alcohol while you are taking Tegretol. Drinking alcohol while you are taking Tegretol can make your sleepiness or dizziness worse.

Do not drive, operate heavy machinery, or engage in dangerous activities until you know how Tegretol affects you. Tegretol can slow your thinking and motor skills.

What are possible food and drug interactions associated with this medication?
If Tegretol is taken with certain other drugs, the effects of either could be increased, decreased, or altered. Tegretol may interact with numerous medications. Therefore, it is very important that you tell your doctor about any other medications you are taking.

What are the possible side effects of this medication?
Please see general statement regarding side effects on page xiii.

> **Side effects may include:** abdominal (stomach) pain, bruising, dark urine, dizziness, drowsiness, fainting, irregular heartbeat, lightheadedness, loss of appetite, nausea, problems with your walking and coordination (unsteadiness), shortness of breath, vomiting, yellowing of your skin or whites of your eyes

Can I receive this medication if I am pregnant or breastfeeding?

Tegretol can harm your unborn baby if you take it during pregnancy. Tegretol can be found in your breast milk if you take it while breastfeeding. Do not breastfeed while you are taking Tegretol. Tell your doctor immediately if you are pregnant, plan to become pregnant, or are breastfeeding.

What should I do if I miss a dose of this medication?

If you miss a dose of Tegretol, take it as soon as you remember. However, if it is almost time for your next dose, skip the one you missed and return to your regular dosing schedule. Do not take two doses at once.

How should I store this medication?

Store at room temperature. Protect from light and moisture.

Telaprevir: *see Incivek, page 463*

Telmisartan: *see Micardis, page 630*

Temazepam: *see Restoril, page 888*

Tekturna

Generic name: Aliskiren

What is this medication?

Tekturna is a medicine used alone or in combination with other medications to treat high blood pressure.

What is the most important information I should know about this medication?

- If you become pregnant while you are taking Tekturna, stop taking it and call your doctor right away. Tekturna can harm your unborn baby. Talk to your doctor about other medicines to treat your high blood pressure if you plan to become pregnant.
- Tekturna can cause a serious allergic reaction. Tell your doctor right away if you experience swelling of your face, lips, tongue, throat, arms and legs, or the whole body.
- Tekturna can cause low blood pressure, especially if you take diuretics (water pills), are on a low-salt diet, receive dialysis, have heart problems, or get sick with vomiting or diarrhea. If you feel faint or dizzy, lie down and call your doctor right away.

Who should not take this medication?

Do not take Tekturna if you are allergic to it or any of its ingredients.

Do not take Tekturna if you have diabetes and are taking blood pressure/heart medications known as angiotensin converting enzyme (ACE) inhibitors (such as enalapril or lisinopril) or angiotensin receptor blockers (ARBs) (such as losartan or olmesartan).

What should I tell my doctor before I take the first dose of this medication?

Tell your doctor about all prescription, over-the-counter, and herbal medications you are taking before beginning treatment with Tekturna. Also, talk to your doctor about your complete medical history, especially if you have kidney problems, heart failure, had a recent heart attack, have ever had an allergic reaction to an ACE inhibitor, or if you are pregnant, plan to become pregnant, or are breastfeeding.

What is the usual dosage?

Please see general statement regarding dosage on page xii.

Adults: The usual starting dose is 150 milligrams once a day. Your doctor will increase your dose as needed, until the desired effect is achieved.

How should I take this medication?
- Take Tekturna exactly as prescribed by your doctor. It is important to take Tekturna on a regular daily basis.
- Take Tekturna once a day, at the same time each day.
- Take Tekturna with or without food.

What should I avoid while taking this medication?
Do not take Tekturna with ARBs or ACE inhibitors if you have kidney impairment.

What are possible food and drug interactions associated with this medication?
If Tekturna is taken with certain other drugs, the effects of either could be increased, decreased, or altered. It is especially important to check with your doctor before combining Tekturna with the following: cyclosporine, itraconazole, nosteroidal anti-inflammatory drugs (NSAIDs) (such as ibuprofen or naproxen), potassium supplements, or salt substitutes that contain potassium.

What are the possible side effects of this medication?
Please see general statement regarding side effects on page xiii.

Side effects may include: back pain, cough, diarrhea, dizziness, "flu-like" symptoms, headache, high blood potassium levels, tiredness

---

Can I receive this medication if I am pregnant or breastfeeding?
Do not take Tekturna if you are pregnant or breastfeeding. Tell your doctor immediately if you are pregnant, plan to become pregnant, or are breastfeeding.

What should I do if I miss a dose of this medication?
If you miss a dose of Tekturna, take it as soon as you remember. However, if it is almost time for your next dose, skip the one you missed and return to your regular dosing schedule. Do not take two doses at once.

How should I store this medication?
Store at room temperature. Protect from moisture.

Keep Tekturna in the original prescription bottle. Do not remove the drying agent from the bottle.

Tenoretic
Generic name: Atenolol/Chlorthalidone

What is this medication?
Tenoretic is a combination medicine used to treat high blood pressure. Tenoretic contains two medicines: atenolol (a beta-blocker) and chlorthalidone (a diuretic [water pill]).

Tenoretic is available as Tenoretic 50, which contains 50 milligrams (mg) of atenolol and 25 mg of chlorthalidone, and Tenoretic 100, which contains 100 mg of atenolol and 25 mg of chlorthalidone.

What is the most important information I should know about this medication?
- Do not stop taking Tenoretic without talking to your doctor. Stopping this medication suddenly can cause harmful effects. Your doctor should reduce your dose gradually when stopping treatment with this medication.
- Tenoretic can worsen heart failure, cause breathing problems, or hide symptoms of low blood sugar levels if you have diabetes. If you have diabetes, monitor your blood sugar frequently, especially when you first start taking Tenoretic.
- Tenoretic can cause fluid and electrolyte imbalances. Signs and symptoms of this include dry mouth, thirst, weakness, fatigue, drowsiness, restlessness, muscle pains or cramps, low blood pressure, decreased urination, fast heart rate, nausea, and vomiting. Your doctor will need to monitor the levels of electrolytes in your blood periodically.

Who should not take this medication?

Do not take Tenoretic if you are allergic to it or any of its ingredients. In addition, do not take Tenoretic if you have a slow heart rate, heart failure, heart block, inability to produce urine, or severe blood circulation disorders.

What should I tell my doctor before I take the first dose of this medication?

Tell your doctor about all prescription, over-the-counter, and herbal medications you are taking before beginning treatment with Tenoretic. Also, talk to your doctor about your complete medical history, especially if you have allergies; heart problems or heart failure; a history of heart attack; breathing problems; pheochromocytoma (tumor of the adrenal gland); diabetes; liver, kidney or thyroid problems; asthma; lupus (disease that affects the immune system); or are planning to have a major surgery.

What is the usual dosage?

Please see general statement regarding dosage on page xii.

Adults: The usual starting dose is 50/25 (50 milligrams [mg] of atenolol and 25 mg of chlorthalidone) once a day. Your doctor will increase your dose as needed until the desired effect is achieved.

If you have kidney impairment, your doctor will adjust your dose appropriately.

How should I take this medication?

• Take Tenoretic exactly as prescribed by your doctor.

What should I avoid while taking this medication?

Do not stop taking Tenoretic without first talking to your doctor.

What are possible food and drug interactions associated with this medication?

If Tenoretic is taken with certain other drugs, the effects of either could be increased, decreased, or altered. It is especially important to check with your doctor before combining Tenoretic with the following: amiodarone, blood pressure medications known as

calcium channel blockers (such as diltiazem and verapamil), clonidine, digoxin, disopyramide, lithium, nonsteroidal anti-inflammatory drugs (such as ibuprofen and indomethacin), norepinephrine,
reserpine, or tubocurarine.

What are the possible side effects of this medication?
Please see general statement regarding side effects on page xiii.

> **Side effects may include:** anemia, cold extremities, constipa-
> tion, depression, diarrhea, dizziness, dreaming, fatigue, itching,
> leg pain, lightheadedness, muscle spasm, nausea, numbness
> or tingling of your skin, rash, restlessness, shortness of breath,
> slow heartbeat, sudden fall in blood pressure, tiredness, vomit-
> ing, weakness, wheezing

Can I receive this medication if I am pregnant or breastfeeding?
Tenoretic can harm your unborn baby if you take it during pregnancy. Tenoretic can be found in your breast milk if you take it while
breastfeeding. Tell your doctor immediately if you are pregnant,
plan to become pregnant, or are breastfeeding.

What should I do if I miss a dose of this medication?
If you miss a dose of Tenoretic, take it as soon as you remember.
However, if it is almost time for your next dose, skip the one you
missed and return to your regular dosing schedule. Do not take
two doses at once.

How should I store this medication?
Store at room temperature.

Tenormin

Generic name: Atenolol

What is this medication?

Tenormin is a medicine known as a beta-blocker, which is used to treat high blood pressure and chest pain. Tenormin is also used after a heart attack to lower the risk of death.

What is the most important information I should know about this medication?

- Do not stop taking Tenormin without talking to your doctor. Abruptly stopping this medication can cause harmful effects. Your doctor should gradually reduce your dose when stopping treatment with this medication.

- Tenormin can worsen heart failure, cause breathing problems, or hide symptoms of low blood sugar levels if you have diabetes. Tell your doctor if you experience weight gain or trouble breathing while you are taking Tenormin. If you have diabetes, monitor your blood sugar frequently, especially when you first start taking Tenormin.

Who should not take this medication?

Do not take Tenormin if you are allergic to it or any of its ingredients. In addition, do not take Tenormin if you have a slow heart rate, heart failure, heart block, or severe blood circulation disorders.

What should I tell my doctor before I take the first dose of this medication?

Tell your doctor about all prescription, over-the-counter, and herbal medications you are taking before beginning treatment with Tenormin. Also, talk to your doctor about your complete medical history, especially if you have allergies, heart problems or heart failure, a history of heart attack, breathing problems, pheochromocytoma (tumor of the adrenal gland), diabetes, or kidney or thyroid problems, or are planning to have a major surgery.

Tell your doctor if you have a history of severe allergic reactions to any allergens, because Tenormin may decrease the effectiveness of epinephrine used to treat the reaction.

What is the usual dosage?

Please see general statement regarding dosage on page xii.

High Blood Pressure

Adults: The usual starting dose is 50 milligrams (mg) once a day, either alone or in combination with other blood pressure-lowering medicines. Full effects should be seen in 1-2 weeks. Your doctor will increase your dose as needed until the desired effect is achieved.

Chest Pain

Adults: The usual starting dose is 50 mg once a day. Your doctor will increase your dose as needed, until the desired effect is achieved.

Heart Attack

Adults: Your doctor will prescribe the appropriate dose for you based on your condition.

If you have kidney impairment, your doctor will adjust your dose appropriately.

How should I take this medication?

• Take Tenormin exactly as prescribed by your doctor.

What should I avoid while taking this medication?

Do not stop taking Tenormin without first talking to your doctor.

What are possible food and drug interactions associated with this medication?

If Tenormin is taken with certain other drugs, the effects of either could be increased, decreased, or altered. It is especially important to check with your doctor before combining Tenormin with the following: amiodarone, blood pressure medications known as calcium channel blockers (such as diltiazem or verapamil), clonidine, disopyramide, nonsteroidal anti-inflammatory drugs (such as ibuprofen or indomethacin), or reserpine.

What are the possible side effects of this medication?
Please see general statement regarding side effects on page xiii.

> **Side effects may include:** dizziness, fatigue, nausea, slow heartbeat

Can I receive this medication if I am pregnant or breastfeeding?
Tenormin can harm your unborn baby if you take it during pregnancy. Tenormin can be found in your breast milk if you take it while breastfeeding. Tell your doctor immediately if you are pregnant, plan to become pregnant, or are breastfeeding.

What should I do if I miss a dose of this medication?
If you miss a dose of Tenormin, take it as soon as you remember. However, if it is almost time for your next dose, skip the one you missed and return to your regular dosing schedule. Do not take two doses at once.

How should I store this medication?
Store at room temperature.

Terazosin HCl: *see Terazosin, page 981*

Terbinafine HCl: *see Lamisil, page 518*

Terazosin
Generic name: Terazosin HCl

What is this medication?
Terazosin is a medicine used alone or in combination with other medications to treat high blood pressure. Terazosin is also used to relieve the signs and symptoms of benign prostatic hyperplasia (enlargement of the prostate gland, which may in turn block the flow of urine).

What is the most important information I should know about this medication?

- Terazosin can cause a sudden drop in your blood pressure, which may cause fainting, dizziness, or lightheadedness. Do not drive or perform other hazardous activities until you know how terazosin affects you.
- Rarely, terazosin can cause painful, prolonged erections (priapism). Tell your doctor right away if this occurs.

Who should not take this medication?

Do not take terazosin if you are allergic to it or any of its ingredients.

What should I tell my doctor before I take the first dose of this medication?

Tell your doctor about all prescription, over-the-counter, and herbal medications you are taking before beginning treatment with terazosin. Also, talk to your doctor about your complete medical history, especially if you have prostate cancer, plan on having cataract surgery, or are pregnant, plan to become pregnant, or are breastfeeding.

What is the usual dosage?

Please see general statement regarding dosage on page xii.

Adults: The recommended starting dose is 1 milligram once a day, at bedtime. Your doctor will prescribe the appropriate dose for you and will increase your dose as needed, until the desired effect is achieved.

How should I take this medication?

- Take terazosin exactly as prescribed by your doctor.
- Take terazosin once a day. Take terazosin with or without food.

What should I avoid while taking this medication?

Do not get up too fast from a sitting or lying position.

Do not drive or perform hazardous tasks for 12 hours after the first dose, after a dose increase, or if your treatment is interrupted then resumed, until you know how terazosin affects you.

What are possible food and drug interactions associated with this medication?

If terazosin is taken with certain other drugs, the effects of either could be increased, decreased, or altered. It is especially important to check with your doctor before combining terazosin with the following: erectile dysfunction medications or other blood pressure/heart medications (such as captopril or verapamil).

What are the possible side effects of this medication?

Please see general statement regarding side effects on page xiii.

Side effects may include: blurred vision, dizziness, impotence, lightheadedness upon standing, nausea, palpitations (fluttery or throbbing heartbeat), runny nose, sleepiness, stuffy nose, swelling, weakness

Can I receive this medication if I am pregnant or breastfeeding?

The effects of terazosin during pregnancy and breastfeeding are unknown. Tell your doctor immediately if you are pregnant, plan to become pregnant, or are breastfeeding.

What should I do if I miss a dose of this medication?

If you miss a dose of terazosin, take it as soon as you remember. However, if it is almost time for your next dose, skip the one you missed and return to your regular dosing schedule. Do not take two doses at once.

How should I store this medication?

Store at room temperature. Protect from light and moisture.

Tessalon

Generic name: Benzonatate

What is this medication?

Tessalon is a medicine used to treat cough.

What is the most important information I should know about this medication?

- Release of the medicine from the Tessalon capsule in your mouth can cause a severe allergic reaction or choking. Swallow the capsule whole. Do not suck or chew it. If you experience numbness or tingling of your tongue, mouth, throat, or face, do not eat or drink anything until the numbness disappears. If these symptoms continue or get worse, call your doctor right away.
- Tessalon can cause bizarre behavior (such as mental confusion or hallucinations) when you take it with other medicines.

Who should not take this medication?

Do not take Tessalon if you are allergic to it or any of its ingredients.

What should I tell my doctor before I take the first dose of this medication?

Tell your doctor about all prescription, over-the-counter, and herbal medications you are taking before beginning treatment with Tessalon. Also, talk to your doctor about your complete medical history, especially if you have ever had an allergic reaction to other anesthetic medicines (such as procaine or tetracaine).

What is the usual dosage?

Please see general statement regarding dosage on page xii.

Adults and children >10 years: The usual dose is 100 milligrams (mg) or 200 mg three times a day as needed. Your doctor will increase your dose as needed until the desired effect is achieved.

How should I take this medication?

- Swallow the Tessalon capsule whole. Do not break, chew, dissolve, cut, or crush it.

What should I avoid while taking this medication?

Do not suck or chew the Tessalon capsule.

What are possible food and drug interactions associated with this medication?

No significant interactions have been reported with Tessalon at this time. However, always tell your doctor about any medicines you take, including over-the-counter medications, vitamins, and herbal supplements.

What are the possible side effects of this medication?

Please see general statement regarding side effects on page xiii.

Side effects may include: allergic reactions, burning sensation in your eyes, confusion, constipation, dizziness, extreme calm, feeling cold, headache, itching, nausea, numbness in your chest, skin rash, stuffy nose, upset stomach, visual hallucinations

---

Can I receive this medication if I am pregnant or breastfeeding?

The effects of Tessalon during pregnancy and breastfeeding are unknown. Tell your doctor immediately if you are pregnant, plan to become pregnant, or are breastfeeding.

What should I do if I miss a dose of this medication?

If you miss a dose of Tessalon, take it as soon as you remember. However, if it is almost time for your next dose, skip the one you missed and return to your regular dosing schedule. Do not take two doses at once.

How should I store this medication?

Store at room temperature.

Testosterone: *see Androgel, page 79*

Thalitone

Generic name: Chlorthalidone

What is this medication?

Thalitone is a diuretic (water pill) used alone or in combination with other medications to treat high blood pressure. Thalitone is also used in combination with other medications to treat edema (swelling) associated with heart, kidney, liver disease, or corticosteroid and estrogen therapy.

What is the most important information I should know about this medication?

- Thalitone can cause a decrease in your blood potassium levels or other electrolyte (chemicals that are important for the cells in your body to function) abnormalities, including low sodium or chloride levels. Your doctor will perform regular blood tests to check your fluids and electrolytes. Tell your doctor if you experience confusion, decreased urination, drowsiness, dry mouth, fast heart rate, low blood pressure, muscle pain or cramps, nausea, restlessness, seizures, tiredness, vomiting, or weakness.

- Thalitone can cause serious side effects, especially if you have kidney or liver problems. Also, you can be at a higher risk of experiencing an allergic reaction to Thalitone if you have a history of allergy or asthma. Tell your doctor if you have kidney or liver problems, allergies, or asthma before you start treatment with Thalitone.

- Thalitone can cause gout (severe and painful inflammation of the joints). Thalitone can also cause an increase in your blood sugar levels and lead to diabetes. Your doctor will monitor you for these conditions.

Who should not take this medication?

Do not take Thalitone if you are allergic to it, any of its ingredients, or to other sulfonamide medications (such as sulfamethoxazole).

Do not take Thalitone if you are unable to produce urine.

What should I tell my doctor before I take the first dose of this medication?

Tell your doctor about all prescription, over-the-counter, and herbal medications you are taking before beginning treatment with Thalitone. Also, talk to your doctor about your complete medical history, especially if you have allergies, asthma, kidney or liver disease, lupus (a chronic condition that affects your immune system), are pregnant, plan to become pregnant, or are breastfeeding.

What is the usual dosage?

Please see general statement regarding dosage on page xii.

High Blood Pressure
Adults: The usual starting dose is 15 milligrams (mg) once a day.

Edema
Adults: The usual starting dose is 30-60 mg a day or 60 mg every other day. The dose may be increased to 90-120 mg a day.

How should I take this medication?
• Take Thalitone exactly as prescribed by your doctor. Do not take extra doses or take more often without asking your doctor.

What should I avoid while taking this medication?

Do not drink alcohol while taking Thalitone. Thalitone can cause dizziness.

What are possible food and drug interactions associated with this medication?

If Thalitone is taken with certain other drugs, the effects of either could be increased, decreased, or altered. It is especially important to check with your doctor before combining Thalitone with any of the following: alcohol, antidiabetic medications (such as insulin), certain blood pressure medications, digoxin, lithium, medications that can cause drowsiness, norepinephrine, or tubocurarine.

What are the possible side effects of this medication?

Please see general statement regarding side effects on page xiii.

Side effects may include: changes in blood sugar, low potassium levels, constipation, cramping, diarrhea, dizziness, headache, impotence, loss of appetite, low blood pressure, muscle spasms, nausea, rash, restlessness, sensitivity to light, stomach irritation, vomiting, weakness, yellowing of your skin or whites of your eyes

---

Can I receive this medication if I am pregnant or breastfeeding?

The effects of Thalitone during pregnancy are unknown. Thalitone can be found in your breast milk if you take it during breastfeeding. Do not take Thalitone while you are breastfeeding. Tell your doctor immediately if you are pregnant, plan to become pregnant, or are breastfeeding.

What should I do if I miss a dose of this medication?

If you miss a dose of Thalitone, take it as soon as you remember. However, if it is almost time for your next dose, skip the one you missed and return to your regular dosing schedule. Do not take two doses at once.

How should I store this medication?

Store at room temperature.

Theophylline ER

Generic name: Theophylline

What is this medication?

Theophylline extended-release (ER) is a medicine used to treat symptoms associated with long-term asthma and other lung diseases, such as emphysema (lung disease that causes shortness of breath) and chronic bronchitis (long-term inflammation of the lungs).

What is the most important information I should know about this medication?

- Your doctor will monitor your blood theophylline levels and will adjust your dose of theophylline ER appropriately.
- Your blood theophylline levels can increase if you take theophylline ER while you have heart diseases, such as heart failure or cor pulmonale (right-sided heart failure); persistent fever; hypothyroidism (an underactive thyroid gland); liver disease, such as cirrhosis (scarring of the liver) or hepatitis; kidney impairment in infants <3 months; sepsis (a bloodstream infection) with failure of multiple organs; shock; or cessation of smoking. Tell your doctor if you have any of these conditions, and he/she will decrease your total daily dose of theophylline ER appropriately.
- Tell your doctor if you develop symptoms of theophylline toxicity (such as nausea, vomiting, persistent headache, insomnia, or rapid heartbeat) while you are taking theophylline ER.
- Theophylline ER can worsen stomach ulcers, seizures, and arrhythmias (life-threatening irregular heartbeats). Tell your doctor if you have any of these conditions.
- Tell your doctor if you develop a new illness, worsening of a long-term illness, start or stop smoking cigarettes or marijuana, start a new medication, or stop using any of your previously prescribed medications while you are taking theophylline ER.

Who should not take this medication?

Do not take theophylline ER if you are allergic to it or any of its ingredients.

What should I tell my doctor before I take the first dose of this medication?

Tell your doctor about all prescription, over-the-counter, and herbal medications you are taking before beginning treatment with theophylline ER. Also, talk to your doctor about your complete medical history, especially if you have certain heart diseases, swelling in your lungs, stomach ulcer, seizures, fever, thyroid problems, liver or kidney problems, or cystic fibrosis (inherited disease that causes your mucus to be thick and sticky, and may result in difficulty breathing).

What is the usual dosage?
Please see general statement regarding dosage on page xii.

Adults and children 12-15 years and >45 kg: The recommended starting dose is 300-400 milligrams (mg) every 24 hours. Your doctor will prescribe the appropriate dose for you and will increase your dose as needed, until the desired effect is achieved.

Children 12-15 years and <45 kg: Your doctor will prescribe the appropriate dose for your child, based on their weight.

How should I take this medication?
• Take theophylline ER exactly as prescribed by your doctor. Do not take extra doses or take more often without asking your doctor. Take theophylline ER in the morning or evening. It is recommended to take this medication with meals consistently. If you choose to take it without food, it should be taken without food consistently.
• When you take theophylline ER, you may see something in your stool that looks like a tablet. This is the empty shell from the tablet after the medicine has been absorbed in your body.

What should I avoid while taking this medication?
Do not chew or crush theophylline ER tablets.

Do not miss your scheduled follow-up appointments with your doctor.

What are possible food and drug interactions associated with this medication?
If theophylline ER is taken with certain other drugs, the effects of either could be increased, decreased, or altered. Theophylline ER may interact with numerous medications. Therefore, it is very important that you tell your doctor about any other medications you are taking.

What are the possible side effects of this medication?
Please see general statement regarding side effects on page xiii.

> **Side effects may include:** arrhythmia, diarrhea, headache, increased urination, insomnia, irritability, nausea, rapid heartbeat, restlessness, seizure, tremor, vomiting

Can I receive this medication if I am pregnant or breastfeeding?
The effects of theophylline ER during pregnancy are unknown. Theophylline ER is excreted into breast milk and may cause irritability in nursing infants. Tell your doctor immediately if you are pregnant, plan to become pregnant, or are breastfeeding.

What should I do if I miss a dose of this medication?
If you miss a dose of theophylline ER, skip the one you missed and return to your regular dosing schedule. Do not take two doses at once.

How should I store this medication?
Store at room temperature.

Theophylline: *see Theophylline ER, page 988*

Thyroid: *see Armour Thyroid, page 92*

Ticagrelor: *see Brilinta, page 156*

Timolol Maleate: *see Timoptic, page 991*

Timoptic
Generic name: Timolol Maleate

What is this medication?
Timoptic is an eye drop used to lower pressure in the eye in people with open-angle glaucoma or high pressure in the eye.

What is the most important information I should know about this medication?

- Even though Timoptic is applied directly to the eye, the medication can still be absorbed in your bloodstream and cause serious adverse reactions, such as breathing difficulties, especially in patients with asthma or heart problems.
- Do not allow the tip of the bottle to touch your eye or any other surface, as serious eye infections may occur if your bottle becomes contaminated. Tell your doctor immediately if you experience any eye injury or infection with Timoptic.
- Do not use other eye medications unless your doctor has prescribed it for you. If you use another eye medication, use it at least 10 minutes before or after using Timoptic.

Who should not take this medication?

Do not use Timoptic if you are allergic to it or any of its ingredients.

Do not use Timoptic if you have or had asthma or severe breathing or lung problems.

Do not use Timoptic if you have heart problems, including a slow or irregular heartbeat or heart failure.

What should I tell my doctor before I take the first dose of this medication?

Tell your doctor about all prescription, over-the-counter, and herbal medications you are taking before beginning treatment with Timoptic. Also, talk to your doctor about your complete medical history, especially if you have problems with muscle weakness; have diabetes; have thyroid problems; are planning to have surgery (including eye surgery); have or have had eye problems; or are pregnant, plan to become pregnant, or are breastfeeding.

What is the usual dosage?

Please see general statement regarding dosage on page xii.

Adults: Apply 1 drop into the affected eye(s) twice a day.

How should I take this medication?

- Apply Timoptic as prescribed by your doctor. Please review the instructions that came with your prescription on how to properly use your eye drops.
- Timoptic contains a preservative that may be absorbed by your contact lenses. Remove your contact lenses prior to the administration of Timoptic and reinsert them after 15 minutes.

What should I avoid while taking this medication?

Do not allow the tip of the bottle to touch your eye or any other surface, as this can contaminate Timoptic.

What are possible food and drug interactions associated with this medication?

If Timoptic is used with certain other drugs, the effects of either could be increased, decreased, or altered. It is especially important to check with your doctor before combining Timoptic with any of the following: blood pressure and heart medications known as beta-blockers (such as propranolol) and calcium channel blockers (such as diltiazem), certain antidepressant medications known as selective serotonin reuptake inhibitors (SSRIs) (such as fluoxetine, paroxetine, or sertraline), clonidine, digitalis, epinephrine, quinidine, or reserpine.

What are the possible side effects of this medication?

Please see general statement regarding side effects on page xiii.

> **Side effects may include:** breathing problems, burning and stinging of your eye, chest pain, diarrhea, dizziness, dry mouth, eye irritation or redness, itching of your eye, hair loss, loss of appetite, muscle weakness, nausea, rash, sweating, weight loss

Can I receive this medication if I am pregnant or breastfeeding?

The effects of Timoptic during pregnancy and breastfeeding are unknown. Timoptic can be found in your breast milk if you use it while breastfeeding. Tell your doctor immediately if you are pregnant, plan to become pregnant, or are breastfeeding.

What should I do if I miss a dose of this medication?

If you miss a dose of Timoptic, apply it as soon as you remember. However, if it is almost time for your next dose, skip the one you missed and return to your regular dosing schedule. Do not apply two doses at once.

How should I store this medication?

Store at room temperature. Do not freeze. Protect from light.

Tiotropium Bromide: *see Spiriva Handihaler, page 942*

Tirofiban HCl: *see Aggrastat, page 41*

Tizanidine HCl: *see Zanaflex, page 1122*

Tobradex

Generic name: Dexamethasone/Tobramycin

What is this medication?

Tobradex is an eye drop used to treat inflammation of the eye and to also prevent and treat bacterial eye infections. Tobradex is available as an ointment, suspension, and as Tobradex ST suspension.

What is the most important information I should know about this medication?

- Prolonged use of Tobradex can lead to glaucoma (high pressure in the eye), visual disturbances, formation of cataracts, and new eye infections.
- Your doctor will monitor the pressure in your eyes if you use Tobradex ST for 10 days or longer.
- Stop using Tobradex ST and tell your doctor if you have pain or inflammation of the eye that lasts longer than 48 hours or worsens.
- The use of Tobradex ST after cataract surgery may delay healing.

Who should not take this medication?

Do not use Tobradex if you are allergic to it or any of its ingredients.

Do not use Tobradex if you have certain fungal or viral eye infections.

What should I tell my doctor before I take the first dose of this medication?

Tell your doctor about all prescription, over-the-counter, and herbal medications you are taking before beginning treatment with Tobradex. Also, talk to your doctor about your complete medical history, especially if you have dry eyes, glaucoma, cataract surgery, or fungal or viral infection of the eyes.

What is the usual dosage?

Please see general statement regarding dosage on page xii.

Tobradex Ointment
Adults and children ≥2 years: Apply a small amount (about 1/2 inch ribbon) into the lower eyelid(s) up to 3 or 4 times a day.

Tobradex Suspension
Adults and children ≥2 years: Apply 1 or 2 drops into the lower eyelid(s) every 4-6 hours. Your doctor will adjust your dose as needed.

Tobradex ST Suspension
Adults and children ≥2 years: Apply 1 drop into the lower eyelid(s) every 4-6 hours. Your doctor will adjust your dose as needed.

How should I take this medication?

- Apply Tobradex exactly as prescribed by your doctor. Shake Tobradex and Tobradex ST suspensions well before use.
- To apply Tobradex ointment, tilt your head back and place a finger on your cheek just under your eye. Gently pull down until a "V" pocket is formed between your eyeball and your lower lid. Place the ointment in the "V" pocket. Do not let the tip of the tube touch your eye. Look downward before closing your eye.

What should I avoid while taking this medication?

Do not touch the dropper tip to your eyelids or any other surface, as this may contaminate Tobradex.

Do not wear contact lenses while you are using Tobradex.

Do not stop using Tobradex without first talking to your doctor.

What are possible food and drug interactions associated with this medication?

No significant interactions have been reported with Tobradex at this time. However, always tell your doctor about any medicines you take, including over-the-counter medications, vitamins, and herbal supplements.

What are the possible side effects of this medication?

Please see general statement regarding side effects on page xiii.

> **Side effects may include:** allergic reaction, eye pain, eyelid itching and swelling, red eye

Can I receive this medication if I am pregnant or breastfeeding?

The effects of Tobradex during pregnancy and breastfeeding are unknown. Tell your doctor immediately if you are pregnant, plan to become pregnant, or are breastfeeding.

What should I do if I miss a dose of this medication?

If you miss a dose of Tobradex, apply it as soon as you remember. However, if it is almost time for your next dose, skip the one you missed and return to your regular dosing schedule. Do not apply two doses at once.

How should I store this medication?

Store at room temperature or in the refrigerator.

Protect Tobradex ST from light.

Tofranil
Generic name: Imipramine HCl

What is this medication?
Tofranil is a medication used to treat depression. It is also used to treat bed-wetting in children ≥6 years.

What is the most important information I should know about this medication?
- Tofranil may increase suicidal thoughts or actions in some children, teenagers, and young adults when it is first started.
- Do not take Tofranil if you are taking another antidepressant drug known as a monoamine oxidase inhibitor (MAOI) or if you have stopped taking an MAOI in the last 14 days. MAOI drugs include phenelzine, tranylcypromine, and isocarboxazid. Taking Tofranil within 2 weeks of an MAOI can result in serious, sometimes fatal, reactions, including abnormally high fever or seizures.

Who should not take this medication?
Do not take Tofranil if you are recovering from a heart attack, if you are allergic or sensitive to it, or if you are using MAOI drugs or have used an MAOI in the last 14 days.

What should I tell my doctor before I take the first dose of this medication?
Tell your doctor about all prescription, over-the-counter, and herbal medications you are taking before beginning treatment with Tofranil. Also, talk to your doctor about your complete medical history, especially if you have a history of heart disease, congestive heart failure, abnormal heart rhythm, have had a heart attack, stroke, rapid heartbeat, glaucoma (increased pressure in the eye), difficulty urinating, an enlarged prostate, overactive thyroid, seizures, schizophrenia, bipolar disorder, kidney or liver disease, diabetes, and if you will be undergoing surgery or electroconvulsive therapy (ECT).

What is the usual dosage?
Please see general statement regarding dosage on page xii.

Depression
Adults: The usual dose is 75 milligrams (mg) a day, but your doctor may increase this to 150 mg a day.

Elderly and adolescents: The usual dose is 30-40 mg a day.

Bed-wetting
Children ≥6 years: The starting dose is 25 mg a day taken 1 hour before bedtime.

How should I take this medication?
- Take Tofranil exactly as prescribed by your doctor. Do not stop taking Tofranil if you feel no immediate effect. It can take anywhere from 1-3 weeks before you feel better. An abrupt decrease in dose could result in general feelings of illness, headache, and nausea.
- Tofranil may be taken with or without food. It may be taken several times a day or in one daily dose at bedtime.

What should I avoid while taking this medication?
Do not drive or operate machinery, or participate in any activities that require full alertness until you know how this medication affects you.

Use alcohol cautiously since it may increase drowsiness and dizziness while you are taking Tofranil.

Tofranil may increase your skin's sensitivity to sunlight which could cause rash, itching, redness, or sunburn. Avoid direct sunlight or wear protective clothing.

What are possible food and drug interactions associated with this medication?
If Tofranil is taken with certain other drugs, the effects of either could be increased, decreased, or altered. It is especially important to check with your doctor before combining Tofranil with the following: albuterol, antidepressants, antipsychotic drugs, barbiturates (such as phenobarbital), benztropine, blood pressure medications, carbamazepine, cimetidine, epinephrine, flecainide, guanethidine,

methylphenidate, narcotic painkillers (such as codeine and oxyco-done), norepinephrine, phenytoin, propafenone, pseudoephedrine, quinidine, thyroid medications, and tranquilizers.

If you are switching from fluoxetine (an antidepressant), wait at least 5 weeks after your last dose of fluoxetine before starting Tofranil.

What are the possible side effects of this medication?
Please see general statement regarding side effects on page xiii.

> **Side effects may include:** breast development in males, breast enlargement in females, breast milk production, confusion, diarrhea, dry mouth, hallucinations, high blood pressure, hives, low blood pressure upon standing, nausea, numbness, tremors, vomiting
>
> *Side effects in children being treated for bed-wetting include:* anxiety, collapse, constipation, emotional instability, fainting, fatigue, nervousness, seizures, sleep disorders, stomach and intestinal problems

Can I receive this medication if I am pregnant or breastfeeding?
The effects of Tofranil during pregnancy and breastfeeding are unknown. Tell your doctor immediately if you are pregnant, plan to become pregnant, or are breastfeeding.

What should I do if I miss a dose of this medication?
If you miss a dose of Tofranil, take it as soon as you remember. However, if it is almost time for your next dose, skip the one you missed and return to your regular dosing schedule. Do not take two doses at once.

How should I store this medication?
Store at room temperature.

Tofranil-PM
Generic name: Imipramine Pamoate

What is this medication?
Tofranil-PM is a medication used to treat depression.

What is the most important information I should know about this medication?
- Tofranil-PM may increase suicidal thoughts or actions in some children, teenagers, and young adults when it is first started.
- Do not take Tofranil-PM if you are taking another antidepressant drug known as a monoamine oxidase inhibitor (MAOI) or if you have stopped taking an MAOI in the last 14 days. MAOI drugs include phenelzine, tranylcypromine, and isocarboxazid. Taking Tofranil within 2 weeks of an MAOI can result in serious, sometimes fatal, reactions, including high body temperature, coma, and seizures.

Who should not take this medication?
Do not take Tofranil-PM if you are recovering from a heart attack, if you are allergic or sensitive to it, or if you are using an MAOI or have used an MAOI in the last 14 days.

What should I tell my doctor before I take the first dose of this medication?
Tell your doctor about all prescription, over-the-counter, and herbal medications you are taking before beginning treatment with Tofranil-PM. Also, talk to your doctor about your complete medical history, especially if you have a history of heart disease, congestive heart failure, abnormal heart rhythm, have had a heart attack, stroke, rapid heartbeat, glaucoma (increased pressure in the eye), difficulty urinating, an enlarged prostate, overactive thyroid, seizures, schizophrenia, bipolar disorder, kidney or liver disease, diabetes, or if you will be undergoing surgery or electroconvulsive therapy (ECT).

What is the usual dosage?
Please see general statement regarding dosage on page xii.

Adults: The usual dose is 75 milligrams (mg) a day. Your doctor may increase this to 150-200 mg a day.

Elderly and adolescents: Effective doses usually do not exceed 100 mg a day.

How should I take this medication?
- Take Tofranil-PM exactly as prescribed by your doctor. Do not stop taking it if you feel no immediate effect. It can take anywhere from 1-3 weeks before you feel better. An abrupt decrease in dose could result in general feelings of illness, headache, and nausea.
- Tofranil-PM may be taken with or without food. It may be taken several times a day or in one daily dose at bedtime.

What should I avoid while taking this medication?
Do not drive or operate machinery, or participate in any activities that require full alertness until you know how this medication affects you.

Use alcohol cautiously since it may increase drowsiness and dizziness while you are taking Tofranil-PM.

Tofranil-PM may increase your skin's sensitivity to sunlight which could cause rash, itching, redness, or sunburn. Avoid direct sunlight or wear protective clothing.

What are possible food and drug interactions associated with this medication?
If Tofranil-PM is taken with certain other drugs, the effects of either could be increased, decreased, or altered. It is especially important to check with your doctor before combining Tofranil-PM with the following: albuterol, antidepressants, antipsychotic drugs, barbiturates (such as phenobarbital), benztropine, blood pressure medications, carbamazepine, cimetidine, epinephrine, flecainide, guanethidine, methylphenidate, narcotic painkillers (such as codeine and oxycodone), norepinephrine, phenytoin, propafenone, pseudoephedrine, quinidine, thyroid medications, or tranquilizers.

If you are switching from fluoxetine (an antidepressant), wait at least 5 weeks after your last dose of fluoxetine before starting Tofranil-PM.

What are the possible side effects of this medication?
Please see general statement regarding side effects on page xiii.

> **Side effects may include:** breast development in males, breast enlargement in females, breast milk production, confusion, diarrhea, dry mouth, hallucinations, high blood pressure, hives, low blood pressure upon standing, nausea, numbness, tremors, vomiting

Can I receive this medication if I am pregnant or breastfeeding?
The effects of Tofranil-PM during pregnancy and breastfeeding are unknown. Tell your doctor immediately if you are pregnant, plan to become pregnant, or are breastfeeding.

What should I do if I miss a dose of this medication?
If you miss a dose of Tofranil-PM, take it as soon as you remember. However, if it is almost time for your next dose, skip the one you missed and return to your regular dosing schedule. Do not take two doses at once.

How should I store this medication?
Store at room temperature.

Tolterodine Tartrate: *see Detrol, page 305*

Tolterodine Tartrate: *see Detrol LA, page 307*

Topamax

Generic name: Topiramate

What is this medication?

Topamax is a medicine used alone or in combination with other medications to treat certain types of seizures. It is also used to prevent migraine headaches. Topamax is available as tablets and Sprinkle capsules.

What is the most important information I should know about this medication?

- Topamax can cause serious eye problems. These include any sudden decrease in vision with or without eye pain and redness, or a blockage of fluid in the eye causing glaucoma (high pressure in the eye). These problems can lead to permanent vision loss if not treated. Tell your doctor right away if you have any new eye symptoms.
- Topamax can cause decreased sweating and fever. Tell your doctor right away if you experience either of these.
- Topamax can cause metabolic acidosis (increased acid in your blood). This can lead to brittle or soft bones, kidney stones, slow the rate of growth in children, and possibly harm your unborn baby if you are pregnant. Tell your doctor if you feel tired, changes in your heartbeat, loss of appetite, or if you have trouble thinking clearly.
- Topamax can cause suicidal thoughts or actions. Tell your doctor immediately if you have thoughts about suicide or dying; attempt to commit suicide; have new or worsening depression, anxiety, or irritability; have panic attacks; have trouble sleeping (insomnia); have an extreme increase in activity and talking (mania); are feeling agitated or restless; acting aggressive; being angry or violent; acting on dangerous impulses; or have other unusual changes in behavior or mood.
- Topamax can harm your unborn baby if you take it while you are pregnant. Your baby has a higher risk for birth defects called cleft lip and cleft palate if you take Topamax during pregnancy. If your doctor decides to prescribe Topamax to you, use an effect birth control. Talk to your doctor about the best kind of birth control to use while you are taking Topamax.

- Topamax can cause high blood ammonia levels or low body temperature when taken alone or in combination with another medicine called valproic acid. Tell your doctor if you experience unexplained changes in your mental status, confusion, tiredness, or vomiting.
- Topamax can cause kidney stones to develop. Drink plenty of fluids while you are taking Topamax to lower your chances of getting kidney stones.
- Topamax can affect your thinking and alertness. You can experience confusion, depression or mood problems, drowsiness, fatigue, or problems with concentration, attention, memory, or speech.

Who should not take this medication?
Do not take Topamax if you are allergic to it or any of its ingredients.

What should I tell my doctor before I take the first dose of this medication?
Tell your doctor about all prescription, over-the-counter, and herbal medications you are taking before beginning treatment with Topamax. Also, talk to your doctor about your complete medical history, especially if you have eye problems (such as glaucoma); growth problems; kidney disease, kidney stones, or are receiving dialysis; diarrhea; liver disease; lung or breathing problems; weak, brittle, or soft bones; or a history of metabolic acidosis, depression, mood problems, or suicidal thoughts or behavior. Tell your doctor if you are on a ketogenic diet (diet high in fat and low in carbohydrates) or if you are planning to have surgery.

What is the usual dosage?
Please see general statement regarding dosage on page xii.

Seizures
Adults: Your doctor will prescribe the appropriate dose for you based on the type of seizures you have.

Children: Your doctor will prescribe the appropriate dose for your child, based on their weight.

Migraine
Adults: Your doctor will prescribe the appropriate dose for you.

How should I take this medication?
- Take Topamax exactly as prescribed by your doctor. Take it with or without food. Drink plenty of fluids during the day to prevent kidney stones.
- Swallow Topamax tablets whole. Do not chew them. They may leave a bitter taste.
- Swallow Topamax Sprinkle capsules whole or open the capsule and sprinkle the medicine on a teaspoonful of soft food. Swallow the medicine and food mixture right away. Do not store any for later use. Drink fluids right after you swallow the mixture to be sure you took all the medicine.

What should I avoid while taking this medication?
Do not drink alcohol while you are taking Topamax.

Do not drive or operate heavy machinery until you know how Topamax affects you.

Do not change your dose or stop taking Topamax without talking to your doctor. Stopping Topamax suddenly can cause serious side effects.

What are possible food and drug interactions associated with this medication?
If Topamax is taken with certain other drugs, the effects of either could be increased, decreased, or altered. It is especially important to check with your doctor before combining Topamax with the following: acetazolamide, alcohol, amitriptyline, birth control pills, carbamazepine, dichlorphenamide, digoxin, hydrochlorothiazide, lithium, metformin, phenytoin, valproic acid, or zonisamide.

What are the possible side effects of this medication?
Please see general statement regarding side effects on page xiii.

> **Side effects may include:** change in taste, diarrhea, loss of appetite, nausea, nervousness, tingling of your arms and legs, upper respiratory tract infection, weight loss

Can I receive this medication if I am pregnant or breastfeeding?

Topamax can harm your unborn baby if you take it during pregnancy. The effects of Topamax during breastfeeding are unknown. Tell your doctor immediately if you are pregnant, plan to become pregnant, or are breastfeeding.

What should I do if I miss a dose of this medication?

If you miss a dose of Topamax, take it as soon as you remember. However, if it is almost time for your next dose, skip the one you missed and return to your regular dosing schedule. Do not take two doses at once.

How should I store this medication?

Store at room temperature. Protect from moisture.

Topiramate: see Topamax, page 1003

Toprol-XL

Generic name: Metoprolol Succinate

What is this medication?

Toprol-XL is a medicine known as a beta-blocker, which is used to treat high blood pressure, chest pain, and heart failure.

What is the most important information I should know about this medication?

• You must take Toprol-XL regularly and continuously for it to be effective. Do not stop taking Toprol-XL without talking to your doctor. Abruptly stopping this medication can cause harmful effects. Your doctor should gradually reduce your dose when stopping treatment with this medication.

- Toprol-XL can worsen heart failure, cause breathing problems, or hide symptoms of low blood sugar levels if you have diabetes. Tell your doctor if you experience weight gain or trouble breathing while you are taking Toprol-XL. If you have diabetes, monitor your blood sugar frequently, especially when you first start taking Toprol-XL.
- Tell your doctor or dentist that you are taking Toprol-XL before undergoing any type of surgery.

Who should not take this medication?

Do not take Toprol-XL if you are allergic to it or any of its ingredients. In addition, do not take Toprol-XL if you have a slow heart rate, heart failure, heart block, or severe blood circulation disorders.

What should I tell my doctor before I take the first dose of this medication?

Tell your doctor about all prescription, over-the-counter, and herbal medications you are taking before beginning treatment with Toprol-XL. Also, talk to your doctor about your complete medical history, especially if you have allergies, heart problems or heart failure, a history of heart attack, breathing problems, pheochromocytoma (tumor of the adrenal gland), diabetes, liver or thyroid problems, or peripheral vascular disease (disease of the blood vessels outside the heart and brain), or are planning to have a major surgery.

Tell your doctor if you have a history of severe allergic reactions to any allergens, because Toprol-XL may decrease the effectiveness of epinephrine used to treat the reaction.

What is the usual dosage?

Please see general statement regarding dosage on page xii.

Blood Pressure

Adults: The usual starting dose is 25-100 milligrams (mg) once a day, either alone or in combination with other blood pressure-lowering medicines. Full effects should be seen in 1 week. Your doctor will increase your dose as needed until the desired effect is achieved.

Children ≥6 years: Your doctor will prescribe the appropriate dose for your child, based on their weight.

Chest Pain
Adults: The usual starting dose is 100 mg once a day. Your doctor will increase your dose as needed until the desired effect is achieved.

Heart Failure
Adults: Your doctor will prescribe the appropriate dose for you based on your condition.

If you have liver impairment, your doctor will adjust your dose appropriately.

How should I take this medication?
- Take Toprol-XL exactly as prescribed by your doctor. Take it with or immediately following meals.
- Toprol-XL tablets can be divided if directed by your doctor. Do not crush or chew the whole or half tablet.

What should I avoid while taking this medication?
Do not drive a car, operate machinery, or engage in other tasks requiring alertness until you know how Toprol-XL affects you.

Do not stop taking Toprol-XL without first talking to your doctor.

What are possible food and drug interactions associated with this medication?
If Toprol-XL is taken with certain other drugs, the effects of either could be increased, decreased, or altered. It is especially important to check with your doctor before combining Toprol-XL with the following: blood pressure medications known as calcium channel blockers (such as diltiazem or verapamil); clonidine; digoxin; fluoxetine; monoamine oxidase inhibitors (such as selegiline or phenelzine), a class of medications used to treat depression and other psychiatric conditions; quinidine; paroxetine; propafenone; or reserpine.

What are the possible side effects of this medication?
Please see general statement regarding side effects on page xiii.

> **Side effects may include:** depression, diarrhea, dizziness, rash, shortness of breath, slow heart beat, tiredness

Can I receive this medication if I am pregnant or breastfeeding?
The effects of Toprol-XL during pregnancy are unknown. Toprol-XL can be found in your breast milk if you take it while breastfeeding. Tell your doctor immediately if you are pregnant, plan to become pregnant, or are breastfeeding.

What should I do if I miss a dose of this medication?
If you miss a dose of Toprol-XL, take it as soon as you remember. However, if it is almost time for your next dose, skip the one you missed and return to your regular dosing schedule. Do not take two doses at once.

How should I store this medication?
Store at room temperature.

Tradjenta
Generic name: Linagliptin

What is this medication?
Tradjenta is a medicine used in addition to diet and exercise to lower blood sugar in adults with type 2 diabetes.

What is the most important information I should know about this medication?
- Do not use Tradjenta if you have type 1 diabetes.
- Tradjenta can cause a serious allergic reaction, including rash, hives, and swelling of your face, lips, tongue, or throat, which may cause difficulty breathing or swallowing. If you have an

allergic reaction, stop taking Tradjenta and call your doctor right away.

- When your body is under some types of stress (such as fever, trauma [for example, a car accident], infection, or surgery), the amount of diabetes medicine that you need may change. Tell your doctor immediately if you have any of these conditions.
- Tradjenta can cause low blood sugar. If you take Tradjenta with another medicine that can cause low blood sugar (such as glipizide or glimepiride), your risk of getting low blood sugar can increase. This can cause confusion, dizziness, drowsiness, fast heartbeat, feeling jittery, headache, hunger, irritability, sweating, or weakness.
- Make sure you stay on your diet and exercise program and check your blood sugar regularly.

Who should not take this medication?
Do not take Tradjenta if you are allergic to it or any of its ingredients.

Do not take Tradjenta if you have type 1 diabetes.

What should I tell my doctor before I take the first dose of this medication?
Tell your doctor about all prescription, over-the-counter, and herbal medications you are taking before beginning treatment with Tradjenta. Also, talk to your doctor about your complete medical history, especially if you are experiencing some type of stress (such as fever, trauma, infection, or surgery), are pregnant, plan to become pregnant, or are breastfeeding.

What is the usual dosage?
Please see general statement regarding dosage on page xii.

Adults: The recommended dose is 5 milligrams once a day.

How should I take this medication?
- Take Tradjenta as prescribed by your doctor.
- Take Tradjenta with or without food.
- Your doctor may prescribe Tradjenta along with other medications that lower your blood sugar.

What should I avoid while taking this medication?
Do not take rifampin while you are taking Tradjenta.

What are possible food and drug interactions associated with this medication?
If Tradjenta is taken with certain other drugs, the effects of either could be increased, decreased, or altered. It is especially important to check with your doctor before combining Tradjenta with the following: other medicines that can lower your blood sugar (such as glipizide or glimepiride) or rifampin.

What are the possible side effects of this medication?
Please see general statement regarding side effects on page xiii.

Side effects may include: allergic reactions, cough, low blood sugar levels, sore throat, stuffy or runny nose, weight gain

Symptoms of low blood sugar: confusion, dizziness, drowsiness, fast heartbeat, feeling jittery, headache, hunger, irritability, sweating, weakness

---

Can I receive this medication if I am pregnant or breastfeeding?
The effects of Tradjenta during pregnancy and breastfeeding are unknown. Tell your doctor immediately if you are pregnant, plan to become pregnant, or are breastfeeding.

What should I do if I miss a dose of this medication?
If you miss a dose of Tradjenta, take it as soon as you remember. However, if it is almost time for your next dose, skip the one you missed and return to your regular dosing schedule. Do not take two doses at once.

How should I store this medication?
Store at room temperature.

Tramadol HCl: *see Rybix ODT, page 913*

Tramadol HCl: *see Ryzolt, page 917*

Tramadol HCl: *see Ultram, page 1038*

Travatan Z
Generic name: Travoprost

What is this medication?
Travatan Z is an eye drop used to lower pressure in the eye in people with open-angle glaucoma or high pressure in the eye.

What is the most important information I should know about this medication?
- Travatan Z can darken the color of your iris (colored part of the eye), eyelid, or eyelashes. The discoloration of your eyelids or eyelashes is usually reversible; however, the discoloration of the iris is most likely permanent.
- Travatan Z can also increase the length, thickness, number of eyelashes, and/or direction of eyelash growth. Tell your doctor if you notice any discoloration or changes in these areas of your eye.
- Do not allow the tip of the bottle to touch your eye or any other surface, as serious eye infections may occur if your bottle becomes contaminated. Tell your doctor immediately if you experience any eye injury, infection, conjunctivitis ("pink eye"), or eyelid reactions with Travatan Z.

Who should not take this medication?
Do not use Travatan Z if you are allergic to it or any of its ingredients.

What should I tell my doctor before I take the first dose of this medication?
Tell your doctor about all prescription, over-the-counter, and herbal medications you are taking before beginning treatment with Travatan Z. Also, talk to your doctor about your complete medical history, especially if you have had eye surgery or other eye disorders.

What is the usual dosage?
Please see general statement regarding dosage on page xii.

Adults and children ≥16 years: Apply 1 drop into the affected eye(s) once a day in the evening.

How should I take this medication?
- Apply Travatan Z exactly as prescribed by your doctor.
- Travatan Z contains a preservative that may be absorbed by your contact lenses. Remove your contact lenses prior to the administration of Travatan Z and reinsert them after 15 minutes.
- If you are using Travatan Z with another eye drop, the drops should be applied at least 5 minutes apart.

What should I avoid while taking this medication?
Do not allow the tip of the bottle to touch your eye or any other surface, as this can contaminate Travatan Z.

What are possible food and drug interactions associated with this medication?
If Travatan Z is used with certain other drugs, the effects of either could be increased, decreased, or altered. It is especially important to check with your doctor before combining Travatan Z with other eye drops.

What are the possible side effects of this medication?
Please see general statement regarding side effects on page xiii.

Side effects may include: blurred vision, cataracts, color changes of your iris, deepening of your eyelids or skin around your eyes, dry eyes, eye discharge and tearing, eye or eyelid redness, growth of eyelashes, itching of your eyes, light sensitivity, pain of your eye, visual disturbances

Can I receive this medication if I am pregnant or breastfeeding?

The effects of Travatan Z during pregnancy and breastfeeding are unknown. Tell your doctor immediately if you are pregnant, plan to become pregnant, or are breastfeeding.

What should I do if I miss a dose of this medication?

If you miss a dose of Travatan Z, apply it as soon as you remember. However, if it is almost time for your next dose, skip the one you missed and return to your regular dosing schedule. Do not apply two doses at once.

How should I store this medication?

Store in the refrigerator or at room temperature.

Travoprost: see Travatan Z, page 1012

Trazodone

Generic name: Trazodone HCl

What is this medication?

Trazodone is a medicine used to treat depression.

What is the most important information I should know about this medication?

- Trazodone can increase suicidal thoughts or actions in some children, teenagers, and young adults within the first few months of treatment.
- Depression and other serious mental illnesses are the most important causes of suicidal thoughts and actions. People with bipolar disorder, or who have a family history of bipolar disorder (also called manic-depressive illness), are at a greater risk. Tell your doctor right away if you experience any changes in your mood, behavior, thoughts, or feelings. This is very important when an antidepressant medicine is first started or when the dose is changed.

- Trazodone can cause a painful, prolonged erection in men. If this occurs, stop taking trazodone and contact your doctor right away.
- Trazodone can cause a decrease in your blood pressure, especially if you are also taking medications for your blood pressure.

Who should not take this medication?

Do not take trazodone if you are allergic to it or any of its ingredients.

What should I tell my doctor before I take the first dose of this medication?

Tell your doctor about all prescription, over-the-counter, and herbal medications you are taking before beginning treatment with trazodone. Also, talk to your doctor about your complete medical history, especially if you have been diagnosed with bipolar disorder, have any heart problems, had a recent heart attack, or are having surgery.

What is the usual dosage?

Please see general statement regarding dosage on page xii.

Adults: The usual starting dose is 150 milligrams (mg) a day in divided doses. Your doctor will increase or decrease your dose as needed.

How should I take this medication?

- Take trazodone shortly after a meal or light snack.
- If you have to break the tablet, your doctor or pharmacist will instruct you on how to do so.

What should I avoid while taking this medication?

Do not drive or operate machinery until you know how trazodone affects you.

Do not start taking any new medicines without first talking to your doctor.

What are possible food and drug interactions associated with this medication?

If trazodone is taken with certain other drugs, the effects of either could be increased, decreased, or altered. It is especially important to check with your doctor before combining trazodone with the following: alcohol, barbiturates (such as phenobarbital), blood pressure medications, carbamazepine, digoxin, indinavir, itraconazole, ketoconazole, antidepressant medications known as monoamine oxidase inhibitors (such as selegiline or phenelzine), nefazodone, phenytoin, ritonavir, or warfarin.

What are the possible side effects of this medication?

Please see general statement regarding side effects on page xiii.

Side effects may include: allergic skin reaction/swelling, anger/hostility, blurred vision, constipation, decreased appetite, diarrhea, dizziness/lightheadedness, drowsiness, dry mouth, excitement, fainting, fast heartbeat, fatigue, headache, incoordination, low blood pressure, muscle pain, nasal congestion, nausea, nervousness, nightmares/vivid dreams, shaking, trouble sleeping, vomiting, weight loss or gain

Can I receive this medication if I am pregnant or breastfeeding?

The effects of trazodone during pregnancy and breastfeeding are unknown. Tell your doctor immediately if you are pregnant, plan to become pregnant, or are breastfeeding.

What should I do if I miss a dose of this medication?

If you miss a dose of trazodone, take it as soon as you remember. However, if it is almost time for your next dose, skip the one you missed and return to your regular dosing schedule. Do not take two doses at once.

How should I store this medication?

Store at room temperature.

Trazodone HCl: *see Trazodone, page 1014*

Tretinoin: *see Retin-A, page 891*

Tricor
Generic name: Fenofibrate

What is this medication?
Tricor is a cholesterol-lowering medicine used, in addition to an appropriate diet, to treat adults with high cholesterol. Tricor reduces bad cholesterol (LDL-C), total cholesterol, triglycerides, and apolipoprotein B; and increases good cholesterol (HDL-C). Tricor is used when diet and exercise alone have not lowered bad cholesterol and triglycerides.

What is the most important information I should know about this medication?
- Tell your doctor if you are taking any other medications while you are taking Tricor. Tricor may have an effect on medicines that help prevent blood clotting (such as the blood thinner warfarin). If you are taking Tricor with a blood thinner, your doctor will monitor your blood-clotting tests. Also, tell your doctor about any cholesterol-lowering medicines you may be taking as he or she will need to determine if the combination of Tricor and one of those medications is right for you.
- Tricor can cause liver problems. Your doctor will monitor your liver function.
- Tricor can increase your risk of developing gallstones. Call your doctor right away if you experience abdominal (stomach) pain, nausea, or vomiting. These may be signs of inflammation of your gallbladder or pancreas. Your doctor will also do studies to check for gallstones.
- Tricor can cause serious muscle conditions that may lead to kidney damage. Your risk can increase if you are also taking other cholesterol-lowering medicines known as statins (atorvastatin, fluvastatin, lovastatin, or pravastatin). Tell your doctor right away if you experience unexplained muscle pain, weakness, or

tenderness, especially if you also have a fever or general body discomfort.
- Tricor can cause pancreatitis (inflammation of the pancreas), severe allergic reactions, and clotting problems.

Who should not take this medication?

Do not take Tricor if you are allergic to it or any of its ingredients.

Do not take Tricor if you have liver, gallbladder, severe kidney problems, or if you are breastfeeding.

What should I tell my doctor before I take the first dose of this medication?

Tell your doctor about all prescription, over-the-counter, and herbal medications you are taking before beginning treatment with Tricor. Also, talk to your doctor about your complete medical history, especially if you have liver, kidney, or gallbladder problems; hypothyroidism (an underactive thyroid gland); diabetes; blood disorders; muscle pain or disease; if you drink large amounts of alcohol; or are pregnant, plan to become pregnant, or are breastfeeding.

What is the usual dosage?

Please see general statement regarding dosage on page xii.

High Cholesterol Levels or a Combination of High Cholesterol and High Triglycerides
Adults: The recommended starting dose is 145 milligrams (mg) once a day.

High Triglyceride Levels
Adults: The recommended starting dose is 48-145 mg once a day. The maximum dose is 145 mg a day.

If you have kidney problems, your doctor will adjust your dose as necessary.

How should I take this medication?

- Take Tricor exactly as prescribed by your doctor. Take Tricor once a day with or without food.

• If you are taking Tricor with another type of cholesterol-lowering medicine called a bile acid sequestrant (such as colestipol and cholestyramine), take Tricor at least 1 hour before or 4-6 hours after you take the other medicine.

What should I avoid while taking this medication?

Do not drink alcohol while you are taking Tricor. Alcohol can raise your triglyceride levels, and may also damage your liver while you are taking Tricor.

What are possible food and drug interactions associated with this medication?

If Tricor is taken with certain other drugs, the effects of either could be increased, decreased, or altered. It is especially important to check with your doctor before combining Tricor with any of the following: bile acid sequestrants, blood thinners, cyclosporine, or statins.

What are the possible side effects of this medication?

Please see general statement regarding side effects on page xiii.

Side effects may include: abdominal pain, back pain, headache, joint pain, liver damage, muscle pain, respiratory problems, runny nose, weakness

---

Can I receive this medication if I am pregnant or breastfeeding?

The effects of Tricor during pregnancy are unknown. Do not take Tricor if you are breastfeeding. Tell your doctor immediately if you are pregnant, plan to become pregnant, or are breastfeeding.

What should I do if I miss a dose of this medication?

If you miss a dose of Tricor, take it as soon as you remember. However, if it is almost time for your next dose, skip the one you missed and return to your regular dosing schedule. Do not take two doses at once.

How should I store this medication?
Store at room temperature. Protect from moisture.

Triglide
Generic name: Fenofibrate

What is this medication?
Triglide is a cholesterol-lowering medicine used, in addition to an appropriate diet, to treat adults with high cholesterol. Triglide reduces LDL ("bad") cholesterol, total cholesterol levels, triglycerides, and apolipoprotein B; and increases HDL ("good") cholesterol.

What is the most important information I should know about this medication?
- Tell your doctor if you are taking any other medications while you are taking Triglide. Triglide should not be used with blood thinners (such as warfarin) or cholesterol-lowering medications known as statins (such as atorvastatin, pravastatin, or simvastatin). If you are taking Triglide with a blood thinner, your doctor will monitor your blood-clotting tests. Also, tell your doctor about any cholesterol-lowering medicines you may be taking as he or she will need to determine if the combination of Triglide and one of those medications is right for you.
- Triglide can cause liver problems. Your doctor will monitor your liver function.
- Triglide can increase your risk of developing gallstones. Call your doctor immediately if you experience abdominal pain, nausea, or vomiting. These may be signs of inflammation of your gallbladder or pancreas. Your doctor will also do studies to test for gallstones.
- Triglide can cause serious muscle conditions that may lead to kidney damage. Your risk can increase if you are also taking statins. Tell your doctor immediately if you experience unexplained muscle pain, weakness, or tenderness, especially if you also have a fever or general body discomfort.

- Triglide can cause pancreatitis (inflammation of the pancreas), severe allergic reactions, blood abnormalities, and clotting problems.

Who should not take this medication?

Do not take Triglide if you are allergic to it or any of its ingredients.

Do not take Triglide if you have liver, gallbladder, or severe kidney problems; if you are receiving dialysis; or are breastfeeding.

What should I tell my doctor before I take the first dose of this medication?

Tell your doctor about all prescription, over-the-counter, and herbal medications you are taking before beginning treatment with Triglide. Also, talk to your doctor about your complete medical history, especially if you have liver, kidney, or gallbladder problems; hypothyroidism (an underactive thyroid gland); diabetes; blood disorders; or have muscle pain or disease. Tell your doctor if you or are pregnant, plan to become pregnant, or are breastfeeding.

What is the usual dosage?

Please see general statement regarding dosage on page xii.

High Cholesterol or a Combination of High Cholesterol and High Triglycerides

Adults: The recommended dose is 160 milligrams (mg) a day.

High Triglyceride

Adults: The recommended dose is 50-160 mg a day.

If you have kidney impairment, your doctor will adjust your dose appropriately.

How should I take this medication?

- Take Triglide exactly as prescribed by your doctor. Take Triglide with or without food.
- Swallow Triglide tablets whole. Do not break, crush, dissolve, or chew the tablets before swallowing.

• If you are taking Triglide with another type of cholesterol-lowering medicine called a bile acid sequestrant (such as colestipol or cholestyramine), take Triglide at least 1 hour before or 4-6 hours after you take the other medicine.

What should I avoid while taking this medication?

Do not breastfeed while you are taking Triglide.

What are possible food and drug interactions associated with this medication?

If Triglide is taken with certain other drugs, the effects of either could be increased, decreased, or altered. It is especially important to check with your doctor before combining Triglide with the following: bile acid sequestrants, blood thinners, cyclosporine, or statins.

What are the possible side effects of this medication?

Please see general statement regarding side effects on page xiii.

Side effects may include: back pain, chest pain, constipation, diarrhea, "flu-like" symptoms, nausea, headache, stomach pain, weakness

If you experience any muscle pain, tenderness or weakness, have stomach pain, or any other new symptoms, contact your doctor right away.

Can I receive this medication if I am pregnant or breastfeeding?

The effects of Triglide during pregnancy are unknown. Do not breastfeed while you are taking Triglide. Tell your doctor immediately if you are pregnant, plan to become pregnant, or are breastfeeding.

What should I do if I miss a dose of this medication?

If you miss a dose of Triglide, take it as soon as you remember. However, if it is almost time for your next dose, skip the one you

missed and return to your regular dosing schedule. Do not take two doses at once.

How should I store this medication?
Store at room temperature away from light and moisture.

Trileptal
Generic name: Oxcarbazepine

What is this medication?
Trileptal is a medication used to treat partial seizures. It is available in tablets and a suspension.

What is the most important information I should know about this medication?
- Trileptal can cause the level of sodium in your blood to be low. This can result in a serious medical condition. Tell your doctor right away if you experience nausea, tiredness, lack of energy, confusion, or more frequent or more severe seizures.
- Trileptal can cause rare but serious skin rashes, allergic reactions, or serious problems affecting organs or other parts of your body, such as your liver or blood cells. Many people who are allergic to carbamazepine are also allergic to Trileptal. Tell your doctor right away if you develop swelling of your face, eyes, lips, or tongue; trouble swallowing or breathing; a skin rash; or hives.
- Trileptal can cause suicidal thoughts or actions. Tell your doctor right away if you have thoughts about suicide or dying; attempt to commit suicide; have new or worse depression, anxiety, or irritability; have panic attacks; have trouble sleeping (insomnia); have an extreme increase in activity and talking (mania); are feeling agitated or restless; acting aggressive; being angry or violent; acting on dangerous impulses; or have other unusual changes in behavior or mood.
- Trileptal can cause rare but serious blood problems. Tell your doctor right away if you experience fever, sore throat, other

infections that come and go or do not go away, easy bruising, unusual bleeding, or severe fatigue or weakness.
• Do not stop taking Trileptal without first talking to your doctor. Stopping Trileptal suddenly can cause serious problems, including seizures that will not stop (status epilepticus).

Who should not take this medication?
Do not take Trileptal if you are allergic to it, any of its ingredients, or carbamazepine.

What should I tell my doctor before I take the first dose of this medication?
Tell your doctor about all prescription, over-the-counter, and herbal medications you are taking before beginning treatment with Trileptal. Also, talk to your doctor about your complete medical history, especially if you have or have had suicidal thoughts or actions, depression or mood problems, have liver or kidney problems, use birth control medicine, are pregnant, plan to become pregnant, or are breastfeeding.

What is the usual dosage?
Please see general statement regarding dosage on page xii.

Adults: The usual starting dose is 300 milligrams (mg) twice a day. Your doctor will increase your dose as appropriate.

Children 4-16 years: Your doctor will prescribe the appropriate dose for your child, based on their weight.

If you have kidney impairment, your doctor will adjust your dose appropriately.

How should I take this medication?
• Take Trileptal exactly as prescribed by your doctor. Do not change your dose or stop taking this medication abruptly without first talking to your doctor. Take Trileptal twice a day. You can take Trileptal with or without food.
• Shake the Trileptal suspension well before use. Use the oral dosing syringe to measure the amount of Trileptal needed. You

can mix the suspension in a small glass of water or swallow it directly from the syringe. After each use, clean the syringe with warm water and let it dry.

What should I avoid while taking this medication?

Do not drive or operate heavy machinery until you know how Trileptal affects you. Trileptal can cause dizziness and sleepiness.

Do not drink alcohol or take other medications that make you sleepy or dizzy while taking Trileptal. Taking these together can make your sleepiness or dizziness worse.

What are possible food and drug interactions associated with this medication?

If Trileptal is taken with certain other drugs, the effects of either could be increased, decreased, or altered. It is especially important to check with your doctor before combining Trileptal with the following: birth control pills, calcium channel blockers (such as felodipine or verapamil), or seizure medications (such as carbamazepine, phenobarbital, phenytoin, or valproic acid).

What are the possible side effects of this medication?

Please see general statement regarding side effects on page xiii.

> **Side effects may include:** confusion, dizziness, double vision or other problems with vision, infections (especially in children), nausea, problems with walking and coordination (unsteadiness), rash, sleepiness, speech problems, stomach pain, tiredness, trembling, trouble concentrating, upset stomach, vomiting, worsening of seizures

Can I receive this medication if I am pregnant or breastfeeding?

The effects of Trileptal during pregnancy are unknown. Trileptal can be found in your breast milk if you take it while breastfeeding. Do not breastfeed while you are taking Trileptal. Tell your doctor immediately if you are pregnant, plan to become pregnant, or are breastfeeding.

What should I do if I miss a dose of this medication?

If you miss a dose of Trileptal, take it as soon as you remember. However, if it is almost time for your next dose, skip the one you missed and return to your regular dosing schedule. Do not take two doses at once.

How should I store this medication?

Store at room temperature. Use the Trileptal suspension within 7 weeks of first opening the bottle.

Trilipix

Generic name: Fenofibric acid

What is this medication?

Trilipix is a cholesterol-lowering medicine used, in addition to an appropriate diet, to treat adults with high cholesterol. Trilipix reduces bad cholesterol (LDL-C), total cholesterol, triglycerides, and apolipoprotein B; and increases good cholesterol (HDL-C). It is also used, in combination with another cholesterol-lowering medicine known as statins (such as atorvastatin, fluvastatin, or pravastatin), to reduce triglycerides and increase HDL-C in patients with high cholesterol and high triglycerides.

What is the most important information I should know about this medication?

- Tell your doctor if you are taking any other medications while you are taking Trilipix. Trilipix may have an effect on medications that help prevent blood clotting (such as the blood thinner warfarin). If you are taking Trilipix with a blood thinner medication, your doctor will monitor your blood-clotting tests. Also, tell your doctor about any cholesterol-lowering medicines you may be taking as he or she will need to determine if the combination of Trilipix and one of those medications is right for you.
- Trilipix can cause liver problems. Your doctor will monitor your liver function.
- Trilipix can increase your risk of developing gallstones. Call your doctor immediately if you experience abdominal pain, nausea,

or vomiting. These may be signs of inflammation of your gall-bladder or pancreas. Your doctor will also do studies to test for gallstones.

• Trilipix can cause serious muscle conditions that may lead to kidney damage. Your risk can increase if you are also taking statins. Tell your doctor immediately if you experience unexplained muscle pain, weakness, or tenderness, especially if you also have a fever or general body discomfort.

• Trilipix can cause pancreatitis (inflammation of the pancreas), severe allergic reactions, blood abnormalities, and clotting problems.

Who should not take this medication?

Do not take Trilipix if you are allergic to it or any of its ingredients; or if you have liver, gallbladder, or severe kidney problems; if you are receiving dialysis; or are breastfeeding.

What should I tell my doctor before I take the first dose of this medication?

Tell your doctor about all prescription, over-the-counter, and herbal medications you are taking before beginning treatment with Trilipix. Also, talk to your doctor about your complete medical history, especially if you have liver, kidney, or gallbladder problems; hypothyroidism (an underactive thyroid gland); diabetes; blood disorders; muscle pain or disease; or are pregnant, plan to become pregnant, or are breastfeeding.

What is the usual dosage?

Please see general statement regarding dosage on page xii.

High Cholesterol Levels or a Combination of High Cholesterol and High Triglycerides

Adults: The recommended dose is 135 milligrams (mg) a day.

High Triglyceride Levels

Adults: The recommended starting dose is 45-135 mg a day.

If you have kidney problems, your doctor will adjust your dose appropriately.

How should I take this medication?
- Take Trilipix exactly as prescribed by your doctor.
- Swallow Trilipix capsules whole. Do not break, crush, dissolve, or chew the capsules before swallowing.
- If you are taking Trilipix with another type of cholesterol-lowering medicine called a bile acid sequestrant (such as colestipol or cholestyramine), take Trilipix at least 1 hour before or 4-6 hours after you take the other medicine.

What should I avoid while taking this medication?
Do not breastfeed while you are taking Trilipix.

What are possible food and drug interactions associated with this medication?
If Trilipix is taken with certain other drugs, the effects of either could be increased, decreased, or altered. It is especially important to check with your doctor before combining Trilipix with the following: bile acid sequestrants, blood thinners, cyclosporine, or statins.

What are the possible side effects of this medication?
Please see general statement regarding side effects on page xiii.

Side effects may include: abdominal pain, back pain, constipation, diarrhea, headache, indigestion, liver damage, muscle pain, nausea, respiratory problems

---

Can I receive this medication if I am pregnant or breastfeeding?
The effects of Trilipix during pregnancy are unknown. Do not breastfeed while you are taking Trilipix. Tell your doctor immediately if you are pregnant, plan to become pregnant, or are breastfeeding.

What should I do if I miss a dose of this medication?
If you miss a dose of Trilipix, take it as soon as you remember. However, if it is almost time for your next dose, skip the one you missed and return to your regular dosing schedule. Do not take two doses at once.

How should I store this medication?
Store at room temperature. Protect from moisture.

Tussionex
Generic name: Chlorpheniramine Polistirex/Hydrocodone Polistirex

What is this medication?
Tussionex Suspension is a medicine used to treat cough and upper respiratory (lung) symptoms you can have with allergies or a cold. Tussionex Suspension contains two medicines: hydrocodone (a mild narcotic cough suppressant) and chlorpheniramine (an antihistamine).

What is the most important information I should know about this medication?
- This medication can cause considerable drowsiness and impair your mental and/or physical abilities required for hazardous tasks, such as driving a car or operating machinery.
- Tussionex Suspension contains a mild narcotic that can cause dependence and tolerance when the medicine is used for several weeks. However, it is unlikely that dependence will develop when Tussionex Suspension is used for the short-term treatment of a cough.
- If you are pregnant and take Tussionex Suspension before your baby is born, your newborn baby may have withdrawal symptoms because his/her body may have become used to the medicine. Check with your doctor before taking this medication while pregnant.

Who should not take this medication?
Do not take Tussionex Suspension if you are allergic to it or any of its ingredients.

Do not give Tussionex Suspension to children <6 years due to an increased risk of respiratory depression (decreased rate of breathing).

What should I tell my doctor before I take the first dose of this medication?

Tell your doctor about all prescription, over-the-counter, and herbal medications you are taking before beginning treatment with Tussionex Suspension. Also, talk to your doctor about your complete medical history, especially if you have glaucoma (high pressure in the eye), kidney, liver, lung or breathing (asthma) problems, underactive thyroid, or urinary tract problems. Also, tell your doctor if you plan to have surgery, have had a head injury, or drink alcohol.

What is the usual dosage?

Please see general statement regarding dosage on page xii.

Adults and children ≥12 years: The usual dose is 5 milliliters (ml) every 12 hours. Do not take more than 10 ml in 24 hours.

Children 6-12 years: The usual dose is 2.5 ml every 12 hours. Do not take more than 5 ml in 24 hours.

How should I take this medication?

- Take Tussionex Suspension exactly as prescribed by your doctor. Do not take extra doses or take it more often without asking your doctor.
- Shake the Tussionex Suspension bottle well before using it. A household teaspoon is not an accurate measuring device; ask your pharmacist to give you an accurate measuring device.
- You can take Tussionex Suspension with or without food.
- Do not mix Tussionex Suspension with other fluids or medications. Mixing can change how the medication works.

What should I avoid while taking this medication?

Tussionex Suspension can cause you to be drowsy. Do not drive a car or use machinery until you know how this medicine affects you.

Do not drink alcohol while you are taking Tussionex Suspension. If you drink alcohol, your chances of having serious side effects can increase.

What are possible food and drug interactions associated with this medication?

If Tussionex Suspension is taken with certain other drugs, the effects of either could be increased, decreased, or altered. It is especially important to check with your doctor before combining Tussionex Suspension with the following: antianxiety agents (such as alprazolam or diazepam), antihistamines (such as diphenhydramine), central nervous system depressants (such as alcohol), certain antidepressants (such as amitriptyline or nortriptyline), medicines for stomach or intestinal problems, monoamine oxidase inhibitors (MAOIs), a class of drugs to treat depression and other psychiatric conditions (such as phenelzine and tranylcypromine), or narcotics (such as oxycodone or meperidine).

What are the possible side effects of this medication?

Please see general statement regarding side effects on page xiii.

Side effects may include: anxiety, chest tightness, confusion, constipation and blockage of your intestines, decreased breathing, decreased mental and physical performance, dependence, difficulty urinating, dizziness, drowsiness, dry throat, exaggerated feeling of depression or sense of well-being, excessive sleepiness, extreme calm, fear, itching, mood changes, nausea, rash, restlessness, tiredness, vomiting

Can I receive this medication if I am pregnant or breastfeeding?

The effects of Tussionex Suspension during pregnancy and breastfeeding are unknown. Tell your doctor immediately if you are pregnant, plan to become pregnant, or are breastfeeding.

What should I do if I miss a dose of this medication?

If you miss a dose of Tussionex Suspension, take it as soon as you remember. However, if it is almost time for your next dose, skip the one you missed and return to your regular dosing schedule. Do not take two doses at once.

How should I store this medication?
Store at room temperature.

Tylenol with Codeine
Generic name: Acetaminophen/Codeine Phosphate

What is this medication?
Tylenol with Codeine is a narcotic analgesic (painkiller) used to treat mild to moderately severe pain. It contains two drugs: acetaminophen and codeine. Acetaminophen, a fever-reducing analgesic, is used to reduce pain and fever. Codeine, a narcotic analgesic, is used to treat pain that is moderate to severe.

What is the most important information I should know about this medication?
- Tylenol with Codeine contains a narcotic (codeine) and, even if taken in prescribed amounts, can cause physical and psychological addiction if taken for a long enough time.
- Tylenol with Codeine tablets contain a sulfite that may cause allergic reactions in some people. These reactions may include shock and severe, possibly life-threatening, asthma attacks. People with asthma are more likely to be sensitive to sulfites.
- Do not exceed the maximum dose of 360 milligrams (mg) of codeine and 4,000 mg of acetaminophen in a 24-hour period.

Who should not take this medication?
You should not use Tylenol with Codeine if you are allergic to acetaminophen or codeine.

What should I tell my doctor before I take the first dose of this medication?
Tell your doctor about all prescription, over-the-counter, and herbal medications you are taking before beginning treatment with Tylenol with Codeine. Also, talk to your doctor about your complete medical history, especially if you have ever had liver, kidney, thyroid, or adrenal disease. Make sure your doctor knows if you have experienced a head injury, difficulty urinating, an enlarged prostate, or

stomach problems such as a stomach ulcer. Also, tell your doctor if you are pregnant, plan to become pregnant, or are breastfeeding.

What is the usual dosage?
Please see general statement regarding dosage on page xii.

Dosage will depend on how severe your pain is and how you respond to the drug.

Adults: A single dose may contain from 15-60 milligrams (mg) of codeine phosphate and from 300-1,000 mg of acetaminophen. Your doctor will determine the amounts of codeine phosphate and acetaminophen taken in each dose.

Adults may also take Tylenol with Codeine elixir (liquid). Tylenol with Codeine elixir contains 120 mg of acetaminophen and 12 mg of codeine phosphate per teaspoonful.

Children 3 to 12 years: Your doctor will prescribe the appropriate dose for your child.

How should I take this medication?
• Tylenol with Codeine may be taken with meals or with milk.

What should I avoid while taking this medication?
If you generally drink three or more alcoholic beverages per day, check with your doctor before using Tylenol with Codeine and other acetaminophen-containing products, and never take more than the recommended dosage. There is a possibility of damage to the liver when large amounts of alcohol and acetaminophen are combined.

This drug may cause drowsiness and impair your ability to drive a car or operate potentially dangerous machinery. Do not participate in any activities that require full attention when using Tylenol with Codeine until you are sure of this medication's effect on you.

What are possible food and drug interactions associated with this medication?

If Tylenol with Codeine is taken with certain other drugs, the effects of either could be increased, decreased, or altered. It is especially important to check with your doctor before combining Tylenol with Codeine with the following: alprazolam, antidepressants, anticholinergics, clozapine, chlorpromazine, diazepam, drugs that control spasms, narcotic painkillers, or tranquilizers.

What are the possible side effects of this medication?

Please see general statement regarding side effects on page xiii.

Side effects may include: dizziness, lightheadedness, nausea, sedation, shortness of breath, vomiting

At high doses, this medication may cause severe breathing problems.

Can I receive this medication if I am pregnant or breastfeeding?

The effects of Tylenol with Codeine during pregnancy and breastfeeding are unknown. Tell your doctor immediately if you are pregnant, plan to become pregnant, or are breastfeeding.

What should I do if I miss a dose of this medication?

If you take Tylenol with Codeine on a regular schedule, take the missed dose as soon as you remember. If it is almost time for your next dose, skip the dose you missed and go back to your regular schedule. Do not take two doses at once.

How should I store this medication?

Store at room temperature, away from heat, light.

Ultracet

Generic name: Acetaminophen/Tramadol HCl

What is this medication?

Ultracet is a pain medicine that contains the narcotic painkiller tramadol and the non-narcotic painkiller acetaminophen. Ultracet is used to treat short-term (5 days or less) sudden pain.

What is the most important information I should know about this medication?

- Ultracet has abuse potential. Mental and physical dependence can occur with the use of Ultracet when it is used improperly.
- Ultracet contains acetaminophen, which can cause severe liver injury. Do not take more than 4000 milligrams (mg) of acetaminophen a day or take other products containing acetaminophen. The risk of liver injury can be higher if you have underlying liver disease or drink alcohol while you are taking Ultracet.
- Ultracet can cause seizures. The risk is greater if you have a history of seizures, are suffering from alcohol or drug withdrawal, or nervous system infections. Your risk of seizures may also be increased if you are taking antidepressants medications such as monoamine oxidase inhibitors (MAOIs) (such as phenelzine), selective serotonin reuptake inhibitors (SSRIs) (such as fluoxetine or paroxetine), selective norepinephrine reuptake inhibitors (SNRIs) (such as venlafaxine), or tricyclic antidepressants (TCAs) (such as amitriptyline); certain migraine products (such as sumatriptan); or other medicines.
- Ultracet can cause serotonin syndrome (a potentially life-threatening drug reaction that causes the body to have too much serotonin, a chemical produced by the nerve cells) when you take it alone or in combination with MAOIs, SSRIs, SNRIs, TCAs, or certain migraine products. Tell your doctor right away if you experience mental status changes, an increase in your heart rate and temperature, lack of coordination, overactive reflexes, nausea, vomiting, or diarrhea.
- Ultracet can cause allergic reactions or anaphylaxis (a serious and rapid allergic reaction that may result in death if not immediately treated). Stop taking Ultracet and tell your doctor right

away if you develop a rash, difficulty breathing, or swelling of
your face, mouth, or throat.
- Ultracet can cause serious breathing problems that can become
life-threatening, especially when it is used in the wrong way.

Who should not take this medication?
Do not take Ultracet if you are allergic to it, any of its ingredients,
or to other narcotic painkillers.

Do not take Ultracet if you have attempted suicide or are addiction
prone.

What should I tell my doctor before I take the first dose of this medication?
Tell your doctor about all prescription, over-the-counter, and herbal
medications you are taking before beginning treatment with Ultracet. Also, talk to your doctor about your complete medical history, especially if you have a history of seizures, difficulty breathing, depression, head injury, kidney or liver disease, brain or spinal
cord infection, stomach problems, attempted suicide, or a history
of alcohol or drug abuse.

What is the usual dosage?
Please see general statement regarding dosage on page xii.

Adults: The recommended dose is 2 tablets every 4-6 hours as
needed for pain relief. Do not take more than 8 tablets a day.

If you have kidney impairment, your doctor will adjust your dose
appropriately.

How should I take this medication?
- Take Ultracet exactly as prescribed by your doctor.

What should I avoid while taking this medication?
Do not drink alcohol while you are taking Ultracet.

Do not drive a car or operate dangerous machinery until you know
how Ultracet affects you.

Do not take Ultracet with other products that contain tramadol or acetaminophen, including over-the-counter products.

What are possible food and drug interactions associated with this medication?

If Ultracet is taken with certain other drugs, the effects of either could be increased, decreased, or altered. It is especially important to check with your doctor before combining Ultracet with the following: alcohol, antidepressants (including MAOIs, SSRIs, SNRIs, or TCAs), carbamazepine, certain migraine products, cyclobenzaprine, digoxin, erythromycin, ketoconazole, linezolid, lithium, phenothiazines (such as promethazine), quinidine, rifampin, sleep aids (such as temazepam), St. John's wort, tranquilizers (such as alprazolam), or warfarin.

What are the possible side effects of this medication?

Please see general statement regarding side effects on page xiii.

> **Side effects may include:** constipation, diarrhea, dizziness, drowsiness, increased sweating, loss of appetite, nausea

Can I receive this medication if I am pregnant or breastfeeding?

The effects of Ultracet during pregnancy and breastfeeding are unknown. Do not breastfeed while you are taking Ultracet. Tell your doctor immediately if you are pregnant, plan to become pregnant, or are breastfeeding.

What should I do if I miss a dose of this medication?

Ultracet should be taken only as needed.

How should I store this medication?

Store at room temperature.

Ultram

Generic name: Tramadol HCl

What is this medication?

Ultram is a pain medicine that contains the narcotic painkiller tramadol. Ultram is used to treat moderate to moderately severe pain. Ultram is also available as extended-release tablets (releases medicine into your body throughout the day) called Ultram ER.

What is the most important information I should know about this medication?

- Ultram has abuse potential. Mental and physical dependence can occur with the use of Ultram when it is used improperly.
- Ultram can cause seizures. The risk is greater if you have a history of seizures, are suffering from alcohol or drug withdrawal, or nervous system infections. Your risk of seizures may also be increased if you are taking antidepressants medications such as monoamine oxidase inhibitors (MAOIs) (such as phenelzine), selective serotonin reuptake inhibitors (SSRIs) (such as fluoxetine or paroxetine), selective norepinephrine reuptake inhibitors (SNRIs) (such as venlafaxine), or tricyclic antidepressants (TCAs) (such as amitriptyline); certain migraine products (such as sumatriptan); or other medicines.
- Ultram can cause serotonin syndrome (a potentially life-threatening drug reaction that causes the body to have too much serotonin, a chemical produced by the nerve cells) when you take it alone or in combination with MAOIs, SSRIs, SNRIs, TCAs, or certain migraine products. Tell your doctor right away if you experience mental status changes, an increase in your heart rate and temperature, lack of coordination, overactive reflexes, nausea, vomiting, or diarrhea.
- Ultram can cause allergic reactions or anaphylaxis (a serious and rapid allergic reaction that may result in death if not immediately treated). Stop taking Ultram and tell your doctor right away if you develop a rash, difficulty breathing, or swelling of your face, mouth, or throat.
- Ultram can cause serious breathing problems that can become life-threatening, especially when it is used in the wrong way.

Who should not take this medication?

Do not take Ultram if you are allergic to it, any of its ingredients, or to other narcotic painkillers.

Do not take Ultram if you have attempted suicide or are addiction prone.

Do not take Ultram ER if you have severe kidney or liver impairment.

What should I tell my doctor before I take the first dose of this medication?

Tell your doctor about all prescription, over-the-counter, and herbal medications you are taking before beginning treatment with Ultram. Also, talk to your doctor about your complete medical history, especially if you have a history of seizures, difficulty breathing, depression, head injury, kidney or liver disease, brain or spinal cord infection, stomach problems, attempted suicide, or a history of alcohol or drug abuse.

What is the usual dosage?

Please see general statement regarding dosage on page xii.

Ultram Tablets

Adults ≥17 years: The recommended starting dose is 25 milligrams (mg) once a day in the morning. Your doctor will increase your dose as needed.

If you are elderly or have kidney or liver impairment, your doctor will adjust your dose appropriately.

Ultram ER Tablets

Adults ≥18 years: Your doctor will prescribed the appropriate dose for you based on your previous pain medication.

How should I take this medication?

- Take Ultram exactly as prescribed by your doctor.
- Swallow Ultram ER tablets whole. Do not chew, crush, or split them.

What should I avoid while taking this medication?
Do not drink alcohol while you are taking Ultram.

Do not drive a car or operate dangerous machinery until you know how Ultram affects you.

Do not stop talking Ultram without first talking to your doctor. Stopping Ultram suddenly can lead to serious side effects.

What are possible food and drug interactions associated with this medication?
If Ultram is taken with certain other drugs, the effects of either could be increased, decreased, or altered. It is especially important to check with your doctor before combining Ultram with the following: alcohol, antidepressants (including MAOIs, SSRIs, SN-RIs, or TCAs), carbamazepine, certain migraine products, cyclobenzaprine, digoxin, erythromycin, ketoconazole, linezolid, lithium, phenothiazines (such as promethazine), quinidine, rifampin, sleep aids (such as temazepam), St. John's wort, tranquilizers (such as alprazolam), or warfarin.

What are the possible side effects of this medication?
Please see general statement regarding side effects on page xiii.

Side effects may include: agitation, anxiety, constipation, diarrhea, dizziness, drowsiness, dry mouth, euphoria (a feeling of extreme happiness and well-being), excessive emotional reactions and frequent mood changes, flushing of your face, hallucination, headache, increased sweating, involuntary muscle contractions, itching, loss of appetite, nausea, nervousness, shaking, sudden fall in your blood pressure, trouble sleeping, upset stomach, vomiting, weakness

---

Can I receive this medication if I am pregnant or breastfeeding?
The effects of Ultram during pregnancy and breastfeeding are unknown. Do not breastfeed while you are taking Ultram. Tell your

doctor immediately if you are pregnant, plan to become pregnant, or are breastfeeding.

What should I do if I miss a dose of this medication?

If you miss a dose of Ultram, take it as soon as you remember. However, if it is almost time for your next dose, skip the one you missed and return to your regular dosing schedule. Do not take two doses at once.

How should I store this medication?

Store at room temperature.

Vagifem
Generic name: Estradiol

What is this medication?

Vagifem is a vaginal tablet that contains the estrogen hormone estradiol. Vagifem is used after menopause to treat menopausal changes in and around the vagina.

What is the most important information I should know about this medication?

- Using estrogen alone may increase your chance of getting cancer of the uterus. Tell your doctor immediately if you experience any unusual vaginal bleeding while you are using Vagifem.
- Do not use Vagifem to prevent heart disease, heart attacks, strokes, or dementia (an illness involving loss of memory, judgment, and confusion). Using Vagifem can increase your chances of heart attacks, strokes, breast cancer, or blood clots.
- Vagifem can also increase your risk of dementia, gallbladder disease, ovarian cancer, visual abnormalities, high blood pressure, pancreatitis (inflammation of your pancreas), or thyroid problems. Talk regularly with your doctor about whether you still need treatment with Vagifem.

Who should not take this medication?

Do not use Vagifem if you are allergic to it or any of its ingredients.

Do not use Vagifem if you have unusual vaginal bleeding, have or have had certain cancers, had a stroke or heart attack, or have or have had blood clots or liver problems.

Do not use Vagifem if you have been diagnosed with a bleeding disorder, or are pregnant or think you may be pregnant.

What should I tell my doctor before I take the first dose of this medication?
Tell your doctor about all prescription, over-the-counter, and herbal medications you are taking before beginning treatment with Vagifem. Also, talk to your doctor about your complete medical history, especially if you have any unusual vaginal bleeding, asthma, seizures, diabetes, migraines, endometriosis (a common gynecological disorder that may result in sores and pain), lupus (disease that affects the immune system), high blood calcium levels, or problems with your heart, liver, thyroid, or kidneys.

Tell your doctor if you are going to have surgery, will be on bed rest, or if you are breastfeeding.

What is the usual dosage?
Please see general statement regarding dosage on page xii.

Adults: The usual dose is 1 tablet inserted inside your vagina once a day for 2 weeks, then 1 tablet is inserted inside your vagina twice a week thereafter.

How should I take this medication?
• Vagifem is a tablet that you place in your vagina with an applicator.
• To use Vagifem, tear off a single applicator. Separate the plastic wrap and remove the tablet-filled applicator from the plastic wrap. Hold the applicator so that the finger of one hand can press the applicator plunger.
• Select a comfortable position for you for vaginal insertion of Vagifem, either lying down or standing. Using the other hand, guide the applicator gently and comfortably through the vaginal opening. If the tablet has come out of the applicator prior to

insertion, do not attempt to replace it. Use a fresh tablet-filled applicator. The applicator should be inserted (without forcing) as far as comfortably possible, or until half of the applicator is inside your vagina, whichever is less.

- Once the tablet-filled applicator has been inserted, gently press the plunger until the plunger is fully depressed. This will eject the tablet inside your vagina where it will dissolve slowly over several hours.
- After depressing the plunger, gently remove the applicator and dispose of it the same way you would a plastic tampon applicator. The applicator is of no further use and should be discarded properly.
- Insertion can be done at any time of the day. Try to use the same time daily for all applications of Vagifem.

What should I avoid while taking this medication?

If the Vagifem tablet has come out of the applicator prior to insertion, do not attempt to replace it. Use a fresh tablet-filled applicator.

Grapefruit juice can increase your risk of side effects with Vagifem. Talk to your doctor before including grapefruit or grapefruit juice in your diet while you are using Vagifem.

What are possible food and drug interactions associated with this medication?

If Vagifem is used with certain other drugs, the effects of either could be increased, decreased, or altered. It is especially important to check with your doctor before combining Vagifem with the following: carbamazepine, clarithromycin, erythromycin, grapefruit juice, itraconazole, ketoconazole, phenobarbital, rifampin, ritonavir, or St. John's wort.

What are the possible side effects of this medication?

Please see general statement regarding side effects on page xiii.

Side effects may include: bloating, breast pain, fluid retention, hair loss, headache, irregular vaginal bleeding or spotting, nausea, stomach or abdominal cramps, vaginal yeast infection, vomiting

Can I receive this medication if I am pregnant or breastfeeding?

Do not use Vagifem if you are pregnant or breastfeeding. The hormone in Vagifem can be found in your breast milk if you use it while you are breastfeeding. Tell your doctor immediately if you are pregnant, plan to become pregnant, or are breastfeeding.

What should I do if I miss a dose of this medication?

If you forget to insert a Vagifem tablet, insert one as soon as you remember. However, if it is almost time for your next dose, skip the dose you missed and return to your regular dosing schedule. Do not take two doses at once.

How should I store this medication?

Store at room temperature.

Valacyclovir HCl: see Valtrex, page 1048

Valium

Generic name: Diazepam

What is this medication?

Valium is an antianxiety medication belonging to a drug class known as benzodiazepines. Valium is used to treat anxiety disorders, the symptoms of sudden alcohol withdrawal, muscle spasms, and seizures.

What is the most important information I should know about this medication?

- Due to the sleepiness and fatigue Valium can cause, you should not drive or operate dangerous machinery until you know how this drug affects you. Do not drink alcohol or take other medications that can make you tired or drowsy while you are taking Valium.
- If you are taking Valium as part of seizure therapy, do not suddenly stop taking it as this may worsen or even cause seizures.

In addition, you may be at increased risk for other certain types of seizures therefore, your doctor may increase the dosage of your other antiseizure medication.

- Use Valium with caution if you have any type of kidney or liver problems. If you take Valium for a long time, your doctor will likely perform blood tests to check your liver health and also the number of disease-fighting cells in your blood.
- Talk to your doctor before increasing your Valium dose or before stopping therapy. Suddenly stopping Valium may cause you to experience symptoms of withdrawal that include shaking, stomach and muscle cramps, vomiting, sweating, insomnia, and seizures.
- You may develop a physical or mental dependence on Valium, especially if you take it for a long time or if you have a history of alcohol or drug abuse.

Who should not take this medication?

Do not take Valium if you are pregnant, have acute narrow-angle glaucoma (high pressure in the eye), or if you are allergic to diazepam or any other ingredient in Valium.

Do not use Valium if you have been diagnosed with psychosis, severe breathing problems, liver disease, sleep apnea (stopping breathing temporarily during sleep), or a condition known as myasthenia gravis (a disease characterized by long-lasting fatigue and muscle weakness).

What should I tell my doctor before I take the first dose of this medication?

Tell your doctor about all prescription, over-the-counter, and herbal medications you are taking before beginning treatment with Valium. Also, talk to your doctor about your complete medical history, especially if you have myasthenia gravis, kidney or liver problems, acute narrow-angle glaucoma, sleeping problems, or if you drink alcohol regularly. Also, tell your doctor if you have a history of drug abuse, breathing problems, or mental disorders and if you are pregnant, plan to become pregnant, or are breastfeeding.

What is the usual dosage?
Please see general statement regarding dosage on page xii.

Anxiety Disorders
Adults: The usual dosage is 2-10 milligrams (mg) taken two to four times a day.

Elderly: The usual starting dosage is 2-2.5 mg taken once or twice daily. Dose may be increased gradually as needed and tolerated.

Children (>6 months): The usual dosage is 1-2.5 mg given three to four times a day. Dose may be increased gradually as needed and tolerated.

Muscle Spasms (in Combination with Other Therapy)
Adults: The usual dosage is 2-10 mg taken three or four times a day.

Elderly: The usual starting dosage is 2-2.5 mg taken once or twice daily. Dose may be increased gradually as needed and tolerated.

Children (>6 months): The usual dosage is 1-2.5 mg given three to four times a day. Dose may be increased gradually as needed and tolerated.

Seizure Disorders (in Combination with Other Therapy)
Adults: The usual dosage is 2-10 mg taken two to four times a day.

Elderly: The usual starting dose is 2-2.5 mg taken once or twice daily. Dose may be increased gradually as needed and tolerated.

Children >6 months: The usual starting dose is 1-2.5 mg given three or four times a day. Dose may be increased gradually as needed and tolerated.

Sudden Alcohol Withdrawal
Adults: The starting dose is 10 mg taken three or four times daily during the first 24 hours. The dose is then reduced to 5 mg, three or four times daily as needed.

How should I take this medication?
- Take Valium exactly the way your doctor prescribed. Valium may work better when taken without food.

What should I avoid while taking this medication?
Do not drink alcohol or take other medications that can make you tired or drowsy while you are taking Valium.

Avoid suddenly stopping Valium therapy without first talking to your doctor. Do not take more than is prescribed without your doctor's approval.

Avoid taking Valium with meals, because food may decrease the effect of Valium and delay the time it takes to work in your body.

What are possible food and drug interactions associated with this medication?
If Valium is taken with certain other drugs, the effects of either could be increased, decreased, or altered. It is especially important to check with your doctor before combining Valium with the following: alcohol, antacids, antianxiety medicines, antidepressants, antipsychotics, barbiturates, cimetidine, fluoxetine, fluvoxamine, ketoconazole, monoamine oxidase inhibitors (MAOIs), narcotics, omeprazole, phenothiazines, phenytoin, and sleep medicines.

What are the possible side effects of this medication?
Please see general statement regarding side effects on page xiii.

Side effects may include: difficulty walking, muscle weakness, loss of coordination, drowsiness, tiredness, constipation, blurred vision

Can I receive this medication if I am pregnant or breastfeeding?

Taking Valium during pregnancy should be avoided. Tell your doctor immediately if you are pregnant or plan to become pregnant. Women taking Valium should not breastfeed because Valium passes into breast milk.

What should I do if I miss a dose of this medication?

If you miss a dose of Valium, take the missed dose as soon as you remember it. However, if it is almost time for your next dose, skip the one you missed and return to your regular dosing schedule. Do not take two doses at once.

How should I store this medication?

Store at room temperature away from light in a tightly closed container.

Valsartan: see Diovan, page 326

Valtrex

Generic name: Valacyclovir HCl

What is this medication?

Valtrex is a medicine used to treat cold sores and shingles (painful rash caused by the chickenpox virus) in adults. Valtrex is also used to treat or control genital herpes outbreaks in adults with healthy immune systems as well as adults with HIV infection (AIDS). In addition, Valtrex is used to treat cold sores and chickenpox in children. Valtrex is available as caplets. Your pharmacist can use the caplets to make an oral suspension.

What is the most important information I should know about this medication?

- Valtrex can cause life-threatening blood disorders, especially when taken at high doses and in patients with advanced HIV disease, or those undergoing bone marrow or kidney transplants.

- Valtrex can cause kidney damage, especially if you already have kidney problems or are elderly. Use caution if you are taking any medications that can harm your kidneys. Stay adequately hydrated while you are taking Valtrex.
- Valtrex can cause nervous system side effects such as aggressive behavior, unsteady movement, shaky movements, confusion, speech problems, hallucinations, seizures, or coma. This occurrence may be more common in persons with kidney problems taking high doses or in the elderly. Tell your doctor right away if you experience any of these symptoms.
- It is not known if Valtrex can reduce the transmission of genital herpes if you have multiple sexual partners. Valtrex does not cure genital herpes. Avoid sexual contact if you have open lesions or an active outbreak.
- Genital herpes can be spread even if you have no symptoms of an outbreak. Always use a condom whenever you have sexual contact. If your doctor advises you to take Valtrex for recurrent outbreaks, start taking it at the first sign or symptom of an outbreak.

Who should not take this medication?
Do not take Valtrex if you are allergic to it or any of its ingredients.

What should I tell my doctor before I take the first dose of this medication?
Tell your doctor about all prescription, over-the-counter, and herbal medications you are taking before beginning treatment with Valtrex. Also, talk to your doctor about your complete medical history, especially if you have HIV or AIDS, kidney problems, have had a bone marrow or kidney transplant, or are pregnant, plan to become pregnant, or are breastfeeding.

What is the usual dosage?
Please see general statement regarding dosage on page xii.

Cold Sores
Adults and children ≥12 years: The recommended dose is 2 grams (g) twice a day (taken 12 hours apart) for 1 day.

Genital Herpes
Adults: Your doctor will prescribe the appropriate dose for you based on the stage of the infection and your other medical conditions.

Shingles
Adults: The recommended dose is 1 g three times a day for 7 days.

Chickenpox
Children 2-18 years: Your doctor will prescribe the appropriate dose for your child, based on their weight.

If you have kidney impairment, your doctor will adjust your dose appropriately.

How should I take this medication?
- Take Valtrex exactly as prescribed by your doctor. Do not change your dose or stop taking Valtrex without talking to your doctor. Take it with or without food.
- If you are taking Valtrex to treat cold sores, chickenpox, shingles, or genital herpes, start taking the medicine as soon as possible after your symptoms start. Valtrex may not help you if you start treatment too late.
- If your child cannot swallow the caplets, your pharmacist will prepare an oral suspension. Shake the suspension well before giving the medicine to your child. Throw away any unused amount of the suspension after 28 days.

What should I avoid while taking this medication?
Do not have sexual contact with your partner when you have any symptoms or outbreak of genital herpes.

Do not become dehydrated. Drink adequate amounts of fluids while you are taking Valtrex.

What are possible food and drug interactions associated with this medication?
No significant interactions have been reported with Valtrex at this time. However, always tell your doctor about any medicines you

take, including over-the-counter medications, vitamins, and herbal supplements.

What are the possible side effects of this medication?
Please see general statement regarding side effects on page xiii.

> **Side effects may include:** dizziness, headache, nausea, rash, stomach pain, tiredness, vomiting

Can I receive this medication if I am pregnant or breastfeeding?
The effects of Valtrex during pregnancy and breastfeeding are unknown. Tell your doctor immediately if you are pregnant, plan to become pregnant, or are breastfeeding.

What should I do if I miss a dose of this medication?
If you miss a dose of Valtrex, take it as soon as you remember. However, if it is almost time for your next dose, skip the one you missed and return to your regular dosing schedule. Do not take two doses at once.

How should I store this medication?
Store the caplets at room temperature.

Store the oral suspension in the refrigerator.

Vardenafil HCl: *see Levitra, page 543*

Varenicline: *see Chantix, page 209*

Vaseretic
Generic name: Enalapril Maleate/Hydrochlorothiazide

What is this medication?
Vaseretic is a combination medicine used to treat high blood pressure. Vaseretic contains two medicines: enalapril (an angiotensin-converting enzyme [ACE] inhibitor) and hydrochlorothiazide (a diuretic [water pill]).

What is the most important information I should know about this medication?
- Vaseretic can cause a rare but serious allergic reaction leading to extreme swelling of your face, lips, tongue, throat, or gut (causing severe abdominal pain). You may have an increased risk of experiencing these symptoms if you have ever had an allergy to angiotensin-converting enzyme (ACE) inhibitor-type medicines or if you are African American. If you experience any of these symptoms, seek emergency medical attention immediately.
- Tell your doctor if you experience lightheadedness, especially during the first few days of Vaseretic therapy. If you faint, stop taking Vaseretic and tell your doctor immediately.
- Vomiting, diarrhea, fever, exercise, hot weather, alcohol, excessive perspiration, and dehydration may lead to an excessive fall in your blood pressure. Tell your doctor if you experience any of these. Make sure to drink plenty of fluids when you are taking Vaseretic.
- Vaseretic may decrease your blood neutrophil (type of blood cells that fight infection) levels, especially if you have a collagen vascular disease (such as lupus [disease that affects the immune system]) or kidney disease. Promptly report any signs of infection (such as sore throat or fever) to your doctor.
- Vaseretic is not recommended in people with severe kidney problems.
- Vaseretic can raise your blood sugar. High blood sugar may make you feel confused, drowsy, or thirsty. It can also make you flush, breathe faster, or have a fruit-like breath odor. If these symptoms occur, tell your doctor right away.

• Vaseretic may not work as well in African Americans and may increase the risk of side effects. Contact your doctor if your symptoms do not improve or if they become worse.

Who should not take this medication?

Do not take Vaseretic if you are allergic to it or any of its ingredients.

Do not take Vaseretic if you have anuria (are unable to produce urine).

Do not take Vaseretic if you have a history of angioedema (a condition involving swelling of the face, extremities, eyes, lips, and tongue) related to previous treatment with similar medicines. Also, do not take Vaseretic if you have a history of certain types of angioedema (such as hereditary or idiopathic).

What should I tell my doctor before I take the first dose of this medication?

Tell your doctor about all prescription, over-the-counter, and herbal medications you are taking before beginning treatment with Vaseretic. Also, talk to your doctor about your complete medical history, especially if you have diabetes, or liver or kidney problems. Tell your doctor if you have bone marrow suppression, heart disease, skin disease, severe immune system problems, lupus, asthma, or are on a sodium-restricted diet. Also, tell your doctor if you have ever had an allergy or sensitivity to ACE inhibitors or sulfonamide-type medications.

What is the usual dosage?

Please see general statement regarding dosage on page xii.

Adults: The usual dose is 5/12.5 (5 milligrams [mg] of enalapril and 12.5 mg of hydrochlorothiazide) or 10/25 (10 mg of enalapril and 25 mg of hydrochlorothiazide) once a day.

Your doctor may give you a higher dose depending on your needs.

How should I take this medication?
- Take Vaseretic at the same time every day. Continue to use Vaseretic even if you feel well.
- Do not take extra doses or take more often without asking your doctor.

What should I avoid while taking this medication?
Do not become pregnant or breastfeed while you are taking Vaseretic.

Do not drive or operate heavy machinery until you know how Vaseretic affects you.

Do not become dehydrated. Drink an adequate amount of fluids while you are taking Vaseretic.

Do not take salt substitutes or supplements containing potassium without consulting your doctor.

Do not stand or sit up quickly when taking Vaseretic, especially in the morning. Sit or lie down at the first sign of dizziness, lightheadedness, or fainting.

What are possible food and drug interactions associated with this medication?
If Vaseretic is taken with certain other drugs, the effects of either could be increased, decreased, or altered. It is especially important to check with your doctor before combining Vaseretic with the following: alcohol, antidiabetic medications, barbiturates (such as phenobarbital), certain diuretics (such as amiloride, spironolactone, or triamterene), cholestyramine, colestipol, corticosteroids, digoxin, injectable gold (sodium aurothiomalate), insulin, lithium, narcotics (such as codeine), nonsteroidal anti-inflammatory medications (such as ibuprofen or naproxen), norepinephrine, other blood pressure-lowering medications, potassium supplements, salt substitutes containing potassium, or skeletal muscle relaxants.

What are the possible side effects of this medication?
Please see general statement regarding side effects on page xiii.

Side effects may include: cough, diarrhea, dizziness, fatigue, headache, low blood pressure, muscle cramps, nausea, weakness

Can I receive this medication if I am pregnant or breastfeeding?
Do not take Vaseretic if you are pregnant or breastfeeding. Vaseretic can harm your unborn baby. It can be found in your breast milk if you take it while breastfeeding. Tell your doctor immediately if you are pregnant, plan to become pregnant, or are breastfeeding.

What should I do if I miss a dose of this medication?
If you miss a dose of Vaseretic, take it as soon as you remember. However, if it is almost time for your next dose, skip the one you missed and return to your regular dosing schedule. Do not take two doses at once.

How should I store this medication?
Store at room temperature. Protect from moisture.

Vasotec
Generic name: Enalapril Maleate

What is this medication?
Vasotec is a medicine known as an angiotensin-converting enzyme (ACE) inhibitor. Vasotec is used alone or in combination with other medications to treat high blood pressure or heart failure.

What is the most important information I should know about this medication?
• Vasotec can cause a rare but serious allergic reaction leading to extreme swelling of your face, lips, tongue, throat, or gut (causing severe abdominal pain). You may have an increased risk of experiencing these symptoms if you have ever had an allergy to ACE inhibitor-type medicines or if you are African American. If you experience any of these symptoms, seek emergency medical attention immediately.

- Tell your doctor if you experience lightheadedness, especially during the first few weeks of Vasotec therapy. If you faint, stop taking Vasotec and tell your doctor immediately.
- Vomiting, diarrhea, fever, exercise, hot weather, alcohol, excessive perspiration, and dehydration may lead to an excessive fall in your blood pressure. Tell your doctor if you experience any of these.
- Vasotec may decrease your blood neutrophil (type of blood cells that fight infections) levels, especially if you have a collagen vascular disease (such as lupus [disease that affects the immune system]) or kidney disease.
- Promptly report any signs of infection (such as sore throat or fever) to your doctor.
- Vasotec may not work as well in African Americans, who may also have a higher risk of side effects. Tell your doctor if your symptoms do not improve or if they become worse.

Who should not take this medication?

Do not take Vasotec if you are allergic to it or any of its ingredients.

Do not take Vasotec if you have a history of angioedema (a condition involving swelling of the face, extremities, eyes, lips, and tongue) related to previous treatment with similar medicines. Also, do not take Vasotec if you have a history of certain types of angioedema (such as hereditary or idiopathic).

What should I tell my doctor before I take the first dose of this medication?

Tell your doctor about all prescription, over-the-counter, and herbal medications you are taking before beginning treatment with Vasotec. Also, talk to your doctor about your complete medical history, especially if you have liver problems, kidney disease, or diabetes. Tell your doctor if you have bone marrow problems or any blood disease, any disease that affects the immune system (such as lupus or scleroderma), collagen vascular disease, narrowing or hardening of the arteries of your brain or heart, chest pain, or if you have ever had an allergy or sensitivity to ACE inhibitors such as Vasotec.

What is the usual dosage?
Please see general statement regarding dosage on page xii.

Blood Pressure
Adults: The usual starting dose is 5 milligrams (mg) once a day. Your doctor may give you a higher dose depending on your needs.

If you are taking a diuretic (water pill), your doctor will prescribe or adjust your dose as needed.

Children: Your doctor will prescribe the appropriate dose for your child, based on their weight.

Heart Failure
Adults: The usual starting dose is 2.5 mg twice a day. Your doctor may give you a higher dose depending on your needs.

If you have kidney impairment, your doctor will adjust your dose appropriately.

How should I take this medication?
- Take Vasotec at the same time every day. Continue to use Vasotec even if you feel well.
- Do not take extra doses or take more often without asking your doctor.

What should I avoid while taking this medication?
Do not become pregnant or breastfeed while you are taking Vasotec.

Do not drive or operate heavy machinery until you know how Vasotec affects you.

Do not take salt substitutes or supplements containing potassium without consulting your doctor.

Do not stand or sit up quickly when you take Vasotec, especially in the morning. Sit or lie down at the first sign of dizziness, lightheadedness, or fainting.

What are possible food and drug interactions associated with this medication?

If Vasotec is taken with certain other drugs, the effects of either could be increased, decreased, or altered. It is especially important to check with your doctor before combining Vasotec with the following: amiloride, auranofin, dextran, diuretics (such as furosemide, hydrochlorothiazide, spironolactone, or triamterene), glyburide, lithium, nonsteroidal anti-inflammatory drugs (NSAIDs) (such as ibuprofen or naproxen), potassium supplements, or salt substitutes containing potassium.

What are the possible side effects of this medication?

Please see general statement regarding side effects on page xiii.

> **Side effects may include:** chest pain, diarrhea, dizziness, dry cough, fatigue, headache, low blood pressure, nausea, rash, vomiting

Can I receive this medication if I am pregnant or breastfeeding?

Do not take Vasotec if you are pregnant or breastfeeding. Vasotec can harm your unborn baby. It can be found in your breast milk if you take it while breastfeeding. Tell your doctor immediately if you are pregnant, plan to become pregnant, or are breastfeeding.

What should I do if I miss a dose of this medication?

If you miss a dose of Vasotec, take it as soon as you remember. However, if it is almost time for your next dose, skip the one you missed and return to your regular dosing schedule. Do not take two doses at once.

How should I store this medication?

Store at room temperature. Store away from heat, moisture, and light.

Venlafaxine HCl: *see Effexor XR, page 355*

Ventolin HFA
Generic name: Albuterol Sulfate

What is this medication?
Ventolin HFA is an inhaled medicine used to prevent and treat airway narrowing associated with certain breathing problems (such as asthma). Ventolin HFA is also used to prevent exercise-induced airway narrowing.

What is the most important information I should know about this medication?
- Do not use Ventolin HFA more frequently than your doctor recommends. Increasing the number of doses can be dangerous and may actually make symptoms of asthma worse. If the dose your doctor recommends does not provide relief of your symptoms, or if your symptoms become worse, tell your doctor right away.
- You can have an immediate, serious allergic reaction to the first dose of Ventolin HFA, with hives, rash, and swelling of your mouth, throat, lips, or tongue. This medication can cause life-threatening breathing problems, especially with the first dose from a new canister. If you experience an allergic reaction or trouble breathing, call your doctor right away.

Who should not take this medication?
Do not use Ventolin HFA if you are allergic to it or any of its ingredients.

What should I tell my doctor before I take the first dose of this medication?
Tell your doctor about all prescription, over-the-counter, and herbal medications you are taking before beginning treatment with Ventolin HFA. Also, talk to your doctor about your complete medical history, especially if you have a heart condition, seizure disorder, high blood pressure, arrhythmia (life-threatening irregular heartbeat), overactive thyroid gland, low blood potassium levels, or diabetes.

What is the usual dosage?
Please see general statement regarding dosage on page xii.

Prevention or Treatment of Airway Narrowing

Adults and children ≥4 years: The usual dose is 2 inhalations every 4-6 hours. Your or your child's doctor will adjust your dose appropriately.

Exercise-Induced Airway Narrowing

Adults and children ≥4 years: The usual dose is 2 inhalations 15-30 minutes before exercise.

How should I take this medication?

- Use Ventolin HFA exactly as prescribed by your doctor. Shake the inhaler well before each use.
- You must prime the inhaler if you are using it for the first time, when it has not been used for more than 2 weeks, or if you drop it. To do this, press the pump 4 times into the air, away from your face.
- Breathe out fully through your mouth, then place the mouthpiece into your mouth and close your lips around it. While breathing in deeply and slowly through your mouth, press down on the top of the metal canister. Hold your breath for 10 seconds if possible.
- If your doctor has prescribed more than one inhalation, wait one minute between inhalations. Clean the mouthpiece without the metal canister at least once a week.
- Please review the instructions that came with your prescription on how to properly use Ventolin HFA.

What should I avoid while taking this medication?

Do not spray Ventolin HFA into your eyes.

Do not inhale extra doses or stop using Ventolin HFA without talking to your doctor.

Do not clean the metal canister or allow it to become wet.

What are possible food and drug interactions associated with this medication?

If Ventolin HFA is used with certain other drugs, the effects of either could be increased, decreased, or altered. It is especially important to check with your doctor before combining Ventolin HFA with the following: blood pressure/heart medications known as beta-blockers (such as metoprolol or propranolol), certain antidepressants (such as amitriptyline or phenelzine), certain diuretics (water pills) (such as furosemide or hydrochlorothiazide), digoxin, or medicines similar to Ventolin HFA (such as terbutaline and epinephrine).

What are the possible side effects of this medication?
Please see general statement regarding side effects on page xiii.

Side effects may include: cough, muscle pain, swelling of your upper respiratory tract, throat irritation, respiratory (lung) tract infections

Can I receive this medication if I am pregnant or breastfeeding?
The effects of Ventolin HFA during pregnancy and breastfeeding are unknown. Do not breastfeed while you are using Ventolin HFA. Tell your doctor immediately if you are pregnant, plan to become pregnant, or are breastfeeding.

What should I do if I miss a dose of this medication?
If you miss a dose of Ventolin HFA, take it as soon as you remember. However, if it is almost time for your next dose, skip the one you missed and return to your regular dosing schedule. Do not take two doses at once.

How should I store this medication?
Store at room temperature. Protect from heat or open flame.

Store the inhaler with the mouthpiece down.

Verapamil HCl: see Calan SR, page 169

Vesicare
Generic name: Solifenacin Succinate

What is this medication?
Vesicare is a medicine used to treat symptoms of overactive bladder, including frequent urination, urgency (increased need to urinate), and urge incontinence (inability to control urination).

What is the most important information I should know about this medication?
- Vesicare can cause blurred vision. Do not drive or operate heavy machinery until you know how Vesicare affects you.
- If you experience severe stomach pain or have constipation for 3 or more days, contact your doctor.

Who should not take this medication?
Do not take Vesicare if you are allergic to it or any of its ingredients. Do not take Vesicare if you have urinary retention (inability to urinate normally). Do not take Vesicare if you have gastric retention (a blockage in the digestive system). Do not take Vesicare if you have narrow-angle glaucoma (high pressure in the eye).

What should I tell my doctor before I take the first dose of this medication?
Tell your doctor about all prescription, over-the-counter, and herbal medications you are taking before beginning treatment with Vesicare. Also, talk to your doctor about your complete medical history, especially if you have any stomach or intestinal problems; problems with constipation; trouble emptying your bladder fully; a weak stream of urine; liver, kidney, or heart problems; narrow-angle glaucoma; or if you are pregnant, plan to become pregnant, or are breastfeeding.

What is the usual dosage?
Please see general statement regarding dosage on page xii.

Adults: The recommended starting dose is 5 milligrams (mg) once a day. Depending on your response, your doctor may increase the dose to 10 mg a day.

If you have severe kidney or moderate liver impairment, your dose should not exceed 5 mg a day.

How should I take this medication?
- Take Vesicare with water and swallow the tablet whole.
- Take Vesicare with or without food.

What should I avoid while taking this medication?
Do not drive or operate heavy machinery until you know how Vesicare affects you.

Avoid hot environments and becoming overheated during activity.

What are possible food and drug interactions associated with this medication?
If Vesicare is taken with certain other drugs, the effects of either could be increased, decreased, or altered. It is especially important to check with your doctor before combining Vesicare with the following: atazanavir, indinavir, itraconazole, ketoconazole, nelfinavir, ritonavir, saquinavir, or voriconazole.

What are the possible side effects of this medication?
Please see general statement regarding side effects on page xiii.

Side effects may include: abdominal (stomach area) pain, blurred vision, constipation, decreased sweating, dizziness, dry mouth, increase in your body temperature, nausea, tiredness, upset stomach, urinary tract infection

---

Can I receive this medication if I am pregnant or breastfeeding?
The effects of Vesicare during pregnancy and breastfeeding are unknown. Tell your doctor immediately if you are pregnant, plan to become pregnant, or are breastfeeding.

What should I do if I miss a dose of this medication?
If you miss a dose of Vesicare, take it again the next day. Do not take two doses the same day.

How should I store this medication?
Store at room temperature.

Viagra
Generic name: Sildenafil Citrate

What is this medication?
Viagra is a medicine used to treat erectile dysfunction in men. It can help men get and keep an erection when they become sexually excited.

What is the most important information I should know about this medication?
- Viagra can help you get an erection only when you are sexually excited. You will not get an erection just by taking this medicine.
- Viagra does not cure erectile dysfunction. It is a treatment for erectile dysfunction.
- Viagra does not protect you or your partner from getting any sexually transmitted diseases.
- Sexual activity can put a strain on your heart, especially if it is already weak from a heart disease. Refrain from further activity and talk to your doctor if you experience chest pain, dizziness, or nausea during sex.
- Viagra can cause a sudden decrease or loss of vision or hearing. Loss of vision can occur in one or both eyes. Loss of hearing can occur with ringing in your ears and dizziness. If you experience these symptoms, stop taking Viagra and call your doctor right away.
- Viagra can cause an erection that lasts many hours. Call your doctor immediately if you ever have an erection that lasts more than 4 hours. If this is not treated right away, permanent damage to your penis can occur.
- Viagra contains the same medicine found in another medicine called Revatio. Do not use these medicines together.

Who should not take this medication?
Do not take Viagra if you are allergic to it or any of its ingredients.

Do not take Viagra if you take any medicines that contain nitrates (such as nitroglycerin, isosorbide mononitrate, or isosorbide dinitrate). If you take Viagra with these medicines, your blood pressure could suddenly drop to an unsafe or life-threatening level.

Do not take Viagra if your doctor told you not to engage in sexual activity due to a heart disease or other heart problems.

What should I tell my doctor before I take the first dose of this medication?

Tell your doctor about all prescription, over-the-counter, and herbal medications you are taking before beginning treatment with Viagra. Also, talk to your doctor about your complete medical history, especially if you have or ever had any heart problems (such as chest pain, heart failure, irregular heartbeats, or heart attack); stroke; low or high blood pressure; severe vision loss or retinitis pigmentosa (eye disease that involves damage to the layer of tissue in the back of the eye, called the retina); kidney, liver, or blood problems (such as sickle cell anemia or leukemia); any deformation of your penis; an erection that lasted more than 4 hours; or stomach ulcers.

What is the usual dosage?

Please see general statement regarding dosage on page xii.

Adults: The recommended dose is 50 milligrams as needed 1 hour before you plan to have sex. Your doctor will increase or decrease your dose as needed.

If you are older than 65 years, or have liver or kidney impairment, your doctor will adjust your dose appropriately.

How should I take this medication?

- Do not take Viagra more than once a day.
- If you take Viagra after a high-fat meal, the medicine may take a little longer to start working.

What should I avoid while taking this medication?

Do not start or stop taking any medicines before talking to your doctor or pharmacist.

What are possible food and drug interactions associated with this medication?

If Viagra is taken with certain other drugs, the effects of either could be increased, decreased, or altered. It is especially important to check with your doctor before combining Viagra with the following: anti-HIV medications called protease inhibitors (such as ritonavir or saquinavir), bosentan, cimetidine, erythromycin, itraconazole, ketoconazole, medications called alpha-blockers (such as doxazosin or tamsulosin) used to treat high blood pressure or prostate problems, nitrates, or rifampin.

What are the possible side effects of this medication?

Please see general statement regarding side effects on page xiii.

> **Side effects may include:** flushing of your face, headache, upset stomach

Can I receive this medication if I am pregnant or breastfeeding?

Viagra is not for use in women.

What should I do if I miss a dose of this medication?

Viagra is not for regular use. Take it only before sexual activity.

How should I store this medication?

Store at room temperature.

Vicodin

Generic name: Acetaminophen/Hydrocodone Bitartrate

What is this medication?

Vicodin is a pain medicine that contains the narcotic painkiller hydrocodone and the non-narcotic painkiller acetaminophen. Vicodin is used to relieve moderate to moderately severe pain.

What is the most important information I should know about this medication?

- Vicodin has abuse potential. Mental and physical dependence can occur with the use of Vicodin when it is used improperly.
- Vicodin can cause serious breathing problems that can become life-threatening, especially when it is used in the wrong way.
- Vicodin contains acetaminophen, which can cause severe liver injury. Do not take more than 4000 milligrams (mg) of acetaminophen a day, or take other products containing acetaminophen while you are taking Vicodin. The risk of liver injury can be higher if you have underlying liver disease or drink alcohol while you are taking Vicodin.
- Vicodin can cause allergic reactions or anaphylaxis (a serious and rapid allergic reaction that may result in death if not treated immediately). Stop taking Vicodin and tell your doctor immediately if you develop a rash, difficulty breathing, or swelling of your face, mouth, or throat.

Who should not take this medication?

Do not take Vicodin if you are allergic to it, any of its ingredients, or other narcotic painkillers.

What should I tell my doctor before I take the first dose of this medication?

Tell your doctor about all prescription, over-the-counter, and herbal medications you are taking before beginning treatment with Vicodin. Also, talk to your doctor about your complete medical history, especially if you have ever had liver or kidney problems, hypothyroidism (an underactive thyroid gland), Addison's disease (adrenal gland failure), an enlarged prostate, urethral stricture (narrowing of the urethra, the tube that connects from the bladder to the genitals to lead urine out of your body), a history of alcohol or drug abuse, or if you have ever had a head injury.

What is the usual dosage?

Please see general statement regarding dosage on page xii.

Adults: The usual dose is one or two tablets every 4-6 hours as needed for pain. Do not take more than eight tablets in one day.

How should I take this medication?
• Take Vicodin exactly as prescribed by your doctor.

What should I avoid while taking this medication?
Do not take any other medications that contain acetaminophen.

Vicodin can impair your mental or physical abilities. Do not drive or operate machinery until you know how Vicodin affects you.

What are possible food and drug interactions associated with this medication?
If Vicodin is taken with certain other drugs, the effects of either could be increased, decreased, or altered. It is especially important to check with your doctor before combining Vicodin with the following: alcohol, antianxiety medications (such as alprazolam or lorazepam), antihistamines (such as chlorpheniramine or diphenhydramine), antipsychotics (such as risperidone or olanzapine), certain antidepressants (such as amitriptyline or selegiline), or other narcotic painkillers.

What are the possible side effects of this medication?
Please see general statement regarding side effects on page xiii.

> **Side effects may include:** dizziness, lightheadedness, nausea, sleepiness, vomiting

Can I receive this medication if I am pregnant or breastfeeding?
The effects of Vicodin during pregnancy and breastfeeding are unknown. Tell your doctor immediately if you are pregnant, plan to become pregnant, or are breastfeeding.

What should I do if I miss a dose of this medication?
Vicodin should be taken only as needed.

How should I store this medication?
Store at room temperature.

Vicoprofen

Generic name: Hydrocodone Bitartrate/Ibuprofen

What is this medication?

Vicoprofen is a pain medicine that contains the narcotic painkiller hydrocodone and the nonsteroidal anti-inflammatory drug (NSAID) ibuprofen. Vicoprofen is used to relieve short-term pain (generally <10 days).

What is the most important information I should know about this medication?

- Vicoprofen has abuse potential. Mental and physical dependence can occur with the use of Vicoprofen when it is used improperly.
- Vicoprofen can cause serious breathing problems that can become life-threatening, especially when it is used in the wrong way.
- Vicoprofen can cause allergic reactions or anaphylaxis (a serious and rapid allergic reaction that may result in death if not treated immediately). Stop taking Vicoprofen and tell your doctor immediately if you develop a rash, difficulty breathing, or swelling of your face, mouth, or throat.
- Do not use Vicoprofen right before or after a heart surgery called a coronary artery bypass graft (CABG).
- Vicoprofen can cause ulcers or bleeding in your stomach and intestines at any time during treatment.
- Stop Vicoprofen and tell your doctor immediately if you experience unexplained weight gain, swelling, shortness of breath, chest pain, weakness in one part or side of your body, slurred speech, or swelling of your face or throat.

Who should not take this medication?

Do not take Vicoprofen if you are allergic to it or any of its ingredients.

Do not take Vicoprofen if you had an asthma attack, hives, or other allergic reaction with aspirin or any other NSAID medicine.

What should I tell my doctor before I take the first dose of this medication?

Tell your doctor about all prescription, over-the-counter, and herbal medications you are taking before beginning treatment with Vicoprofen. Also, talk to your doctor about your complete medical history, especially if you have ever had liver or kidney problems, heart disease, hypothyroidism (an underactive thyroid gland), Addison's disease (adrenal gland failure), an enlarged prostate, urethral stricture (narrowing of the urethra, the tube that connects from the bladder to the genitals to lead urine out of your body), a history of alcohol or drug abuse, or if you have ever had a head injury.

What is the usual dosage?

Please see general statement regarding dosage on page xii.

Adults: The recommended dose is one tablet every 4-6 hours, as needed for pain. Do not take more than 5 tablets in one day.

How should I take this medication?

- Take Vicoprofen exactly as prescribed by your doctor. Do not take extra doses or take more often without asking your doctor.

What should I avoid while taking this medication?

Vicoprofen can impair your mental or physical abilities. Do not drive or operate machinery until you know how Vicoprofen affects you.

What are possible food and drug interactions associated with this medication?

If Vicoprofen is taken with certain other drugs, the effects of either could be increased, decreased, or altered. It is especially important to check with your doctor before combining Vicoprofen with the following: alcohol, angiotensin-converting enzyme (ACE) inhibitors (such as enalapril or lisinopril), antianxiety medications (such as alprazolam or lorazepam), antihistamines (such as chlorpheniramine or diphenhydramine), antipsychotics (such as risperidone or olanzapine), certain antidepressants (such as amitriptyline or

selegiline), other narcotic painkillers, or water pills (such as furosemide or hydrochlorothiazide).

What are the possible side effects of this medication?

Please see general statement regarding side effects on page xiii.

> **Side effects may include:** constipation, difficulty sleeping, diz-
> ziness, diarrhea, dry mouth, gas, headache, heartburn, itching,
> nausea, nervousness, sleepiness, sweating, swelling, vomiting

Can I receive this medication if I am pregnant or breastfeeding?

The effects of Vicoprofen during pregnancy and breastfeeding are
unknown. Do not take Vicoprofen late in your pregnancy. Tell your
doctor immediately if you are pregnant, plan to become pregnant,
or are breastfeeding.

What should I do if I miss a dose of this medication?

Vicoprofen should be taken only as needed.

How should I store this medication?

Store at room temperature.

Victrelis

Generic name: Boceprevir

What is this medication?

Victrelis is a medicine used with peginterferon alfa and ribavirin to
treat long-term hepatitis C infection in adults who have not been
treated before or who have failed previous treatment.

What is the most important information I should know about this medication?

• Do not take Victrelis alone to treat long-term hepatitis C infection. Victrelis must be used with peginterferon alfa and ribavirin.

- Victrelis, in combination with peginterferon alfa and ribavirin, can cause harm or death to your unborn baby. You, or your female sexual partner, should not become pregnant while taking these medications, and for 6 months after treatment is over. You must have a negative pregnancy test before starting treatment, each month during treatment, and for 6 months after your treatment ends. You must use two forms of effective birth control during treatment and for 6 months after treatment is over.
- Your doctor will perform blood tests before you start treatment, and at other times as needed during treatment, to see how well the medicines are working and to check for side effects.

Who should not take this medication?

Do not take Victrelis if you are allergic to it or any of its ingredients.

Do not take Victrelis if you or your female sexual partner is pregnant or may become pregnant.

What should I tell my doctor before I take the first dose of this medication?

Tell your doctor about all prescription, over-the-counter, and herbal medications you are taking before beginning treatment with Victrelis. Also, talk to your doctor about your complete medical history, especially if you have low red blood cell counts (anemia), have liver problems other than hepatitis C infection, have human immunodeficiency virus (HIV) infection (AIDS), have had an organ transplant, plan to have surgery, are pregnant, plan to become pregnant, or are breastfeeding.

What is the usual dosage?

Please see general statement regarding dosage on page xii.

Adults: The usual dose is 800 milligrams (mg), (four 200-mg capsules), 3 times a day.

How should I take this medication?

- Take Victrelis exactly as prescribed by your doctor.
- Always take Victrelis with a meal or light snack.

- Each bottle has your entire day's worth of medicine. Make sure you are taking the correct amount of medicine each time.

What should I avoid while taking this medication?

You, or your sexual partner, should avoid becoming pregnant while taking Victrelis.

Do not give Victrelis to other people, even if they have the same symptoms that you have. It may harm them.

Do not stop taking Victrelis without first talking to your doctor.

What are possible food and drug interactions associated with this medication?

If Victrelis is taken with certain other drugs, the effects of either could be increased, decreased, or altered. It is especially important to check with your doctor before combining Victrelis with any other medication.

What are the possible side effects of this medication?

Please see general statement regarding side effects on page xiii.

> **Side effects may include:** anemia, change in your taste, headache, low white blood cell counts, nausea, tiredness

Can I receive this medication if I am pregnant or breastfeeding?

Do not take Victrelis if you are pregnant or plan to become pregnant. Victrelis, in combination with peginterferon alfa and ribavirin, may cause harm or even death to your unborn baby. The effects of Victrelis during breastfeeding are unknown. Tell your doctor immediately if you are pregnant, plan to become pregnant, or are breastfeeding.

What should I do if I miss a dose of this medication?

If you miss a dose of Victrelis and it is more than 2 hours before the next dose, take your missed dose with food as soon as you remember. However, if it is less than 2 hours before the next dose, skip the one you missed and return to your regular dosing schedule. Do not take two doses at once.

How should I store this medication?
Store in the refrigerator until expiration date. It may also be stored at room temperature for 3 months.

Keep in a tightly closed container and away from heat.

Vigamox
Generic name: Moxifloxacin HCl

What is this medication?
Vigamox is an antibiotic known as a quinolone that comes as eye drops. Vigamox is used to treat bacterial infections in your eyes, such as pink eye.

What is the most important information I should know about this medication?
- Vigamox is for use only in your eyes.
- If you have an allergic reaction, such as a rash or difficulty breathing, stop using this medication and contact your doctor.
- If you use Vigamox for a long period of time, it can cause infections, including fungal infections.
- Do not touch the applicator tip to the eye, fingers, or other source as this can contaminate Vigamox.

Who should not take this medication?
Do not use Vigamox if you are allergic to it or any of its ingredients, or if you are allergic to other quinolone antibiotics (such as levofloxacin).

What should I tell my doctor before I take the first dose of this medication?
Tell your doctor about all prescription, over-the-counter, and herbal medications you are taking before beginning treatment with Vigamox. Also, talk to your doctor about your complete medical

history, especially if you are allergic to quinolone antibiotics, are pregnant, plan to become pregnant, or are breastfeeding.

What is the usual dosage?
Please see general statement regarding dosage on page xii.

Adults and children >1 year: Apply 1 drop in the affected eye(s) 3 times a day for 7 days.

How should I take this medication?
- Apply Vigamox as prescribed by your doctor. Please review the instructions that came with your prescription on how to properly use your eye drops.

What should I avoid while taking this medication?
Do not wear contact lenses while you are using Vigamox.

Do not touch the applicator tip to your eyes, fingers, or other source as this can contaminate Vigamox.

What are possible food and drug interactions associated with this medication?
No significant interactions have been reported with Vigamox at this time. However, always tell your doctor about any medicines you take, including over-the-counter medications, vitamins, and herbal supplements.

What are the possible side effects of this medication?
Please see general statement regarding side effects on page xiii.

> **Side effects may include:** decreased vision accuracy, dry eye, eye pain, eye redness, fever, infection, rash

Can I receive this medication if I am pregnant or breastfeeding?
The effects of Vigamox during pregnancy and breastfeeding are unknown. Tell your doctor immediately if you are pregnant, plan to become pregnant, or are breastfeeding.

What should I do if I miss a dose of this medication?

If you miss a dose of Vigamox, apply it as soon as you remember. However, if it is almost time for your next dose, skip the one you missed and return to your regular dosing schedule. Do not apply two doses at once.

How should I store this medication?

Store at room temperature.

Viibryd

Generic name: Vilazodone HCl

What is this medication?

Viibryd is an antidepressant medicine used to treat major depressive disorder (MDD).

What is the most important information I should know about this medication?

- Viibryd can increase suicidal thoughts or actions in some children, teenagers, or young adults within the first few months of treatment or when the dose is changed. Call your doctor right away if you have any of the following symptoms, especially if they are new, worse, or worry you: attempts to commit suicide, acting on dangerous impulses, acting aggressive or violent, thoughts about suicide or dying, new or worse depression, new or worse anxiety or panic attacks, feeling agitated, restless, angry or irritable, trouble sleeping, an increase in activity or talking more than what is normal for you (mania), or other unusual changes in behavior or mood develop.
- Viibryd can cause a severe, possibly life-threatening condition called serotonin syndrome (a drug reaction that causes the body to have too much serotonin, a chemical produced by the nerve cells) or neuroleptic malignant syndrome (a life-threatening brain disorder). Contact your doctor immediately if you experience agitation, hallucinations, fast heartbeat, changes in your blood pressure, fever, lack of coordination, overactive reflexes, nausea, vomiting, or diarrhea.

- Viibryd can increase your risk of bleeding, especially if you take it with aspirin, nonsteroidal anti-inflammatory drugs (NSAIDs) (such as ibuprofen) or blood thinners (such as warfarin).
- Contact your doctor if you develop symptoms of a manic episode such as greatly increased energy, severe trouble sleeping, racing thoughts, reckless behavior, unusually grand ideas, excessive happiness or irritability, or talking more or faster than usual.
- Viibryd can cause low blood sodium levels. Contact your doctor immediately if you experience headache, difficulty concentrating, confusion, weakness, unsteadiness, hallucinations, falls, or seizures.
- Do not suddenly stop taking Viibryd without first talking to your doctor, as this can cause serious side effects.

Who should not take this medication?
Do not take Viibryd if you are taking an MAOI (such as selegiline or phenelzine), a class of medications used to treat depression and other conditions, or if you stopped taking an MAOI in the last 14 days.

Do not take Viibryd if you have had an allergic reaction or sensitivity to it or any of its ingredients.

What should I tell my doctor before I take the first dose of this medication?
Tell your doctor about all prescription, over-the-counter, and herbal medications you are taking before beginning treatment with Viibryd. Also, talk to your doctor about your complete medical history, especially if you have bleeding, liver, or kidney problems; seizures or convulsions; bipolar disorder (manic depression) or mania; low blood sodium levels; drink alcohol; or are pregnant, plan to become pregnant, or are breastfeeding or plan to breastfeed.

What is the usual dosage?
Please see general statement regarding dosage on page xii.

Adults: The usual starting dose is 10 milligrams (mg) once a day. Your doctor will increase your dose as appropriate.

How should I take this medication?

- Take Viibryd exactly as prescribed by your doctor. Your doctor may need to change the dosage until it is the right dose for you.
- Take Viibryd with food. It may not work as well if taken on an empty stomach.

What should I avoid while taking this medication?

Viibryd can cause sleepiness or may affect your ability to make decisions, think clearly, or react quickly. Do not drive, operate heavy machinery, or engage in other dangerous activities until you know how Viibryd affects you.

Do not drink alcohol while you are taking Viibryd.

What are possible food and drug interactions associated with this medication?

If Viibryd is taken with certain other drugs, the effects of either could be increased, decreased, or altered. It is especially important to check with your doctor before combining Viibryd with the following: alcohol; aspirin; buspirone; erythromycin; diuretics (water pills) (such as furosemide); ketoconazole; lithium; medicines used to treat migraine headaches (such as sumatriptan or solmitriptan); medicines used to treat mood, psychotic, or thought disorders (such as citalopram, paroxetine, or fluoxetine); MAOIs (such as selegiline or phenelzine); mephenytoin; NSAIDs (such as ibuprofen); blood thinners (such as warfarin); over-the-counter supplements (such as tryptophan or St. John's wort); or tramadol.

What are the possible side effects of this medication?

Please see general statement regarding side effects on page xiii.

Side effects may include: diarrhea, nausea, trouble sleeping, vomiting

Can I receive this medication if I am pregnant or breastfeeding?

The effects of Viibryd during pregnancy and breastfeeding are unknown. Tell your doctor immediately if you are pregnant, plan to become pregnant, or are breastfeeding.

What should I do if I miss a dose of this medication?

If you miss a dose Viibryd, take it as soon as you remember. However, if it is almost time for your next dose, skip the one you missed and return to your regular dosing schedule. Do not take two doses at once.

How should I store this medication?

Store at room temperature.

Vilazodone HCl: see Viibryd, page 1076

Vivelle-Dot

Generic name: Estradiol

What is this medication?

Vivelle-Dot is a transdermal patch (applied to your skin) that contains the estrogen hormone, estradiol. It is used to treat moderate to severe symptoms of menopause, such as hot flashes or severe dryness, itching, and burning in or around your vagina. Also, Vivelle-Dot is used to treat certain conditions in which a young woman's ovaries do not produce enough estrogens naturally, and to reduce your chances of getting postmenopausal osteoporosis (thin, weak bones).

What is the most important information I should know about this medication?

- Estrogens increase your risk of developing cancer of the uterus. Tell your doctor immediately if you experience any unusual vaginal bleeding while you are using Vivelle-Dot.

- Do not use Vivelle-Dot to prevent heart disease, heart attacks, strokes, or dementia. Using Vivelle-Dot can increase your chances of getting heart attacks, strokes, breast cancer, or blood clots.
- Vivelle-Dot can also increase your risk of dementia, gallbladder disease, ovarian cancer, visual abnormalities, high blood pressure, pancreatitis (inflammation of your pancreas), or thyroid problems. Talk regularly with your doctor about whether you still need treatment with Vivelle-Dot.
- You can lower your changes of serious side effects with Vivelle-Dot by having a breast exam and mammogram (breast x-ray) every year, unless directed by your doctor to have it more often. See your doctor immediately if you get vaginal bleeding while you are using Vivelle-Dot. Also, ask your doctor for ways to lower your chances of getting heart disease, especially if you have high blood pressure, high cholesterol, or diabetes, if you are overweight, or if you use tobacco.

Who should not take this medication?
Do not use Vivelle-Dot if you are allergic to it or any of its ingredients, or if you are pregnant or think you may be pregnant.

Do not use Vivelle-Dot if you have a history of stroke or heart attack, blood clots, liver problems, unusual vaginal bleeding, or certain cancers, including cancer of your breast or uterus.

What should I tell my doctor before I take the first dose of this medication?
Tell your doctor about all prescription, over-the-counter, and herbal medications you are taking before beginning treatment with Vivelle-Dot. Also, talk to your doctor about your complete medical history, especially if you are pregnant or breastfeeding, or have any unusual vaginal bleeding, asthma, seizures, diabetes, migraine headaches, endometriosis (a common gynecological disorder that may result in sores and pain), lupus (disease that affects the immune system), high blood calcium levels, or problems with your heart, liver, thyroid, or kidneys. Also, tell your doctor if you are going to have surgery or will be on bed rest.

What is the usual dosage?
Please see general statement regarding dosage on page xii.

Adults: Apply 1 patch to your skin, and replace the patch twice a week.

How should I take this medication?
- Use Vivelle-Dot exactly as prescribed by your doctor. Talk to your doctor regularly (every 3-6 months) about whether you still need treatment with Vivelle-Dot.
- Each patch is individually sealed in a protective pouch. Tear open at the tear notch (do not use scissors). Remove the patch. Holding the patch with the rigid protective liner facing you, remove half of the liner, which covers the sticky surface of the patch. Using the other half of the rigid protective liner as a handle, apply the sticky side of the patch to the selected area of your abdomen.
- When changing your patch, apply your new patch to a different area of your body. Do not apply a new patch to that same area for at least 1 week.
- Please review the instructions that came with your prescription on how to properly use Vivelle-Dot.

What should I avoid while taking this medication?
Do not apply Vivelle-Dot onto your breasts; waistline; or onto areas of your skin that are oily, damaged, or irritated.

Do not touch the sticky side of the patch with your fingers.

Grapefruit juice can increase your risk of side effects with Vivelle-Dot. Talk to your doctor before including grapefruit or grapefruit juice in your diet while you are using Vivelle-Dot.

What are possible food and drug interactions associated with this medication?
If Vivelle-Dot is used with certain other drugs, the effects of either could be increased, decreased, or altered. It is especially important to check with your doctor before combining Vivelle-Dot with the following: carbamazepine, clarithromycin, erythromycin, grapefruit

juice, itraconazole, ketoconazole, phenobarbital, rifampin, ritonavir, or St. John's wort.

What are the possible side effects of this medication?
Please see general statement regarding side effects on page xiii.

> **Side effects may include:** abdominal pain, application-site redness, back pain, bloating, breast pain, constipation, dizziness, fluid retention, hair loss, headache, indigestion, infection, irregular vaginal bleeding or spotting, joint pain or inflammation, muscle pain, nausea, pain, rash, vaginal yeast infection, vomiting
>
> If you experience symptoms of breast lumps, changes in your speech, changes in your vision, chest pain, dizziness and faintness, pain in your legs, severe headaches, shortness of breath, unusual vaginal bleeding, or vomiting, contact your doctor immediately.

Can I receive this medication if I am pregnant or breastfeeding?
Do not use Vivelle-Dot if you are pregnant. The hormone in Vivelle-Dot can be found in your breast milk if you use it while you are breastfeeding. Tell your doctor immediately if you are pregnant, plan to become pregnant, or are breastfeeding.

What should I do if I miss a dose of this medication?
Vivelle-Dot should be used under special circumstances determined by your doctor. If you miss your scheduled dose, contact your doctor or pharmacist for advice.

How should I store this medication?
Store at room temperature. Do not store the patch outside of the pouch.

Voltaren-XR

Generic name: Diclofenac Sodium

What is this medication?

Voltaren-XR is a nonsteroidal anti-inflammatory drug (NSAID) used to treat osteoarthritis and rheumatoid arthritis.

What is the most important information I should know about this medication?

- Voltaren-XR can cause serious problems (such as heart attack or stroke). Your risk can increase when this medication is used for long periods of time and if you have heart disease. Tell your doctor if you experience chest pain, shortness of breath, weakness, or slurred speech.
- Voltaren-XR can cause high blood pressure and heart failure or worsen existing high blood pressure. Tell your doctor if you experience weight gain or swelling.
- Voltaren-XR can cause discomfort, ulcers, or bleeding in your stomach or intestines. Your risk can increase with long-term use, smoking, drinking alcohol, older age, or with certain medications. Tell your doctor immediately if you experience stomach pain or if you have bloody vomit or stools.
- Long-term use of Voltaren-XR can cause kidney injury. Your risk can increase if you have kidney impairment; heart failure; liver problems; are taking certain medications, including diuretics (water pills) (such as furosemide or hydrochlorothiazide) or blood/heart medications known as angiotensin-converting enzyme (ACE) inhibitors (such as lisinopril); or are elderly.
- Voltaren-XR can also cause liver injury. Stop taking Voltaren-XR and call your doctor if you experience nausea, tiredness, weakness, itchiness, yellowing of your skin or whites of your eyes, right upper abdominal tenderness, or "flu-like" symptoms.
- Voltaren-XR can cause a serious allergic reaction. Stop taking Voltaren-XR and tell your doctor right away if you experience difficulty breathing or swelling of your face or throat.
- Stop taking Voltaren-XR and tell your doctor right away if you experience serious skin reactions, such as rash, blisters, fever, or itchiness.

Who should not take this medication?
Do not take Voltaren-XR if you are allergic to it or any of its ingredients.

Do not take Voltaren-XR if you have experienced asthma, hives, or allergic-type reactions after taking aspirin or other NSAIDs (such as ibuprofen or naproxen).

Do not take Voltaren-XR right before or after a heart surgery called a coronary artery bypass graft (CABG).

What should I tell my doctor before I take the first dose of this medication?
Tell your doctor about all prescription, over-the-counter, and herbal medications you are taking before beginning treatment with Voltaren-XR. Also, talk to your doctor about your complete medical history, especially if you have any of the following: allergies to medications, heart problems, history of asthma, high blood pressure, kidney or liver disease, or stomach problems, or are pregnant, plan to become pregnant, or are breastfeeding.

What is the usual dosage?
Please see general statement regarding dosage on page xii.

Osteoarthritis
Adults: The recommended dose is 100 milligrams (mg) once a day.

Rheumatoid Arthritis
Adults: The recommended dose is 100 mg once a day. Your doctor will increase your dose as needed until the desired effect is achieved.

How should I take this medication?
• Take Voltaren-XR exactly as prescribed by your doctor.
• Swallow Voltaren-XR tablets whole. Do not crush, cut, or chew them.

What should I avoid while taking this medication?

Do not take aspirin or other NSAIDs in combination with Voltaren-XR.

What are possible food and drug interactions associated with this medication?

If Voltaren-XR is taken with certain other drugs, the effects of either could be increased, decreased, or altered. It is especially important to check with your doctor before combining Voltaren-XR with the following: ACE inhibitors, aspirin, blood thinners (such as warfarin), cyclosporine, diuretics, lithium, methotrexate, rifampin, steroids, or voriconazole.

What are the possible side effects of this medication?

Please see general statement regarding side effects on page xiii.

Side effects may include: constipation, diarrhea, dizziness, gas, heartburn, nausea, stomach pain, vomiting

Can I receive this medication if I am pregnant or breastfeeding?

Do not take Voltaren-XR if you are in the late stage of your pregnancy or if you are breastfeeding. The effects of Voltaren-XR during early pregnancy are unknown. Tell your doctor immediately if you are pregnant, plan to become pregnant, or are breastfeeding.

What should I do if I miss a dose of this medication?

If you miss a dose of Voltaren-XR, take it as soon as you remember. However, if it is almost time for your next dose, skip the one you missed and return to your regular dosing schedule. Do not take two doses at once.

How should I store this medication?

Store at room temperature. Protect from moisture.

Vytorin
Generic name: Ezetimibe/Simvastatin

What is this medication?
Vytorin is a combination medicine used to lower your cholesterol when a low-fat diet is not enough. Vytorin contains two cholesterol-lowering medicines: simvastatin and ezetimibe.

What is the most important information I should know about this medication?
- Taking Vytorin is not a substitute for following a healthy low-fat and low-cholesterol diet and exercising to lower your cholesterol.
- Do not take Vytorin if you are pregnant, think you may be pregnant, if you are planning to become pregnant, or if you are breastfeeding.
- Vytorin can cause serious muscle conditions or liver problems. Call your doctor right away if you experience unexplained muscle pain, weakness, or tenderness, feeling tired or weak, loss of appetite, pain in the upper right part of your stomach, dark urine, or yellowing of your skin or the whites of your eyes.

Who should not take this medication?
Do not take Vytorin if you are allergic to it or any of its ingredients, or if you currently have liver disease. Also, do not take Vytorin in combination with anti-HIV medications (such as indinavir), boceprevir, clarithromycin, cyclosporine, danazol, erythromycin, gemfibrozil, itraconazole, ketoconazole, nefazodone, posaconazole, telaprevir, or telithromycin.

Do not take Vytorin if you are pregnant, plan to become pregnant, or are breastfeeding.

What should I tell my doctor before I take the first dose of this medication?
Tell your doctor about all prescription, over-the-counter, and herbal medications you are taking before beginning treatment with Vytorin. Also, talk to your doctor about your complete medical history, especially if you drink excessive amounts of alcohol, have liver or kidney problems, muscle aches or weakness, diabetes, or

thyroid problems. Tell your doctor if you are pregnant, plan to become pregnant, or are breastfeeding.

What is the usual dosage?
Please see general statement regarding dosage on page xii.

Adults: The usual starting dose is 10/10 (10 milligrams [mg] of ezetimibe and 10 mg of simvastatin) once a day or 10/20 (10 mg of ezetimibe and 20 mg of simvastatin) once a day. Your doctor may give you a higher dose, depending on your needs.

How should I take this medication?
- Your doctor will likely start you on a low-cholesterol diet before giving you Vytorin. Stay on this diet while you are taking Vytorin.
- Take Vytorin exactly as prescribed by your doctor. Take Vytorin once a day, in the evening. Take it with or without food.

What should I avoid while taking this medication?
Do not drink large amounts of grapefruit juice (>1 quart a day) while you are taking Vytorin.

What are possible food and drug interactions associated with this medication?
If Vytorin is taken with certain other drugs, the effects of either could be increased, decreased, or altered. It is especially important to check with your doctor before combining Vytorin with the following: alcohol, amiodarone, blood pressure medications known as calcium channel blockers (such as amlodipine, diltiazem, or verapamil), blood thinners (such as warfarin), cholesterol-lowering medicines known as fibrates (such as fenofibrate), cholestyramine, colchicine, digoxin, grapefruit juice, niacin, ranolazine, or voriconazole.

What are the possible side effects of this medication?
Please see general statement regarding side effects on page xiii.

Side effects may include: diarrhea, headache, muscle pain

Can I receive this medication if I am pregnant or breastfeeding?

Do not take Vytorin during pregnancy or breastfeeding. Tell your doctor immediately if you are pregnant, plan to become pregnant, or are breastfeeding.

What should I do if I miss a dose of this medication?

If you miss a dose of Vytorin, take it as soon as you remember. However, if it is almost time for your next dose, skip the one you missed and return to your regular dosing schedule. Do not take two doses at once.

How should I store this medication?

Store at room temperature.

Vyvanse

Generic name: Lisdexamfetamine Dimesylate

What is this medication?

Vyvanse is a medicine used to treat attention-deficit hyperactivity disorder (ADHD). This medicine can help to increase attention and decrease impulsiveness and hyperactivity in people with ADHD.

What is the most important information I should know about this medication?

• Vyvanse has a high potential for abuse. Taking Vyvanse for long periods of time may lead to extreme emotional and physical dependence. Your doctor will monitor your response and make sure you receive the correct dose. Tell your doctor if you have a history of drug or alcohol abuse.

• Vyvanse can cause serious heart-related and mental problems, stroke and heart attacks in adults, and increased blood pressure and heart rate. It can also cause new or worsening behavior and thought problems, bipolar illness, and aggressive or hostile behavior.

• In addition, new symptoms (such as hearing voices, believing things that are not true, being suspicious, or manic symptoms)

can occur. Call your doctor right away if you or your child experiences chest pain, shortness of breath, fainting, or new mental problems while taking Vyvanse.
- The doctor will check your child's height and weight while he/she is taking Vyvanse. If your child is not growing in height or gaining weight as expected, the doctor may stop this medicine.
- Vyvanse can cause eyesight changes or blurred vision. If this occurs, tell your doctor.

Who should not take this medication?
Do not take Vyvanse if you are allergic to it or any of its ingredients.

Do not take Vyvanse if you are taking antidepressant medications known as monoamine oxidase inhibitors (MAOIs) (such as phenelzine or tranylcypromine) or have taken them within the past 14 days.

What should I tell my doctor before I take the first dose of this medication?
Tell your doctor about all prescription, over-the-counter, and herbal medications you are taking before beginning treatment with Vyvanse. Also, talk to your doctor about your complete medical history, including heart problems, heart defects, high blood pressure, or a family history of these problems. Tell your doctor if you have a history of mental problems or a family history of psychosis, mania, bipolar disorder, or depression; tics or Tourette's syndrome; or seizures or an abnormal brain wave test (EEG).

What is the usual dosage?
Please see general statement regarding dosage on page xii.

Adults and children ≥6 years: The usual starting dose is 30 milligrams once a day. Your or your child's doctor may increase the dose as appropriate.

How should I take this medication?
- Take Vyvanse exactly as prescribed by your doctor. Take Vyvanse once a day in the morning. Do not take Vyvanse in the afternoon to avoid having trouble sleeping. Take it with or without food.

• If you or your child have difficulty swallowing the capsule, open it and dissolve the entire contents of the capsule in a glass of water. Drink the entire glass of water right away. Do not store it for later use.

What should I avoid while taking this medication?

Use caution when driving, operating heavy machinery, or performing activities that require alertness.

Do not start any new medicine while you are taking Vyvanse without first talking to your doctor.

What are possible food and drug interactions associated with this medication?

If Vyvanse is taken with certain other drugs, the effects of either could be increased, decreased, or altered. It is especially important to check with your doctor before combining Vyvanse with the following: acetazolamide, ammonium chloride, antihistamines (such as cetirizine or loratadine), blood pressure medications, certain antidepressants (such as desipramine or protriptyline), certain diuretics (water pills) (such as hydrochlorothiazide), chlorpromazine, cryptenamine, ethosuximide, haloperidol, lithium, MAOIs, meperidine, methenamine, norepinephrine, propoxyphene, seizure medications (such as phenobarbital or phenytoin), or sodium acid phosphate.

What are the possible side effects of this medication?

Please see general statement regarding side effects on page xiii.

> **Side effects may include:** anxiety, decreased appetite, diarrhea, dizziness, dry mouth, irritability, loss of appetite, nausea, trouble sleeping, upper stomach pain, vomiting, weight loss

Can I receive this medication if I am pregnant or breastfeeding?

The effects of Vyvanse during pregnancy are unknown. Vyvanse can be found in your breast milk if you take it while breastfeeding. Do not breastfeed while you are taking Vyvanse. Tell your doctor immediately if you are pregnant, plan to become pregnant, or are breastfeeding.

What should I do if I miss a dose of this medication?
If you miss a dose of Vyvanse, take it as soon as you remember. However, if it is almost time for your next dose, skip the one you missed and return to your regular dosing schedule. Do not take two doses at once.

How should I store this medication?
Store at room temperature.

Warfarin Sodium: *see Coumadin, page 276*

Wellbutrin
Generic name: Bupropion HCl

What is this medication?
Wellbutrin is a medicine used to treat adults with major depressive disorder.

What is the most important information I should know about this medication?
- Wellbutrin can increase the risk of suicidal thoughts and behavior in children, adolescents, and young adults. Your doctor will monitor you closely for clinical worsening, suicidal or unusual behaviour after you start taking Wellbutrin or a new dose of Wellbutrin. Tell your doctor immediately if you experience anxiety, hostility, sleeplessness, restlessness, impulsive or dangerous behavior, or thoughts about suicide or dying; or if you have new symptoms or seem to be feeling worse.
- Wellbutrin can cause seizures or changes in your appetite or weight. Stop taking Wellbutrin and call your doctor right away if you have a seizure.

- Wellbutrin can increase your blood pressure. The risk of high blood pressure may be higher if you are also using nicotine patches to help you stop smoking.
- Wellbutrin can cause severe allergic reactions. Stop taking this medication and tell your doctor right away if you develop a rash, itching, hives, fever, painful sores in your mouth or around your eyes, swelling of your lips or tongue, chest pain, or trouble breathing.
- Wellbutrin can cause unusual thoughts or behaviors. Tell your doctor if you believe you are someone else, see or hear things that are not there, feel that people are against you, or feel confused.

Who should not take this medication?

Do not take Wellbutrin if you are allergic to it or any of its ingredients. Do not take Wellbutrin if you have or had a seizure disorder or epilepsy, or if you have or had an eating disorder (such as anorexia or bulimia).

Do not take Wellbutrin if you are currently taking other medicines known as a monoamine oxidase inhibitors (MAOI), a class of medications used to treat depression and other psychiatric conditions (such as phenelzine, tranylcypromine, or isocarboxazid). You must stop taking your MAOI at least 14 days before beginning treatment with Wellbutrin.

Do not take Wellbutrin if you are taking a medication called Zyban, which is used to help quit smoking, since both medicines contain the same active ingredient.

Do not take Wellbutrin if you drink a lot of alcohol or use sedatives (medicines that make you sleepy) and you stop them suddenly.

What should I tell my doctor before I take the first dose of this medication?

Tell your doctor about all prescription, over-the-counter, and herbal medications you are taking before beginning treatment with Wellbutrin. Also, talk to your doctor about your complete medical history, especially if you have kidney or liver problems, an eating disorder, a head injury, have had a seizure, have a tumor in the spine or brain, have had a heart attack, heart problems, or high blood pressure, or if you are diabetic and you are taking insulin or other medicines to control your blood sugar.

What is the usual dosage?
Please see general statement regarding dosage on page xii.

Adults: The usual starting dose is 100 milligrams twice a day. Your doctor will increase your dose as needed until the desired effect is achieved.

If you have liver or kidney impairment, your doctor will adjust your dose appropriately.

How should I take this medication?
• Take Wellbutrin exactly as prescribed by your doctor. Take it at the same time every day, at least 6 hours apart. You can take Wellbutrin with or without food.

What should I avoid while taking this medication?
Do not drink alcohol while you are taking Wellbutrin.

Do not drive a car or operate heavy machinery until you know how Wellbutrin affects you.

Do not increase, decrease, or stop taking Wellbutrin without first talking to your doctor.

What are possible food and drug interactions associated with this medication?
If Wellbutrin is taken with certain other drugs, the effects of either could be increased, decreased, or altered. It is especially important to check with your doctor before combining Wellbutrin with the following: alcohol, amantadine, carbamazepine, cimetidine, clopidogrel, cyclophosphamide, desipramine, efavirenz, flecainide, fluoxetine, fluvoxamine, haloperidol, imipramine, levodopa, MAOIs, metoprolol, nelfinavir, nicotine patches, norfluoxetine, nortriptyline, orphenadrine, paroxetine, phenobarbital, phenytoin,

propafenone, risperidone, ritonavir, sertraline, steroids, theophylline, thioridazine, thiotepa, or ticlopidine.

What are the possible side effects of this medication?
Please see general statement regarding side effects on page xiii.

> **Side effects may include:** constipation, dry mouth, headache, nausea, nervousness, shaking, trouble sleeping, vomiting

Can I receive this medication if I am pregnant or breastfeeding?
The effects of Wellbutrin during pregnancy are unknown. Wellbutrin can be found in your breast milk if you take it while breastfeeding. Do not breastfeed while you are taking Wellbutrin. Tell your doctor immediately if you are pregnant, plan to become pregnant, or are breastfeeding.

What should I do if I miss a dose of this medication?
If you miss a dose of Wellbutrin, take it as soon as you remember. However, if it is almost time for your next dose, skip the one you missed and return to your regular dosing schedule. Do not take two doses at once.

How should I store this medication?
Store at room temperature, away from light and moisture.

Wellbutrin SR
Generic name: Bupropion HCl

What is this medication?
Wellbutrin SR is a medicine used to treat adults with major depressive disorder.

What is the most important information I should know about this medication?

- Wellbutrin SR can increase the risk of suicidal thoughts and behavior in children, adolescents, and young adults. Your doctor will monitor you closely for clinical worsening, suicidal or unusual behavior after you start taking Wellbutrin SR or a new dose of Wellbutrin SR. Tell your doctor immediately if you experience anxiety, hostility, sleeplessness, restlessness, impulsive or dangerous behavior, or thoughts about suicide or dying; or if you have new symptoms or seem to be feeling worse.
- Wellbutrin SR can cause seizures or changes in your appetite or weight. Stop taking Wellbutrin SR and call your doctor right away if you have a seizure.
- Wellbutrin SR can increase your blood pressure. The risk of high blood pressure may be higher if you are also using nicotine patches to help you stop smoking.
- Wellbutrin SR can cause severe allergic reactions. Stop taking this medication and tell your doctor right away if you develop a rash, itching, hives, fever, painful sores in your mouth or around your eyes, swelling of your lips or tongue, chest pain, or trouble breathing.
- Wellbutrin SR can cause unusual thoughts or behaviors. Tell your doctor if you believe you are someone else, see or hear things that are not there, feel that people are against you, or feel confused.

Who should not take this medication?

Do not take Wellbutrin SR if you are allergic to it or any of its ingredients. Do not take Wellbutrin SR if you have or had a seizure disorder or epilepsy, or if you have or had an eating disorder (such as anorexia or bulimia).

Do not take Wellbutrin SR if you are currently taking other medicines known as monoamine oxidase inhibitors (MAOIs), a class of medications used to treat depression and other psychiatric conditions (such as phenelzine, tranylcypromine, or isocarboxazid). You must stop taking your MAOI at least 14 days before beginning treatment with Wellbutrin SR.

Do not take Wellbutrin SR if you are taking a medication called Zyban, which is used to help quit smoking, since both medicines contain the same active ingredient.

Do not take Wellbutrin SR if you drink a lot of alcohol or use sedatives (medicines that make you sleepy) and you stop them suddenly.

What should I tell my doctor before I take the first dose of this medication?
Tell your doctor about all prescription, over-the-counter, and herbal medications you are taking before beginning treatment with Wellbutrin SR. Also, talk to your doctor about your complete medical history, especially if you have kidney or liver problems, an eating disorder, a head injury, have had a seizure, have a tumor in the spine or brain, have had a heart attack, heart problems, or high blood pressure, or if you are diabetic and you are using insulin or other medicines to control your blood sugar.

What is the usual dosage?
Please see general statement regarding dosage on page xii.

Adults: The usual starting dose is 150 milligrams once a day, in the morning. Your doctor will increase your dose as needed until the desired effect is achieved.

If you have liver or kidney impairment, your doctor will adjust your dose appropriately.

How should I take this medication?
- Take Wellbutrin SR exactly as prescribed by your doctor. Take it at the same time every day. You can take Wellbutrin SR with or without food.
- Swallow Wellbutrin SR tablets whole. Do not chew, cut, or crush them.

What should I avoid while taking this medication?
Do not drink alcohol while you are taking Wellbutrin SR.

Do not drive a car or operate heavy machinery until you know how Wellbutrin SR affects you.

Do not increase, decrease, or stop taking Wellbutrin SR without first talking to your doctor.

Do not take any other medicines while you are taking Wellbutrin SR without first talking to your doctor.

What are possible food and drug interactions associated with this medication?

If Wellbutrin SR is taken with certain other drugs, the effects of either could be increased, decreased, or altered. It is especially important to check with your doctor before combining Wellbutrin SR with the following: alcohol, amantadine, carbamazepine, cimetidine, citalopram, clopidogrel, cyclophosphamide, desipramine, efavirenz, flecainide, fluoxetine, fluvoxamine, haloperidol, imipramine, levodopa, lopinavir, MAOIs, metoprolol, nelfinavir, nicotine patches, norfluoxetine, nortriptyline, orphenadrine, paroxetine, phenobarbital, phenytoin, propafenone, risperidone, ritonavir, sertraline, steroids, tamoxifen, theophylline, thioridazine, thiotepa, or ticlopidine.

What are the possible side effects of this medication?

Please see general statement regarding side effects on page xiii.

> **Side effects may include:** agitation, anxiety, dizziness, dry mouth, fast heartbeat, loss of appetite, muscle pain, nausea, ringing in your ears, shakiness, skin rash, sore throat, stomach pain, sweating, trouble sleeping, urinating more often

Can I receive this medication if I am pregnant or breastfeeding?

The effects of Wellbutrin SR during pregnancy are unknown. Wellbutrin SR can be found in your breast milk if you take it while breastfeeding. Do not breastfeed while you are taking Wellbutrin SR. Tell your doctor immediately if you are pregnant, plan to become pregnant, or are breastfeeding.

What should I do if I miss a dose of this medication?

If you miss a dose of Wellbutrin SR, take it as soon as you remember. However, if it is almost time for your next dose, skip the one you missed and return to your regular dosing schedule. Do not take two doses at once.

How should I store this medication?

Store at room temperature.

Xalatan

Generic name: Latanoprost

What is this medication?

Xalatan is an eye drop used to lower pressure in the eye in people with open-angle glaucoma or ocular hypertension (high pressure in the eye).

What is the most important information I should know about this medication?

- Xalatan can darken the color of your iris (colored part of the eye), eyelid, or eyelashes. The discoloration of your eyelids or eyelashes is usually reversible; however the discoloration of the iris is most likely permanent.
- Xalatan can also increase the length, thickness, number of eyelashes, and/or direction of eyelash growth. Tell your doctor if you notice any discoloration or changes in these areas of your eye.
- Do not allow the tip of the bottle to touch your eye or any other surface, as serious eye infections may occur if your bottle becomes contaminated. Tell your doctor immediately if you experience any eye injury, infection, conjunctivitis ("pink eye"), or eyelid reactions with Xalatan.

Who should not take this medication?

Do not use Xalatan if you are allergic to it or any of its ingredients.

What should I tell my doctor before I take the first dose of this medication?

Tell your doctor about all prescription, over-the-counter, and herbal medications you are taking before beginning treatment with Xalatan. Also, talk to your doctor about your complete medical history, especially if you have had eye surgery or other eye disorders.

What is the usual dosage?

Please see general statement regarding dosage on page xii.

Adults: The recommended dose is 1 drop in the affected eye(s) once a day in the evening.

How should I take this medication?

- Apply Xalatan exactly as prescribed by your doctor.
- Xalatan contains a preservative that may be absorbed by your contact lenses. Remove your contact lenses prior to the administration of Xalatan and reinsert them after 15 minutes.
- If you are using Xalatan with another eye drop, the drops should be applied at least 5 minutes apart.

What should I avoid while taking this medication?

Do not allow the tip of the bottle to touch your eye or any other surface, as this can contaminate the medication.

What are possible food and drug interactions associated with this medication?

If Xalatan is used with certain other drugs, the effects of either could be increased, decreased, or altered. It is especially important to check with your doctor before combining Xalatan with other eye drops.

What are the possible side effects of this medication?

Please see general statement regarding side effects on page xiii.

Side effects may include: blurred vision; burning, stinging, or itching of your eye; feeling of something in your eye; red eye

---

Can I receive this medication if I am pregnant or breastfeeding?

The effects of Xalatan during pregnancy and breastfeeding are unknown. Tell your doctor immediately if you are pregnant, plan to become pregnant, or are breastfeeding.

What should I do if I miss a dose of this medication?

If you miss a dose of Xalatan, apply it as soon as you remember. However, if it is almost time for your next dose, skip the one you missed and return to your regular dosing schedule. Do not apply two doses at once.

How should I store this medication?

Store unopened bottles in the refrigerator.

Once opened, Xalatan may be stored at room temperature for up to 6 weeks.

Protect Xalatan from light.

Xanax

Generic name: Alprazolam

What is this medication?

Xanax is a medicine used for the management of anxiety disorder, short-term relief of anxiety symptoms, and treatment of panic disorder.

What is the most important information I should know about this medication?

- Xanax has abuse potential. Mental and physical dependence can occur with the use of Xanax.
- Do not stop taking Xanax or decrease the dose without first talking to your doctor. Stopping or reducing the dose of Xanax suddenly can cause withdrawal symptoms, including seizures.
- Early-morning anxiety and anxiety symptoms between doses of Xanax can occur in patients with panic disorder.

Who should not take this medication?
Do not take Xanax if you are allergic to it or any of its ingredients.

Do not take Xanax if you have an eye condition called acute narrow-angle glaucoma (high pressure in the eye) or if you are taking the medications itraconazole or ketoconazole.

What should I tell my doctor before I take the first dose of this medication?
Tell your doctor about all prescription, over-the-counter, and herbal medications you are taking before beginning treatment with Xanax. Also, talk to your doctor about your complete medical history, especially if you have a history of alcohol or drug abuse; liver, kidney, or breathing problems; glaucoma; muscle problems; or depression or suicidal tendencies. Also, tell your doctor if you are pregnant, plan to become pregnant, or are breastfeeding.

What is the usual dosage?
Please see general statement regarding dosage on page xii.

<u>Anxiety Disorders and Temporary Symptoms of Anxiety</u>
Adults: The usual starting dose is 0.25-0.5 milligrams (mg) three times a day.

<u>Panic Disorder</u>
Adults: The usual starting dose is 0.5 mg three times a day.

Your doctor will increase your dose as needed until the desired effect is achieved.

If you are elderly or have liver impairment, your doctor will adjust your dose appropriately.

How should I take this medication?
- Take Xanax exactly as prescribed by your doctor.
- Do not increase, decrease, or stop taking Xanax without first talking to your doctor.

What should I avoid while taking this medication?

Do not drink alcohol while you are taking Xanax.

Do not drive a car or operate dangerous machinery until you know how Xanax affects you.

What are possible food and drug interactions associated with this medication?

If Xanax is taken with certain other drugs, the effects of either could be increased, decreased, or altered. It is especially important to check with your doctor before combining Xanax with the following: alcohol, amiodarone, antihistamines (such as cetirizine or loratadine), birth control pills, carbamazepine, certain antibiotics (such as clarithromycin or erythromycin), certain antipsychotics (such as amitriptyline or olanzapine), cimetidine, cyclosporine, desipramine, diltiazem, ergotamine, fluoxetine, fluvoxamine, grapefruit juice, imipramine, isoniazid, itraconazole, ketoconazole, nefazodone, nicardipine, nifedipine, paroxetine, propoxyphene, seizure medicines (such as valproate or phenytoin), or sertraline.

What are the possible side effects of this medication?

Please see general statement regarding side effects on page xiii.

Side effects may include: anxiety, blurred vision, changes in your appetite or sexual desire, chest pain, confusion, constipation, depression, diarrhea, difficulty speaking, dizziness, drowsiness, dry mouth, fainting, fast heartbeat, fatigue, headache, impaired coordination, increased or decreased salivation, increased rate of breathing, irritability, lightheadedness, low blood pressure, memory impairment, menstrual disorders, muscle stiffness or twitching, nasal congestion, nausea, nervousness, rash, restlessness, ringing in your ears, sexual dysfunction, shaking, skin irritation, stomach pain, sweating, swelling, tiredness, trouble sleeping or urinating, upper respiratory tract infection, vomiting, weakness, weight gain or loss

Can I receive this medication if I am pregnant or breastfeeding?

Do not take Xanax if you are pregnant or breastfeeding. Xanax can harm your unborn baby. Tell your doctor immediately if you are pregnant, plan to become pregnant, or are breastfeeding.

What should I do if I miss a dose of this medication?

If you miss a dose of Xanax, take it as soon as you remember. However, if it is almost time for your next dose, skip the one you missed and return to your regular dosing schedule. Do not take two doses at once.

How should I store this medication?

Store at room temperature.

Xanax XR

Generic name: Alprazolam

What is this medication?

Xanax XR is a medicine used for the management of anxiety disorder, short-term relief of anxiety symptoms, and treatment of panic disorder.

What is the most important information I should know about this medication?

- Xanax XR has abuse potential. Mental and physical dependence can occur with the use of Xanax XR.
- Do not stop taking Xanax XR or decrease the dose without first talking to your doctor. Stopping or reducing the dose of Xanax XR suddenly can cause withdrawal symptoms, including seizures.
- Early-morning anxiety and anxiety symptoms between doses of Xanax XR can occur in patients with panic disorder.

Who should not take this medication?

Do not take Xanax XR if you are allergic to it or any of its ingredients.

Do not take Xanax XR if you have an eye condition called acute narrow-angle glaucoma (high pressure in the eye) or if you are taking the medications itraconazole or ketoconazole.

What should I tell my doctor before I take the first dose of this medication?

Tell your doctor about all prescription, over-the-counter, and herbal medications you are taking before beginning treatment with Xanax XR. Also, talk to your doctor about your complete medical history, especially if you have a history of alcohol or drug abuse; liver, kidney, or breathing problems; glaucoma; muscle problems; depression or suicidal tendencies; or have ever been physically or mentally dependent on a benzodiazepine medication. Also, tell your doctor if you are pregnant, plan to become pregnant, or are breastfeeding.

What is the usual dosage?
Please see general statement regarding dosage on page xii.

Adults: The usual starting dose is 0.5-1 milligram once a day. Your doctor will increase your dose as needed until the desired effect is achieved.

If you are elderly or have liver impairment, your doctor will adjust your dose appropriately.

How should I take this medication?
- Take Xanax XR exactly as prescribed by your doctor.
- Take Xanax XR every day, preferably in the morning.
- Swallow the Xanax XR tablet whole. Do not chew, crush, or break the tablet.
- Do not increase, decrease, or stop taking Xanax XR without first talking to your doctor.

What should I avoid while taking this medication?
Do not drink alcohol while you are taking Xanax XR.

Do not drive a car or operate dangerous machinery until you know how Xanax XR affects you.

What are possible food and drug interactions associated with this medication?

If Xanax XR is taken with certain other drugs, the effects of either could be increased, decreased, or altered. It is especially important to check with your doctor before combining Xanax XR with the following: alcohol, amiodarone, antihistamines (such as cetirizine or loratadine), birth control pills, carbamazepine, certain antibiotics (such as clarithromycin or erythromycin), certain antipsychotics (such as amitriptyline or olanzapine), cimetidine, cyclosporine, desipramine, diltiazem, ergotamine, fluoxetine, fluvoxamine, grapefruit juice, imipramine, isoniazid, itraconazole, ketoconazole, nefazodone, nicardipine, nifedipine, paroxetine, propoxyphene, seizure medicines (such as valproate or phenytoin), or sertraline.

What are the possible side effects of this medication?

Please see general statement regarding side effects on page xiii.

Side effects may include: constipation, decrease or increase in your appetite, depression, drowsiness, dry mouth, memory impairment, sleepiness, sexual dysfunction, tiredness

Can I receive this medication if I am pregnant or breastfeeding?

Do not take Xanax XR if you are pregnant or breastfeeding. Xanax XR can harm your unborn baby. Tell your doctor immediately if you are pregnant, plan to become pregnant, or are breastfeeding.

What should I do if I miss a dose of this medication?

If you miss a dose of Xanax XR, take it as soon as you remember. However, if it is almost time for your next dose, skip the one you missed and return to your regular dosing schedule. Do not take two doses at once.

How should I store this medication?

Store at room temperature.

Xarelto

Generic name: Rivaroxaban

What is this medication?

Xarelto is a medicine used to reduce your risk of stroke and blood clots if you have a medical condition called atrial fibrillation (an irregular, fast heartbeat). Xarelto is also used to reduce your risk of forming a blood clot in your legs and lungs if you have just had a hip or knee replacement surgery.

What is the most important information I should know about this medication?

- If you have atrial fibrillation and are taking Xarelto, do not stop taking it without first talking to your doctor. Stopping Xarelto can increase your risk of having a stroke. If you have to stop taking Xarelto, your doctor may prescribe another blood thinner medicine to prevent a blood clot from forming.
- Xarelto can cause bleeding which can be serious. While you are taking Xarelto, you are likely to bruise more easily and it may take longer for bleeding to stop.
- Call your doctor or get medical help immediately if you develop unexpected bleeding or bleeding that lasts a long time; bleeding that is severe or you cannot control; red, pink, or brown urine; bright red or black stools; if you cough up blood or blood clots; if you vomit blood or your vomit looks like "coffee grounds;" if you develop headaches, feel dizzy, or weak; or if you experience pain, swelling, or new drainage at wound sites.
- Tell all your doctors and dentists that you are taking Xarelto. They should talk to the doctor who prescribed Xarelto for you before you have any surgery, medical, or dental procedure.

Who should not take this medication?

Do not take Xarelto if you currently have certain types of abnormal bleeding. Talk to your doctor before taking Xarelto if you currently have unusual bleeding.

Do not take Xarelto if you are allergic to it or any of its ingredients.

What should I tell my doctor before I take the first dose of this medication?

Tell your doctor about all prescription, over-the-counter, and herbal medications you are taking before beginning treatment with Xarelto. Also, talk to your doctor about your complete medical history, especially if you have ever had bleeding problems, have liver or kidneys problems, are pregnant, plan to become pregnant, if you are breastfeeding, or plan to breastfeed.

What is the usual dosage?

Please see general statement regarding dosage on page xii.

Atrial Fibrillation
Adults: The recommended dose is 20 milligrams (mg) taken once a day. If you have kidney impairment, your doctor will adjust your dose appropriately.

Hip or Knee Replacement Surgery
Adults: The recommended dose is 10 mg taken once a day.

If you are receiving any other blood thinner, your doctor will instruct you on how to start taking Xarelto.

How should I take this medication?
- Take Xarelto exactly as prescribed by your doctor.
- *Atrial Fibrillation:* Take Xarelto once a day with your evening meal.
- *Hip or Knee Replacement Surgery:* Take Xarelto once a day with or without food.

What should I avoid while taking this medication?
Do not change your dose or stop taking Xarelto unless your doctor tells you to.

What are possible food and drug interactions associated with this medication?
If Xarelto is taken with certain other drugs, the effects of either could be increased, decreased, or altered. It is especially important to check with your doctor before combining Xarelto with the

following: aspirin, blood thinners (such as enoxaparin, heparin, or warfarin), carbamazepine, clarithromycin, clopidogrel, conivaptan, erythromycin, medicines to treat fungal infections (such as fluconazole, itraconazole, or ketoconazole), indinavir, lopinavir, nonsteroidal anti-inflammatory drugs (NSAIDs) (such as ibuprofen or naproxen), ritonavir, phenytoin, prasugrel, rifampin, St. John's wort, or ticagrelor.

What are the possible side effects of this medication?
Please see general statement regarding side effects on page xiii.

> **Side effects may include:** bleeding

Can I receive this medication if I am pregnant or breastfeeding?
The effects of Xarelto during pregnancy and breastfeeding are unknown. Tell your doctor immediately if you are pregnant, plan to become pregnant, or are breastfeeding.

What should I do if I miss a dose of this medication?
If you miss a dose of Xarelto, take it as soon as you remember on the same day, and return to your regular dosing schedule on the following day. Do not apply two doses at once.

How should I store this medication?
Store at room temperature.

Xopenex HFA
Generic name: Levalbuterol Tartrate

What is this medication?
Xopenex HFA is an inhaled medicine used to prevent and treat airway narrowing associated with certain breathing problems (such as asthma).

What is the most important information I should know about this medication?

- Do not use Xopenex HFA more frequently than your doctor rec-ommends. Increasing the number of doses can be dangerous and may actually make symptoms of asthma worse. If the dose your doctor recommends does not provide relief of your symp-toms, or if your symptoms become worse, tell your doctor right away.
- You can have an immediate, serious allergic reaction to the first dose of Xopenex HFA, with hives, rash, and swelling of your mouth, throat, lips, or tongue. This medication can cause life-threatening breathing problems, especially with the first dose from a new canister. If you experience an allergic reaction or trouble breathing, call your doctor right away.

Who should not take this medication?

Do not use Xopenex HFA if you are allergic to it or any of its ingredients.

What should I tell my doctor before I take the first dose of this medication?

Tell your doctor about all prescription, over-the-counter, and herbal medications you are taking before beginning treatment with Xopenex HFA. Also, talk to your doctor about your complete medi-cal history, especially if you have a heart condition, seizure dis-order, high blood pressure, arrhythmia (life-threatening irregular heartbeat), overactive thyroid gland, low blood potassium levels, or diabetes.

What is the usual dosage?

Please see general statement regarding dosage on page xii.

Adults and children ≥4 years: The usual dose is 2 inhalations every 4-6 hours. Your or your child's doctor will adjust your dose appropriately.

How should I take this medication?

- Use Xopenex HFA exactly as prescribed by your doctor. Shake the inhaler well before each use.

- You must prime the inhaler if you are using it for the first time and when it has not been used for more than 3 days. To do this, press the pump 4 times into the air, away from your face.
- Breathe out fully through your mouth, then place the mouthpiece into your mouth and close your lips around it. While breathing in deeply and slowly through your mouth, press down on the top of the metal canister. Hold your breath for 10 seconds if possible.
- If your doctor has prescribed more than one inhalation, wait one minute between inhalations. Clean the mouthpiece without the metal canister at least once a week.
- Please review the instructions that came with your prescription on how to properly use Xopenex HFA.

What should I avoid while taking this medication?
Do not spray Xopenex HFA into your eyes.

Do not inhale extra doses or stop using Xopenex HFA without talking to your doctor.

Do not clean the metal canister or allow it to become wet.

What are possible food and drug interactions associated with this medication?
If Xopenex HFA is used with certain other drugs, the effects of either could be increased, decreased, or altered. It is especially important to check with your doctor before combining Xopenex HFA with the following: blood pressure/heart medications known as beta-blockers (such as metoprolol or propranolol), certain antidepressants (such as amitriptyline or phenelzine), certain diuretics (water pills) (such as furosemide or hydrochlorothiazide), digoxin, or medicines similar to Xopenex HFA (such as terbutaline and epinephrine).

What are the possible side effects of this medication?
Please see general statement regarding side effects on page xiii.

Side effects may include: chest pain, fluttery or throbbing heartbeat, nervousness, rapid heart rate, shaking

Can I receive this medication if I am pregnant or breastfeeding?

The effects of Xopenex HFA during pregnancy and breastfeeding are unknown. Do not breastfeed while you are using Xopenex HFA. Tell your doctor immediately if you are pregnant, plan to become pregnant, or are breastfeeding.

What should I do if I miss a dose of this medication?

If you miss a dose of Xopenex HFA, take it as soon as you remember. However, if it is almost time for your next dose, skip the one you missed and return to your regular dosing schedule. Do not take two doses at once.

How should I store this medication?

Store at room temperature. Protect from heat, open flame, or direct sunlight.

Store the inhaler with the mouthpiece down.

Xyzal

Generic name: Levocetirizine Dihydrochloride

What is this medication?

Xyzal is an antihistamine used to relieve the symptoms of seasonal and year-round allergies, such as watery and itchy eyes, runny nose, and sneezing. It is also used to treat the symptoms of hives. Xyzal is available as tablets and liquid.

What is the most important information I should know about this medication?

- Xyzal can make you feel tired, drowsy, and weak. Do not drive or perform other potentially hazardous activities until you know how Xyzal affects you.
- Do not consume alcohol or take other medicines that affect your central nervous system while on Xyzal. This can decrease your mental alertness.

Who should not take this medication?

Do not take Xyzal if you are allergic to it or any of its ingredients.

Do not take Xyzal if you have end-stage kidney disease or if you are on dialysis.

Do not give Xyzal to your child if they have impaired kidney function.

What should I tell my doctor before I take the first dose of this medication?

Tell your doctor about all prescription, over-the-counter, and herbal medications you are taking before beginning treatment with Xyzal. Also, talk to your doctor about your complete medical history, especially if you have kidney problems, are pregnant, plan to become pregnant, or are breastfeeding.

What is the usual dosage?

Please see general statement regarding dosage on page xii.

Adults and children ≥12 years: The usual dose is 5 milligrams (mg) once a day in the evening.

Children 6-11 years: The usual dose is 2.5 mg once a day in the evening.

Children 6 months-5 years: The usual dose is 1.25 mg once a day in the evening.

If you or your child have kidney impairment, your doctor will adjust the dose appropriately.

How should I take this medication?

• Take Xyzal exactly as prescribed by your doctor. Do not take extra doses or take more often without asking your doctor.
• Xyzal can be taken with or without food.

What should I avoid while taking this medication?

Do not drink alcoholic beverages while on Xyzal.

Do not drive or engage in potentially hazardous activities until you know how Xyzal affects you.

What are possible food and drug interactions associated with this medication?

If Xyzal is taken with certain other drugs, the effects of either could be increased, decreased, or altered. It is especially important to check with your doctor before combining Xyzal with the following: antipyrine, azithromycin, cimetidine, erythromycin, ketoconazole, pseudoephedrine, ritonavir, and theophylline.

What are the possible side effects of this medication?

Please see general statement regarding side effects on page xiii.

> **Side effects may include:** allergic reactions, cough, diarrhea, drowsiness, dry mouth, ear infection, fatigue, fever, sleepiness, vomiting

Can I receive this medication if I am pregnant or breastfeeding?

The effects of Xyzal during pregnancy and breastfeeding are unknown. Xyzal can be found in your breast milk if you take it while breastfeeding. Tell your doctor immediately if you are pregnant, plan to become pregnant, or are breastfeeding.

What should I do if I miss a dose of this medication?

If you miss a dose of Xyzal, take it as soon as you remember. However, if it is almost time for your next dose, skip the one you missed and return to your regular dosing schedule. Do not take two doses at once.

How should I store this medication?

Store at room temperature.

Yasmin

Generic name: Drospirenone/Ethinyl Estradiol

What is this medication?

Yasmin is a birth control pill used to prevent pregnancy. Yasmin contains the hormones drospirenone and ethinyl estradiol.

What is the most important information I should know about this medication?

- Cigarette smoking increases the risk of serious heart-related side effects (such as blood clots, stroke, and heart attack) from use of birth control pills, such as Yasmin. The risk increases with age (especially if you are >35 years old and smoke). Do not smoke while you are taking birth control pills.
- Birth control pills increase your risk of serious blood clots, especially if you smoke, are obese, or are >35 years old. This increased risk is highest when you first start taking birth control pills and when you restart the same or different birth control pills after not using them for a month or more. This risk is higher if you take birth control pills with drospirenone (like Yasmin) than if you take birth control pills that do not contain drospirenone.
- Tell your doctor if you plan to have a major surgery. Your doctor will tell you when to stop taking Yasmin before the surgery and when to restart it after the surgery.
- Yasmin does not protect against HIV infection (AIDS) and other sexually transmitted diseases.
- Some women miss periods or have light periods when they take birth control pills, even when they are not pregnant. Contact your doctor for advice if you think you are pregnant, miss one period and have not taken your birth control pills on time every day, or if you miss two periods in a row.
- Yasmin contains the progestin drospirenone. Women who use birth control pills with drospirenone may have a higher risk of getting a blood clot.
- Drospirenone may increase your potassium levels. During the first month that you take Yasmin, your doctor will order a blood test to check your potassium levels.
- If you have vomiting or diarrhea, your birth control pills may not work as well. Take another pill if you vomit within 3-4 hours

after taking your pill, or use another birth control method, like condoms or spermicide, until you check with your doctor.

Who should not take this medication?

Do not take Yasmin if you smoke cigarettes and are >35 years old. Do not take Yasmin if you have a history of blood clots in your legs, lungs, or eyes; stroke; heart attack; certain types of headaches; or breast or cervical cancer. Also, do not take Yasmin if you have certain heart valve problems or heart rhythm abnormalities that can cause blood clots to form in your heart. Do not take Yasmin if you have an inherited problem that makes your blood clot more than normal; high blood pressure that medication cannot control; diabetes with kidney, eye, nerve, or blood vessel damage; liver disease, including liver tumors; or kidney or adrenal disease.

What should I tell my doctor before I take the first dose of this medication?

Tell your doctor about all prescription, over-the-counter, and herbal medications you are taking before beginning treatment with Yasmin. Also, talk to your doctor about your complete medical history, especially if you have ever had any of the health conditions listed above; or depression; diabetes; high triglycerides; history of jaundice (yellowing of your skin or whites of your eyes) caused by pregnancy; you smoke; or if you are pregnant, plan to become pregnant, or are breastfeeding.

What is the usual dosage?

Please see general statement regarding dosage on page xii.

Adults: Yasmin may be taken in one of two ways: On the Sunday after your period begins or during the first 24 hours of your period, as outlined below.

Sunday Start: Take the first yellow pill of the pack on the Sunday after your period begins, even if you are still bleeding. If your period begins on Sunday, start the pack that same day. Take one pill at the same time every day until the pack is empty. When you finish the pack, start the next pack on the day after your last white pill. Do not wait any days between packs.

Day 1 Start: Take the first yellow pill of the pack during the first 24 hours of your period. Take one pill at the same time every day until the pack is empty. When you finish the pack, start the next pack on the day after your last white pill. Do not wait any days between packs.

How should I take this medication?

- Before you start taking Yasmin, be sure to read the directions. Take Yasmin once a day, at the same time every day in the order directed on the package. Take the pill after the evening meal or at bedtime, with some liquid, as needed. You can take it with meals. The Yasmin pill pack has 21 yellow pills (with hormones) to be taken for three weeks, followed by 7 white pills (without hormones) to be taken for one week.
- For the *Sunday Start*, use another method of birth control (such as a condom or spermicide) as a back-up method if you have sex anytime from the Sunday you start your first pack until the next Sunday (7 days). This also applies if you start Yasmin after having been pregnant and you have not had a period since your pregnancy.
- You will not need to use a back-up method of birth control for the *Day 1 Start*, because you are starting the pill at the beginning of your period. However, if you start Yasmin later than the first day of your period, you should use another method of birth control as a back-up method until you have taken 7 yellow pills.

What should I avoid while taking this medication?

Do not smoke or become pregnant while you are taking Yasmin. Do not skip pills even if you have spotting or bleeding between monthly periods, feel sick to your stomach, or if you do not have sex very often.

What are possible food and drug interactions associated with this medication?

If Yasmin is taken with certain other drugs, the effects of either could be increased, decreased, or altered. It is especially important to check with your doctor before combining Yasmin with the following: antibiotics; blood pressure/heart medications known as angiotensin-converting enzyme (ACE) inhibitors (such as captopril and enalapril), angiotensin-II receptor antagonists (such as losartan, irbesartan, or valsartan), or aldosterone antagonists (such as eplerenone); barbiturates (such as phenobarbital); bosentan; carbamazepine; certain diuretics (water pills) (such as spironolactone); felbamate; griseofulvin; heparin; lamotrigine; nonsteroidal anti-inflammatory drugs (NSAIDs) (such as ibuprofen and naproxen); oxcarbazepine; phenytoin; potassium supplements; rifampin; St. John's wort; or topiramate.

What are the possible side effects of this medication?
Please see general statement regarding side effects on page xiii.

Side effects may include: acne (pimples), bloating or fluid retention, blotchy darkening of the skin, breast tenderness, depression, headache, high blood sugar, high cholesterol, less sexual desire, nausea, problems tolerating contact lenses, spotting or bleeding between menstrual periods, weight changes

Can I receive this medication if I am pregnant or breastfeeding?
Do not take Yasmin if you are pregnant or breastfeeding. Tell your doctor immediately if you are pregnant, plan to become pregnant, or are breastfeeding.

What should I do if I miss a dose of this medication?
If you miss one yellow pill, take it as soon as you remember. Take the next pill at your regular time. This means you can take two pills in one day. You do not need to use a back-up birth control method if you have sex.

If you miss two or more yellow pills, consult the patient information that accompanied your prescription or call your doctor or pharmacist for advice.

How should I store this medication?
Store at room temperature.

Yaz
Generic name: Drospirenone/Ethinyl Estradiol

What is this medication?
Yaz is a birth control pill used to prevent pregnancy. Yaz is also used to treat premenstrual dysphoric disorder (PMDD) (a severe condition that consists of physical and emotional symptoms, such as depression and irritability, before menstruation) in women who choose to use Yaz for birth control. Yaz is also used to treat moderate acne in women ≥14 years who are able to and wish to use Yaz for birth control.

What is the most important information I should know about this medication?
- Cigarette smoking increases the risk of serious heart-related side effects (such as blood clots, stroke, and heart attack) from use of birth control pills, such as Yaz. The risk increases with age (especially if you are >35 years old and smoke). Do not smoke while you are taking birth control pills.
- Use of birth control pills is associated with increased risk of heart attack, clotting disorders, stroke, liver tumors, and gallbladder disease. These risks increase in people with a history of high blood pressure, high cholesterol, obesity, diabetes, clotting disorders, heart attack, stroke, chest pain, cancer of the breast or sex organs, or liver tumors.
- Birth control pills may increase your cholesterol levels. Women with high cholesterol should be monitored closely.
- Yaz does not protect against HIV infection (AIDS) and other sexually transmitted diseases.
- You can experience breakthrough bleeding or spotting while you are taking birth control pills, especially during the first 3 months of use. You may also have irregular periods. If you have missed more than two periods in a row, take a pregnancy test to determine if you are pregnant. Do not use Yaz if you are pregnant.
- Yaz is different from other birth control pills because it contains the progestin (a type of hormone) drospirenone. Drospirenone may increase your potassium levels. During the first month that you take Yaz, your doctor will order a blood test to check your potassium levels.

Who should not take this medication?

Do not use Yaz if you are >35 years old and smoke cigarettes.

Do not use Yaz if you have a history of heart attack or stroke; heart disease; blood clots in your legs, lungs, or eyes; chest pain (angina); diabetes with kidney, eye, nerve or blood vessel damage; history of breast cancer; cancer of the lining of the uterus, cervix, or vagina; unexplained vaginal bleeding; yellowing of your skin or the whites of your eyes during pregnancy or during previous use of oral birth control pills; liver tumors; high blood pressure uncontrolled by medication; certain types of headaches; are allergic to any of the ingredients in Yaz; or if you plan to have surgery with prolonged bed rest. Do not take Yaz if you think you may be pregnant or if you have not had your first period.

What should I tell my doctor before I take the first dose of this medication?

Tell your doctor about all prescription, over-the-counter, and herbal medications you are taking before beginning treatment with Yaz. Tell your doctor if you have ever had any of the health conditions listed above. Also, talk to your doctor about your complete medical history, especially if you have or have had breast nodules, fibrocystic disease of the breast (lumpy and painful breasts), an abnormal breast x-ray or mammogram, high triglycerides, water retention, depression, migraines or other headaches, seizures, gallbladder disease, history of irregular menstrual bleeding or periods, wear contact lenses, smoke, plan to have surgery with prolonged bed rest, or if you are pregnant, plan to become pregnant, or are breastfeeding.

What is the usual dosage?

Please see general statement regarding dosage on page xii.

   Adults: Each pink "active" pill of Yaz contains 3 milligrams (mg) of drospirenone and 0.02 mg of ethinyl estradiol. Each white "reminder" pill contains inactive ingredients.
   Sunday Start: Take the first pink "active" pill on the Sunday after your period begins, even if you are still bleeding. Take one pink "active" pill a day for 24 days followed by one white "reminder"

pill a day for 4 days. After all 28 pills have been taken, start a new course the next day (Sunday).

Day 1 Start: Take the first pink "active" pill of the first pack during the first 24 hours of your period. Take one pink "active" pill a day from the 1st day through the 24th day of the menstrual cycle (counting the day your period starts as Day 1) followed by one white "reminder" pill a day for 4 days. Take the pills without interruption for 28 days. After all 28 tablets have been taken, start a new course the next day.

How should I take this medication?

- Before you start taking Yaz, be sure to read the directions. Take Yaz once a day at the same time every day until the pack is empty. When you finish a pack, start the next pack on the day after your last white "reminder" pill. Do not wait any days between packs. If you are switching from another birth control pill, start Yaz on the same day that a new pack of the previous pills should have been started.

- For the first cycle of a *Sunday Start* regimen, use another method of birth control (such as condoms or spermicide) as a back-up method if you have sex anytime from the Sunday you start your first pack until you have been taking the pills for 7 days. You will not need to use a back-up method of birth control for the first cycle of a Day 1 regimen, since you are starting the pill at the beginning of your period.

What should I avoid while taking this medication?

Do not smoke or become pregnant while you are taking Yaz. Do not skip pills, even if you are spotting or bleeding between monthly periods, feel sick to your stomach (nausea), or if you do not have sex very often.

What are possible food and drug interactions associated with this medication?

If Yaz is taken with certain other drugs, the effects of either could be increased, decreased, or altered. It is especially important to check with your doctor before combining Yaz with the following: acetaminophen; antibiotics; blood pressure/heart medications known as angiotensin-converting enzyme (ACE) inhibitors (such as

captopril, enalapril, or lisinopril) or angiotensin-II receptor antagonists (such as losartan, valsartan, or irbesartan); bosentan; griseofulvin; heparin; nonsteroidal anti-inflammatory drugs (NSAIDs)
(such as ibuprofen and naproxen) when taken long-term and daily;
potassium-sparing diuretics (water pills) (such as spironolactone);
potassium supplements; rifampin; seizure medications (such as
carbamazepine, felbamate, phenobarbital, topiramate, or phenytoin); St. John's wort; or vitamin C.

What are the possible side effects of this medication?
Please see general statement regarding side effects on page xiii.

Side effects may include: abdominal cramps and bloating, absence of a period, allergic reactions, blotchy darkening of the
skin (especially on your face), breakthrough bleeding or spotting,
breast tenderness, change in your appetite, change in your vision
or inability to wear your contact lenses, depression, dizziness,
gallbladder disease, headache, high blood pressure, irregular
vaginal bleeding, nausea, nervousness, vomiting, water retention
causing swelling of the fingers or ankles, or weight change

Can I receive this medication if I am pregnant or breastfeeding?
Do not take Yaz if you are pregnant or breastfeeding. Tell your doctor immediately if you are pregnant, plan to become pregnant, or
are breastfeeding.

What should I do if I miss a dose of this medication?
If you miss one pink "active" pill, take it as soon as you remember.
Take the next pill at your regular time. This means you can take two
pills in one day. You do not need a back-up birth control method if
you have sex.

If you miss two or more pills, consult the patient information that
accompanied your prescription or call your pharmacist for advice.

How should I store this medication?
Store at room temperature.

Zanaflex
Generic name: Tizanidine HCl

What is this medication?
Zanaflex is a medicine used to manage muscle spasms that interfere with daily activities. Zanaflex is available as capsules and
tablets.

What is the most important information I should know about this medication?
- Zanaflex can cause low blood pressure, especially if you take
  blood pressure lowering medicines. Tell your doctor if you feel
  lightheaded or dizzy while you are taking Zanaflex.
- Zanaflex can cause liver damage. Tell your doctor if you experience nausea, vomiting, loss of appetite, or yellowing of your
  skin or whites of your eyes.
- Zanaflex can cause drowsiness or hallucinations. Do not drive
  or operate machinery until you know how Zanaflex affects you.
- Do not stop taking Zanaflex without first talking to your doctor.
  Stopping Zanaflex suddenly can cause withdrawal symptoms,
  including muscle rigidity, anxiety, and shaking. These symptoms can occur with a sudden rise in your blood pressure and
  heart rate.

Who should not take this medication?
Do not take Zanaflex if you are allergic to it or any of its ingredients.

Also, do not take Zanaflex in combination with fluvoxamine or
ciprofloxacin.

What should I tell my doctor before I take the first dose of this medication?
Tell your doctor about all prescription, over-the-counter, and herbal
medications you are taking before beginning treatment with Zanaflex. Also, talk to your doctor about your complete medical history,
especially if you have liver or kidney disease, heart problems, or
are pregnant, plan to become pregnant, or are breastfeeding.

What is the usual dosage?
Please see general statement regarding dosage on page xii.

Adults: The recommended starting dose is 4 milligrams every 6-8 hours as needed. Do not take more than 3 doses in 24 hours. Your doctor will increase your dose as needed, until the desired effect is achieved.

If you have kidney impairment, your doctor will adjust your dose appropriately.

How should I take this medication?
• Take Zanaflex exactly as prescribed by your doctor. Food can affect the amount of Zanaflex absorbed by your body. Talk to your doctor about the best way for you to take Zanaflex.

What should I avoid while taking this medication?
Do not drive or operate machinery until you know how Zanaflex affects you.

Do not change your dose or stop taking Zanaflex without first talking to your doctor.

What are possible food and drug interactions associated with this medication?
If Zanaflex is taken with certain other drugs, the effects of either could be increased, decreased, or altered. It is especially important to check with your doctor before combing Zanaflex with the following: acetaminophen, acyclovir, alcohol, baclofen, benzodiazepines (such as alprazolam or lorazepam), birth control pills, certain antibiotics (such as ciprofloxacin or levofloxacin), cimetidine, famotidine, fluvoxamine, heart medications (such as amiodarone, mexiletine, propafenone, or verapamil), ticlopidine, or zileuton.

What are the possible side effects of this medication?
Please see general statement regarding side effects on page xiii.

Side effects may include: dizziness, drowsiness, dry mouth, fatigue, sedation, tiredness, weakness

---

Can I receive this medication if I am pregnant or breastfeeding?

The effects of Zanaflex during pregnancy and breastfeeding are unknown. Tell your doctor immediately if you are pregnant, plan to become pregnant, or are breastfeeding.

What should I do if I miss a dose of this medication?

Zanaflex should be taken only as needed.

How should I store this medication?

Store at room temperature.

Zantac

Generic name: Ranitidine HCl

What is this medication?

Zantac is a medicine that reduces the amount of acid in your stomach. It is used to treat stomach and duodenal ulcers (ulcer in the upper intestine), gastroesophageal reflux disease (GERD), and erosive esophagitis (inflammation of the esophagus [tube that connects your mouth and stomach] due to excess acid). Zantac is also used to prevent a relapse of esophagitis or stomach or duodenal ulcers and for treatment of conditions where your stomach makes too much acid, such as Zollinger-Ellison syndrome. Zantac is available as tablets, syrup, or effervescent tablets called Zantac 25 EFFERdose.

What is the most important information I should know about this medication?

- Zantac can cause a sudden attack of porphyria (a blood disorder that interferes with how your body produces heme, which is the oxygen-carrying component of your red blood cells). Tell your doctor if you have ever had this condition.
- If you have a condition known as phenylketonuria (an inability to process phenylalanine, a protein in your body), be aware that Zantac 25 EFFERdose tablets contain phenylalanine.

Who should not take this medication?

Do not take Zantac if you are allergic to it or any of its ingredients.

What should I tell my doctor before I take the first dose of this medication?

Tell your doctor about all prescription, over-the-counter, and herbal medications you are taking before beginning treatment with Zantac. Also, talk to your doctor about your complete medical history, especially if you have kidney or liver problems, phenylketonuria, or a history of porphyria. Tell your doctor if you are pregnant, plan to become pregnant, or are breastfeeding.

What is the usual dosage?

Please see general statement regarding dosage on page xii.

Treatment of Stomach Ulcer, Duodenal Ulcer, and GERD

Adults: The recommended dose is 150 milligrams (mg) or 10 milliliters (mL) of syrup (2 teaspoonfuls) twice a day.

Children 1 month-16 years: Your doctor will prescribe the appropriate dose for your child, based on their weight.

Maintenance of a Healed Stomach and Duodenal Ulcer

Adults: The recommended dose is 150 mg or 10 mL of syrup (2 teaspoonfuls) at bedtime.

Children 1 month-16 years: Your doctor will prescribe the appropriate dose for your child, based on their weight.

Erosive Esophagitis

Adults: The recommended dose is 150 mg or 10 mL of syrup (2 teaspoonfuls) four times a day.

Children 1 month-16 years: Your doctor will prescribe the appropriate dose for your child, based on their weight.

Maintenance of a Healed Erosive Esophagitis

Adults: The recommended dose is 150 mg or 10 mL of syrup (2 teaspoonfuls) twice a day.

Treatment of Excess Stomach Acid (Such as Zollinger-Ellison Syndrome)

Adults: The recommended dose is 150 mg or 10 mL of syrup (2 teaspoonfuls) twice a day. Your doctor may increase your dose as needed.

If you have kidney impairment, your doctor will adjust your dose appropriately.

How should I take this medication?
- Take Zantac exactly as prescribed by your doctor.
- You can continue to take antacids for pain relief while you are taking Zantac.
- To prepare Zantac 25 EFFERdose tablets, dissolve 1 tablet in no less than 5 mL (1 teaspoonful) of water in an appropriate measuring cup. Wait until the tablet is completely dissolved before giving the solution to your child. If your child is an infant, use a medicine dropper or oral syringe to give him/her the medicine.

What should I avoid while taking this medication?
Do not chew, swallow whole, or dissolve Zantac 25 EFFERdose tablets on your or your child's tongue.

What are possible food and drug interactions associated with this medication?
If Zantac is taken with certain other drugs, the effects of either could be increased, decreased, or altered. It is especially important to check with your doctor before combining Zantac with the following: atazanavir, delavirdine, gefitinib, glipizide, ketoconazole, midazolam, procainamide, triazolam, or warfarin.

What are the possible side effects of this medication?
Please see general statement regarding side effects on page xiii.

Side effects may include: allergic reaction, blurred vision, changes in blood counts, changes in heart rate, confusion, constipation, diarrhea, headache, impotence, joint and muscle pain, loss of libido, rash, tiredness, weakness

---

Can I receive this medication if I am pregnant or breastfeeding?

The effects of Zantac during pregnancy are unknown. Zantac can be found in your breast milk if you take it while breastfeeding. Tell your doctor immediately if you are pregnant, plan to become pregnant, or are breastfeeding.

What should I do if I miss a dose of this medication?

If you miss a dose of Zantac, take it as soon as you remember. However, if it is almost time for your next dose, skip the one you missed and return to your regular dosing schedule. Do not take two doses at once.

How should I store this medication?

Store at room temperature. Zantac syrup and Zantac 25 EFFERdose tablets can also be stored in the refrigerator.

Protect Zantac tablets from light.

Zebeta

Generic name: Bisoprolol Fumarate

What is this medication?

Zebeta is a medicine known as a beta-blocker, which is used to treat high blood pressure alone or in combination with other blood pressure lowering medicines.

What is the most important information I should know about this medication?

- Do not stop taking Zebeta without talking to your doctor. Stopping this medication suddenly can cause harmful effects. Your doctor should gradually reduce your dose when stopping treatment with this medication.
- Zebeta can worsen heart failure, cause breathing problems, or hide symptoms of low blood sugar levels if you have diabetes. Tell your doctor if you experience trouble breathing while you are taking Zebeta. If you have diabetes, monitor your blood sugar frequently, especially when you first start taking Zebeta.

Who should not take this medication?

Do not take Zebeta if you are allergic to it or any of its ingredients. In addition, do not take Zebeta if you have a slow heart rate, heart failure, heart block, or severe blood circulation disorders.

What should I tell my doctor before I take the first dose of this medication?

Tell your doctor about all prescription, over-the-counter, and herbal medications you are taking before beginning treatment with Zebeta. Also, talk to your doctor about your complete medical history, especially if you have allergies; heart problems or heart failure; a history of heart attack; breathing problems (such as asthma); diabetes; liver, kidney, or thyroid problems; peripheral vascular disease (disease of the blood vessels outside the heart and brain); or are planning to have a major surgery.

Tell your doctor if you have a history of severe allergic reactions to any allergens, because Zebeta may decrease the effectiveness of epinephrine used to treat the reaction.

What is the usual dosage?

Please see general statement regarding dosage on page xii.

Adults: The usual starting dose is 5 milligrams once a day. Your doctor will increase your dose as needed until the desired effect is achieved.

If you have liver or kidney impairment, your doctor will adjust your dose appropriately.

How should I take this medication?

• Take Zebeta exactly as prescribed by your doctor.

What should I avoid while taking this medication?

Do not drive a car, operate machinery, or engage in other tasks requiring alertness until you know how Zebeta affects you.

Do not stop taking Zebeta without first talking to your doctor.

What are possible food and drug interactions associated with this medication?

If Zebeta is taken with certain other drugs, the effects of either could be increased, decreased, or altered. It is especially important to check with your doctor before combining Zebeta with the following: blood pressure/heart medications known as calcium channel blockers (such as diltiazem or verapamil), clonidine, diabetes medicines (such as insulin), digoxin, disopyramide, guanethidine, other beta-blockers (such as metoprolol), reserpine, or rifampin.

What are the possible side effects of this medication?

Please see general statement regarding side effects on page xiii.

> **Side effects may include:** cough, dizziness, headache, runny and stuffy nose, swelling of your arms and legs, upper respiratory infection

Can I receive this medication if I am pregnant or breastfeeding?

The effects of Zebeta during pregnancy and breastfeeding are unknown. Tell your doctor immediately if you are pregnant, plan to become pregnant, or are breastfeeding.

What should I do if I miss a dose of this medication?

If you miss a dose of Zebeta, take it as soon as you remember. However, if it is almost time for your next dose, skip the one you missed and return to your regular dosing schedule. Do not take two doses at once.

How should I store this medication?

Store at room temperature. Protect from moisture.

Zestril

Generic name: Lisinopril

What is this medication?

Zestril is a medicine known as an angiotensin-converting enzyme (ACE) inhibitor. Zestril is used alone or in combination with other medications to treat high blood pressure or heart failure. Also, it is used after a heart attack to improve survival in some people.

What is the most important information I should know about this medication?

- Zestril can cause a rare but serious allergic reaction leading to extreme swelling of your face, lips, tongue, throat, or gut (causing severe abdominal pain). You may have an increased risk of experiencing these symptoms if you have ever had an allergy to ACE inhibitor-type medicines or if you are African American. If you experience any of these symptoms, seek emergency medical attention immediately.
- Tell your doctor if you experience lightheadedness, especially during the first few weeks of Zestril therapy. If you faint, stop taking Zestril and tell your doctor immediately.
- Vomiting, diarrhea, fever, exercise, hot weather, drinking alcohol, excessive perspiration, and dehydration may lead to an excessive fall in your blood pressure. Tell your doctor if you experience any of these.
- Zestril may decrease your blood neutrophil (type of blood cells that fight infections) levels, especially if you have a collagen vascular disease (such as lupus [disease that affects the immune system]) or kidney disease.
- Promptly report any signs of infection (such as sore throat or fever) to your doctor.
- Zestril may not work as well in African Americans, who may also have a higher risk of side effects. Contact your doctor if your symptoms do not improve or if they become worse.

Who should not take this medication?

Do not take Zestril if you are allergic to it or any of its ingredients.

Do not take Zestril if you have a history of angioedema (a condition involving swelling of the face, extremities, eyes, lips, and tongue) related to previous treatment with similar medicines. Also, do not take Zestril if you have a history of certain types of angioedema (such as hereditary or idiopathic).

What should I tell my doctor before I take the first dose of this medication?

Tell your doctor about all prescription, over-the-counter, and herbal medications you are taking before beginning treatment with Zestril. Also, talk to your doctor about your complete medical history, especially if you have liver problems, kidney disease, or diabetes. Tell your doctor if you have bone marrow problems or any blood disease, any disease that affects the immune system (such as lupus or scleroderma), collagen vascular disease, narrowing or hardening of the arteries of your brain or heart, chest pain, or if you have ever had an allergy or sensitivity to ACE inhibitors such as Zestril.

What is the usual dosage?
Please see general statement regarding dosage on page xii.

High Blood Pressure
Adults: The usual starting dosage is 10 milligrams (mg) once a day. Your doctor will adjust your dose based on your previous blood pressure medication and will increase your dose as needed until the desired effect is achieved.

Children ≥6 years: Your doctor will prescribe the appropriate dose for your child, based on their weight.

Heart Failure
Adults: The usual starting dose is 5 mg once a day. Your doctor may give you a higher dose depending on your needs.

Heart Attack
Adults: The usual starting dose is 5 mg, then increased to 10 mg once a day for 6 weeks. Your doctor will prescribe the appropriate dose for you based on your condition.

If you have kidney impairment, your doctor will adjust your dose appropriately.

How should I take this medication?
- Take Zestril at the same time every day. Continue to take Zestril even if you feel well.
- Do not take extra doses or take more often without asking your doctor.

What should I avoid while taking this medication?
Do not become pregnant or breastfeed while you are taking Zestril.

Do not drive or operate heavy machinery until you know how Zestril affects you.

Do not take salt substitutes or supplements containing potassium without consulting your doctor.

Do not stand or sit up quickly when you take Zestril, especially in the morning. Sit or lie down at the first sign of dizziness, lightheadedness, or fainting.

What are possible food and drug interactions associated with this medication?
If Zestril is taken with certain other drugs, the effects of either could be increased, decreased, or altered. It is especially important to check with your doctor before combining Zestril with the following: amiloride, dextran, diuretics (water pills) (such as furosemide, hydrochlorothiazide, spironolactone, or triamterene), lithium, nonsteroidal anti-inflammatory drugs (such as ibuprofen or naproxen), potassium supplements, or salt substitutes containing potassium.

What are the possible side effects of this medication?
Please see general statement regarding side effects on page xiii.

Side effects may include: cough, diarrhea, dizziness, fatigue, headache, low blood pressure, upper respiratory infection

---

Can I receive this medication if I am pregnant or breastfeeding?

Do not take Zestril if you are pregnant or breastfeeding. Zestril can harm your unborn baby. Tell your doctor immediately if you are pregnant, plan to become pregnant, or are breastfeeding.

What should I do if I miss a dose of this medication?

If you miss a dose of Zestril, take it as soon as you remember. However, if it is almost time for your next dose, skip the one you missed and return to your regular dosing schedule. Do not take two doses at once.

How should I store this medication?

Store at room temperature.

Zetia

Generic name: Ezetimibe

What is this medication?

Zetia is a medicine used to lower your cholesterol when a low-fat diet is not enough. Zetia is used alone or in combination with other cholesterol-lowering medicines known as "statins" (such as atorvastatin or rosuvastatin) or fenofibrate to lower your total cholesterol and the "bad" low-density lipoprotein (LDL) cholesterol.

What is the most important information I should know about this medication?

- Taking Zetia is not a substitute for following a healthy low-fat and low-cholesterol diet and exercising to lower your cholesterol.
- Zetia can cause serious muscle conditions or liver problems. Your risk can increase if you are also taking statins. Tell your doctor right away if you experience unexplained muscle pain, weakness, or tenderness. Your doctor will monitor your liver function.
- Zetia can cause serious allergic reactions. Tell your doctor right away if you experience swelling of your face, lips, tongue, or throat; difficulty breathing or swallowing; rash; or hives.

Who should not take this medication?
Do not take Zetia if you are allergic to it or any of its ingredients.

Do not take Zetia with a statin if you currently have liver disease or if you are pregnant, plan to become pregnant, or are breastfeeding.

What should I tell my doctor before I take the first dose of this medication?
Tell your doctor about all prescription, over-the-counter, and herbal medications you are taking before beginning treatment with Zetia. Also, talk to your doctor about your complete medical history, especially if you have allergies, liver problems, or muscle aches or weakness. Tell your doctor if you are pregnant, plan to become pregnant, or are breastfeeding.

What is the usual dosage?
Please see general statement regarding dosage on page xii.

> ***Adults and children ≥10 years:*** The recommended dose is 10 milligrams once a day.

If you are taking other medications, your doctor will adjust your dose appropriately.

How should I take this medication?
- Your doctor will likely start you on a low-cholesterol diet before prescribing Zetia. Stay on this diet while you are taking Zetia.
- Take Zetia at the same time every day, with or without food.

What should I avoid while taking this medication?
Do not stop taking Zetia without first talking to your doctor, even if you feel well.

What are possible food and drug interactions associated with this medication?
If Zetia is taken with certain other drugs, the effects of either could be increased, decreased, or altered. It is especially important to check with your doctor before combining Zetia with the following: blood thinners (such as warfarin), cholesterol-lowering medicines

known as fibrates (such as gemfibrozil), cholestyramine, or cyclosporine.

What are the possible side effects of this medication?
Please see general statement regarding side effects on page xiii.

> **Side effects may include:** diarrhea, feeling tired, joint pain

Can I receive this medication if I am pregnant or breastfeeding?
The effects of Zetia alone during pregnancy and breastfeeding are unknown. However, do not take Zetia with a statin if you are pregnant or breastfeeding. Tell your doctor immediately if you are pregnant, plan to become pregnant, or are breastfeeding.

What should I do if I miss a dose of this medication?
If you miss a dose of Zetia, take it as soon as you remember. However, if it is almost time for your next dose, skip the one you missed and return to your regular dosing schedule. Do not take two doses at once.

How should I store this medication?
Store at room temperature. Protect from moisture.

Ziac
Generic name: Bisoprolol Fumarate/Hydrochlorothiazide

What is this medication?
Ziac is a combination medicine used to treat high blood pressure. Ziac contains two medicines: bisoprolol (a beta-blocker) and hydrochlorothiazide (a diuretic [water pill]).

What is the most important information I should know about this medication?
- Do not stop taking Ziac without talking to your doctor. Stopping this medication suddenly can cause harmful effects. Your

doctor should gradually reduce your dose when stopping treatment with this medication.

- Ziac can worsen heart failure, cause breathing problems, or hide symptoms of low blood sugar levels if you have diabetes. Tell your doctor if you experience trouble breathing while you are taking Ziac. If you have diabetes, monitor your blood sugar frequently, especially when you first start taking Ziac.
- Ziac can cause temporary problems to see objects farther away or glaucoma (high pressure in the eye). Symptoms of these include changes in your vision or eye pain.
- Ziac can cause imbalances in fluids and electrolytes (chemicals that are important for the cells in your body to function, such as sodium and potassium). Signs and symptoms of this include dry mouth, thirst, weakness, fatigue, drowsiness, restlessness, muscle pains or cramps, low blood pressure, decreased urination, fast heart rate, nausea, or vomiting. Your doctor will monitor your blood electrolyte levels periodically during treatment with Ziac.

Who should not take this medication?

Do not take Ziac if you are allergic to it or any of its ingredients. In addition, do not take Ziac if you have a slow heart rate, heart failure, heart block, inability to produce urine, or severe blood circulation disorders.

What should I tell my doctor before I take the first dose of this medication?

Tell your doctor about all prescription, over-the-counter, and herbal medications you are taking before beginning treatment with Ziac. Also, talk to your doctor about your complete medical history, especially if you have allergies; heart problems or heart failure; a history of heart attack; breathing problems (such as asthma); diabetes; liver, kidney, or thyroid problems; peripheral vascular disease (disease of the blood vessels outside the heart and brain); asthma; lupus (disease that affects the immune system); or are planning to have a major surgery.

Tell your doctor if you have a history of severe allergic reactions to any allergens, because Ziac may decrease the effectiveness of epinephrine used to treat the reaction.

What is the usual dosage?

Please see general statement regarding dosage on page xii.

Adults: The usual starting dose is 2.5/6.25 (2.5 milligrams [mg] of bisoprolol and 6.25 mg of hydrochlorothiazide) once a day. Your doctor will increase your dose as needed until the desired effect is achieved.

If you have liver or kidney impairment, your doctor will adjust your dose appropriately.

How should I take this medication?

• Take Ziac exactly as prescribed by your doctor.

What should I avoid while taking this medication?

Do not drive a car, operate machinery, or engage in other tasks requiring alertness until you know how Ziac affects you.

Do not stop taking Ziac without first talking to your doctor.

What are possible food and drug interactions associated with this medication?

If Ziac is taken with certain other drugs, the effects of either could be increased, decreased, or altered. It is especially important to check with your doctor before combining Ziac with the following: alcohol, barbiturates (such as phenobarbital), blood pressure medications known as calcium channel blockers (such as diltiazem or verapamil), cholestyramine, clonidine, colestipol, diabetes medicines (such as insulin), digoxin, disopyramide, guanethidine, lithium, narcotic painkillers (such as morphine or oxycodone), nonsteroidal anti-inflammatory drugs (such as ibuprofen or naproxen), norepinephrine, reserpine, rifampin, or steroids (such as prednisone).

What are the possible side effects of this medication?
Please see general statement regarding side effects on page xiii.

> **Side effects may include:** diarrhea, dizziness, fatigue, headache, sensitivity to sunlight

Can I receive this medication if I am pregnant or breastfeeding?
The effects of Ziac during pregnancy are unknown. Ziac can be found in your breast milk if you take it while breastfeeding. Do not take Ziac if you are breastfeeding. Tell your doctor immediately if you are pregnant, plan to become pregnant, or are breastfeeding.

What should I do if I miss a dose of this medication?
If you miss a dose of Ziac, take it as soon as you remember. However, if it is almost time for your next dose, skip the one you missed and return to your regular dosing schedule. Do not take two doses at once.

How should I store this medication?
Store at room temperature.

Ziprasidone HCl: see Geodon, page 417

Zithromax
Generic name: Azithromycin

What is this medication?
Zithromax is an antibiotic used in adults to treat infections of the urethra and cervix, skin, and infections associated with chronic obstructive pulmonary disease (COPD) (narrowing of the lungs that makes it hard to breath). Zithromax is also used to treat adults with genital ulcer disease, as well as prevent and treat *Mycobacterium avium complex* (MAC) (a number of bacterial infections that are usually associated with HIV infections). In addition, Zithromax is

used in adults and children to treat certain types of pneumonia and infections of the throat/tonsils and sinuses. It is also used to treat ear infections in children. Zithromax is available as tablets, an oral suspension, and 1-gram single dose packets.

What is the most important information I should know about this medication?

- Zithromax only works against bacteria; it does not work against viruses like the common cold.
- Diarrhea is a common problem caused by antibiotics, and usually ends when the antibiotic is stopped. Sometimes after starting treatment with antibiotics, people may develop watery and bloody stools (with or without stomach cramps and fever) even as late as two or more months after having taken the last dose of the antibiotic. Contact your doctor immediately if this occurs.
- Not taking the complete dose of Zithromax may decrease the effectiveness of the treatment and may increase the possibility that bacteria will develop resistance and will not be treatable by Zithromax or other antibiotics in the future.
- Zithromax may cause serious allergic reactions or serious skin reactions. Get emergency help if you or your child has hives, a skin rash, mouth sores, skin blistering or peeling, trouble swallowing, wheezing, trouble breathing, or swelling of the face, eyes, lips, tongue or throat.
- Zithromax can cause liver impairment. Tell your doctor if you experience loss of appetite, right upper abdominal discomfort, dark urine, or yellowing of your skin or whites of your eyes.
- Tell your doctor if you or your child feel an abnormal heartbeat, dizziness, or feel faint. This has been seen with other antibiotics similar to Zithromax.
- Zithromax can cause or worsen myasthenia gravis (a disease characterized by long-lasting fatigue and muscle weakness). Tell your doctor if you have this condition.

Who should not take this medication?

Do not take Zithromax if you are allergic to it, any of its ingredients, or antibiotics such as erythromycin or telithromycin. Also, do not take Zithromax if you have a history of jaundice (yellowing of your skin or whites of your eyes) or liver impairment associated with previous treatment with azithromycin.

What should I tell my doctor before I take the first dose of this medication?

Tell your doctor about all prescription, over-the-counter, and herbal medications you are taking before beginning treatment with Zithromax. Also, talk to your doctor about your complete medical history, especially if you have liver problems, long QT syndrome (very fast or abnormal heart beats), low blood potassium or magnesium levels, very low heart rate, or myasthenia gravis, are pregnant, plan to become pregnant, or are breastfeeding. Tell your doctor if you are taking medications to treat arrhythmias (irregular heartbeats) (such as amiodarone, dofetilide, procainamide, quinidine, or sotalol).

What is the usual dosage?
Please see general statement regarding dosage on page xii.

Infection of the Urethra and Cervix
Adults: The recommended dose is a single 1-gram (g) or 2-g dose. Your doctor will prescribe the appropriate dose for you based on your condition.

Genital Ulcer Disease
Adults: The recommended dose is a single 1-g dose.

Prevention of MAC Infection
Adults: The recommended dose is 1200 milligrams (mg) once a week.

Treatment of MAC Infection
Adults: The recommended dose is 600 mg once a day.

Skin Infection
Adults: The recommended dose is 500 mg as a single dose on Day 1, followed by 250 mg once a day for 4 days.

Infection Associated with COPD
Adults: The recommended dose is 500 mg once a day for 3 days or 500 mg as a single dose on Day 1, followed by 250 mg once a day for 4 days.

Community-Acquired Pneumonia and Infection of the Throat/Tonsils
Adults: The recommended dose is 500 mg as a single dose on Day 1, followed by 250 mg once a day for 4 days.

Children ≥6 months (pneumonia): Your doctor will prescribe the appropriate dose for your child, based on their weight.

Children ≥2 years (throat/tonsils): Your doctor will prescribe the appropriate dose for your child, based on their weight.

Sinus Infection
Adults: The recommended dose is 500 mg once a day for 3 days.

Children ≥6 months: Your doctor will prescribe the appropriate dose for your child, based on their weight.

Ear Infection
Children ≥6 months: Your doctor will prescribe the appropriate dose for your child, based on their weight.

How should I take this medication?
- Take Zithromax exactly as prescribed by your doctor. Take it with or without food.
- To prepare the 1-gram single dose packet, empty the entire contents of the packet in 2 ounces (about 60 milliliters [mL]) of water and mix thoroughly. Drink the entire mixture immediately. Add another 2 ounces of water, mix, and drink to be sure you took all the medicine. This packet is not for use in children.
- If you receive Zithromax oral suspension in liquid form, it is ready to take. Shake the oral suspension well before you take it or give it to your child. Use it within 10 days. If you receive Zithromax as dry powder, your pharmacist will tell you how to prepare the medicine.

What should I avoid while taking this medication?

Do not use the 1-gram single dose packets to treat infections in children.

Do not take antacids that contain aluminum and magnesium with Zithromax.

What are possible food and drug interactions associated with this medication?

If Zithromax is taken with certain other drugs, the effects of either could be increased, decreased, or altered. It is especially important to check with your doctor before combining Zithromax with the following: antacids containing aluminum or magnesium, blood thinners (such as warfarin), carbamazepine, cyclosporine, digoxin, ergotamine or dihydroergotamine, hexobarbital, nelfinavir, phenytoin, terfenadine, theophylline, or triazolam.

What are the possible side effects of this medication?

Please see general statement regarding side effects on page xiii.

Side effects may include: diarrhea or loose stools, nausea, stomach pain

Can I receive this medication if I am pregnant or breastfeeding?

The effects of Zithromax during pregnancy and breastfeeding are unknown. Tell your doctor immediately if you are pregnant, plan to become pregnant, or are breastfeeding.

What should I do if I miss a dose of this medication?

If you miss a dose of Zithromax, take it as soon as you remember. However, if it is almost time for your next dose, skip the one you missed and return to your regular dosing schedule. Do not take two doses at once.

Zithromax may require only a single dose. If you forget to take your dose, take it as soon as you remember.

How should I store this medication?
Store at room temperature.

Zocor
Generic name: Simvastatin

What is this medication?
Zocor belongs to a class of medicines called "statins", which are used to lower your cholesterol when a low-fat diet is not enough. Zocor lowers your total cholesterol and the "bad" low-density lipoprotein (LDL) cholesterol, thereby helping to lower your risk of a heart attack or stroke, death from coronary heart disease (narrowing of small blood vessels that supply blood and oxygen to the heart), or the need for procedures to restore the blood flow back to the heart or to another part of the body.

What is the most important information I should know about this medication?
- Taking Zocor is not a substitute for following a healthy low-fat and low-cholesterol diet and exercising to lower your cholesterol.
- Do not take Zocor if you are pregnant, think you may be pregnant, if you are planning to become pregnant, or if you are breastfeeding.
- Zocor can cause muscle pain, tenderness, weakness, fatigue, loss of appetite, right upper abdominal discomfort, dark urine, or yellowing of your skin or whites of your eyes. Call your doctor right away if you notice any of these symptoms.

Who should not take this medication?
Do not take Zocor if you are allergic to it or any of its ingredients, or if you currently have liver disease. Also, do not take Zocor in combination with anti-HIV medications (such as indinavir), boceprevir, clarithromycin, cyclosporine, danazol, erythromycin, gemfibrozil, itraconazole, ketoconazole, nefazodone, posaconazole, telaprevir, or telithromycin.

Do not take Zocor if you are pregnant, plan to become pregnant, or are breastfeeding.

What should I tell my doctor before I take the first dose of this medication?

Tell your doctor about all prescription, over-the-counter, and herbal medications you are taking before beginning treatment with Zocor. Also, talk to your doctor about your complete medical history, especially if you drink excessive amounts of alcohol or you have liver, kidney, or heart problems; muscle aches or weakness; diabetes; or thyroid problems. Tell your doctor if you are pregnant, plan to become pregnant, or are breastfeeding.

What is the usual dosage?

Please see general statement regarding dosage on page xii.

Adults: The usual starting dose is 10-20 milligrams (mg) once a day in the evening. Your doctor will check your blood cholesterol levels during treatment with Zocor and will change your dose based on the results.

Adolescents 10-17 years: The usual starting dose is 10 mg once a day in the evening. Your doctor will check your blood cholesterol levels during treatment with Zocor and will change your dose based on the results.

If you have kidney impairment or you are taking other medications, your doctor will adjust your dose appropriately.

How should I take this medication?

• Your doctor will likely start you on a low-cholesterol diet before giving you Zocor. Stay on this diet while you are taking Zocor.

What should I avoid while taking this medication?

Do not drink large amounts of grapefruit juice (>1 quart a day) while you are taking Zocor.

What are possible food and drug interactions associated with this medication?

If Zocor is taken with certain other drugs, the effects of either could be increased, decreased, or altered. It is especially important to check with your doctor before combining Zocor with the following: alcohol, amiodarone, blood pressure medications known as calcium channel blockers (such as amlodipine, diltiazem, or verapamil), blood thinners (such as warfarin), cholesterol-lowering medicines known as fibrates (such as fenofibrate), colchicine, digoxin, grapefruit juice, nelfinavir, niacin, ranolazine, or voriconazole.

What are the possible side effects of this medication?

Please see general statement regarding side effects on page xiii.

> **Side effects may include:** abdominal pain, constipation, headache, nausea, upper respiratory infections

Can I receive this medication if I am pregnant or breastfeeding?

Do not take Zocor during pregnancy or breastfeeding. Tell your doctor immediately if you are pregnant, plan to become pregnant, or are breastfeeding.

What should I do if I miss a dose of this medication?

If you miss a dose of Zocor, take it as soon as you remember. However, if it is almost time for your next dose, skip the one you missed and return to your regular dosing schedule. Do not take two doses at once.

How should I store this medication?

Store at room temperature.

Zofran
Generic name: Ondansetron HCl

What is this medication?
Zofran is a medicine used to prevent nausea or vomiting in patients who are receiving chemotherapy or radiation. Zofran is also used to prevent nausea and vomiting after surgery. Zofran is administered intravenously (through a vein in your arm) and it is also available as a tablet or oral solution.

What is the most important information I should know about this medication?
- Taking Zofran after you have had abdominal surgery, or to prevent nausea or vomiting from chemotherapy, may hide the signs and symptoms of stomach distension (bloating). It may also hide signs and symptoms of a disorder of the intestines known as progressive ileus (obstruction of the intestines).
- Zofran may cause irregular heartbeats or rhythms. Tell your doctor immediately if you experience a change in your heart rate, feel lightheaded, or if you have a fainting episode.
- If you have phenylketonuria (an inability to process phenylalanine, a protein in your body), it is important to know that Zofran ODT (orally disintegrating tablets) contains phenylalanine.

Who should not take this medication?
Do not take Zofran if you are allergic to it, any of its ingredients or any other similar medications known as 5HT-3 antagonists.

Do not take Zofran if you are taking apomorphine.

What should I tell my doctor before I take the first dose of this medication?
Tell your doctor about all prescription, over-the-counter, and herbal medications you are taking before beginning treatment with Zofran. Also, talk to your doctor about your complete medical history, especially if you have heart, stomach, intestinal, or liver problems.

Tell your doctor if you have phenylketonuria.

What is the usual dosage?
Please see general statement regarding dosage on page xii.

Injection
Adults and children ≥1 month: Your doctor will administer this medicine to you or your child intravenously.

Tablets and Oral Solution
Adults and children ≥4 years: Your doctor will prescribe the appropriate dose for you or your child based on the condition.

How should I take this medication?
- Take Zofran exactly as prescribed by your doctor.
- Your doctor will administer Zofran injection to you.
- Zofran ODT should not be pushed through the foil wrapping. With dry hands, carefully peel back the foil. Place the tablet on the tip of the tongue, where it will dissolve, then swallow. Do not remove the foil packaging until it is time to take the medication.

What should I avoid while taking this medication?
Do not take more Zofran than prescribed by your doctor.

Do not miss any scheduled follow-up appointments with your doctor.

What are possible food and drug interactions associated with this medication?
If Zofran is used with certain other drugs, the effects of either could be increased, decreased, or altered. It is especially important to check with your doctor before combining Zofran with the following: apomorphine, carbamazepine, phenytoin, rifampicin, or tramadol.

What are the possible side effects of this medication?
Please see general statement regarding side effects on page xiii.

Side effects may include: constipation, diarrhea, drowsiness, headache, itching, fever

---

Can I receive this medication if I am pregnant or breastfeeding?
The effects of Zofran during pregnancy and breastfeeding are unknown. Tell your doctor immediately if you are pregnant, plan to become pregnant, or are breastfeeding.

What should I do if I miss a dose of this medication?
Zofran should be given under special circumstances determined by your doctor. If you miss your scheduled dose, contact your doctor for advice.

How should I store this medication?
Store oral solution, ODT, and tablets at room temperature and protect from light. Your doctor will store Zofran injection.

Zoloft
Generic name: Sertraline HCl

What is this medication?
Zoloft is an antidepressant medication known as a selective serotonin reuptake inhibitor (SSRI). It is used to treat major depressive disorder, obsessive compulsive disorder, panic disorder, post-traumatic stress disorder, premenstrual dysphoric disorder, and social anxiety disorder. Zoloft is available in tablets and an oral solution.

What is the most important information I should know about this medication?
- Zoloft can increase the risk of suicidal thoughts and behavior in children, adolescents, and young adults. Your doctor will monitor you closely for clinical worsening, suicidal or unusual behavior after you start taking Zoloft or start a new dose of Zoloft. Tell your doctor immediately if you experience anxiety, hostility, sleeplessness, restlessness, impulsive or dangerous behavior, or thoughts about suicide or dying; or if you have new symptoms or seem to be feeling worse.
- Zoloft can cause serotonin syndrome (a potentially life-threatening drug reaction that causes the body to have too much

serotonin, a chemical produced by the nerve cells) or neuroleptic malignant syndrome (a brain disorder) when you take it alone or in combination with other medicines. You can experience mental status changes, an increase in your heart rate and temperature, lack of coordination, overactive reflexes, muscle rigidity, nausea, vomiting, or diarrhea. Tell your doctor immediately if you experience any of these signs or symptoms.

- Zoloft can cause severe allergic reactions. Stop taking this medication and tell your doctor immediately if you develop a rash, trouble breathing, or swelling of your face, tongue, eyes, or mouth.
- Your risk of abnormal bleeding or bruising can increase if you take Zoloft, especially if you also take blood thinners (such as warfarin), nonsteroidal anti-inflammatory drugs (NSAIDs) (such as ibuprofen or naproxen), or aspirin.
- You can experience manic episodes while you are taking Zoloft. Tell your doctor if you experience greatly increased energy, severe trouble sleeping, racing thoughts, reckless behavior, unusually grand ideas, excessive happiness or irritability, or talking more or faster than usual.
- Zoloft can cause seizures or changes in your appetite or weight. Your doctor will monitor you for these effects during treatment.
- Zoloft can decrease your blood sodium levels, especially if you are elderly. Tell your doctor if you have a headache, weakness, an unsteady feeling, confusion, problems concentrating or thinking, or memory problems while you are taking Zoloft.
- Do not stop taking Zoloft without first talking to your doctor. Stopping Zoloft suddenly can cause serious symptoms, including anxiety, irritability, high or low mood, feeling restless, changes in your sleep habits, headache, sweating, nausea, dizziness, electric shock-like sensations, shaking, or confusion.

Who should not take this medication?
Do not take Zoloft if you are allergic to it or any of its ingredients.

Do not take Zoloft while you are taking other medicines known as monoamine oxidase inhibitors (MAOIs) (such as phenelzine), a class of medications used to treat depression and other conditions. In addition, do not take Zoloft if you are taking pimozide.

Do not take the liquid form of Zoloft while you are taking disulfiram.

What should I tell my doctor before I take the first dose of this medication?

Tell your doctor about all prescription, over-the-counter, and herbal medication you are taking before beginning treatment with Zoloft. Also, talk to your doctor about your complete medical history, especially if you have high blood pressure; heart, liver, or kidney problems; history of stroke; glaucoma; bleeding problems; seizures; mania or bipolar disorder; or low sodium levels in your blood. Also, tell your doctor if you are pregnant, plan to become pregnant, or are breastfeeding.

What is the usual dosage?

Please see general statement regarding dosage on page xii.

Major Depressive Disorder and Premenstrual Dysphoric Disorder

Adults: The usual starting dose is 50 milligrams (mg) once a day.

Obsessive-Compulsive Disorder

Adults and children 13-17 years: The usual starting dose is 50 mg once a day.

Children 6-12 years: The usual starting dose is 25 mg once a day.

Panic Disorder, Post-Traumatic Stress Disorder, and Social Anxiety Disorder

Adults: The usual starting dose is 25 mg once a day.

Your doctor will increase your dose as needed until the desired effect is achieved.

If you have liver impairment, your doctor will adjust your dose appropriately.

How should I take this medication?

- Take Zoloft exactly as prescribed by your doctor. Take Zoloft once a day, in the morning or in the evening. Take it with or without food.
- To prepare Zoloft solution, use the dropper provided to remove the amount prescribed by your doctor and mix it with 4 ounces (1/2 cup) of water, ginger ale, lemon-lime soda, lemonade, or orange juice. Do not mix it with anything other than these liquids. Take the dose immediately; do not prepare the mix for later use.

What should I avoid while taking this medication?

Do not drive, operate heavy machinery, or do other dangerous activities until you know how Zoloft affects you.

Do not drink alcohol while you are taking Zoloft.

Do not stop taking Zoloft suddenly without first talking to your doctor, as this can cause serious side effects.

Do not take Zoloft and MAOIs together or within 14 days of each other. Combining these medicines with Zoloft can cause serious and even life-threatening reactions.

What are possible food and drug interactions associated with this medication?

If Zoloft is taken with certain other drugs, the effects of either could be increased, decreased, or altered. Zoloft may interact with numerous medications. Therefore, it is very important that you tell your doctor about any other medications you are taking.

What are the possible side effects of this medication?

Please see general statement regarding side effects on page xiii.

> **Side effects may include:** abnormal ejaculation, agitation, decreased sexual desire, diarrhea, feeling tired or fatigued, increased sleepiness, indigestion, loss of appetite, nausea, shaking, sweating, trouble sleeping

Can I receive this medication if I am pregnant or breastfeeding?

The effects of Zoloft during pregnancy and breastfeeding are unknown. Tell your doctor immediately if you are pregnant, plan to become pregnant, or are breastfeeding.

What should I do if I miss a dose of this medication?

If you miss a dose of Zoloft, take it as soon as you remember. However, if it is almost time for your next dose, skip the one you missed and return to your regular dosing schedule. Do not take two doses at once.

How should I store this medication?

Store at room temperature.

Zolpidem Tartrate: *see Ambien, page 64*

Zolpidem Tartrate: *see Intermezzo, page 473*

Zostavax

Generic name: Zoster Vaccine Live

What is this medication?

Zostavax is a vaccine that is used for adults to prevent shingles (painful rash caused by chickenpox virus).

What is the most important information I should know about this medication?

- Zostavax may not protect everyone who receives the vaccine and it cannot be used to treat shingles once you have it. If you do get shingles, see your doctor within the first few days of getting the rash.

Who should not take this medication?

You should not receive Zostavax if you are allergic to it or any of its ingredients; have a disease or condition that causes a weakened immune system, such as an immune deficiency, leukemia, lymphoma, or HIV/AIDS; or are taking high doses of steroids by injection or by mouth. Also, pregnant women should not receive Zostavax.

What should I tell my doctor before I take the first dose of this medication?

Tell your doctor about all prescription, over-the-counter, and herbal medications you are taking before beginning treatment with Zostavax. Also, talk to your doctor about your complete medical history, especially if you have had shingles, are currently exposed to chickenpox, have tuberculosis (a bacterial infection that affects the lungs), are pregnant, plan to become pregnant, or are breastfeeding.

What is the usual dosage?

Please see general statement regarding dosage on page xii.

Adults ≥50 years: Your doctor will prescribe the appropriate dose for you.

How should I take this medication?

- Zostavax is given as an injection, directly under the skin, by your doctor.

What should I avoid while taking this medication?

Avoid becoming pregnant for 3 months following administration of Zostavax.

What are possible food and drug interactions associated with this medication?

No significant interactions have been reported with Zostavax at this time. However, always tell your doctor about any medicines you take, including over-the-counter drugs, vitamins, and herbal supplements.

What are the possible side effects of this medication?

Please see general statement regarding side effects on page xiii.

> **Side effects may include:** bruising, itching, pain, redness, swelling, or warmth at the injection site; headache

Can I receive this medication if I am pregnant or breastfeeding?

The effects of Zostavax during pregnancy and breastfeeding are unknown. Tell your doctor immediately if you are pregnant, plan to become pregnant, or are breastfeeding.

What should I do if I miss a dose of this medication?

If you miss your scheduled appointment, contact your doctor.

How should I store this medication?

This medication will be stored by your doctor.

Zoster Vaccine Live: *see Zostavax, page 1152*

Zovirax Cream

Generic name: Acyclovir

What is this medication?

Zovirax Cream is a topical cream (applied directly on the skin) used to treat herpes labialis (cold sores) that occur on your face or lips.

What is the most important information I should know about this medication?

- Zovirax Cream is not a cure for cold sores.
- Zovirax Cream is for external use only. Do not use it in your eyes, inside your mouth or nose, or on your genitals.
- Zovirax Cream can cause irritation or allergic reactions when it is applied. Tell your doctor immediately if this occurs.

Who should not take this medication?

Do not use Zovirax Cream if you are allergic to it or any of its ingredients, or to valacyclovir.

What should I tell my doctor before I take the first dose of this medication?

Tell your doctor about all prescription, over-the-counter, and herbal medications you are taking before beginning treatment with Zovirax Cream. Also, talk to your doctor about your complete medical history, especially if you have a weak immune system (become sick very easily).

What is the usual dosage?

Please see general statement regarding dosage on page xii.

Adults and children ≥12 years: Apply a layer of the cream to the affected area(s) 5 times a day for 4 days.

How should I take this medication?

• Apply Zovirax Cream exactly as prescribed by your doctor. Begin using Zovirax Cream early, at the first sign of a cold sore (such as tingle, redness, bump, or itch) for best results. Wash your hands before and after using Zovirax Cream. Clean and dry the skin before applying it. Apply a layer of cream to cover only the cold sore or the area of tingling (or other symptoms) before the cold sore appears.

What should I avoid while taking this medication?

Do not use Zovirax Cream in your eyes, inside your mouth or nose, on your genitals, or on unaffected skin.

Do not cover the cold sore area with a bandage or dressing unless otherwise instructed by your doctor.

Do not use other skin products (such as cosmetics, sunscreen, or lip balm) or skin medicines on the cold sore area while you are using Zovirax Cream unless otherwise instructed by your doctor.

Do not bathe, shower, or swim immediately after applying Zovirax Cream.

What are possible food and drug interactions associated with this medication?

No significant interactions have been reported with Zovirax Cream at this time. However, always tell your doctor about any medicines you take, including over-the-counter medications, vitamins, and herbal supplements.

What are the possible side effects of this medication?

Please see general statement regarding side effects on page xiii.

Side effects may include: burning or stinging feeling; dry or cracked lips; dryness, flakiness, or itching of your skin

Can I receive this medication if I am pregnant or breastfeeding?

The effects of Zovirax Cream during pregnancy and breastfeeding are unknown. Tell your doctor immediately if you are pregnant, plan to become pregnant, or are breastfeeding.

What should I do if I miss a dose of this medication?

If you miss a dose of Zovirax Cream, apply it as soon as you remember. However, if it is almost time for your next dose, skip the one you missed and return to your regular dosing schedule. Do not apply two doses at once.

How should I store this medication?

Store at room temperature. Do not leave Zovirax Cream in your car in cold or hot weather. Tightly close the tube with the cap.

Zovirax Ointment

Generic name: Acyclovir

What is this medication?

Zovirax Ointment is a topical ointment (applied directly on the skin) used for the management of genital herpes and in herpes simplex virus infections in people with a weak immune system (become sick very easily).

What is the most important information I should know about this medication?

- Zovirax Ointment does not reduce your risk of passing the infection to others. Also, Zovirax Ointment does not prevent recurrent herpes simplex virus infections when applied in the absence of signs and symptoms.
- Zovirax Ointment is for external use only. Do not use it in your eyes.

Who should not take this medication?

Do not use Zovirax Ointment if you are allergic to it or any of its ingredients, or to valacyclovir.

What should I tell my doctor before I take the first dose of this medication?

Tell your doctor about all prescription, over-the-counter, and herbal medications you are taking before beginning treatment with Zovirax Ointment. Also, talk to your doctor about your complete medical history, especially if you have a weak immune system.

What is the usual dosage?

Please see general statement regarding dosage on page xii.

Adults: Apply a sufficient quantity of the ointment to adequately cover all lesions every 3 hours, 6 times a day for 7 days.

How should I take this medication?

- Apply Zovirax Ointment exactly as prescribed by your doctor. Begin using Zovirax Ointment as early as possible following onset of signs and symptoms. Use a finger cot or rubber glove when applying Zovirax Ointment to prevent transmission to other body sites and transmission of the infection to other persons.

What should I avoid while taking this medication?

Do not use Zovirax Ointment in your eyes.

Do not exceed the dose, frequency of applications, and length of treatment prescribed by your doctor.

What are possible food and drug interactions associated with this medication?

No significant interactions have been reported with Zovirax Ointment at this time. However, always tell your doctor about any medicines you take, including over-the-counter medications, vitamins, and herbal supplements.

What are the possible side effects of this medication?

Please see general statement regarding side effects on page xiii.

> **Side effects may include:** burning or stinging feeling, itching of your skin, mild pain, rash, swelling

Can I receive this medication if I am pregnant or breastfeeding?

The effects of Zovirax Ointment during pregnancy and breastfeeding are unknown. Tell your doctor immediately if you are pregnant, plan to become pregnant, or are breastfeeding.

What should I do if I miss a dose of this medication?

If you miss a dose of Zovirax Ointment, apply it as soon as you remember. However, if it is almost time for your next dose, skip the one you missed and return to your regular dosing schedule. Do not apply two doses at once.

How should I store this medication?

Store at room temperature in a dry place.

Zyloprim

Generic name: Allopurinol

What is this medication?

Zyloprim is a medicine used to treat the signs and symptoms of gout (severe and painful inflammation of the joints). Zyloprim is also used to manage elevated uric acid levels caused by certain cancer therapy for leukemia, lymphoma, and other cancers. In addition, Zyloprim is used to treat recurrent kidney stones in people with elevated uric acid levels.

What is the most important information I should know about this medication?

- Zyloprim can cause serious allergic reactions. Tell your doctor right away if you develop a skin rash, painful urination, blood in your urine, eye irritation, or swelling of your lips or mouth.
- Zyloprim can cause an increase in the frequency of gout attacks when you first start taking the medicine. If this happens, continue taking Zyloprim since the medicine does not take effect for about 2-6 weeks.
- Zyloprim can cause liver damage. Tell your doctor if you experience a loss in appetite, weight loss, or itching. If you have liver disease, your doctor will perform periodic liver function tests early during Zyloprim treatment.
- Drink adequate amounts of fluid while you are taking Zyloprim to prevent kidney stones.
- Zyloprim can cause bone marrow suppression (a decrease in the production of blood cells).

Who should not take this medication?

Do not take Zyloprim if you are allergic to it or any of its ingredients.

What should I tell my doctor before I take the first dose of this medication?

Tell your doctor about all prescription, over-the-counter, and herbal medications you are taking before beginning treatment with Zyloprim. Also, talk to your doctor about your complete medical history, especially if you have kidney or liver problems, heart disease, or are pregnant, plan to become pregnant, or are breastfeeding.

What is the usual dosage?

Please see general statement regarding dosage on page xii.

Gout

Adults: The recommended starting dose is 100 milligrams (mg) once a day.

Increased Uric Acid Due to Cancer

Adults: The recommended dose is 600-800 mg a day for 2 or 3 days.

Children 6-10 years: The recommended dose is 300 mg a day.

Children <6 years: The recommended dose is 150 mg a day.

Recurrent Kidney Stones

Adults: The recommended dose is 200-300 mg a day in divided doses or as a single dose.

Your doctor will adjust your dose as needed, until the desired effect is achieved.

If you have kidney impairment, your doctor will adjust your dose appropriately.

How should I take this medication?

- Take Zyloprim exactly as prescribed by your doctor. If Zyloprim upsets your stomach, take it after a meal.

What should I avoid while taking this medication?

Do not miss your scheduled follow-up appointments with your doctor.

Do not drive or operate machinery until you know how Zyloprim affects you.

What are possible food and drug interactions associated with this medication?

If Zyloprim is taken with certain other drugs, the effects of either could be increased, decreased, or altered. It is especially important to check with your doctor before combing Zyloprim with the following: amoxicillin, ampicillin, azathioprine, chlorpropamide, cyclophosphamide, cyclosporine, dicumarol, diuretics (water pills) (such as chlorthalidone or hydrochlorothiazide), mercaptopurine, or sulfinpyrazone.

What are the possible side effects of this medication?

Please see general statement regarding side effects on page xiii.

> **Side effects may include:** diarrhea, liver problems, nausea, rash, sudden gout attacks

Can I receive this medication if I am pregnant or breastfeeding?

The effects of Zyloprim during pregnancy are unknown. Zyloprim can be found in your breast milk if you take it while breastfeeding. Tell your doctor immediately if you are pregnant, plan to become pregnant, or are breastfeeding.

What should I do if I miss a dose of this medication?

If you miss a dose of Zyloprim, take it as soon as you remember. However, if it is almost time for your next dose, skip the one you missed and return to your regular dosing schedule. Do not take two doses at once.

How should I store this medication?

Store at room temperature in a dry place. Protect from light.

Zyprexa
Generic name: Olanzapine

What is this medication?
Zyprexa is a medicine used to treat schizophrenia. This medication can also be used to treat manic or depressive episodes associated with bipolar disorder alone or in combination with lithium or valproate. Also, Zyprexa is used to treat episodes of depression that have not improved after taking two other medicines. Zyprexa is available in tablets or tablets that dissolve in your mouth called Zyprexa Zydis.

What is the most important information I should know about this medication?
- Zyprexa can be life-threatening when used in elderly people with mental problems caused by dementia (an illness involving loss of memory, judgment, and confusion). Zyprexa is not approved to treat mental problems caused by dementia.
- Zyprexa can increase the risk of suicidal thoughts and behavior in children, adolescents, and young adults. Your doctor will monitor you closely for clinical worsening, suicidality, or unusual behavior after you start taking Zyprexa or a new dose. Tell your doctor right away if you experience anxiety, hostility, sleeplessness, restlessness, impulsive or dangerous behavior, or thoughts about suicide or dying; or if you have new symptoms or seem to be feeling worse.
- In rare cases, Zyprexa can cause neuroleptic malignant syndrome (NMS) (a life-threatening brain disorder). NMS is a medical emergency, get medical help right away. Tell your doctor right away if you experience high fever, muscle rigidity, confusion, fast or irregular heartbeat, changes in your blood pressure, or increased sweating.
- Zyprexa can cause tardive dyskinesia (abnormal muscle movements, including tremor, shuffling and uncontrolled, involuntary movements). Tell your doctor if you experience uncontrollable muscle movements.
- Zyprexa can cause an increase in your blood sugar levels or diabetes. Tell your doctor if you experience excessive thirst, an increase in urination, an increase in appetite, or weakness.

If you have diabetes or are at risk for diabetes, monitor your blood sugar regularly, as determined by your doctor. Also, you can experience an increase in your blood cholesterol levels or weight gain while you are taking Zyprexa. Monitor your weight regularly.

- Zyprexa can cause sudden decrease in your blood pressure with dizziness, rapid heartbeat, and faintness. Zyprexa can also cause seizures, problems with your body temperature regulation, difficulty swallowing, or impairment of your judgment, thinking, or motor skills.
- Zyprexa can also cause hyperprolactinemia (an increase in a hormone called prolactin, which can affect lactation, menstruation, and fertility). Tell your doctor right away if you experience missed menstrual periods, leakage of milk from your breasts, development of the breasts in men, or problems with erections.
- Zyprexa can lower the ability of your body to fight infections. Tell your doctor if you notice any signs of infection such as fever, sore throat, rash, or chills.

Who should not take this medication?
Do not take Zyprexa if you are allergic to it or any of its ingredients.

Zyprexa is not approved to treat mental problems caused by dementia in the elderly.

What should I tell my doctor before I take the first dose of this medication?
Tell your doctor about all prescription, over-the-counter, and herbal medications you are taking before beginning treatment with Zyprexa. Also, talk to your doctor about your complete medical history, especially if you have heart, liver, or thyroid problems; seizures; diabetes; high cholesterol; high or low blood pressure; strokes; Alzheimer's disease; glaucoma (high pressure in the eye); enlarged prostate in men; bowel obstruction; breast cancer; or are pregnant, plan to become pregnant, or are breastfeeding.

What is the usual dosage?
Please see general statement regarding dosage on page xii.

Schizophrenia
Adults: The recommended starting dose is 5-10 milligrams (mg) once a day. Your doctor will increase your dose as needed, until the desired effect is achieved.

Adolescents 13-17 years: The recommended starting dose is 2.5-5 mg once a day. Your doctor will increase your dose as needed, until the desired effect is achieved.

Bipolar Disorder (Manic)
Adults: The recommended starting dose is 10-15 mg once a day. Your doctor will increase your dose as needed, until the desired effect is achieved.

Adolescents 13-17 years: The recommended starting dose is 2.5-5 mg once a day. Your doctor will increase your dose as needed, until the desired effect is achieved.

Depression
Adults: The recommended starting dose is 5 mg given in combination with 20 mg of fluoxetine. Your doctor will increase your dose as needed, until the desired effect is achieved.

How should I take this medication?
- Take Zyprexa exactly as prescribed by your doctor. Do not take extra doses or take more often without asking your doctor.
- Take Zyprexa tablets once a day. You can take Zyprexa with or without food.
- Zyprexa Zydis comes as a tablet that should be placed under your tongue and left to dissolve completely. Immediately after opening the blister packet, remove the tablet and place it in your mouth. Use dry hands when handling the tablet. The tablet will dissolve quickly in your saliva so you can easily swallow it with or without liquids.
- If you feel you need to stop Zyprexa, talk to your doctor first.

What should I avoid while taking this medication?
Do not drink alcohol while you are taking Zyprexa.

Do not drive or operate machinery until you know how Zyprexa affects you.

Do not expose yourself to extreme heat or dehydration while you are taking Zyprexa.

What are possible food and drug interactions associated with this medication?

If Zyprexa is taken with certain other drugs, the effects of either could be increased, decreased, or altered. It is especially important to check with your doctor before combining Zyprexa with the following: alcohol, blood pressure medications, carbamazepine, diazepam, fluvoxamine, levodopa, lorazepam, omeprazole, or rifampin.

What are the possible side effects of this medication?

Please see general statement regarding side effects on page xiii.

Side effects may include: changes in your behavior, difficulty swallowing, dizziness, dry mouth, feeling very hot or thirsty, headache, hard or infrequent stools, impaired judgment, increased appetite, infections, lack of energy, restlessness, sleepiness, strokes, tremor, upset stomach, weight gain

---

Can I receive this medication if I am pregnant or breastfeeding?

The effects of Zyprexa during pregnancy are unknown. Zyprexa can be found in your breast milk if you take it while breastfeeding. Do not breastfeed while you are taking Zyprexa. Tell your doctor immediately if you are pregnant, plan to become pregnant, or are breastfeeding.

What should I do if I miss a dose of this medication?

If you miss a dose of Zyprexa, take it as soon as you remember. However, if it is almost time for your next dose, skip the one you missed and return to your regular dosing schedule. Do not take two doses at once.

How should I store this medication?
Store at room temperature.

Zytiga
Generic name: Abiraterone Acetate

What is this medication?
Zytiga is a medicine used to treat men with castration-resistant prostate cancer (prostate cancer that is resistant to medical or surgical treatments that lower testosterone) that has spread to other parts of the body and who have received treatment with docetaxel. Zytiga is used in combination with prednisone.

What is the most important information I should know about this medication?
- Zytiga can cause serious side effects, including high blood pressure, low blood potassium levels, or fluid retention. Tell your doctor if you experience dizziness, fast heartbeats, feel faint or lightheaded, headache, confusion, muscle weakness, pain in your legs, or swelling in your legs or feet.
- Zytiga can cause adrenal problems if you get an infection or are under stress, or if you stop taking prednisone.
- Zytiga can cause liver problems. Your doctor will order blood tests to check your liver function before treatment and during treatment.
- Men who are sexually active with a pregnant woman must use a condom during and for one week after treatment with Zytiga. If your sexual partner becomes pregnant, you should use a condom and another form of birth control during and for one week after treatment with Zytiga. Talk with your doctor if you have questions about birth control.

Who should not take this medication?
Zytiga is not for use in women. Zytiga may harm your unborn baby. Women who are pregnant or who may become pregnant should not touch Zytiga without protection, such as gloves.

What should I tell my doctor before I take the first dose of this medication?

Tell your doctor about all prescription, over-the-counter, and herbal medications you are taking before beginning treatment with Zytiga. Also, talk to your doctor about your complete medical history, especially if you have heart problems, a history of adrenal and/or pituitary problems, or liver problems.

What is the usual dosage?

Please see general statement regarding dosage on page xii.

Adults: The usual dose is 1000 milligrams (4 tablets) once a day.

If you have liver impairment, your doctor will adjust your dose appropriately.

How should I take this medication?

- Take Zytiga exactly as prescribed by your doctor.
- Take Zytiga on an empty stomach. Do not take Zytiga with food. If you take Zytiga with food, more of the medication can be absorbed by your body than is needed and this can cause side effects. Do not eat 2 hours before and 1 hour after you take Zytiga.
- Swallow Zytiga tablets whole, and take it with water. Do not crush or chew tablets.

What should I avoid while taking this medication?

Do not take Zytiga with food.

What are possible food and drug interactions associated with this medication?

If Zytiga is taken with certain other drugs, the effects of either could be increased, decreased, or altered. It is especially important to check with your doctor before combining Zytiga with the following: atazanavir, carbamazepine, clarithromycin, indinavir, itraconazole, ketoconazole, nefazodone, nelfinavir, phenobarbital, phenytoin, rifabutin, rifampin, rifapentine, ritonavir, saquinavir, telithromycin, thioridazine, or voriconazole.

What are the possible side effects of this medication?
Please see general statement regarding side effects on page xiii.

Side effects may include: bone fractures, cold-like symptoms, cough, diarrhea, heartburn, hot flushes, irregular heartbeats, joint swelling or pain, muscle aches, need to get up at night to urinate, urinary tract infection, urinating more often than normal

Can I receive this medication if I am pregnant or breastfeeding?
Zytiga is not for use in women.

What should I do if I miss a dose of this medication?
If you miss a dose of Zytiga or prednisone, take your prescribed dose the following day. If you miss more than 1 dose, tell your doctor immediately.

How should I store this medication?
Store at room temperature.

Poison Control Centers

The American Association of Poison Control Centers (AAPCC) uses a single, nationwide emergency number to automatically link callers with their regional poison center. This toll-free number, 800-222-1222, also works for teletype lines (TTY) for the hearing-impaired and telecommunication devices (TDD) for individuals who are deaf. However, a few local poison centers and the ASPCA/Animal Poison Control Center are not part of this nationwide system and continue to use separate numbers.

Most of the centers listed below are accredited by the AAPCC. Certified centers are marked by an asterisk after the name. Each has to meet certain criteria. It must, for example, serve a large geographic area; it must be open 24 hours a day and provide direct-dial or toll-free access; it must be supervised by a medical director; and it must have registered pharmacists or nurses available to answer questions from the public.

Within each state, centers are listed alphabetically by city. Some state poison centers also list their original emergency numbers (including TDD/TTY) that only work within that state. For these listings, callers may use either the state number or the nationwide 800 number.

ALABAMA

BIRMINGHAM

Regional Poison Control Center (*)
Children's Hospital of Alabama

1600 7th Ave South
Birmingham AL 35233-1711
Business: 205-939-9201
Emergency: 800-222-1222
www.chsys.org

TUSCALOOSA

Alabama Poison Center (*)

2503 Phoenix Dr
Tuscaloosa AL 35405
Business: 205-345-0600
Emergency: 800-222-1222
                   800-462-0800 (AL)
www.alapoisoncenter.org

ALASKA

JUNEAU

Alaska Poison Control System
Section of Injury Prevention and EMS

410 Willoughby Ave – Room 109
Box 110616
Juneau AK 99811-0616
Business: 907-465-3027
Emergency: 800-222-1222
www.chems.alaska.gov

(PORTLAND, OR)

Oregon Poison Center (*)
Oregon Health and Science University

3181 SW Sam Jackson Park Rd –
Suite CB550
Portland OR 97239
Business: 503-494-8600
Emergency: 800-222-1222
www.ohsu.edu/poison

(Continued)

ARIZONA

PHOENIX

Banner Poison Control Center (*)
Banner Good Samaritan Medical Center

901 E Willetta St
Phoenix AZ 85006
Business: 602-495-6360
Emergency: 800-222-1222
                   800-362-0101 (AZ)
                   800-253-3334 (AZ)
www.bannerpoisoncontrol.com

TUCSON

Arizona Poison and Drug Information Center (*)
Arizona Health Sciences Center

1501 N Campbell Ave – Room 1156
Tucson AZ 85724
Business: 520-626-7899
Emergency: 800-222-1222
www.pharmacy.arizona.edu/outreach/
poison

ARKANSAS

LITTLE ROCK

Arkansas Poison and Drug Information Center (*)
College of Pharmacy – UAMS

4301 W Markham St – MS 522-2
Little Rock AR 72205
Business: 501-686-5540
Emergency: 800-222-1222
                   800-376-4766
(AR)
TDD/TTY: 800-641-3805
www.uams.edu/cop/

ASPCA/Animal Poison Control Center

1717 S Philo Rd – Suite 36
Urbana IL 61802
Business: 217-337-5030
Emergency: 888-426-4435
                   800-548-2423
www.aspcapro.org/
animal-poison-control.php

CALIFORNIA

FRESNO/MADERA

California Poison Control System
Fresno/Madera Division (*)
Children's Hospital Central California

9300 Valley Children's Place – MB 15
Madera CA 93636
Business: 559-622-2300
Emergency: 800-222-1222
                   800-876-4766 (CA)
TDD/TTY: 800-972-3323
www.calpoison.org

SACRAMENTO

California Poison Control System
Sacramento Division (*)
UC Davis Medical Center

2315 Stockton Blvd –
Room HSF 1024
Sacramento CA 95817
Business: 916-227-1400
Emergency: 800-222-1222
                   800-876-4766 (CA)
TDD/TTY: 800-972-3323
www.calpoison.org

SAN DIEGO

California Poison Control System
San Diego Division (*)
UC San Diego Medical Center

200 W Arbor Dr
San Diego CA 92103-8925
Business: 858-715-6300
Emergency: 800-222-1222
           800-876-4766 (CA)
TDD/TTY: 800-972-3323
www.calpoison.org

SAN FRANCISCO

California Poison Control System
San Francisco Division (*)

UCSF Box 1369
San Francisco CA 94143
Business: 415-502-6000
Emergency: 800-222-1222
           800-876-4766 (CA)
TDD/TTY: 800-972-3323
www.calpoison.org

COLORADO

DENVER

Rocky Mountain Poison and Drug
Center (*)

777 Bannock St – MC 0180
Denver CO 80204-4507
Business: 303-389-1100
Emergency: 800-222-1222
TDD/TTY: 303-739-1127
(CO)
www.rmpdc.org

CONNECTICUT

FARMINGTON

Connecticut Poison Control Center (*)
University of Connecticut Health
Center

263 Farmington Ave
Farmington CT 06030-5365
Business: 860-679-4540
Emergency: 800-222-1222
TDD/TTY: 866-218-5372
http://poisoncontrol.uchc.edu

DELAWARE

(PHILADELPHIA, PA)

The Poison Control Center (*)
Children's Hospital of Philadelphia

34th St & Civic Center Blvd
Philadelphia PA 19104-4399
Business: 215-590-2003
Emergency: 800-222-1222
           800-722-7112 (DE)
TDD/TTY: 215-590-8789
www.chop.edu/service/
poison-control-center/home.html

DISTRICT OF COLUMBIA

WASHINGTON, DC

National Capital Poison Center (*)

3201 New Mexico Ave NW
Suite 310
Washington DC 20016
Business: 202-362-3867
Emergency: 800-222-1222
www.poison.org

(Continued)

FLORIDA

JACKSONVILLE

Florida Poison Information Center-Jacksonville (*)
SHANDS Hospital

655 W 8th St
Jacksonville FL 32209
Business: 904-244-4465
Emergency: 800-222-1222
http://fpicjax.org

MIAMI

Florida/USVI Poison Information Center-Miami (*)
University of Miami, Department of Pediatrics

PO Box 016960 (R-131)
Miami FL 33101
Business: 305-585-5250
Emergency: 800-222-1222
www.med.miami.edu/poisoncontrol

TAMPA

Florida Poison Information Center-Tampa (*)
Tampa Division

PO Box 1289
Tampa FL 33601-1289
Business: 813-844-7044
Emergency: 800-222-1222
www.poisoncentertampa.org

GEORGIA

ATLANTA

Georgia Poison Center (*)
Hughes Spalding Children's Hospital
Grady Health System

80 Jesse Hill Jr. Dr SE
PO Box 26066
Atlanta GA 30303
Business: 404-616-9237
Emergency: 800-222-1222
                       404-616-9000
(Atlanta)
TDD: 404-616-9287
www.georgiapoisoncenter.org

HAWAII

(DENVER, CO)

Rocky Mountain Poison and Drug Center (*)

777 Bannock St – MC 0180
Denver CO 80204-4507
Business: 303-389-1100
Emergency: 800-222-1222
www.rmpdc.org

IDAHO

(DENVER, CO)

Rocky Mountain Poison and Drug Center (*)

777 Bannock St – MC 0180
Denver CO 80204-4507
Business: 303-739-1100
Emergency: 800-222-1222
www.rmpdc.org

ILLINOIS

CHICAGO

Illinois Poison Center (*)

222 S Riverside Plaza – Suite 1900
Chicago IL 60606
Business:　　　　312-906-6136
Emergency:　　800-222-1222
TDD/TTY:　　　　312-906-6185
www.illinoispoisoncenter.org/

INDIANA

INDIANAPOLIS

Indiana Poison Center (*)
Clarian Health Partners Methodist Hospital

I-65 at 21st Street
Indianapolis, IN 46206-1367
Business:　　　　317-962-2335
Emergency:　　800-222-1222
　　　　　　　　800-382-9097 (IN)
317-962-2323 (Indianapolis)
www.clarian.org/poisoncontrol

IOWA

SIOUX CITY

Iowa Statewide Poison Control Center (*)
Iowa Health System and the University of Iowa Hospitals and Clinics

2910 Hamilton Blvd – Suite 101
Sioux City IA 51101
Business:　　　　712-279-3710
Emergency:　　800-222-1222
　　　　　　　　712-277-2222 (IA)
www.iowapoison.org

KANSAS

KANSAS CITY

Mid-America Poison Control
University of Kansas Medical Center

3901 Rainbow Blvd
Room B-400
Kansas City KS 66160-7231
Business:　　　　913-588-6638
Emergency:　　800-222-1222
　　　　　　　　800-332-6633 (KS)
TDD:　　　　　　913-588-6639
www.kumed.com/poison

KENTUCKY

LOUISVILLE

Kentucky Regional Poison Center (*)

PO Box 35070
Louisville KY 40232-5070
Business:　　　　502-629-7264
Emergency:　　800-222-1222
　　　　　　　　502-589-8222
　　　　　　　　(Louisville)
www.krpc.com

LOUISIANA

MONROE

Louisiana Drug and Poison
Information Center (*)
University of Louisiana at Monroe

700 University Ave
Monroe LA 71209-6430
Business:　　　　318-342-3648
Emergency:　　800-222-1222
www.ulm.edu

(Continued)

MAINE

PORTLAND

Northern New England Poison Center (*)

Maine Medical Center
22 Bramhall St
Portland ME 04102
Business: 207-662-7220
Emergency: 800-222-1222
TDD/TTY   877-299-4447
(ME)
www.nnepc.org

MARYLAND

BALTIMORE

Maryland Poison Center (*)
University of Maryland at Baltimore
School of Pharmacy

20 North Pine St, PH 772
Baltimore MD 21201
Business: 410-706-7604
Emergency: 800-222-1222
TDD: 410-706-1858
www.mdpoison.com

(WASHINGTON, DC)

National Capital Poison Center (*)
3201 New Mexico Ave NW
Suite 310
Washington DC 20016
Business: 202-362-3867
Emergency: 800-222-1222
www.poison.org

MASSACHUSETTS

BOSTON

**Regional Center for Poison Control
and Prevention (*)
(Serving Massachusetts and Rhode
Island)**

300 Longwood Ave
Boston MA 02115
Business: 617-355-6609
Emergency: 800-222-1222
TDD/TTY   888-244-5313
www.maripoisoncenter.com

MICHIGAN

DETROIT

Regional Poison Control Center (*)
Children's Hospital of Michigan

4160 John R Harper Professional Office Bldg – Suite 616
Detroit MI 48201
Business: 313-745-5335
Emergency: 800-222-1222
                 313-745-5711
[Detroit]
www.mitoxic.org/pcc

MINNESOTA

MINNEAPOLIS

Minnesota Poison Control System (*)
Hennepin County Medical Center

701 Park Avenue, Mail Code RL
Minneapolis, MN 55415
Business: 612-873-3144
Emergency: 800-222-1222
www.mnpoison.org

MISSISSIPPI

JACKSON

Mississippi Regional Poison Control Center
University of Mississippi Medical Center

2500 N State St
Jackson MS 39216
Business: 601-984-1680
Emergency: 800-222-1222
http://poisoncontrol.umc.edu

MISSOURI

ST. LOUIS

Missouri Regional Poison Center (*)
Cardinal Glennon Children's Medical Center

1465 S Grand Blvd
St Louis MO 63104-1095
Business: 314-577-5610
Emergency: 800-222-1222
www.cardinalglennon.com

MONTANA

(DENVER, CO)

Rocky Mountain Poison and Drug Center (*)

777 Bannock St – MC 0180
Denver CO 80204-4507
Business: 303-389-1100
Emergency: 800-222-1222
www.rmpdc.org

NEBRASKA

OMAHA

The Poison Center (*)
Children's Hospital

8200 Dodge St
Omaha NE 68114
Business: 402-390-5555
Emergency: 800-222-1222
www.nebraskapoison.com

NEVADA

(DENVER, CO)

Rocky Mountain Poison and Drug Center (*)

777 Bannock St – MC 0180
Denver CO 80204-4507
Business: 303-389-1100
Emergency: 800-222-1222
www.rmpdc.org

(PORTLAND, OR)

Oregon Poison Center (*)
Oregon Health Sciences University

33181 SW Sam Jackson Park Rd
Portland OR 97201
Business: 503-494-8600
Emergency: 800-222-1222
www.ohsu.edu/poison

NEW HAMPSHIRE

(PORTLAND, ME)

Northern New England Poison Center (*)

22 Bramhall St
Portland ME 04102
Business: 207-662-7220
Emergency: 800-222-1222
www.nnepc.org

NEW JERSEY

NEWARK

New Jersey Poison Information and Education System (*)
UMDNJ

65 Bergen St
Newark NJ 07101
Business: 973-972-9280
Emergency: 800-222-1222
TDD/TTY: 973-926-8008
www.njpies.org

(Continued)

NEW MEXICO

ALBUQUERQUE

New Mexico Poison and Drug Information Center (*)

1 University of New Mexico
Albuquerque NM 87131-0001
Business: 505-272-4261
Emergency: 800-222-1222
http://hsc.unm.edu/pharmacy/poison

NEW YORK

MINEOLA

Long Island Regional Poison and Drug Information Center (*)
Winthrop University Hospital

259 First St
Mineola NY 11501
Business: 516-663-2650
Emergency: 800-222-1222
TDD: 516-747-3323
(Nassau)

                        516-924-8811
(Suffolk)
www.winthrop.org

NEW YORK CITY

New York City Poison Control Center (*)
NYC Bureau of Public Health

455 1st Ave – Room 123
New York NY 10016
Business: 212-447-8152
English
Emergency: 800-222-1222
                        212-340-4494
                        212-POISONS
                        (212-764-7667)
Spanish
Emergency: 212-venenos
                        (212-836-3667)
www.nyc.gov/html/doh/html/poison/
poison.shtml

ROCHESTER

Fingerlakes Regional Poison and Drug Information Center (*)
University of Rochester Medical Center

601 Elmwood Ave
Box 321
Rochester NY 14642
Business: 585-273-4155
Emergency: 800-222-1222
TTY: 585-273-3854
www.fingerlakespoison.org

SYRACUSE

Upstate New York Poison Center (*)
SUNY Upstate Medical University

750 E Adams St
Syracuse NY 13210
Business: 315-464-7078
Emergency: 800-222-1222
TTY: 315-464-5424
www.upstate.edu/poison/contactus

NORTH CAROLINA

CHARLOTTE

Carolinas Poison Center (*)
Carolinas Medical Center

PO Box 32861
Charlotte NC 28232
Business: 704-395-3795
Emergency: 800-222-1222
TDD: 800-735-8262
TYY: 800-735-2962
www.ncpoisoncenter.org

NORTH DAKOTA

(MINNEAPOLIS, MN)

Minnesota Poison Control System (*)
Hennepin County Medical Center

701 Park Avenue, Mail Code RL
Minneapolis, MN 55415
Business: 612-873-3144
Emergency: 800-222-1222
www.mnpoison.org

OHIO

CINCINNATI

Cincinnati Drug and Poison
Information Center (*)
Regional Poison Control System

3333 Burnett Ave
Vermon Place, 3rd Floor
Cincinnati OH 45229
Business: 513-636-5111
Emergency: 800-222-1222
TTY: 800-253-7955
www.cincinnatichildrens.org/dpic

CLEVELAND

Greater Cleveland Poison Control
Center
University Hospitals

11100 Euclid Ave – B261 MP6007
Cleveland OH 44106
Business: 216-844-1573
Emergency: 800-222-1222
     216-231-4455
(OH)
www.uhhospitals.org/rainbow
children/tabid/195/default.aspx

COLUMBUS

Central Ohio Poison Center (*)
Nationwide Children's Hospital

700 Children's Dr
Room L032
Columbus OH 43205
Business: 614-722-2635
Emergency: 800-222-1222
     614-228-1323
     937-222-2227
     (Dayton region)
www.nationwidechildrens.org/
poison-center

OKLAHOMA

OKLAHOMA CITY

Oklahoma Poison Control Center (*)
Children's Hospital at OU Health
Science Center

940 NE 13th St – Room 3510
Oklahoma City OK 73104
Business: 405-271-5062
Emergency: 800-222-1222
www.oklahomapoison.org

OREGON

PORTLAND

Oregon Poison Center (*)
Oregon Health and Science
University

3181 SW Sam Jackson Park Rd –
Suite CB550
Portland OR 97239
Business: 503-494-8600
Emergency: 800-222-1222
www.ohsu.edu/poison

(Continued)

PENNSYLVANIA

PHILADELPHIA

The Poison Control Center (*)
Children's Hospital of Philadelphia

34th St & Civic Center Blvd
Philadelphia PA 19104-4399
Business: 215-590-2003
Emergency: 800-222-1222
TDD/TTY: 215-590-8789
http://www.chop.edu/service/
poison-control-center/

PITTSBURGH

Pittsburgh Poison Center (*)
**University of Pittsburgh Medical
Center**

200 Lothrop Street
Pittsburgh PA 15213
Business: 412-390-3300
Emergency: 800-222-1222
                       412-681-6669
                       (Pittsburgh)
www.upmc.com/services/poison-center

RHODE ISLAND

(BOSTON, MA)

**Regional Center for Poison Control
and Prevention (*)**

300 Longwood Ave
Boston MA 02115
Business: 617-355-6609
Emergency: 800-222-1222
TDD/TTY   888-244-5313
www.maripoisoncenter.com

SOUTH CAROLINA

COLUMBIA

Palmetto Poison Center (*)
**University of South Carolina College
of Pharmacy**

USC Columbia SC 29208
Business: 803-777-7909
Emergency: 800-222-1222
http://poison.sc.edu

SOUTH DAKOTA

(MINNEAPOLIS, MN)

Minnesota Poison Control System (*)
Hennepin County Medical Center

701 Park Ave, Mail Code RL
Minneapolis MN 55415
Business: 612-873-3144
Emergency: 800-222-1222
www.mnpoison.org

(SIOUX FALLS)

Sanford Poison Center
Sanford Health USD Medical Center

1305 W 18th St - PO box 5039
Sioux Falls SD 57117
Business: 605-333-6638
Emergency: 800-222-1222
www.sdpoison.org

TENNESSEE

NASHVILLE

Tennessee Poison Center (*)

1161 21st Ave South
501 Oxford House
Nashville TN 37232-4632
Business: 615-936-0760
Emergency: 800-222-1222
www.tnpoisoncenter.org

TEXAS

AMARILLO

Texas Panhandle Poison Center (*)
Texas Poison Center Network

1501 S Coulter Dr
Amarillo TX 79106
Business: 806-354-1630
Emergency: 800-222-1222
www.poisoncontrol.org

DALLAS

North Texas Poison Center (*)
Texas Poison Center Network
Parkland Health & Hospital System

5201 Harry Hines Blvd
Dallas TX 75235
Business: 214-589-0911
Emergency: 800-222-1222
www.poisoncontrol.org

EL PASO

West Texas Regional Poison
Center (*)
Thomason Hospital

4815 Alameda Ave
El Paso TX 79905
Business: 915-534-3802
Emergency: 800-222-1222
www.poisoncontrol.org

GALVESTON

Southeast Texas Poison Center (*)
The University of Texas Medical
Branch

201 University Blvd
3.112 Trauma Bldg
Galveston TX 77555-1175
Business: 409-766-4403
Emergency: 800-222-1222
www.utmb.edu/setpc

SAN ANTONIO

South Texas Poison Center (*)
The University of Texas Health
Science Center-San Antonio

7703 Floyd Curl Dr-MSC 7849
Trauma Bldg
San Antonio TX 78229-3900
Business: 210-567-5762
Emergency: 800-222-1222
www.texaspoison.com

TEMPLE

Central Texas Poison Center (*)
Scott & White Memorial Hospital

2401 S 31st St
Temple TX 76508-0001
Business: 254-724-2111
Emergency: 800-222-1222
http://www.sw.org/poison-center/
poison-landing

UTAH

SALT LAKE CITY

Utah Poison Control Center (*)
University of Utah

585 Komas Dr – Suite 200
Salt Lake City UT 84108-1234
Business: 801-581-7504
Emergency: 800-222-1222
http://uuhsc.utah.edu/poison

VERMONT

(PORTLAND, ME)

Northern New England Poison Center
(*)
Maine Medical Center

22 Bramhall St
Portland ME 04102
Business: 207-662-7220
Emergency: 800-222-1222
www.nnepc.org

(Continued)

VIRGINIA

CHARLOTTESVILLE

Blue Ridge Poison Center (*)
University of Virginia School of Medicine

PO Box 800774
Charlottesville VA 22908
Business: 434-924-5118
Emergency: 800-222-1222
         800-451-1418 (VA)
www.healthsystem.virginia.edu/brpc

RICHMOND

Virginia Poison Center (*)
Virginia Commonwealth University Medical Center

PO Box 980522
Richmond VA 23298-0522
Business: 804-828-4780
Emergency: 800-222-1222
         804-828-9123
TDD/TYY: 804-828-9123
www.poison.vcu.edu

WASHINGTON

SEATTLE

Washington Poison Control Center (*)

155 NE 100th St, Suite 400
Seattle WA 98125-8007
Business: 206-517-2351
Emergency: 800-222-1222
         206-517-2394
(WA)
TDD: 800-572-0638
(WA)
         206-517-2394
(Seattle)
www.wapc.org

WEST VIRGINIA

CHARLESTON

West Virginia Poison Center (*)
WVU Robert C. Byrd Health Sciences Center

3110 MacCorkle Ave SE
Charleston WV 25304
Business: 304-347-1212
Emergency: 800-222-1222
www.wvpoisoncenter.org

WISCONSIN

MILWAUKEE

Wisconsin Poison Center
Children's Hospital of Wisconsin

9000 W Wisconsin Ave
PO Box 1997, Mail Station 677A
Milwaukee WI 53201
Business: 414-266-2000
Emergency: 800-222-1222
TDD/TYY: 414-964-3497
www.wisconsinpoison.org

WYOMING

(OMAHA, NE)

Nebraska Regional Poison Center (*)

8401 W Dodge Rd, Suite 115
Omaha NE 68114
Business: 402-955-5555
Emergency: 800-222-1222
www.nebraskapoison.com

Lactose- and Galactose-Free Medicines

The following is a selection of lactose- and galactose-free products. This is not a complete list. Generic and alternate brands may exist. Always check with your doctor if you have questions about specific ingredients.

BRAND (OTC)	FORM	BRAND (OTC)	FORM
Advil	Tablets, Caplets, Gel Caplets, Liquigels	Benadryl Allergy Kapgels	Caplets
Advil Cold and Sinus	Caplets, Liquigels	Benadryl Allergy Plus Cold	Kapgels
Advil PM	Liquigels	Benadryl Allergy Plus Sinus	Caplets
Aleve	Tablets	Benadryl Allergy Ultratab	Tablets
Aleve Smooth Gels	Gel Tablets	Benadryl Children's Allergy	Liquid
Alka-Seltzer	Effervescent Tablets	Benadryl Children's Dye-Free Allergy	Liquid
Alka-Seltzer Plus Cold	Effervescent Tablets, Softgels	Benadryl Children's Perfect Measure	Liquid
Alka-Seltzer Plus Cold and Cough Formula	Effervescent Tablets, Liquigels	Benadryl-D Allergy Plus Sinus	Tablets
Alka-Seltzer Plus Day and Night Cold Formula	Effervescent Tablets, Liquigels	Benadryl-D Children's Allergy and Sinus	Liquid
Alka-Seltzer Plus Flu Formula	Effervescent Tablets	Benadryl Dye-Free Allergy	Liquigels
Alka-Seltzer Plus Mucus and Congestion	Liquigels	Benadryl Quick Dissolve Strips	Oral Films
Alka-Seltzer Plus Night Cold Formula	Effervescent Tablets, Liquigels	Benadryl Severe Allergy Plus Sinus Headache	Caplets
Alka-Seltzer Plus Sinus Formula	Effervescent Tablets	Caltrate 600	Tablets
Ascriptin	Tablets	Caltrate 600 PLUS	Tablets
Axid	Tablets	Caltrate 600+D Plus Minerals	Tablets, Chewables
Axid AR	Tablets	Claritin-D 24	Tablets
Benadryl	Liquid	Claritin Reditabs	Tablets (disintegrating)

(Continued)

BRAND (OTC)	FORM	BRAND (OTC)	FORM
Colace	Capsules	Jevity	Liquid
Dramamine Chewable	Tablets	Kaopectate Advanced Formula	Suspension
Elecare	Powder	Kaopectate Cherry	Liquid
Enfamil ProSobee	Liquid, Powder	Kaopectate Peppermint	Liquid
Ensure	Liquid, Powder	Kaopectate Vanilla	Liquid
Ensure Bone Health	Liquid	Konsyl	Powder
Ensure Clinical Strength	Liquid	Konsyl Bladder Control	Capsules
Ensure Fiber	Liquid	Lactaid	Tablets
Ensure High Calcium	Liquid	Lactaid Fast Act	Caplets, Chewables
Ensure High Protein	Liquid		
Ensure Immune Health	Liquid	MCT Oil	Oil
		Medi-Lyte	Tablets
Ensure Muscle Health	Liquid	Metamucil	Capsules, Powder, Wafers
Ensure Plus	Liquid		
Excedrin Back and Body	Caplets	Motrin Children's	Suspension
Excedrin Extra-Strength	Caplets, Capsules, Tablets	Motrin IB	Tablets
		Motrin Infants'	Drops
Excedrin Menstrual Complete	Capsules	Motrin Junior Strength	Caplets, Tablets
Excedrin Migraine	Capsules, Tablets, Gel Tablets	Mylanta Gas Maximum Strength	Softgels
Excedrin PM	Caplets, Gel Tablets	Mylanta Maximum Strength	Tablets, Chewables
Excedrin Tension Headache	Caplets, Capsules, Tablets	Mylanta Regular Strength	Liquid
Ex-Lax Maximum Strength	Tablets	Mylanta Supreme	Liquid
Ex-Lax Regular Strength	Tablets	Mylanta Ultimate Strength	Liquid
Fergon	Tablets	Mylicon Infants'	Drops
Gaviscon Regular Strength	Tablets	Ocuvite Vitamin and Mineral Supplement	Tablets
Imodium A-D	Liquid, Tablets		

BRAND (OTC)	FORM	BRAND (OTC)	FORM
One-A-Day Cholesterol Plus	Tablets	Prilosec OTC	Tablets
		Promote	Liquid
One-A-Day Energy	Tablets	Promote with Fiber	Liquid
One-A-Day Essential	Tablets	Pulmocare	Liquid
One-A-Day Maximum	Tablets	RCF	Liquid
One-A-Day Men's	Tablets	Simply Sleep	Caplets
One-A-Day Men's 50+ Advantage	Tablets	St. Joseph Adult Low Strength Aspirin	Tablets
One-A-Day Men's Health Formula	Tablets	Sucrets Children's	Lozenges
One-A-Day Men's Pro Edge	Tablets	Sucrets Complete	Lozenges
		Sucrets Cough	Lozenges
One-A-Day Menopause Formula	Tablets	Sucrets Herbal	Lozenges
		Sucrets Liquid	Liquid
One-A-Day Teen Advantage	Tablets	Sucrets Maximum Strength	Lozenges
One-A-Day VitaCraves Gummies	Gummies	Sudafed	Tablets
One-A-Day Women's	Tablets	Sudafed 12 Hour	Tablets
One-A-Day Women's 50+ Advantage	Tablets	Sudafed 24 Hour	Tablets
		Sudafed Children's	Liquid
One-A-Day Women's Active Metabolism	Tablets	Sudafed Congestion	Tablets
One-A-Day Women's Active Mind & Body	Tablets	Sudafed OM Sinus Congestion Spray	Liquid
One-A-Day Women's Prenatal	Tablets	Sudafed PE Cold and Cough	Caplets
Pepto-Bismol	Suspension, Caplets	Sudafed PE Congestion	Tablets
Pepto-Bismol Instacool Chewable	Tablets	Sudafed PE Day and Night Cold	Caplets
Pepto-Bismol Max. Strength	Suspension	Sudafed PE Day and Night Congestion	Tablets
Pepto Children's Chewable	Tablets	Sudafed PE Non-Drying Sinus	Caplets
Percy Medicine	Suspension	Sudafed PE Sinus and Allergy	Tablets
Polycose	Liquid, Powder		

(Continued)

BRAND (OTC)	FORM
Sudafed PE Pressure and Pain	Caplets
Sudafed PE Severe Cold Formula	Caplets
Sudafed PE Sinus and Allergy	Tablets
Sudafed PE Triple Action	Caplets
Sudafed Triple Action	Caplets
Titralac	Tablets
Titralac Plus	Tablets
Tums	Tablets
Tums E-X 750	Tablets
Tums E-X- Sugar Free	Tablets
Tums Kids	Tablets
Tums Ultra 1000	Tablets
Tylenol	Tablets
Tylenol Children's Plus Cold	Liquid
Tylenol Children's Plus Cold & Allergy	Liquid
Tylenol Children's Plus Cold & Cough	Liquid
Tylenol Children's Plus Cold & Stuffy Nose	Liquid
Tylenol Children's Plus Cough & Runny Nose	Liquid
Tylenol Children's Plus Cough & Sore Throat	Liquid
Tylenol Children's Plus Flu	Liquid
Tylenol Children's Plus Multi- Symptom Cold	Suspension

BRAND (OTC)	FORM
Tylenol Infants'	Suspension
Tylenol Meltaways Jr.	Tablets
Unisom SleepTabs	Gels, Melts, Tablets
Unisom PM Pain SleepCaps	Caplets
Zantac 75	Tablets
Zantac 150	Tablets
Zantac 150 Cool Mint	Tablets

BRAND (Rx)	FORM
Actigall	Capsules
Advicor	Tablets
Aldactazide	Tablets
Aldactone	Tablets
Allegra Children's Oral	Suspension
Allegra	Suspension, Tablets
Allegra-D 12 Hr, 24 Hr	Tablets
Altace	Capsules
Amicar	Solution, Tablets
Amnesteem	Capsules
Antivert	Tablets
Aplenzin	Tablets
Apriso	Capsules
Aromasin	Tablets
Augmentin Chewable	Tablets
Augmentin ES 600	Powder
Augmentin XR	Tablets
Augmentin	Suspension, Tablets
Axid	Solution

BRAND (Rx)	FORM	BRAND (Rx)	FORM
Bactrim	Tablets	DiaBeta	Tablets
Bactrim DS	Tablets	Diovan HCT	Tablets
Biaxin Filmtab	Tablets	Diovan	Tablets
Biaxin Granules	Suspension	E.E.S	Suspension, Tablets
Calan SR	Tablets	Edluar	Tablets
Cambia	Solution	Embeda	Capsules
Carafate	Suspension, Tablets	Enwgereg	Capsules
Cardizem CD	Capsules	Epivir	Solution, Tablets
Cardizem LA	Tablets	Epivir-HBV	Solution, Tablets
Ceftin	Suspension, Tablets	Ery-Tab	Tablets
		Esgic-Plus	Capsules, Tablets
Cefzil	Suspension, Tablets	Exelon	Capsules, Solution
Cipro	Suspension, Tablets	Exforge	Tablets
Cipro XR	Tablets	Exforge HCT	Tablets
Citranatal RX	Tablets	Fibricor (fenofibric acid)	Tablets
Clinoril	Tablets		
Coartem	Tablets	Fioricet	Tablets
Combivir	Tablets	Fioricet with Codeine	Capsules
Comtan	Tablets	Flomax	Capsules
Covera-HS	Tablets	Gleevec	Tablets
Creon	Capsules	Glucotrol XL	Tablets
Cytotec	Tablets	Glucovance	Tablets
Daypro	Tablets	Glyset	Tablets
Demerol	Tablets	GoLYTELY	Powder
Depakene	Capsules, Solution	Grifulvin V	Suspension, Tablets
Depakote	Tablets	Inderal LA	Capsules
Depakote Sprinkle	Capsules	Isoptin SR	Tablets
Detrol	Tablets	Kaletra	Solution, Tablets
Detrol LA	Capsules	Kapidex	Capsules

(Continued)

BRAND (Rx)	FORM	BRAND (Rx)	FORM
Keppra	Solution, Tablets	Onsolis	Buccal Film
K-Lor	Powder	Pamelor	Capsules
K-Phos Neutral	Tablets	Pamine Forte	Tablets
K-Phos Original Formula	Tablets	Patanase	Liquid
K-Tab	Tablets	Paxil	Suspension, Tablets
Lamisil	Tablets, Oral Granules	Pepcid	Suspension, Tablets
Lescol	Capsules	Percocet	Tablets
Lescol XL	Tablets	Percodan	Tablets
Levaquin	Solution, Tablets	Plaquenil	Tablets
Levothroid	Tablets	Pletal	Tablets
Levoxyl	Tablets	PrandiMet	Tablets
Lexapro	Solution, Tablets	Prandin	Tablets
Lomotil	Tablets	Precose	Tablets
Lopid	Tablets	Prevacid	Capsules
Lysteda	Tablets	Prinivil	Tablets
Malarone	Tablets	Pristiq	Tablets
Malarone Pediatric	Tablets	Procardia	Capsules
Maxzide	Tablets	Procardia XL	Tablets
Methylin ER	Tablets	Promacta	Tablets
Micardis	Tablets	Prometrium	Capsules
Micro-K	Capsules	Protonix	Suspension, Tablets
Micronase	Tablets	Prozac	Capsules
Minipress	Capsules	Qualaquin	Capsules
Minocin	Capsules	Questran	Powder
Moxatag	Tablets	Questran Light	Powder
Niaspan	Tablets	Rapaflo	Capsules
Norpramin	Tablets	Remeron SolTab	Tablets
Norvasc	Tablets	Rifadin	Capsules, Solution
Omnicef	Capsules, Suspension		

BRAND (Rx)	FORM	BRAND (Rx)	FORM
Robaxin	Tablets	Trizivir	Tablets
Ryzolt	Tablets	Twynsta	Tablets
Sabril	Solution, Tablets	Tyvaso	Liquid
Saphris	Tablets	Uniphyl	Tablets
Sarafem	Tablets	Urex	Tablets
Savella	Tablets	Valcyte	Solution, Tablets
Sectral	Capsules	Valtrex	Caplets
Sinemet	Tablets	Valturna	Tablets
Sinemet CR	Tablets	Vibramycin Hyclate	Capsules, Suspension
Soma	Tablets	Vicodin	Tablets
Stalevo	Tablets	Vicodin ES	Tablets
Stavzor	Capsules	Vicodin HP	Tablets
Sucraid	Solution	Vicoprofen	Tablets
Tamiflu	Capsules, Suspension	Videx EC	Capsules, Delayed Release Tablets
Tegretol/Tegretol-XR	Suspension, Tablets	Vimpat	Solution, Tablets
Tenoretic	Tablets	Visicol	Tablets
Tenormin	Tablets	Vistaril	Capsules
Tessalon	Capsules	Votrient	Tablets
Tiazac	Capsules	Welchol	Suspension, Tablets
Ticlid	Tablets	Wellbutrin	Tablets
Tikosyn	Capsules	Wellbutrin SR	Tablets
Tofranil	Tablets	Wellbutrin XL	Tablets
Tofranil-PM	Capsules	Xenical	Capsules
Toprol-XL	Tablets	Zantac	Efferdose Tablets, Syrup, Tablets
Treanda	Powder	Zarontin	Capsules, Solution
Trental	Tablets	Zebeta	Tablets
Treximet	Tablets	Zenpep	Capsules
Trileptal	Suspension, Tablets	Zestril	Tablets
Trilipix	Capsules		

(Continued)

BRAND (Rx)	FORM	BRAND (Rx)	FORM
Ziac	Tablets	Zonegran	Capsules
Ziagen	Solution, Tablets	Zyban	Tablets
Zipsor	Capsules	Zyvox	Suspension, Tablets
Zofran	Solution		
Zoloft	Oral Concentrate, Tablets		

Abbreviations:
OTC = over-the-counter
Rx = prescription

Sugar-Free Products

The following is a selection of sugar-free products, grouped by class. If you are diabetic, keep in mind that many of these medications may contain sorbitol, alcohol, or other sources of carbohydrates. This list is not a complete list. Generic and alternate brands may be available. Check with your doctor if you have questions about inactive ingredients.

Analgesics

Addaprin Tablets	Dover
Aminofen Tablets	Dover
Back Pain-Off Tablets ‡	Medique
Children's Silapap Liquid	Silarx
I-Prin Tablets ‡	Medique
Medi-Seltzer Effervescent Tablets	Medique
Methadose Sugar Free Oral Concentrate	Covidien
Ms.-Aid Tablets ‡	Medique

Antacids/Antiflatulants

Alcalak Chewable Tablets*† ‡ §	Medique
Diotame Chewable Tablets*† ‡ §	Medique
Pepto-Bismol Caplets † ‡	Procter & Gamble
Tums Extra Sugar Free Tablets* §	GlaxoSmithKline Consumer

Anti-Asthmatic/Respiratory Agent

Jay-Phyl Syrup	JayMac

Antidiarrheal

Imogen Liquid	Pharm Generic

Blood Modifier/Iron Preparation

I.L.X. B-12 Elixir	Kenwood

Corticosteroid

Pediapred Solution* §	UCB

Cough/Cold/Allergy Preparations

Bromhist-DM Solution	Cypress
Bromhist Pediatric Solution	Cypress
Bromphenex DM Solution*† §	Breckenridge
Bromplex DM Solution*† §	Prasco
Broncotron Liquid	Seyer Pharmatec
Broncotron-D Suspension	Seyer Pharmatec
Carbaphen 12 Ped Suspension	Gil
Carbaphen 12 Suspension	Gil
Carbatuss-12 Suspension	GM
Carbatuss-CL Solution	GM
Cetafen Cold Tablets ‡	Hart Health and Safety
Cetafen Cough & Cold Tablets ‡	Hart Health and Safety
Cheratussin DAC Liquid	Qualitest
Coldcough PD Syrup* §	Breckenridge
Coldcough Syrup* §	Breckenridge
Coldonyl Tablets	Medique

(Continued)

* Contains sorbitol.
† May contain other sugar alcohols (eg, glycerol, isomalt, maltitol, mannitol, xylitol).
‡ May contain other sources of carbohydrates (eg, cellulose, lactose, maltodextrin, polydextrose, starch).
§ May contain natural or artificial flavors.

Cough/Cold/Allergy Preparations
(Continued)

Corfen DM Solution	Cypress
Crantex Syrup	Breckenridge
De-Chlor DM Solution	Cypress
Despec Liquid	International Ethical
Despec-SF Liquid	International Ethical
Diabetic Siltussin DAS-Na	Silarx
Diabetic Siltussin-DM DAS-Na	Silarx
Diabetic Tussin	Health Care Products
Diabetic Tussin DM Liquid §	Health Care Products
Diabetic Tussin Solution§	Health Care Products
Diphen Capsules ‡	Medique
Double Tussin DM Liquid	Reese
Dytan-CS Tablets	Hawthorn
Emagrin Forte Tablets	Medique
Gilphex TR Tablets	Gil
Giltuss Ped-C Solution§	Gil
Neo DM Syrup*† §	Laser
Neotuss-D Liquid † §	A.G. Marin
Neotuss S/F Liquid † §	A.G. Marin
Phena-HC Solution	GM
Phena-S 12 Suspension	GM
Phena-S Liquid	GM
Poly Hist PD Solution	Poly
Scot-Tussin Diabetes CF Liquid	Scot-Tussin
Scot-Tussin Expectorant Solution	Scot-Tussin
Scot-Tussin Senior Solution	Scot-Tussin
Siladryl Allergy Solution* §	Silarx
Siltussin DAS Liquid*† §	Silarx
Siltussin DM DAS Cough Formula Syrup*† §	Silarx
Siltussin SA Liquid*† §	Silarx
Children's Sudafed PE Cough & Cold Liquid*† §	McNeil Consumer
Children's Sudafed Nasal	McNeil Consumer
Supress DX Pediatric Drops † §	Kramer-Novis
Suttar-SF Syrup	Gil
Vazol Solution	Wraser
Z-Tuss DM Syrup † §	Magna
Z-Tuss Expectorant Solution † §	Magna

Fluoride Preparations

Fluor-A-Day Liquid	Arbor
Fluor-A-Day Tablets*† §	Arbor
Sensodyne Tartar Control with Whitening † ‡ §	GlaxoSmithKline Consumer
Sensodyne with Fluoride Cool Gel*† ‡ §	GlaxoSmithKline Consumer
Sensodyne with Fluoride Toothpaste Original Flavor*† ‡ §	GlaxoSmithKline Consumer

Laxatives

Benefiber Powder	Novartis
Citrucel Powder ‡ §	GlaxoSmithKline Consumer
Colace Solution	Purdue Products
Fiber Choice Tablets * ‡ §	GlaxoSmithKline Consumer
Fibro-XL Capsules	Key
Konsyl Easy Mix Formula Powder ‡	Konsyl

* Contains sorbitol.
† May contain other sugar alcohols (eg, glycerol, isomalt, maltitol, mannitol, xylitol).
‡ May contain other sources of carbohydrates (eg, cellulose, lactose, maltodextrin, polydextrose, starch).
§ May contain natural or artificial flavors.

Konsyl Orange Powder ‡ §	Konsyl
Konsyl Powder ‡	Konsyl
Metamucil Smooth Texture Powder ‡	Procter & Gamble
Reguloid Powder Orange Flavor ‡ §	Rugby
Reguloid Powder Regular Flavor ‡	Rugby

Mouth/Throat Preparations

Cepacol Dual Relief Sore Throat Spray † §	Combe
Cepacol Sore Throat + Coating Relief Lozenge † §	Combe
Cepacol Sore Throat Lozenges † §	Combe
Cheracol Sore Throat Spray †	Lee
Chloraseptic Spray*† §	Prestige
Diabetic Tussin Cough Drops † §	Health Care Products
Fisherman's Friend Sugar Free Mint Lozenges*	Lofthouse of Fleetwood
Fresh N Free Liquid	Geritrex
Listerine Pocketpaks Film ‡ §	Johnson & Johnson
Luden's Sugar Free & Wild Cherry Throat Drops † §	McNeil Consumer
Medikoff Sugar Free Drops †	Medique
N'ice Lozenges* §	Heritage/Insight
Oragesic Solution* §	Parnell
Orajel Dry Mouth Moisturizing Gel*† ‡ §	Del
Orajel Dry Mouth Moisturizing Spray † ‡ §	Del
Sepasoothe Lozenges* ‡ §	Medique

Vitamins/Minerals/Supplements

Adaptosode For Stress Liquid	HVS
Adaptosode R+R For Acute Stress Liquid	HVS
Alamag Tablets*† ‡ §	Medique
Alcalak Tablets*† ‡	Medique
Apetigen Elixir*†	Kramer-Novis
Apptrim Capsules	Physician Therapeutics
Apptrim-D Capsules	Physician Therapeutics
Bevitamel Tablets	Westlake
Biosode Liquid	HVS
Bugs Bunny Complete	Bayer
C&M Caps-375 Capsules	Key
Cal-Cee Tablets	Key
Calcet Plus Tablets	Mission Pharmacal
Calcimin-300 Tablets	Key
Cerefolin NAC Tablets	Pamlab
Chromacaps ‡	Key
Delta D3 Tablets ‡	Freeda Vitamins
Detoxosode Liquids	HVS
DHEA Capsules	ADH Health Products
Diatx ZN Tablets ‡	Centrix
Diucaps Capsules	Legere
DL-Phen-500 Capsules	Key
Enterex Diabetic Liquid ‡	Victus
Evening Primose Oil Capsules †	Nature's Bounty
Ex-L Tablets ‡	Key
Extress Tablets	Key
Eyetamins Tablets ‡	Rexall Consumer
Fem-Cal Citrate Tablets ‡	Freeda Vitamins
Fem-Cal Plus Tablets	Freeda Vitamins
Fem-Cal Tablets ‡	Freeda Vitamins
Ferrocite Plus Tablets ‡	Breckenridge
Folacin-800 Tablets ‡	Key
Folbee Plus Tablets ‡	Breckenridge
Folbee Tablets ‡	Breckenridge

(Continued)

Vitamins/Minerals/Supplements
(Continued)

Folplex 2.2 Tablets ‡	Breckenridge
Foltx Tablets ‡	Pamlab
Gabadone Capsules	Physician Therapeutics
Gram-O-Leci Tablets*†‡	Freeda Vitamins
Herbal Slim Complex Capsules	ADH Health Products
Hypertensa Capsules ‡	Physician Therapeutics
Lynae Calcium/Vitamin C Chewable Tablets	Boscogen
Lynae Chondroitin/ Glucosamine Capsules	Boscogen
Lynae Ginse-Cool Chewable Tablets	Boscogen
Magimin Tablets ‡	Key
Magnacaps Capsules ‡	Key
Mag-Ox 400 Tablets	Health Care Products
Medi-Lyte Tablets ‡	Medique
Metanx Tablets ‡	Pamlab
Multi-Delyn with Iron Liquid †	Silarx
New Life Hair Tablets ‡	Rexall Consumer
Niferex Elixir* ‡ §	Ther-Rx
Nutrisure OTC Tablets	Westlake
Nutrivit Solution*†§	Llorens
Ob Complete Tablets	Vertical
O-Cal Fa Tablets ‡	Pharmics
Os-Cal 500 + D Tablets ‡	GlaxoSmithKline Consumer
Powervites Tablets ‡	Green Turtle Bay Vitamin
Prostaplex Herbal Complex Capsules	ADH Health Products
Protect Plus Liquid	Gil
Protect Plus Liquid NR Softgels	Gil
Pulmona Capsules	Physician Therapeutics
Quintabs-M Tablets ‡	Freeda Vitamins
Replace w/o Iron Capsules ‡	Key
Samolinic Softgels †	Key
Sea Omega 30 Softgels †	Rugby
Sea Omega 50 Softgels †	Rugby
Sentra AM Capsules	Physician Therapeutics
Sentra PM Capsules	Physician Therapeutics
Soy Care for Menopause Capsules	Inverness Medical
Span C Tablets ‡	Freeda Vitamins
Strovite Forte Syrup	Everett
Sunnie Tablets	Green Turtle Bay Vitamin
Sunvite Tablets † ‡	Rexall Naturalist
Super Dec B100 Tablets ‡	Freeda Vitamins
Super Quints B-50 Tablets ‡	Freeda Vitamins
Supervite Liquid	Seyer Pharmatec
Theramine Capsules	Physician Therapeutics
Triamin Tablets	Key
Triamino Tablets* ‡	Freeda Vitamins
Ultramino Powder	Freeda Vitamins
Uro-Mag Capsules ‡	Health Care Products
Vitafol Tablets † ‡	Everett
Vitamin C/Rose Hips Tablets	ADH Health Products
Xtramins Tablets	Key
Ze Plus Softgels	Everett

* Contains sorbitol.
† May contain other sugar alcohols (eg, glycerol, isomalt, maltitol, mannitol, xylitol).
‡ May contain other sources of carbohydrates (eg, cellulose, lactose, maltodextrin, polydextrose, starch).
§ May contain natural or artificial flavors.

Miscellaneous

Acidoll Capsules	Key
Alka-Gest Tablets	Key
Cafergot Tablets ‡	Sandoz
Cytra-2 Solution* §	Cypress
Cytra-K Crystals	Cypress
Cytra-K Solution* §	Cypress
Melatin Tablets ‡	Mason Vitamins
Namenda Solution*† §	Forest
Prosed/DS Tablets ‡	Ferring
Questran Light Powder ‡ §	Par

Medicines That Should Not Be Crushed

Some medicines are manufactured to be released into your system slowly, or some time after you actually take them. It may be dangerous to crush such products before taking them.

This section lists various "slow-release" and "enteric-coated" products that should not be crushed or chewed. Slow-release (sr) products are controlled-release, extended-release, long-acting, or timed-release. Enteric-coated (ec) products are delayed-release.

In general, capsules containing slow-release or enteric-coated particles may be opened and their contents sprinkled on a spoonful of soft food that you can swallow without chewing. You should never chew the particles. In fact, you should not chew any medication unless it is specifically made to be taken that way.

This is not a complete list of all products that should not be crushed; generic or alternate brands of some products may exist. Tablets intended for sublingual (dissolved under the tongue) or buccal (dissolved in the mouth or cheek) administrations are not included in this list and should only be taken according to the directions. Be sure to ask your doctor or pharmacist if you have questions about how to take any medication.

MEDICINE	MANUFACTURER	FORM
AcipHex	Eisai	ec
Actoplus Met XR	Takeda	sr
Adalat CC	Bayer Healthcare	sr
Adderall XR	Shire U.S.	sr
Adenovirus Type 4 and Type 7 Vaccine	Teva Women's Health, Inc.	ec
Advicor	Abbott	sr
Afeditab CR	Watson	sr
Aggrenox	Boehringer Ingelheim	sr
Aleve Cold & Sinus	Bayer Healthcare	sr
Aleve Sinus & Headache	Bayer Healthcare	sr
Allegra-D 12 Hour	sanofi-aventis	sr
Allegra-D 24 Hour	sanofi-aventis	sr
AlleRx	Cornerstone	sr
Allfen	MCR American	sr
Allfen-DM	MCR American	sr
Alophen	Numark	ec
Altoprev	Watson	sr
Ambien CR	sanofi-aventis	sr

ec = Enteric-coated   sr = Slow-released

(Continued)

MEDICINE	MANUFACTURER	FORM
Ampyra ER	Acorda Therapeutics	sr
Amrix	Cephalon	sr
Aplenzin	sanofi-aventis	sr
Apriso	Salix	sr
Arthrotec	Pfizer	ec
Asacol	Procter & Gamble	ec
Asacol HD	Procter & Gamble	ec
Ascriptin Enteric	Novartis Consumer	ec
Augmentin XR	GlaxoSmithKline	sr
Avinza	King	sr
Azulfidine Entabs	Pfizer	ec
Bayer Aspirin Regimen	Bayer Healthcare	ec
Biaxin XL	Abbott	sr
Bidex-A	SJ Pharmaceuticals	sr
Blanex-A	Blansett	sr
Bontril Slow-Release	Valeant	sr
Bromfed-PD	Victory	sr
Bromfenex PD	Quality Care	sr
Budeprion SR	Teva	sr
Budeprion XL	Teva	sr
Buproban	Teva	sr
Calan SR	Pfizer	sr
Campral	Forest	ec
Carbatrol	Shire U.S.	sr
Cardene SR	EKR Therapeutics	sr
Cardizem CD	Biovail	sr
Cardizem LA	Abbott	sr
Cardura XL	Pfizer	sr
Cartia XL	Watson	sr
Cemill 500	Miller	sr
Cemill 1000	Miller	sr
Certuss-D	Capellon	sr
Chlorex-A	Cypress	sr
Chlor-Phen	Truxton	sr
Chlor-Trimeton Allergy	Schering-Plough	sr
Cipro XR	Schering-Plough	sr
Clarinex-D 24 Hour	Schering-Plough	sr
Claritin-D	Schering-Plough	sr
Claritin-D 12 Hour	Schering-Plough	sr

MEDICINE	MANUFACTURER	FORM
Claritin-D 24 Hour	Schering-Plough	sr
Concerta	Ortho-McNeil-Janssen	sr
Contac 12-Hour	GlaxoSmithKline	sr
Correctol	Schering-Plough	ec
Coreg CR	GlaxoSmithKline	sr
Covera-HS	Pfizer	sr
CPM 8/PE 20/MSC 1.25	Cypress	sr
Creon 5	Solvay	ec
Creon 10	Solvay	ec
Creon 20	Solvay	ec
Cymbalta	Eli Lilly	ec
Dairycare	Plainview	ec
Deconsal II	Cornerstone	sr
Deconex DM	Poly	sr
Depakote	Abbott	ec
Depakote ER	Abbott	sr
Depakote Sprinkles	Abbott	ec
Despec SR	International Ethical	sr
Detrol LA	Pfizer	sr
Dexedrine Spansules	GlaxoSmithKline	sr
Dexilant	Takeda	sr
Diamox Sequels	Duramed	sr
Dilacor XR	Watson	sr
Dilantin	Pfizer	sr
Dilantin Kapseals	Pfizer	sr
Dilatrate-SR	UCB	sr
Diltia XT	Watson	sr
Dilt-CD	Apotex	sr
Ditropan XL	Ortho-McNeil-Janssen	sr
Donnatal Extentabs	PBM	sr
Doryx	Warner Chilcott	ec
D-Phen 1000	Midlothian	sr
Dulcolax	Boehringer Ingelheim	ec
Duomax	Capellon	sr
Duratuss	Physicians Total Care	sr
Duratuss DA	Victory	sr
Dynacirc CR	GlaxoSmithKline	sr
Dynex LA	Athlon	sr
Dynex VR	Athlon	sr

(Continued)

MEDICINE	MANUFACTURER	FORM
Dytan-CS	Hawthorn	sr
Easprin	Rosedale	ec
EC Naprosyn	Genentech	ec
Ecotrin	GlaxoSmithKline	ec
Ecotrin Adult Low Strength	GlaxoSmithKline	ec
Ecotrin Maximum Strength	GlaxoSmithKline	ec
Ecpirin	Prime Marketing	ec
Ed A-Hist	Edwards	sr
Effexor-XR	Wyeth	sr
Embeda	King	sr
Enablex	Novartis Consumer	sr
Entercote	Global Source	ec
Entocort EC	Prometheus	ec
Equetro	Validus	sr
ERYC	Warner Chilcott	sr
Ery-Tab	Abbott	ec
Exalgo	Mallinckrodt	sr
Extress-30	Key	sr
Extress-60	Key	sr
Feen-A-Mint	Schering-Plough	ec
Femilax	G & W	ec
Fero-Folic-500	Abbott	sr
Fero-Grad-500	Abbott	sr
Ferro-Sequels	Inverness Medical	sr
Ferrous Fumarate DS	Vita-Rx	sr
Fetrin	Lunsco	sr
Flagyl ER	Pharmacia	sr
Fleet Bisacodyl	Fleet, C.B.	ec
Focalin XR	Novartis	sr
Folitab 500	Rising	sr
Fortamet	Shionogi Pharma	sr
Forfivo XL	IntelGenx	sr
Fumatinic	Laser	sr
Genacote	Teva	ec
GFN 600/Phenylephrine 20	Cypress	sr
Gilphex TR	Gil	sr
Glucophage XR	Bristol-Myers Squibb	sr
Glucotrol XL	Pfizer	sr
Glumetza	Depomed	sr

MEDICINE	MANUFACTURER	FORM
Guaifenex GP	Ethex	sr
Guaifenex PSE 60	Ethex	sr
Guaifenex PSE 80	Ethex	sr
Guaifenex PSE 85	Ethex	sr
Guaifenex PSE 120	Ethex	sr
Halfprin	Kramer	ec
Hemax	Pronova	sr
Histacol LA	Breckenridge	sr
Horizant	GlaxoSmithKline	sr
Iberet-500	Abbott	sr
Iberet-Folic-500	Abbott	sr
Icar-C Plus SR	Hawthorn	sr
Inderal LA	Akrimax	sr
Indocin SR	Forte Pharma	sr
Innopran XL	GlaxoSmithKline	sr
Intuniv	Shire	sr
Invega	Ortho-McNeil-Janssen	sr
Isochron	Forest	sr
Isoptin SR	Ranbaxy	sr
Janumet XR	Merck Sharp & Dohme Corp.	sr
Kadian	Actavis	sr
Kapvay ER	Shionogi	sr
Kaon-Cl 10	Savage	sr
Keppra XR	UCB	sr
Klor-Con 8	Upsher-Smith	sr
Klor-Con 10	Upsher-Smith	sr
Klor-Con M10	Upsher-Smith	sr
Klor-Con M15	Upsher-Smith	sr
Klor-Con M20	Upsher-Smith	sr
Kombiglyze ER	BMS/AstraZeneca	sr
K-Tab	Abbott	sr
K-Tan	Prasco	sr
Lamictal XR	GlaxoSmithKline	sr
Lescol XL	Novartis	sr
Levall G	Auriga	sr
Levbid	Alaven	sr
Levsinex	Alaven	sr
Lialda	Shire	ec
Lipram 4500	Global	ec

(Continued)

MEDICINE	MANUFACTURER	FORM
Lipram-PN10	Global	ec
Lipram-PN16	Global	ec
Lipram-PN20	Global	ec
Liquibid-D	Capellon	sr
Liquibid-D 1200	Capellon	sr
Lithobid	Noven Therapeutics	sr
Lohist-12	Larken	sr
Luvox CR	Jazz Pharmaceuticals	sr
Mag Delay	Major	ec
Mag 64	Rising	ec
Mag-Tab SR	Niche	sr
Maxifed	MCR American	sr
Maxifed DM	MCR American	sr
Maxifed DMX	MCR American	sr
Maxifed-G	MCR American	sr
Medent PE	SJ Pharmaceuticals	sr
Mega-C	Merit	sr
Menopause Trio	Mason Vitamins	sr
Mestinon Timespan	Valeant	sr
Metadate CD	UCB	sr
Metadate ER	UCB	sr
Methylin ER	Mallinckrodt	sr
Micro-K	Ther-Rx	sr
Micro-K 10	Ther-Rx	sr
Mild-C	Carlson, J.R.	sr
Mirapex ER	Boehringer Ingelheim	sr
Moxatag	Victory	sr
MS Contin	Purdue	sr
Mucinex	Reckitt Benckiser	sr
Mucinex D	Reckitt Benckiser	sr
Mucinex DM	Reckitt Benckiser	sr
Mydocs	Centurion	sr
Myfortic	Novartis	ec
Nalex-A	Blansett	sr
Namenda XR	Forest	sr
Naprelan	Victory	sr
New Ami-Tex LA	Actavis	sr
Nexium	AstraZeneca	ec
Nexiclon XR	Next Wave	sr

MEDICINE	MANUFACTURER	FORM
Niaspan	Abbott	sr
Nifediac CC	Teva	sr
Nifedical XL	Teva	sr
Nitro-Time	Time-Cap	sr
Norel SR	U.S. Pharmaceutical	sr
Norpace CR	Pfizer	sr
Nucynta ER	Janssen	sr
Obstetrix EC	Seyer Pharmatec	ec
Oleptro	LaboPharm	sr
Opana ER	Endo	sr
Oramorph SR	Xanodyne	sr
Oracea	Galderma	sr
Oxecta	King Pharmaceuticals	sr
Oxycontin	Purdue	sr
Palcaps 10	Breckenridge	ec
Palcaps 20	Breckenridge	ec
Pancreaze	Ortho-McNeil-Janssen	ec
Pancrecarb MS-4	Digestive Care	ec
Pancrecarb MS-8	Digestive Care	ec
Pancrecarb MS-16	Digestive Care	ec
Pangestyme CN-10	Ethex	ec
Pangestyme CN-20	Ethex	ec
Pangestyme EC	Ethex	ec
Pangestyme MT16	Ethex	ec
Pangestyme UL12	Ethex	ec
Pangestyme UL18	Ethex	ec
Pangestyme UL20	Ethex	ec
Panocaps	Breckenridge	ec
Panocaps MT 16	Breckenridge	ec
Panocaps MT 20	Breckenridge	ec
Paser	Jacobus	sr
Pavacot	Truxton	sr
Paxil CR	GlaxoSmithKline	sr
PCE Dispertab	Abbott	sr
PCM LA	Cypress	sr
Pendex	Cypress	sr
Pentasa	Shire U.S.	sr
Pentoxil	Upsher-Smith	sr
Phenavent D	Ethex	sr

(Continued)

MEDICINE	MANUFACTURER	FORM
Phenytek	Mylan	sr
Phlemex-PE	Cypress	sr
Poly Hist Forte	Poly	sr
Poly-Vent	Poly	sr
Prehist D	Marnel	sr
Prevacid	Takeda	ec
Prilosec	AstraZeneca	ec
Prilosec OTC	Procter & Gamble	sr
Pristiq	Wyeth	sr
Procardia XL	Pfizer	sr
Prolex PD	Blansett	sr
Prolex-D	Blansett	sr
Proquin XR	Depomed	sr
Protid	Lunsco	sr
Protonix	Wyeth	ec
Prozac Weekly	Eli Lilly	ec
Pseudocot-C	Truxton	sr
Pseudocot-G	Truxton	sr
Pseudovent DM	Ethex	sr
Ralix	Cypress	sr
Ranexa	Gilead	sr
Razadyne ER	Ortho-McNeil-Janssen	sr
Requip XL	GlaxoSmithKline	sr
Rescon-Jr	Capellon	sr
Respa-AR	Respa	sr
Respa-BR	Respa	sr
Respaire-120 SR	Laser	sr
Rhinacon A	Breckenridge	sr
Ritalin LA	Novartis	sr
Ritalin-SR	Novartis	sr
Rodex Forte	Legere	sr
Ru-Tuss	Carwin	sr
Rythmol SR	GlaxoSmithKline	sr
Ryzolt	Purdue	sr
SAM-e	Pharmavite	ec
Sanctura XR	Allergan	sr
Seroquel XR	AstraZeneca	sr
Simcor	Abbott	sr
Sinemet CR	Bristol-Myers Squibb	sr

MEDICINE	MANUFACTURER	FORM
Slo-Niacin	Upsher-Smith	sr
Slow Fe	Novartis Consumer	sr
Slow Fe With Folic Acid	Novartis Consumer	sr
Slow-Mag	Purdue	ec
Solodyn	Medicis	sr
St. Joseph Pain Reliever	McNeil Consumer	ec
Stahist	Magna	sr
Stavzor	Noven	sr
Sudafed 12 hour	McNeil Consumer	sr
Sudafed 24 hour	McNeil Consumer	sr
Sular	Shionogi Pharma	sr
Sulfazine EC	Qualitest	ec
Symax Duotab	Capellon	sr
Symax-SR	Capellon	sr
Tarka	Abbott	sr
Taztia XT	Watson	sr
Tegretol-XR	Novartis	sr
Theo-24	UCB	sr
Theocron	Carac	sr
Theo-Time	Major	sr
Tiazac	Forest	sr
Toprol XL	AstraZeneca	sr
Totalday	National Vitamin	sr
Toviaz	Pfizer	sr
Trental	sanofi-aventis	sr
Treximet	GlaxoSmithKline	ec
Trilipix	Abbott	ec
Tussicaps	Mallinckrodt	sr
Tylenol Arthritis	McNeil Consumer	sr
Ultram ER	Valeant	sr
Urocit-K 5	Mission	sr
Urocit-K 10	Mission	sr
Uroxatral	sanofi-aventis	sr
Utira	Hawthorn	sr
Veracolate	Numark	ec
Verelan	UCB	sr
Verelan PM	UCB	sr
Videx EC	Bristol-Myers Squibb	ec
Vimovo	AstraZeneca	ec

(Continued)

MEDICINE	MANUFACTURER	FORM
Vivitrol	Alkermes	sr
Voltaren-XR	Novartis	sr
Vospire ER	Dava	sr
Votrient	GlaxoSmithKline	ec
Wellbutrin SR	GlaxoSmithKline	sr
Wellbutrin XL	GlaxoSmithKline	sr
Wobenzym N	Marlyn	ec
Xanax ER	Pfizer	sr
Xedec II	Cypress	sr
Xpect-AT	Hawthorn	sr
Xpect-HC	Hawthorn	sr
Xpect-PE	Hawthorn	sr
Zenpep	Eurand	ec
Zmax	Pfizer	sr
Zyban	GlaxoSmithKline	sr
Zyflo CR	Cornerstone	sr
Zyrtec-D	McNeil Consumer	sr

Common Equivalent Measurements

We learn common measurements starting in grade school, but that may not prepare you for precisely measuring the right dose of medication to give a sick loved one. While it's always best to use a measuring device that came with a medication, knowing the equivalent measurements below may help you ensure proper dosing when one is not available.

Common Measures	
1 teaspoon	5 milliliters
1 tablespoon	15 milliliters
	3 teaspoons
1 wineglass	2 ounces
	60 milliliters
1 teacup	4 ounces
	120 milliliters
1 cup	8 ounces
	240 milliliters
1 gallon	4 quarts
	128 ounces
	3800 milliliters
1 quart	2 pints
	32 ounces
	960 milliliters
1 pint	16 ounces
	480 milliliters
8 ounces	240 milliliters
4 ounces	120 milliliters
1 pound	16 ounces
2.2 pounds	1 kilogram

(Continued)

Metric Measures	
1 kilogram	1000 grams
1 gram	1000 milligrams
1 milligram	0.001 grams
1 microgram	0.001 milligrams
	0.000001 grams
1 liter	1000 milliliters
1 milliliter	0.001 liters

US Fluid Measures	
1 pint	16 ounces
1 quart	2 pints
	32 ounces
1 gallon	4 quarts
	128 ounces

Metric Liquid Measures	
30 milliliters	1 ounce
50 milliliters	1 ¾ ounces
100 milliliters	3 ½ ounces
200 milliliters	7 ounces
230 milliliters	8 ounces
500 milliliters	1 pint
750 milliliters	1 ½ pints
1000 milliliters	1 quart

Common Abbreviations	
kg	kilogram
g	gram
mg	milligram
mcg	microgram
L	liter
mL	milliliter

Common Abbreviations *(Continued)*	
oz	ounce
qt	quart
pt	pint
lb	pound
tsp	teaspoon

How to Apply Eye Drops and Ointment

How to apply eye drops:

1. Wash your hands thoroughly.

2. Tilt your head back.

3. Gently pull the lower eyelid away from your eye to create a pocket.

4. Hold the bottle upside down and look up just before instilling a single drop. **NOTE:** To prevent contamination, do not let the tip of the eye drop applicator touch any surface (including the eye or eyelid). When you are not using it, keep the container tightly closed.

5. After instilling the drop, look down for several seconds (still holding the eyelid away from your eye).

6. Slowly release the eyelid and close your eyes for 1 to 2 minutes. Do not blink.

7. Gently press on the inside corner of your eye (where the eyelid meets your nose) with a finger.

8. Blot excessive solution from around the eye with a tissue.

How to apply eye ointment:

1. Wash your hands thoroughly.

2. Tilt your head back.

3. Gently grasp the lower outer eyelid below your lashes, and pull the eyelid away from your eye.

4. Place the ointment tube over your eye by directly looking at it. With a sweeping motion, place 1/4- to 1/2-inch of your ointment inside your lower eyelid by gently squeezing the tube. **NOTE:** To prevent contamination, do not let the tip of the tube touch any surface (including your eye or eyelid). When you are not using it, keep the tube tightly closed.

(Continued)

5. Slowly the release eyelid and close your eyes for 1 to 2 minutes.

6. Blot excessive ointment from around your eye with a tissue.

7. Your vision may be temporarily blurred. Until your vision clears, avoid activities requiring good visual ability.

Tips for user:

• If you have difficulty determining whether an eye dropper has touched the eye surface, keep the dropper in a refrigerator (not in a freezer).

• If more than one drop is needed, wait at least 5 minutes before instilling the next drop to prevent flushing away or diluting the first drop.

• If both eye drops and ointment therapy is needed, instill the eye drop at least 10 minutes before the ointment.

• If you wear contact lenses, remove them unless the product is designed specifically for use with contact lenses.

How to Use Metered-Dose Inhalers

General Guidelines

1. Remove the dust cap and hold the inhaler upright.

2. Shake the canister well before each use.

3. Prime (release into the air the dose already in the device) the inhaler before you use it for the first time and in cases where you haven't used it for extended periods of time.*

4. Tilt your head back slightly and breathe out slowly and completely.

5. For **closed mouth technique**: Place the mouthpiece in your mouth and close your lips tightly around (not recommended for steroid inhaler).

For **open mouth technique**: Hold the inhaler 1 to 2 inches from open your mouth (about the width of 2 fingers).

6. Inhale slowly and deeply, and press down on the inhaler to release the medication. (The slower you breathe, the greater the chance that the medication will reach the smaller airways.) **NOTE:** Children or elderly patients having difficulty with coordination of technique can use a spacer or holding chamber. If you use a spacer, put the mouthpiece of the spacer between your teeth and into your mouth. Then, close your mouth around the spacer. With the device in place, actuate the inhaler once and inhale the medication immediately after actuating the aerosol.

7. Breathe in slowly and hold your breath for about 10 seconds to allow the medication to go into your lungs.

8. Breathe out slowly and wait about 30 seconds to 1 minute before administering a second inhalation. **NOTE:** You can expect relief of your symptoms within 5 to 15 minutes. Seek medical attention if you still have symptoms after 20 minutes (this should occur with short-acting medications like albuterol).

9. If you use a steroid inhaler, rinse your mouth with water after use. **NOTE:** Spit out the water after the last puff. Do not swallow it.

(Continued)

Tips for the User:

• Rinse only the inhaler mouthpiece and cap with warm running water, then air dry. Do not wash the canister or immerse it in water.

• Keep the dust cap over the mouthpiece of the inhaler when it is not in use.

• Do not puncture the canister. The contents are under pressure.

• Store the canister at room temperature (15°C to 30°C), away from heat (48.9°F) or open flames.

---

*Refer to the instructions that came with your prescription.

Adapted from http://www.nhlbi.nih.gov/guidelines/asthma/asthgdln.htm

Basic Laboratory Values for Cholesterol, High Blood Pressure, and Diabetes

Cholesterol

LDL, HDL, and Total Cholesterol Lab Values (mg/dL)*	
LDL[a] cholesterol ("bad" cholesterol)	
<100	Best
100-129	Near best
130-159	Borderline high
160-189	High
≥190	Very high
HDL[b] cholesterol ("good" cholesterol)	
<40	Low
≥60	High
Total cholesterol	
<200	Best
200-239	Borderline high
≥240	High

*milligrams per deciliter (mg/dL)
[a] low-density lipoprotein
[b] high-density lipoprotein

High Blood Pressure (Hypertension)

Blood Pressure Levels for Adults (mm Hg)*			
Systolic[a] BP[b]		**Diastolic[c] BP**	
<120	and	<80	Normal
120-139	or	80-89	Prehypertension
140-159	or	90-99	Stage 1 hypertension
≥160	or	≥100	Stage 2 hypertension

*millimeters of mercury (mm Hg)
[a] The blood pressure in the arteries while your heart beats
[b] Blood pressure (BP)
[c] The blood pressure in the arteries between heartbeats

Diabetes

Lab Values for Prediabetes and Diabetes

Prediabetes[a]

Fasting[b] blood sugar level	100-125 mg/dL
or	
2-hr sugar level OGTT[c]	140-199 mg/dL
or	
A1C[d]	5.7-6.4%

Diabetes

Fasting[b] blood sugar level	≥126 mg/dL
or	
2-hr sugar level OGTT[c]	≥200 mg/dL
or	
Random blood sugar level with symptoms of high blood sugar (increased thirst, increased urination, increased appetite, unexplained weight loss)	≥200 mg/dL
or	
A1C[d]	≥6.5%

[a] Prediabetes means that you are at a higher risk for diabetes
[b] Fasting means that you cannot eat for at least 8 hours
[c] Oral glucose tolerance test (OGTT): Test in which a patient, after fasting for at least 8 hours, drinks 75 g of sugar dissolved in water. The blood sugar level is measured 2 hours later
[d] The A1C test shows your average blood sugar level for the past 2-3 months

Sources:

1. Third Report of the National Cholesterol Education Program (NCEP) Expert Panel on Detection, Evaluation, and Treatment of High Blood Cholesterol in Adults (Adult Treatment Panel III). *JAMA*. 2001.

2. The Seventh Report of the Joint National Committee on Prevention, Detection, Evaluation, and Treatment of High Blood Pressure: the JNC 7 report. *Hypertension*. 2003.

3. MedlinePlus. High Blood Pressure. http://www.nlm.nih.gov/medlineplus/highbloodpressure.html. Posted on August 2012. Accessed August 1, 2012.

4. American Diabetes Association. Standards of Medical Care in Diabetes – 2012. *Diabetes Care*. 2012.

5. Chapter 18. Disorders of the Endocrine Pancreas. *Pathophysiology of Disease: An Introduction to Clinical Medicine*. 6th ed. New York: McGraw-Hill; 2010.

Are My Numbers in the Normal Range?

What is a comprehensive metabolic panel?

A comprehensive metabolic panel is a group of chemical tests performed on the blood serum (the part of blood that does not contain cells).

The test will provide an overall picture of your body's metabolism. Metabolism refers to all the physical and chemical processes in the body that use energy.

How is the test performed?

A blood sample is needed.

How should I prepare for the test?

You should not eat or drink for 8 hours before the test.

Why is the test performed?

The test will give your doctor information about:
  • how your kidney and liver are working
  • blood sugar, cholesterol, and calcium levels
  • sodium, potassium, and chloride levels (called electrolytes)
  • protein levels.

Your doctor may order this test during a yearly exam or routine checkup.

Normal Results

		Normal Range*
Electrolytes**	Sodium	136-144 mEq/L
	Potassium	3.7-5.2 mEq/L
	Calcium	8.5-10.9 mg/dL
	Chloride	96-106 mmol/L
	Blood sugar	100 mg/dL
Liver Function Test	Alkaline phosphatase	44-147 IU/L
	Alanine aminotransferase (ALT)	8-37 IU/L
	Aspartate aminotransferase (AST)	10-34 IU/L
	Bilirubin	0.2-1.9 mg/dL

(Continued)

		Normal Range*
Kidney Function Test	Blood urea nitrogen (BUN)	7-20 mg/dL
	Creatinine	0.8-1.4 mg/dL
Proteins	Álbumin	3.9-5.0 g/dL
	Protein	6.3-7.9 g/dL

* Creatinine values could be different with age. Different laboratories may use ranges. Please ask your doctor about specific test results.

** Electrolytes are chemicals that are important for the cells in your body to function.

This list in not comprehensive; always check with your doctor regarding what is normal and abnormal.

Abbreviations:

IU = international unit
L = liter
dL = deciliter=0.1 liter
g/dL = gram per deciliter
mg/dL = milligram per deciliter
mg = milligram
mmol = millimole
mEq = milliequivalents

Source:
Zieve D, Eltz DR. Comprehensive metabolic panel. MedlinePlus.
www.nlm.nih.gov/medlineplus/ency/article/003468.htm. Posted August 30, 2011.
Accessed August 1, 2012.

What Is Your BMI? and How Can You Calculate It?

What is the Body Mass Index?	How can I use it?	Why use it?
• The Body Mass Index (BMI) is a number calculated from your weight and height • The BMI is used to assess your body fat • The BMI formula is the same for both adults and children	• You can use the BMI as a screening method to detect any health problems that may be related to your weight • The BMI is not a diagnostic tool	• It is inexpensive and an easy tool to assess your body fat • Allows you to compare your weight with the general population

Calculation

$\text{BMI} = \dfrac{\text{weight (pounds)} \times 703}{[\text{height (inches)}]^2}$	$\text{or BMI} = \dfrac{\text{weight (kg)}}{[\text{height (m)}]^2}$

Categories

BMI	Weight Status
18.5	• Underweight
18.5 -24.9	• Normal
25-29.9	• Overweight
>30	• Obese

What are some of the risks if you are overweight?

- High blood pressure
- High cholesterol
- Type 2 diabetes
- Stroke
- Gallbladder disease

- Breathing problem
- Heart disease
- Arthritis
- Certain forms of cancers

Assess Your Weight and Height

Height (inches)	Normal (pounds)	Overweight (pounds)	Obese (pounds)
58	89-119	120-143	>144
59	92-123	124-148	>149
60	95-127	128-153	>154
61	97-132	133-158	>159
62	101-136	137-163	>164
63	104-140	141-169	>170
64	108-145	146-174	>175
65	111-150	150-179	>180
66	115-154	155-185	>186
67	118-159	160-191	>192
68	122-164	165-196	>197
69	125-169	169-202	>203
70	129-174	174-208	>209
71	133-179	179-214	>215
72	136-184	184-220	>221
73	140-189	190-227	>228
74	144-194	195-233	>234
75	148-199	200-239	>240
76	152-204	205-246	>247

Sources:
Healthy Weight—It's Not a Diet, It's a Lifestyle. Centers for Disease Control and Prevention.
www.cdc.gov/healthyweight/assessing/bmi/adult_bmi/index.html. Posted September 13, 2011.
Accessed August 1, 2012.
Body Mass Index Table. National Heart Lung and Blood Institute.
www.nhlbi.nih.gov/guidelines/obesity/bmi_tbl.htm. Accessed August 1, 2012.

Healthy Lifestyle Choices for Men and Women of All Ages

Stop using tobacco products	• If you smoke or chew tobacco, stop! • Call 1-800-227-2345 for help.
Maintain a healthy weight	• Being overweight can increase your risk for many types of cancer. • Control your weight with the choices you make every day for healthy eating and exercise by: – Avoiding excessive weight gain. – Watch your portion sizes and eat more fruits, vegetables, and whole grains instead of higher calorie foods. – Balance how much you eat with the amount of physical activity you do. – Get to a healthy weight and stay there.
Exercise	• Adults: Get at least 150 minutes of moderate-intensity or 75 minutes of vigorous-intensity activity each week (or a combination of these), preferably spread out over the week. • Adolescents and children: Get at least 1 hour of moderate- or vigorous-intensity activity each day, with vigorous activity on at least 3 days each week.
Eat healthy	• Eat at least 2½ cups of fruits and vegetables each day. They contain many vitamins, fiber, minerals, and antioxidants, and are low in fat and calories. • Choose whole grain rice, bread, pasta, and cereal instead of processed (refined) grains. Look for whole wheat, pumpernickel, rye, or oats as the first ingredient on the food label. • Limit the amount of processed meats (bacon or cold cuts) and red meats (beef or lamb) you eat. • Eat lean meats (look for "loin" or "round" in the name and the amount of fat on the meat) in smaller portions, skinless poultry breasts, fish, or legumes (beans and peas) as healthier sources of protein.

(Continued)

| Limit alcohol | • Men should not have more than 2 drinks a day.
• Women should not have more than 1 drink a day.
• (A drink is 12 ounces of regular beer, 5 ounces of wine, or 1½ ounces of 80-proof distilled spirits). |

Source:
American Cancer Society. 2012. Screening Recommendations by Age.
http://www.cancer.org/Healthy/ToolsandCalculators/Reminders/screening-recommendations-by-age. Accessed August 8, 2012.

Cancer Screening Recommendations by Age and Gender

Age: 20-29 years	
WOMEN	
Breast Cancer	• Have a breast exam by a doctor or nurse **every 3 years**. • Tell your doctor right away if you notice any breast changes. • Find out if you are at a higher risk of developing breast cancer. • Talk to your doctor about when to start getting mammograms.
Cervical Cancer	• Starting at the age of 21, have a Pap test **every 3 years**. • Follow testing recommendations even if you have been vaccinated against human papilloma virus (HPV).
Colon Cancer	• Find out if you have a higher risk of developing colon cancer because of family history or other factors. • Talk to your doctor about when to start testing and what tests are right for you.
MEN	
Colon Cancer	• If you have a higher risk of developing colon cancer because of family history or other factors, talk to your doctor about when to start testing and what tests are right for you.
Age: 30-39 years	
WOMEN	
Breast Cancer	• Have a breast exam by a doctor or nurse **every 3 years**. • Tell your doctor right away if you notice any breast changes. • Find out if you are at a higher risk of developing breast cancer. • Talk to your doctor about when to start getting mammograms.

(Continued)

Age: 30-39 years *(Continued)*	
WOMEN *(Continued)*	
Cervical Cancer	• Have a Pap test and HPV test **every 5 years** (preferred) or just a Pap test **every 3 years**. • Follow testing recommendations even if you have been vaccinated against HPV. • No testing is needed if you had a hysterectomy that removed the uterus and cervix if it was done for reasons not related to cervical cancer.
Colon Cancer	• Find out if you have a higher risk of developing colon cancer because of family history or other factors. • Talk to your doctor about when to start testing and what tests are right for you.
MEN	
Colon Cancer	• If you have a higher risk of developing colon cancer because of family history or other factors, talk to your doctor about when to start testing and what tests are right for you.
Age: 40-49 years	
WOMEN	
Breast Cancer	• Have a breast exam by a doctor or nurse **every year**. • Tell your doctor right away if you notice any breast changes. • Have a mammogram **every year**.
Cervical Cancer	• Have a Pap test and HPV test **every 5 years** (preferred) or just a Pap test **every 3 years**. • No testing is needed if you had a hysterectomy that removed the uterus and cervix if it was done for reasons not related to cervical cancer.
Colon Cancer	• Find out if you have a higher risk of developing colon cancer because of family history or other factors. • Talk to your doctor about when to start testing and what tests are right for you.

MEN	
Prostate Cancer	• If you are at a higher risk of developing prostate cancer, talk to your doctor about the potential benefits of testing beginning at the age of 45. • Men at risk include African Americans and men with a close family member (father, brother, son) with prostate cancer. • If you have several close family members with prostate cancer before the age of 65, talk to your doctor about starting testing at the age of 40.
Colon Cancer	• If you have a higher risk of developing colon cancer because of family history or other factors, talk to your doctor about when to start testing and what tests are right for you.
Age: 50-65 years	
WOMEN	
Breast Cancer	• Have a breast exam by a doctor or nurse **every year**. • Tell your doctor right away if you notice any breast changes. • Have a mammogram **every year**.
Cervical Cancer	• Have a Pap test and HPV test **every 5 years** (preferred) or just a Pap test **every 3 years**. • No testing is needed if you had a hysterectomy that removed the uterus and cervix if it was done for reasons not related to cervical cancer.
Colon Cancer	• Start testing **at the age of 50**. Talk to your doctor to decide which test is right for you and how often to have it done.
MEN	
Prostate Cancer	• **At the age of 50**, talk to your doctor about potential benefits of starting testing early.
Colon Cancer	• Start testing **at the age of 50**. Talk to your doctor to decide which test is right for you and how frequently tests should be done.

(Continued)

Age: >65 years	
WOMEN	
Breast Cancer	• Have a breast exam by a doctor or nurse **every year**. • Tell your doctor right away if you notice any breast changes. • Medicare recommends and covers **yearly** mammograms.
Cervical Cancer	• No testing is needed if you have had regular testing with normal results. • No testing is needed if you had a hysterectomy that removed the uterus and cervix if it was done for reasons not related to cervical cancer. • Women with a history of cervical precancer should continue to test for 20 years after the diagnosis.
Colon Cancer	• Medicare **recommends** and covers testing. Talk to your doctor about which tests are best for you and how frequently tests should be done.
MEN	
Prostate Cancer	• Medicare **recommends** and covers testing. • If your life expectancy is greater than 10 years, talk to your doctor about the potential benefits of yearly testing.
Colon Cancer	• Medicare **recommends** and covers testing. • Talk to your doctor about which tests are best for you and how frequently tests should be done.

Sources:
American Cancer Society. 2012. Screening Recommendations by Age.
http://www.cancer.org/Healthy/ToolsandCalculators/Reminders/screening-recommendations-by-age.
Accessed August 8, 2012.
HPV Test Beats Pap Long-Term: Study. HealthDay News. July 30, 2012. Copyright 2012.
http://www.nlm.nih.gov/medlineplus/news/fullstory_127738.html. Posted July 31, 2012.
Accessed August 8, 2012.

Cancer Prevention Checklist for Men and Women

Evaluate and Decrease Your Risk for Cancer

MEN

Type of Cancer	Risk Factors	Risk Reduction

Skin Cancer	• Have you ever sunbathed?
	• Have you used tanning beds or sunlamps?
	• Do you have pale skin and blond or red hair?
	• Do you sunburn easily or have many freckles?
	• Did you have severe sunburns as a child?
	• Do you have many or unusually shaped moles?
	• Do you live in a southern climate or at a high altitude?
	• Do you spend a lot of time outdoors (for work or recreation)?
	• Have you ever had radiation treatment?
	• Has anyone in your family had skin cancer?
	• Do you have a weakened immune system due to an organ transplant, HIV infection, or other condition?
	• Were you born with xeroderma pigmentosum, basal cell nevus syndrome, or dysplastic nevus syndrome?
	• Have you been exposed to any of the following chemicals?
	  –Arsenic
	  –Radium
	  –Industrial tar
	  –Paraffin
		• Stay out of the sun as much as possible, especially between 10 a.m. and 4 p.m.
		• Wear a broad-brimmed hat, a shirt, and UV-protective sunglasses when out in the sun.
		• Use a sunscreen with an SPF of 15 or higher, and reapply it often.
		• Wear wrap-around sunglasses with at least 99% UV absorption, labeled as blocking UVA and UVB light; or "UV absorption to 400 nm," which means UVA and UVB protection.
		• Do not use tanning beds or sunlamps.
		• Protect young children from excessive sun exposure.
		• Check your skin often for abnormal or changing areas, especially moles, and have them checked by a doctor.

(Continued)

MEN		
Type of Cancer	**Risk Factors**	**Risk Reduction**
Prostate Cancer	• Are you older than 50? • Are you African American? • Do you have a father, brother, or son who was diagnosed with prostate cancer before they were 65? • Do you eat a lot of red meat or high-fat dairy products and tend to eat fewer fruits and vegetables? • Are you overweight?	• Eat plenty of fruits, vegetables, and whole grains, and limit your intake of red meats (beef, pork, or lamb), especially high fat or processed meats (like deli meats, hot dogs, and bacon). • Get to and stay at a healthy weight. • Be physically active. • Talk to your doctor about whether medicine to reduce prostate cancer risk may be right for you.

Lung Cancer	• Do you smoke tobacco?
	• Do you now or have you ever worked around asbestos?
	• Are you or have you been exposed to radon?
	• Have you been exposed to any of these in your workplace?
	  –Uranium
	  –Arsenic
	  –Vinyl chloride
	• Do you smoke marijuana?
	• Are you now or have you been regularly exposed to secondhand smoke?
	• Do you have family members who have had lung cancer?
		• Quit smoking.
		• Encourage those you live or work with to quit smoking.
		• Avoid areas where people are smoking around you.
		• Contact your state's radon office or the U.S. Environmental Protection Agency to learn about having your home checked for radon.
		• Use precautions when working with cancer-causing chemicals, or avoid them altogether.

Colorectal Cancer	• Have you ever had colon or rectal cancer? • Has anyone in your family had colon or rectal cancer? • Do you have a colorectal cancer syndrome in your family, such as familial adenomatous polyposis or hereditary nonpolyposis colon cancer, also called Lynch syndrome?	• Follow early detection (screening) guidelines to find and remove adenomatous polyps before they become cancer. • Increase the intensity and amount of physical activity you get each week. • Get to and stay at a healthy weight.

MEN

Type of Cancer	Risk Factors	Risk Reduction
Colorectal Cancer *(Cont.)*	• Have you ever had a type of intestinal polyp called an adenomatous polyp? • Have you had a chronic inflammatory bowel disease such as Crohn's disease or ulcerative colitis for several years? • Are you older than 50? • Do you eat a lot of red meat (beef, pork, lamb) or processed meats (deli meat, hot dogs, bacon)? • Are you physically inactive? • Are you overweight? • Do you use tobacco? • Do you drink more than 2 alcoholic drinks per day?	• Eat plenty of fruits, vegetables, and whole-grain foods, and limit processed meats and red meats. • Quit smoking. • Cut back to no more than 2 alcoholic drinks per day, if you drink at all.

WOMEN

Type of Cancer	Risk Factors	Risk Reduction
Skin Cancer	• Have you ever sunbathed? • Have you used tanning beds or sunlamps? • Do you have pale skin and blond or red hair? • Do you sunburn easily or have many freckles? • Did you have severe sunburns as a child? • Do you have many or unusually shaped moles? • Do you live in a southern climate or at a high altitude? • Do you spend a lot of time outdoors (for work or recreation)?	• Stay out of the sun as much as possible, especially between 10 a.m. and 4 p.m. • Wear a broad-brimmed hat, a shirt, and UV-protective sunglasses when out in the sun. • Use a sunscreen with an SPF of 15 or higher, and reapply it often. • Wear wrap-around sunglasses with at least 99% UV absorption, labeled as blocking UVA and UVB light; or "UV absorption to 400 nm," which means UVA and UVB protection.

(Continued)

WOMEN		
Type of Cancer	**Risk Factors**	**Risk Reduction**

Skin Cancer *(Cont.)*	• Have you ever had radiation treatment?
	• Has anyone in your family had skin cancer?
	• Do you have a weakened immune system due to an organ transplant, HIV infection, or other condition?
	• Were you born with xeroderma pigmentosum, basal cell nevus syndrome, or dysplastic nevus syndrome?
	• Have you been exposed to any of the following chemicals?
	  –Arsenic
	  –Radium
	  –Industrial tar
	  –Paraffin
		• Do not use tanning beds or sunlamps.
		• Protect young children from excess sun exposure.
		• Check your skin often for abnormal or changing areas, especially moles, and have them checked by a doctor.

Breast Cancer	• Are you older than 40?
	• Have you had radiation to the chest as treatment for another cancer?
	• Are you or other family members known to have a gene mutation that carries high breast cancer risk, such as BRCA?
	• Has anyone in your family had breast cancer (especially mother, sister, or daughter)?
	• Have you had breast cancer?
	• Did you have your first child after you were 30 or have no children?
	• Did you begin menstruating before you were 12 or go through menopause after you were 55?
	• Have you been on hormone-replacement therapy?
	• Do you drink 2 or more alcoholic drinks per day?
		• Talk to your doctor about the risks and benefits of hormone-replacement therapy for your specific situation.
		• Get regular physical activity.
		• Get to and stay at a healthy weight.
		• Cut back to not more than 1 alcoholic drink per day, if you drink at all.
		• If you think you may be at high risk for breast cancer:
		  –Talk to your doctor about genetic counseling,
		  –ask about taking tamoxifen or raloxifene, or
		  –ask about enrolling in a chemoprevention study.

WOMEN		
Type of Cancer	**Risk Factors**	**Risk Reduction**
Breast Cancer *(Cont.)*	• Are you physically inactive? • If you are past menopause, have you gained weights, especially around your waist?	

Lung Cancer	• Do you smoke tobacco?
	• Do you now or have you ever worked around asbestos?
	• Are you or have you been exposed to radon?
	• Have you been exposed to any of these in your workplace?
	  –Uranium
	  –Arsenic
	  –Vinyl chloride
	• Do you smoke marijuana?
	• Are you now or have you been regularly exposed to secondhand smoke?
	• Do you have family members who have had lung cancer?
		• Quit smoking.
		• Encourage those you live or work with to quit smoking.
		• Avoid areas where people are smoking around you.
		• Contact your state's radon office or the U.S. Environmental Protection Agency to learn about having your home checked for radon.
		• Use precautions when working with cancer-causing chemicals, or avoid them altogether.

Colorectal Cancer	• Have you ever had colon or rectal cancer? • Has anyone in your family had colon or rectal cancer? • Do you have a colorectal cancer syndrome in your family, such as familial adenomatous polyposis or hereditary nonpolyposis colon cancer, also called Lynch syndrome? • Have you ever had a type of intestinal polyp called an adenomatous polyp? • Have you had a chronic inflammatory bowel disease such as Crohn's disease or ulcerative colitis for several years?	• Follow early detection (screening) guidelines to find and remove adenomatous polyps before they become cancer. • Increase the intensity and amount of physical activity you get each week. • Get to and stay at a healthy weight. • Eat plenty of fruits, vegetables, and whole-grain foods, and limit processed meats and red meats. • Quit smoking. • Cut back to no more than 1 alcoholic drink per day, if you drink at all.

(Continued)

WOMEN		
Type of Cancer	**Risk Factors**	**Risk Reduction**
Colorectal Cancer *(Cont.)*	• Are you older than 50? • Do you eat a lot of red meat (beef, pork, lamb) or processed meats (deli meat, hot dogs, bacon)? • Are you physically inactive? • Are you overweight? • Do you use tobacco? • Do you drink more than 1 alcoholic drink per day?	
Endometrial Cancer	• Do you or does anyone in your family have hereditary nonpolyposis colorectal cancer, also called Lynch syndrome? • Are you over 40? • Did you begin menstruating before age 12, or go through menopause after age 55? • Do you have a history of infertility or never giving birth? • Are you obese (very overweight)? • Do you have diabetes? • Have you taken tamoxifen or long-term estrogen-replacement therapy without progesterone (if you still have your uterus)? • Have you had breast or ovarian cancer? • Have you had radiation therapy to your pelvis?	• Talk to your doctor about the risks and benefits of hormone therapy for your specific situation. • Get to and stay at a healthy weight. • If you are taking hormone therapy for symptoms of menopause and you still have your uterus, talk to your doctor about using estrogen with progestin rather than estrogen alone. • If you think you may be at higher risk, talk to a doctor about other ways to reduce your risk.
Ovarian Cancer	• Are you older than 40? • Have you already gone through menopause? • Are you obese (very overweight)? • Do you have no children?	• Use oral contraceptives for several years. • Talk to your doctor about the risks and benefits of hormone-replacement therapy for your specific situation.

WOMEN		
Type of Cancer	**Risk Factors**	**Risk Reduction**
Ovarian Cancer *(Cont.)*	• Has your mother, sister, or daughter had ovarian or breast cancer? • Do you or does anyone in your family have hereditary nonpolyposis colorectal cancer, also called Lynch syndrome, or are you at risk for this syndrome? • Do you or does anyone in your family have a BRCA gene mutation? • Have you had breast cancer? • Have you been on estrogen-replacement therapy without progesterone for more than 5 years?	• Talk to your doctor about having your ovaries removed, if you are at high risk. (This surgery causes sudden menopause.)

Cervical Cancer	• Have you ever had sex?
	• Have you ever been told that you had human papilloma virus (HPV)?
	• Have you ever been told that you had Chlamydia?
	• Have you ever had genital warts?
	• Do you smoke?
	• Do you have human immunodeficiency virus (HIV) infection or AIDS?
	• Did your mother take diethylstilbestrol (DES) when she was pregnant with you?
	• Do you have a sister or mother who has or had cervical cancer?
		• If you are sexually active, you can reduce your risk of getting HPV and cervical cancer by:
		  –Having sex with only one other person who only has sex with you.
		  –Practicing safer sex by using condoms each time you have sex.
		• Quit smoking.
		• Have regular screening for cervical cancer.
		Vaccination: The HPV vaccines are given in a 3-dose series to fight HPV infection. The vaccine must be given before the woman is infected.
		The HPV vaccines:
		• Are best given to girls between ages 11 and 13 (may be given as young as 9).
		• May be given between ages 13 and 18 to "catch up."

(Continued)

WOMEN		
Type of Cancer	**Risk Factors**	**Risk Reduction**
Cervical Cancer *(Cont.)*		• Are of uncertain value for women aged 19-26. • Do not replace regular cervical cancer screening because they cannot fight all strains of HPV.

Sources:

Adapted from American Cancer Society Inc.; 2012. Prevention Checklist for Men. http://www.cancer.org/acs/groups/content/@nho/documents/webcontent/acsq-009104.pdf Posted March 2012. Accessed August 8, 2012.

American Cancer Society Inc.; 2012. Prevention Checklist for Women. http://www.cancer.org/acs/groups/content/@editorial/documents/webcontent/acsq-009098.pdf. Posted March 2012. Accessed August 8, 2012.

How Much Calcium Do I Need in My Diet?

Calcium is the most abundant mineral in your body. It is found in some foods, added to others, available as a dietary supplement, and present in some medicines (such as antacids). Many parts of your body, such as your veins and arteries, muscles, nerves, and cells, require calcium to function properly. Only 1% of the total calcium in your body is needed for these functions. Your blood calcium level is very tightly regulated and does not fluctuate with changes in your diet. Your body uses bone as a reservoir for, and source of, calcium to maintain constant levels of calcium in your blood, muscle, and fluids.

The remaining 99% of your body's calcium supply is stored in your bones and teeth, where it supports their structure and function. Bone undergoes continuous changes with age. Bone formation is predominant in periods of growth in children and adolescents. In aging adults, particularly post-menopausal women, bone breakdown is more common than formation, resulting in bone loss that increases the risk of osteoporosis over time.

How Much Calcium Do I Need to Take?

Recommended Daily Calcium Intake to Meet the Nutrient Requirements of Nearly All Healthy Persons				
Age	Men	Women	Pregnant	Lactating
0–6 months*	200 mg	200 mg		
7–12 months*	260 mg	260 mg		
1–3 years	700 mg	700 mg		
4–8 years	1000 mg	1000 mg		
9–13 years	1300 mg	1300 mg		
14–18 years	1300 mg	1300 mg	1300 mg	1300 mg
19–50 years	1000 mg	1000 mg	1000 mg	1000 mg
51–70 years	1000 mg	1200 mg		
71+ years	1200 mg	1200 mg		

*Adequate Intake (AI)
Adapted from the Office of Dietary Supplement. National Institutes of Health.
http://ods.od.nih.gov/factsheets/Calcium-HealthProfessional. Accessed August 17, 2012.

Nutrients with a % Daily Value but No Weight Listed— Spotlight on Calcium

Calcium: Look at the % Daily Value (DV) for calcium on food packages so you know how much one serving contributes to the total amount you need per day. Remember, a food with 20% DV or more contributes a lot of calcium to your daily total, while one with 5% DV or less contributes a little.

Nutrition Facts	
Serving Size 1 cup (236ml)	
Servings Per Container 1	
Amount Per Serving	
Calories 80	Calories from Fat 0
	% Daily Value*
Total Fat 0g	0%
Saturated Fat 0g	0%
Trans Fat 0g	
Cholesterol Less than 5mg	0%
Sodium 120mg	5%
Total Carbohydrate 11g	4%
Dietary Fiber 0g	0%
Sugars 11g	
Protein 9g	17%
Vitamin A 10%	Vitamin C 4%
Calcium 30% Iron 0%	Vitamin D 25%
*Percent Daily Values are based on a 2,000 calorie diet. Your daily values may be higher or lower depending on your calorie needs	

Experts advise adult consumers to consume adequate amounts of calcium—that is, 1000 mg or 100% DV in a daily 2000 calorie diet. This advice is often given in milligrams (mg), but the Nutrition Facts label only lists a % DV for calcium.

Experts also advise that adolescents, especially girls, consume 1300 mg (130% DV) and postmenopausal women consume 1200 mg (120% DV) of calcium daily. The DV for calcium on food labels is 1000 mg.

Don't be fooled—always check the label for calcium because you cannot make assumptions about the amount of calcium in specific food categories. For example, the amount of calcium in milk, whether skim or

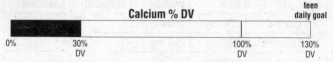

Calcium % DV

0%   30% DV   100% DV   130% DV   teen daily goal

whole, is generally the same per serving, whereas the amount of calcium in the same size yogurt container (8 oz) can vary from 20-45% DV.

Equivalencies
30% DV = 300 mg calcium = one cup of milk
100% DV = 1000 mg calcium
130% DV = 1300mg calcium

Source:
U.S. Food and Drug Administration. How to Understand and Use the Nutrition Facts Label. http://www.fda.gov/Food/ResourcesForYou/Consumers/NFLPM/ucm274593.htm#dvs. Posted February 15, 2012. Accessed August 17, 2012.

Osteoporosis

Osteoporosis is a silent disease; it makes your bones weak and more likely to break. Anyone can develop osteoporosis, but it is most common in older women. As many as half of all women and a quarter of men older than 50 will break a bone due to osteoporosis.

Evaluate and Decrease Your Risk for Osteoporosis

Risk Factors	Risk Reduction
Are you older than 50? • More common in older people than younger people. • Bone density loss is more common with age. **Are you a woman?** • A woman over the age of 50 has increased risk of breaking a bone. • Women have lighter, thinner bones than men. • Women may also lose bone quickly after menopause. • However, osteoporosis isn't just a woman's disease. Men over the age of 50 may also break a bone due to osteoporosis. **If you are a woman, have you already gone through menopause?** • In women, the sex hormone estrogen protects bones. • Bone loss increases after menopause when estrogen levels drop sharply. • If you go through menopause early, your risk of osteoporosis increases.	• Get enough calcium and vitamin D. • If you are under age 50, get at least 1000 mg of calcium and 400-800 international units (IU) of vitamin D each day. • If you are over age 50, get at least 1200 mg of calcium and 800-1000 IU of vitamin D each day. • Eat more fruits and vegetables (or take a multivitamin or supplement) to get other important vitamins and minerals. • Limit the amount of salt and caffeine you consume. • Limit the amount of protein (eg, animal protein) you eat that comes from sources other than milk products. • Get regular exercise, including fast walking and muscle-strengthening exercise such as lifting weights. • Quit smoking.

(Continued)

Risk Factors	Risk Reduction
Do either of your parents have osteoporosis? • Family history (heredity and genetics play a major role in osteoporosis and broken bones). **Do you have a small or thin body type?** • Women and men with small bones are more likely than larger people to have osteoporosis. • This doesn't mean heavier and larger people can't get it. **Did you have one or more broken bones as an adult, or does your spine curve forward?** • People who have broken one or more bones during their adult years may have osteoporosis and not know it. • Broken bones in the spine may occur with no noticeable pain. These breaks can cause height loss and can go unnoticed until a person becomes aware that a significant loss of height of an inch or more has occurred.	• Limit alcohol intake. Drinking heavily can reduce bone formation. • If you are trying to lose weight, protect your bones by exercising and eating a healthy diet that provides enough calcium and vitamin D.

Medicines That May Cause Bone Loss

Some medicines can be harmful to your bones, even if you need to take these medicines for another condition. Bone loss is usually greater if you take them in high doses or for a long time. One risky type of medicine for bones is corticosteroid medicines. Many people need to take these medicines to relieve inflammation in conditions like rheumatoid arthritis, asthma, and for other reasons.

It is important to talk with your doctor about the risks and benefits of any medicines you take and about how they may affect your bones. Do not stop any treatment or change the dose of your medicines unless your doctor says it is safe to do so. If you need to take a medicine that causes bone loss, work with your doctor to take the lowest possible dose to control your symptoms.

Below is a list of medicines that may cause bone loss.
- Aluminum-containing antacids
- Antiseizure medicines (only some), such as Dilantin or Phenobarbital
- Aromatase inhibitors, such as Arimidex, Aromasin, and Femara
- Cancer chemotherapeutic medicines
- Cyclosporine A and FK506 (Tacrolimus)
- Gonadotropin-releasing hormone, such as Lupron and Zoladex
- Heparin
- Lithium
- Medroxyprogesterone acetate for contraception (Depo-Provera)
- Methotrexate
- Proton pump inhibitors, such as Nexium, Prevacid, and Prilosec
- Selective serotonin reuptake inhibitors, such as Lexapro, Prozac, and Zoloft
- Corticosteroids, such as cortisone and prednisone
- Tamoxifen (premenopausal use)
- Thiazolidinediones, such as Actos and Avandia
- Thyroid hormones in excess

Note: This list may not include all medicines that may cause bone loss.

Diseases and Conditions That May Cause Bone Loss

Many health problems can increase your chance of having osteoporosis. Ask your doctor if you have any diseases or conditions that can cause bone loss. If you do, it is important to take action to keep your bones healthy. Here are some examples of the diseases and conditions that may cause bone loss.

Autoimmune Disorders

Rheumatoid arthritis (RA). RA is a form of arthritis that is associated with an increased risk for osteoporosis. Corticosteroid medicines used to treat it, as well as the condition on its own, can increase the risk of osteoporosis.

Lupus. People with lupus may need to take medicines, including corticosteroids, to control their symptoms. These medicines can lead to bone loss and osteoporosis.

Digestive and Gastrointestinal Disorders

Celiac disease. People with celiac disease have trouble digesting foods with gluten. Gluten is found in grains such as wheat, rye, and barley. People with celiac disease also have problems absorbing nutrients, including calcium and vitamin D. Celiac disease doesn't always cause noticeable symptoms. Ask your doctor if you should have a test for celiac disease.

Inflammatory bowel disease (IBD). Different forms of IBD, such as Crohn's disease and ulcerative colitis, can cause bone loss. People with IBD often take corticosteroid medicines to treat these conditions. People with IBD may also have trouble absorbing the calcium and vitamin D needed for healthy bones.

Weight loss surgery. Weight loss procedures, such as gastric bypass surgery, can help people lose a large amount of weight in a short period of time. This weight loss may lead to bone loss. These procedures can also interfere with the body's ability to properly absorb the vitamins and minerals needed for bone health.

Endocrine and Hormonal Disorders

Diabetes. People with diabetes have a higher risk of developing osteoporosis. While type 1 diabetes seems to cause the greatest amount of bone loss, people with both type 1 and type 2 diabetes have an increased risk of breaking bones.

Hyperparathyroidism. This is a condition in which the parathyroid glands (two pairs of small glands located behind the thyroid in the neck) produce too much parathyroid hormone (PTH). Having too much PTH causes bone loss. This condition is more common in women after menopause. A simple blood test can tell your doctor if this is a problem.

Hyperthyroidism. In people with this condition, the thyroid gland produces too much thyroid hormone. This can lead to weak muscles and fragile bones. Bone loss can also occur if a person takes too much thyroid hormone medicine for an underactive thyroid.

Missing periods. If you are a young woman and do not have regular periods, this could mean low estrogen levels. There could be many reasons for this, such as exercising too much or eating so little that you become too thin. Other causes of irregular periods could include disorders of the ovaries or pituitary. Loss of estrogen and extreme thinness can harm bones and affect other body systems. Young women who don't have regular periods should talk to their doctor about their bone health.

Testosterone levels. In men, testosterone protects bone. Very low levels of testosterone suggest that there is an underlying disorder that needs to be evaluated. Estrogen levels in men are also important. Low levels of these hormones can lead to bone loss. A number of factors can cause levels to be low, such as an eating disorder or drinking too much alcohol. A blood test can tell you if your hormone levels are normal.

Hematologic and Blood Disorders

Leukemia and lymphoma. Many of the medicines, including chemo-therapy, used to treat these two forms of cancer can lead to bone loss and osteoporosis.

Multiple myeloma. Multiple myeloma is a cancer of the bone marrow. Its first symptoms may be back pain and broken bones in the spine. Blood and urine tests can detect the problem. Other forms of cancer that affect bones or bone marrow can also cause broken bones.

Sickle cell disease. People with sickle cell disease may need to take medicines, including steroids, to control their symptoms. These medicines can lead to bone loss and osteoporosis.

Neurological and Nervous System Disorders

Stroke, Parkinson's disease, and multiple sclerosis. These conditions reduce mobility. People with these conditions are more likely to be inactive, fall, and have low vitamin D levels.

Other Diseases and Medical Conditions

Many health problems, including genetic disorders and diseases of the kidneys, lungs, and digestive system, can cause osteoporosis and broken bones. Below are some other common causes of bone loss.

- Breast cancer
- Depression
- Eating disorders
- Organ transplant
- Prostate cancer

Source:
Factors That Put You at Risk. National Osteoporosis Foundation. Washington, DC; copyright 2011. www.nof.org/node/51. Accessed Aug 16, 2012.

Is It a Cold, the Flu, or an Allergy?

	COLD	FLU	AIRBORNE ALLERGY
SYMPTOMS			
Chest discomfort	Mild to moderate	Common; can become severe	Sometimes
Cough	Common (hacking cough)	Sometimes	Sometimes
Diarrhea	Never	Sometimes (more common in children)	Never
Duration	3-14 days	Days to weeks	Weeks (eg, 6 weeks for ragweed or grass pollen seasons)
Extreme exhaustion	Never	Early and prominent	Never
Fatigue, weakness	Sometimes	Usual; can last up to 2-3 weeks	Sometimes
Fever	Rare	Characteristic; high (100-102°F; occasionally higher, especially in young children); lasts 3-4 days	Never
General aches, pains	Slight	Usual; often severe	Never
Headache	Rare	Common	Sometimes
Itchy eyes	Rare or never	Rare or never	Common
Runny nose	Common	Common	Common
Sneezing	Usual	Sometimes	Usual
Sore throat	Common	Sometimes	Sometimes
Stuffy nose	Common	Sometimes	Common
Vomiting	Never	Sometimes (more common in children)	Never
TREATMENT			
	Antihistamines*	Amantadine	Antihistamines*
	Decongestants*	Rimantadine	Nasal steroids*
	Nonsteroidal anti-inflammatories*	Oseltamivir	Decongestants*
		Zanamivir	

(Continued)

	COLD	FLU	AIRBORNE ALLERGY
PREVENTION			
	Wash your hands often; avoid close contact with anyone with a cold	• Annual vaccination • Amantadine • Rimantadine • Oseltamivir	Avoid allergens such as pollen, house flies, dust mites, mold, pet dander, cockroaches
COMPLICATIONS			
	Sinus infection	Bronchitis	Sinus infections
	Middle ear infection	Pneumonia	Asthma
	Asthma	Can be life-threatening	
		Can worsen chronic conditions	
		Complications more likely in the elderly, those with chronic conditions, young children, and pregnant women	

Adapted from the National Institute of Allergy and Infectious Diseases, November 2008 and CDC.gov.
*Used only for temporary relief of cold symptoms.

Things I Should Know About Seasonal Influenza (Flu) Vaccines

Influenza vaccine

An influenza vaccine protects people against the flu. A new form of the flu vaccine needs to be developed most years to protect people against the exact strains that are expected to be most common.

The flu is a contagious respiratory disease caused by an influenza virus. Flu vaccines are generally given at the beginning of the "flu" season—usually late October or early November in the United States.

Following are questions you may have about seasonal flu—and, more importantly, answers that may help you make important decisions regarding your and your family's health.

Should I get vaccinated?

Everyone 6 months and older should get the flu shot, according to the Centers for Disease Control and Prevention (CDC). Some people are at serious risk; thus, the CDC strongly recommends a vaccination in the following circumstances:

- If you are pregnant or plan to become pregnant during the flu season
- If you are 65 years and older, or live in a nursing home or extended care facility
- For children younger than 5 years—especially those under 2 years (but 6 months or older)
- If you have household contact and are caregivers of children under the age of 6 months, including breastfeeding women
- If you have or currently live with people who have chronic health problems
- If you are a healthcare worker or live with a healthcare worker
- If you live in a nursing home or extended care facility
- If you have anemia, asthma, diabetes, kidney disease, or a weakened immune system (including cancer or HIV/AIDS)
- If you receive long-term treatment with steroids for any condition
- If you have chronic lung or heart disease
- If you have sickle cell anemia or other hemoglobinopathies

Who should not get the vaccine?

Always talk to your doctor first before getting vaccinated. The vaccine is not approved for people less than 6 months of age. In general, you should not get a flu shot if you:

• Have or had a severe allergic reaction to chicken or egg protein

• Have or had a moderate to severe reaction to a previous flu vaccine

• Have or had a fever or illness that is more than "just a cold"

• Developed Guillain-Barre syndrome (a rare disorder that causes your immune system to attack your peripheral nervous system) within 6 weeks after receiving a flu vaccine

If you meet any of the above criteria, ask your doctor if a flu vaccine is safe for you.

What kinds of flu vaccines are available for me?

The "flu shot" is an inactivated vaccine (containing killed virus) that is given with a needle, usually in the arm. There are three different flu shots available, plus a nasal spray flu vaccine:

• A regular flu shot approved for people 6 months of age and older

• A high dose flu shot approved for people 65 years of age and older

• An intradermal flu shot approved for people 18-64 years of age

Listed below are flu vaccines available for the 2012-2013 season:

Afluria®

Agriflu®

Fluarix®

FluLaval®

Fluvirin®

Fluzone®

The nasal spray flu vaccine is a vaccine made with a live, weakened flu virus that is given as a nasal spray. The viruses in the nasal spray vaccine do not cause the flu. This vaccine is approved for use in healthy people 2-49 years of age who are not pregnant.

FluMist®

What kind of side effects can I expect from the flu vaccine?

The flu shot:

- soreness, redness, or swelling where the shot was given
- fever (low grade)
- aches

The nasal spray flu vaccine:

- runny nose
- wheezing
- headache
- vomiting
- muscle aches
- fever
- cough
- sore throat

Sources:

Influenza Vaccine. MedlinePlus. www.nlm.nih.gov/medlineplus/ency/article/002025.htm. Posted September 16, 2011. Accessed August 16, 2012.

Seasonal Influenza (Flu). Centers for Disease Control and Prevention. www.cdc.gov/flu/protect/keyfacts.htm. Posted July 6, 2012. Accessed August 16, 2012.

Vaccines, Blood & Biologics. U.S. Food and Drug Administration. www.fda.gov/BiologicsBloodVaccines/GuidanceComplianceRegulatoryInformation/Post-MarketActivities/LotReleases/ucm310644.htm. Posted August 15, 2012. Accessed August 16, 2012.

Brand and Generic Name Index

Organized alphabetically, this index includes the brand and generic names of each medication covered in the profiles. Brand names appear in regular type; *generic names are shown in italics.*

D

U

V

W

Disease and Disorder Index

Organized alphabetically by disease and disorder, this index lists which medications are available for a specific medical condition. Only medications covered in the profiles are included. Brand names appear in regular type, and *generic names in italics.*

Personal Information

Name, First and Last	
Date of Birth	
Address	
Phone Number	
Cell Number	

Emergency Contact

Name	
Relationship	
Address	
Phone Number	
Cell Number	

Primary Care Physician

Name	
Address	
Phone Number	

Pharmacy/Drugstore

Pharmacy Name	
Address	
Phone Number	

Allergic Reactions or Other Problems I've had with any medication, dietary supplement, food, etc.

My Current Medical Condition(s)

Personal Information

Name, First and Last	
Date of Birth	
Address	
Phone Number	
Cell Number	

Emergency Contact

Name	
Relationship	
Address	
Phone Number	
Cell Number	

Primary Care Physician

Name	
Address	
Phone Number	

Pharmacy/Drugstore

Pharmacy Name	
Address	
Phone Number	

Allergic Reactions or Other Problems I've had with any medication, dietary supplement, food, etc.

My Current Medical Condition(s)

Personal Information

Name – First and Last	
Date of Birth	
Address	
Phone Number	
Cell Number	

Emergency Contact

Name	
Relationship	
Address	
Phone Number	
Cell Number	

Primary Care Physician

Name	
Address	
Phone Number	

Pharmacy Information

Pharmacy Name	
Address	
Phone Number	

Medical Conditions

Personal Information

Name, First and Last	
Date of Birth	
Address	
Phone Number	
Cell Number	

Emergency Contact

Name	
Relationship	
Address	
Phone Number	
Cell Number	

Primary Care Physician

Name	
Address	
Phone Number	

Pharmacy/Drugstore

Pharmacy Name	
Address	
Phone Number	

Allergic Reactions or Other Problems I've had with any medication, dietary supplement, food, etc.

My Current Medical Condition(s)

MY MEDICINE TRACKER

Name of Medicine	Dose I am Taking	What is the Medicine for?	How Do I take the Medicine?	Special Instructions	Date Started	When to Stop or Review with my Doctor	Who Told me to Take the Medicine/ Contact Information

MY MEDICINE TRACKER

Name of Medicine	Dose I am Taking	What is the Medicine for?	How Do I take the Medicine?	Special Instructions	Date Started	When to Stop or Review with my Doctor	Who Told me to Take the Medicine/ Contact Information